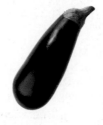

### SIXTH EDITION

# NUTRITION ESSENTIALS *for* NURSING PRACTICE

▲

## Susan G. Dudek, RD, CDN, BS

Nutrition Instructor, Dietetic Technology Program
Erie Community College
Williamsville, New York

Consultant Dietitian for Employee Assistance
Program of Child and Family Services
West Seneca, New York

. Wolters Kluwer | Lippincott Williams & Wilkins
Health

Philadelphia · Baltimore · New York · London
Buenos Aires · Hong Kong · Sydney · Tokyo

*Acquisitions Editor:* Elizabeth Nieginski
*Product Manager:* Mary Kinsella
*Editorial Assistant:* Laura Scott
*Design Coordinator:* Holly Reid McLaughlin
*Illustration Coordinator:* Brett McNaughton
*Manufacturing Coordinator:* Karin Duffield
*Prepress Vendor:* Macmillan Publishing Solutions

Sixth Edition

9  8  7  6  5  4  3

Printed in China

**Library of Congress Cataloging-in-Publication Data**
Dudek, Susan G.
    Nutrition essentials for nursing practice / Susan G. Dudek.—6th ed.
        p. ; cm.
    Includes bibliographical references and index.
    ISBN 978-0-7817-8454-2 (alk. paper)
  1. Diet therapy. 2. Nutrition. 3. Nursing.  I. Title.
    [DNLM: 1. Diet Therapy—Handbooks. 2. Diet Therapy—Nurses' Instruction.
3. Nutritional Physiological Phenomena—Handbooks. 4. Nutritional Physiological
Phenomena—Nurses' Instruction.  WB 39 D845n 2010]
    RM216.D8627 2010
    615.8'54—dc22

                                                                    2009028370

CCS0311

*Dedicated, with gratitude, to old friends,*
*new friends, compassionate friends,*
*and my family—I could not have written this edition*
*without your love and support*

# REVIEWERS

▲

**Zita Allen, RN, MSN**
Professor of Nursing
Alverno College
Milwaukee, Wisconsin

**Lisette Barton, RN, FNP-BC, CNE**
Assistant Professor
Houston Baptist University
Houston Texas

**Terri Blevins, RN, BSN, MSEd**
Practical Nursing Director
Tennessee Technology Center
Elizabethton, Tennessee

**Josephine Cumberbatch-Tate**
Atlanta Technical College
Atlanta, Georgia

**Karen Dolk, RN, MSN**
Nursing Department Chair
Ivy Tech Community College
Lafayette, Indiana

**Sherlyn A. Farrish-Barner, RN, MSN**
Nursing Educator
Germanna Community College
Locust Grove, Virginia

**Amy Hall, RN, PhD**
Professor and Chair
Department of Nursing and Health Sciences
University of Evansville
Evansville, Indiana

**Phyllis S. Hayes, BS, BSN**
Nursing Instructor
Halifax Community College
Weldon, North Carolina

**Penelope Hennessy, MS, RN**
Director, Practical Nursing Program
Tri-County Vocational Regional Technical High School
Franklin, Massachusetts

**Barbara Hulsman**
South College
Knoxville, Tennessee

**Donna J. Jones, MSN**
Associate Professor
Missouri State University, West Plains
Missouri

**James Kane**
Rensselaer Educational Center
Troy, New York

**Claudette Kelly, RN, PhD**
Nurse Educator Researcher
Thompson Rivers University
Kamloops, British Columbia

**Karen Lincoln, RNC, MSN**
Nursing Instructor
Montcalm Community College
Sidney, Michigan

**Joseph Morris, CNS, GNP, PhD**
Associate Dean
West Coast University
Anaheim, California

**Teak Nelson, MS, RN, NP-C**
Assistant Professor of Nursing
Truman State University
Kirksville, Missouri

**Marilyn Obiecunas, RD, MSEd, CDE, LDN**
Adjunct Faculty
Medical Nutrition Consultant, Certified Diabetes Educator
Chatham University
Pittsburgh, Pennsylvania

**Nancy Schlapman**
Indiana University
Kokomo, Indiana

**Tracy Slemp, MSN, RN**
Assistant Professor
King College
Bristol, Tennessee

**Margaret Wilson, RN, MSN, EdD**
Professor/Clinical Instructor in Nursing
California State University, Fullerton
California

# PREFACE

▲

Like air and sleep, nutrition is a basic human need, essential for survival. Nutrition can help keep people healthy, propel them toward wellness, or aid in recovery. It is a complex blend of science and art, evolving over time and in response to technology. Nutrition at its most basic level is food—for the mind, body, and soul.

Although considered the realm of the dietitian, nutrition is a vital and integral component of nursing care. Today's nurses need to know, understand, apply, analyze, synthesize, and evaluate nutrition throughout the life cycle and along the wellness–illness continuum. They incorporate nutrition into all aspects of nursing care plans, from assessment and nursing diagnoses to implementation and evaluation. By virtue of their close contact with patients and families, nurses are often on the front line in facilitating nutrition.

## ▶ New to This Edition

This text strives to illuminate how nutrition is intimately intertwined in nursing practice. Popular features of the fifth edition have been retained, such as How Do You Respond?, True/False questions at the beginning of each chapter, the definition of key terms in the margin, Quick Bites, and Key Concepts summarized at the end of each chapter. A more valuable sixth edition has been created by

- Changing the Nursing Process sections into a table format to make application more accessible to the reader.
- Including a Case Study in each chapter. Real life scenarios challenge the reader to demonstrate application and analysis of nutrition knowledge.
- Including NCLEX-style study questions at the end of each chapter. The answers are listed in Appendix 4.
- Updating the content to reflect the latest evidence-based practice with more extensive references noted in the text. I am always amazed by how much nutrition changes between editions. Updates to this edition include MyPyramid for Moms and revised nutrition recommendations from the American Diabetes Association and the World Cancer Research Fund/American Institute for Cancer Research.
- Streamlining the content to more narrowly focus on what the nurse needs to know. Chapter 7 reflects this change; Energy Metabolism has been renamed Energy Balance and the interesting-but-not-essential biochemistry of metabolism has been deleted.
- Dividing the chapter on gastrointestinal disorders into two separate chapters to coincide with how they are presented in nursing curricula.
- Critically evaluating my writing to improve its precision and strength. I am grateful for the review that challenged my self-perception as author.

## ▶ Additional Resources

Students and instructors will find valuable resources to accompany the book by accessing thePoint at http://thePoint.lww.com, including PowerPoint presentations and a Test Generator for instructors!

## ▶ Chapter Organization

Unit One is entitled "Principles of Nutrition." It begins with Chapter 1, "Nutrition in Nursing," which focuses on why and how nutrition is important to nurses in all settings. Chapters that address carbohydrates, protein, lipids, vitamins, fluids and minerals, and energy balance present a foundation for wellness. The second part of each chapter highlights health promotion topics and demonstrates practical application of essential information, such as how to increase fiber intake, criteria to consider when buying a vitamin supplement, and the risks and benefits of a vegetarian diet.

Unit Two, "Nutrition in Health Promotion," begins with Chapter 8, "Guidelines for Healthy Eating." This chapter features the Dietary Reference Intakes, the Dietary Guidelines for Americans, and MyPyramid. Other chapters in this unit are Chapter 9, "Consumer Issues," and Chapter 10, "Cultural and Religious Influences on Food and Nutrition." The nutritional needs associated with the life cycle are discussed in chapters devoted to pregnant and lactating women, children and adolescents, and older adults.

Unit Three, "Nutrition in Clinical Practice," presents nutrition therapy for obesity and eating disorders, enteral and parenteral nutrition, metabolic and respiratory distress, gastrointestinal disorders, diabetes, cardiovascular disorders, renal disorders, and cancer and HIV/AIDS. Pathophysiology is tightly focused within the context of nutrition.

I hope this text provides the impetus to improve nutrition on both a personal and professional level.

*Susan G. Dudek*

# ACKNOWLEDGMENTS

▲

I am truly humbled to be still writing this book after five editions and extend my heartfelt thanks to all the dedicated and creative professionals at Lippincott Williams & Wilkins. Because of their support and talents, I am able to do what I love—write, create, teach, and learn. I especially thank

❧ Elizabeth Nieginski, Senior Acquisitions Editor, who provided the spark to ignite the project.
  • Helen Kogut, Senior Managing Editor, for her painstaking attention to detail and her ability to see what I did not. I am grateful for her patience.
  • Brett MacNaughton, Art Director, an artistic master of color and style.
  • All the behind-the-scene production staff for their creative talent.

❧ The reviewers of the fifth edition, whose insightful comments and suggestions helped shape this text into a new and improved edition. I am grateful they were willing to share their time and expertise.

❧ My daughters Kaitlyn and Kara, and my late son Christopher, for all they have taught me about work and play, faith and hope, love and life.

❧ And my husband, Joe. Thanks for being here—literally and figuratively.

# CONTENTS

▲

## UNIT THREE
## Nutrition in Clinical Practice  325

## APPENDICES  563

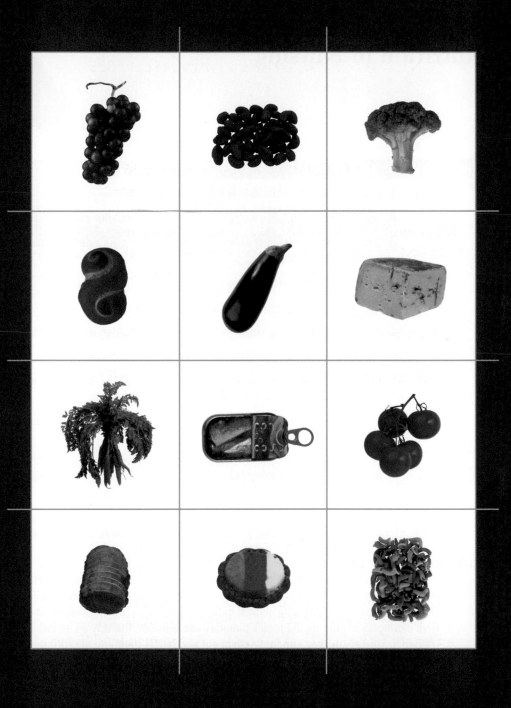

UNIT ONE

Principles of Nutrition

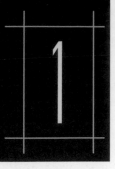

# 1 Nutrition in Nursing

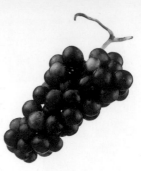

| TRUE | FALSE | |
|------|-------|---|
| ☐ | ☐ | **1** The nurse's role in nutrition is to call the dietitian. |
| ☐ | ☐ | **2** Nutrition screening is used to identify clients at risk for malnutrition. |
| ☐ | ☐ | **3** The Joint Commission stipulates the criteria to be included on a nutritional screen for hospitalized patients. |
| ☐ | ☐ | **4** Changes in weight reflect acute changes in nutritional status. |
| ☐ | ☐ | **5** A person can be malnourished without being underweight. |
| ☐ | ☐ | **6** The only cause of a low serum albumin concentration is protein malnutrition. |
| ☐ | ☐ | **7** "Significant" weight loss is 5% of body weight in 1 month. |
| ☐ | ☐ | **8** People who take five or more prescription or over-the-counter medications or dietary supplements are at risk for nutritional problems. |
| ☐ | ☐ | **9** Obtaining reliable and accurate information on what the client usually eats can help identify intake as a source of nutrition problems. |
| ☐ | ☐ | **10** Physical signs and symptoms of malnutrition develop only after other signs of malnutrition are apparent (e.g., abnormal lab values, weight change). |

## UPON COMPLETION OF THIS CHAPTER, YOU WILL BE ABLE TO

- Compare nutrition screening to nutrition assessment.
- Calculate ideal body weight based on height for men and women using the Hamwi method.
- Evaluate weight loss for its significance over a 1-month or 6-month interval.
- Debate the usefulness of using clinical data to support a nutritional diagnosis of malnutrition.
- Give examples of nursing diagnosis that may use nutrition therapy as an intervention.
- Demonstrate how nurses can facilitate client and family teaching of nutrition therapy.
- Explain why an alternative term to "diet" is useful.

Based on Maslow's hierarchy of needs, food and nutrition rank on the same level as air in the basic necessities of life. Obviously, death eventually occurs without food. But unlike air, food does so much more than simply sustain life. Food is loaded with personal, social, and cultural meanings that define our food values, beliefs, and customs. That food nourishes the mind as well as the body broadens nutrition to an art as well as a science. For most people, nutrition is not simply a matter of food or no food but rather a question of what kind, how much, and how often. Merging want with need and pleasure with health is key to feeding the body, mind, and soul.

Although the dietitian is the nutrition and food expert, nurses play a vital role in nutrition care. Nurses may be responsible for screening hospitalized patients to determine the existing level of risk. They often serve as the liaison between the dietitian and physician, as well as with other members of the health-care team. Nurses also have far more contact with the patient and family and are often available as a nutrition resource when dietitians are not, such as during the evening, on weekends, and during discharge instructions. In home care and wellness settings, dietitians may be available only on a consultative basis. Nurses may reinforce nutrition counseling provided by the dietitian and may be responsible for basic nutrition counseling in hospitalized clients with low to mild nutritional risk. Nurses are intimately involved in all aspects of nutritional care.

This chapter discusses nutrition within the context of nursing, including nutrition screening and how nutrition can be integrated into the nursing care process. Real-life scenarios show practical application.

## ▶ NUTRITION SCREENING

**Nutritional Screen:** a quick look at a few variables to judge a client's relative risk for nutritional problems. Can be custom designed for a particular population (e.g., pregnant women) or for a specific disorder (e.g., cardiac disease).

**Nutrition screening** is a quick look at a few variables associated with nutrition problems to determine if individuals are malnourished or are at risk for malnutrition. To be efficient and quick, screening relies on information that is readily available within the given setting and associated with nutrition risks of the specific population screened. For instance, a nutrition screen to identify malnutrition in noninstitutionalized people over the age of 80 focuses mostly on intake problems common to that population; lab values and weight measurements are not used because they are generally unavailable (Fig. 1.1). In comparison, a nutrition screen for a general hospital population may range from only looking at significant weight loss and change in appetite to a more broad view that includes difficulty eating, use of enteral or parenteral nutrition, certain diagnoses, and other factors (Box 1.1). There is no universally agreed upon tool that is valid and reliable at identifying risk of malnutrition in all populations at all times.

**Nutritional Assessment:** an in-depth analysis of a person's nutritional status. In the clinical setting, nutritional assessments focus on moderate- to high-risk patients with suspected or confirmed protein–energy malnutrition.

The Joint Commission, a nonprofit organization that sets health-care standards and accredits health-care facilities that meet those standards, specifies that nutrition screening be conducted within 24 hours after admission to a hospital or other health-care facility—even on weekends and holidays. The Joint Commission allows facilities to determine what factors are used on the screen and what defines risk. For instance, a hospital may use serum creatinine level as a screening criterion, with a level greater than 2.5 mg/dL defined as "high risk" because the majority of their patients are elderly and the prevalence of chronic renal problems is high. The Joint Commission also leaves the decision of who performs the screening up to individual facilities. Because the standard applies 24 hours a day, 7 days a week, staff nurses are often responsible for completing the screen as part of the admission process. Clients who "pass" the initial screen are rescreened after a specified amount of time to determine if their status has changed.

## ▶ COMPREHENSIVE NUTRITIONAL ASSESSMENT

Clients considered to be at moderate or high risk for malnutrition through screening are usually referred to a dietitian for a comprehensive **nutritional assessment**. Nutritional assessment is more accurately called the nutritional care process that includes four steps: assessment, nutritional diagnosis, implementation, and monitoring and evaluation. While nurses use the same problem-solving model to develop nursing or multidisciplinary care

## DETERMINE YOUR NUTRITIONAL HEALTH

*The warning signs of poor nutritional health are often overlooked. Use this checklist to find out if you or someone you know is at nutritional risk.*

Read the statements below. Circle the number in the "yes" column for those that apply to you or someone you know. For each "yes" answer, score the number in the box. Total your nutritional score.

|  | YES |
|---|---|
| I have an illness or condition that made me change the kind and/or amount of food I eat. | 2 |
| I eat fewer than two meals per day. | 3 |
| I eat few fruits or vegetables, or milk products. | 2 |
| I have three or more drinks of beer, liquor or wine almost every day. | 2 |
| I have tooth or mouth problems that make it hard for me to eat. | 2 |
| I don't always have enough money to buy the food I need. | 4 |
| I eat alone most of the time. | 1 |
| I take three or more different prescribed or over-the-counter drugs a day. | 1 |
| Without wanting to, I have lost or gained 10 pounds in the last six months. | 2 |
| I am not always physically able to shop, cook and/or feed myself. | 2 |
| TOTAL | |

Total your nutritional score. If it's –

0-2      Good! Recheck your nutritional score in six months.

3-5      You are at moderate nutritional risk. See what can be done to improve your eating habits and lifestyle. Your office on aging, senior nutrition program, senior citizens center or health department can help. Recheck your nutritional score in three months.

6 or more      You are at high nutritional risk. Bring this checklist the next time you see your doctor, dietitian or other qualified health or social service professional. Talk with them about any problems you may have. Ask for help to improve your nutritional health.

*Remember that warning signs suggest risk, but do not represent diagnosis of any condition.*

**FIGURE 1.1** Determine your nutritional health. American Academy of Family Physicians, the American Dietetic Association, the National Council on the Aging, Inc. The Nutrition Screening Initiative.

---

**BOX 1.1**      **CRITERIA FREQUENTLY USED IN SCREENING HOSPITALIZED PATIENTS**

- Height
- Weight
- Weight change
- Diet
- Albumin, hematocrit

- Change in appetite
- Nausea/vomiting
- Bowel habits
- Chewing/swallowing
- Diagnosis

*Source:* Charney, P. & Malone, A. (Ed.). (2004) *ADA Pocket Guide to Nutrition Assessment.* Chicago: American Dietetic Association.

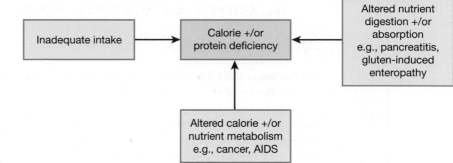

**FIGURE 1.2** Factors that may be involved in the etiology of calorie and/or protein deficiency.

plans that may also integrate nutrition, the nutritional plan of care devised by dietitians is specific for nutrition problems that dietetics professionals are responsible for treating independently (American Dietetic Association Evidence Library, 2006). Some obvious differences in focus are described below:

• Dietitians may obtain much of their preliminary information about the patient from the nursing history and physical, such as height and weight; skin integrity; usual diet prior to admission; difficulty chewing, swallowing, or self-feeding; chief complaint; medications, supplements, and over-the-counter drugs used prior to admission; and living situation.

• Dietitians interview patients and/or families to obtain a nutrition history, which may include information on current dietary habits; recent changes in intake or appetite; intake of snacks; alcohol consumption; food allergies and intolerances; ethnic, cultural, or religious diet influences; and use of supplements. A nutrition history can help differentiate nutrition problems caused by inadequate intake from those caused by illness or its treatments (Fig. 1.2).

• Dietitians usually calculate estimated calorie and protein requirements based on the assessment data and determine whether the diet ordered is adequate and appropriate for the individual.

• Dietitians determine nutritional diagnoses that define the nutritional problem, etiology, and signs and symptoms. While a nursing diagnosis statement may begin with "Imbalanced nutrition: less than body requirements," a nutritional diagnosis would be more specific, such as "Inadequate protein–energy intake."

• Dietitians may also determine the appropriate malnutrition diagnosis code for the patient for hospital reimbursement purposes.

• Nutrition interventions may include requesting a diet order change, requesting additional laboratory tests to monitor nutritional repletion, and performing nutrition counseling or education.

## ▶ INTEGRATING NUTRITION

The remainder of this chapter describes how nurses can use the nursing care process to integrate nutrition into nursing practice. The goal is to help nurses provide quality nursing care that includes basic nutrition, not to help nurses become dietitians.

### Assessment

Assessment data can be classified as ABCD: anthropometric, biochemical, clinical, and dietary data. A client's medical–psychosocial history is also evaluated for its impact on nutritional status.

## Anthropometric Data

**Body Mass Index:** an
index of weight in
relation to height that is
calculated
mathematically by
dividing weight in
kilograms by the square
of height in meters.

**"Ideal" Body Weight:**
the formula given here is
a universally used
standard in clinical
practice to quickly
estimate a person's
reasonable weight based
on height, even though
this and all other
methods are not
absolute.

Anthropometric measurements are physical measurements of the body, most commonly, height and weight. Measuring height and weight is relatively quick and easy and requires little skill; therefore, *measures* not *estimates* should be used whenever possible to ensure accuracy and reliability. A patient's *stated* height and weight should be used only when there are no other options.

After height and weight are obtained, weight can be evaluated (Table 1.1). **Body mass index** (BMI), an index of a person's weight in relation to height, estimates relative risk of health problems related to weight. "Healthy" or "normal" BMI is defined as 18.5 to 24.9. Values above and below this range are associated with increased health risks. Although BMI can be calculated with a mathematical formula, tables and nomograms are available for convenience (Chapter 14). One drawback of using BMI is that a person can have a high BMI and still be undernourished in one or more nutrients if intake is unbalanced or if nutritional needs are high and intake is low.

Another way to assess weight is to calculate **"ideal" body weight** (IBW) using the Hamwi method. From a person's ideal weight, the percentage of ideal weight can be calculated and evaluated (Table 1.1). Like BMI, IBW does not measure body composition or evaluate distribution of body fat, both of which impact health risk. Other problems are that edema or dehydration skews accurate weight measurements.

Recent weight change is another factor that may indicate nutritional risk, particularly if weight loss occurs rapidly or unintentionally. The formula for determining percent weight change and the criteria for defining the severity of weight loss appear in Box 1.2.

| TABLE 1.1 | Evaluating Weight for Height | | |
| --- | --- | --- | --- |
| **Standard** | **Calculate** | | **Interpretation** |
| Body mass index (BMI) | $\dfrac{\text{Weight (kg)}}{\text{Height (m}^2)}$ | | <18.5 may ↑ health risk<br>18.5–24.9 healthy weight<br>25–29.9 overweight<br>30–34.9 obesity class 1<br>35–39.9 obesity class 2<br>≥40 obesity class 3 |
| Percentage of "ideal" body weight (% IBW) | First calculate IBW using the Hamwi method:<br>For women:<br>Allow 100 pounds for the first 5 ft of height, and add 5 pounds for each additional in.<br>For men:<br>Allow 106 pounds for the first 5 ft of height, and add 6 pounds for each additional in.<br>IBW may be adjusted up or down by 10% based on body frame size.<br>Then calculate % IBW.<br>$\% \text{ IBW} = \dfrac{\text{current weight}}{\text{IBW}} \times 100$ | | <69% severe malnutrition<br>70–79% moderate malnutrition<br>80–89% mild malnutrition<br>90–110% within normal range<br>110–119% overweight<br>>120% obese<br>>200% morbidly obese |

| BOX 1.2 | CALCULATING AND EVALUATING PERCENT WEIGHT CHANGE |

**Calculating percent weight change**

$$\% \text{ weight change} = \frac{(\text{usual body weight} - \text{current body weight})}{\text{usual body weight}} \times 100$$

**Evaluating Weight Change**

| Time Period | Significant Weight Loss (%) | Severe Weight Loss (%) |
| --- | --- | --- |
| 1 week | 1–2 | >2 |
| 1 month | 5 | >5 |
| 3 months | 7.5 | >7.5 |
| 6 months | 10 | >10 |
| Unlimited | 10–20 | >20 |

*Source:* Charney, P. & Malone, A. (Ed.). (2004) *ADA Pocket Guide to Nutrition Assessment*. Chicago: American Dietetic Association.

## Biochemical Data

Blood and urine tests can measure a variety of proteins and components that *may* reflect nutrition status; however, there is no single test that is both sensitive and specific for protein–calorie malnutrition (Charney & Malone, 2004). Disease, treatments, hydration, pregnancy, or exercise can profoundly alter lab values. However, combined with other assessment information, biochemical data may help support the diagnosis of a nutritional problem.

**Albumin.** Albumin is often used to assess protein status, even though albumin values are more likely to be altered during critical illness from factors other than protein malnutrition, such as from injury, infection, dehydration, liver disease, renal disease, and congestive heart failure. Albumin is degraded slowly, so serum levels may be maintained until malnutrition is in a chronic stage. Although hypoalbuminemia (<3.5 g/dL) is not a sensitive indicator of protein malnutrition, it has been associated with increased length of hospital stay, complications, morbidity, and mortality because it reflects severity of illness (Charney & Malone, 2004). Therefore a low albumin may indirectly identify patients who may benefit from nutrition assessment and intervention.

**Prealbumin.** Prealbumin, also known as thyroxin-binding protein, is a more sensitive indicator of protein status than albumin but not entirely specific for malnutrition; it is affected by metabolic stress and other medical conditions. Prealbumin is more expensive to measure than albumin and is frequently not available, so it is not a routine part of nutritional assessment. Guidelines for interpreting prealbumin are listed in Box 1.3.

| BOX 1.3 | GENERAL GUIDELINES FOR INTERPRETING PREALBUMIN LEVELS |

| | Prealbumin (mg/dL) |
| --- | --- |
| Normal | 23–43 |
| Mild depletion | 10–15 |
| Moderate depletion | 5–9 |
| Severe depletion | <5 |

*Source:* Charney, P. & Malone, A. (Ed.). (2004) *ADA Pocket Guide to Nutrition Assessment*. Chicago: American Dietetic Association.

| BOX 1.4 | PHYSICAL SIGNS AND SYMPTOMS SUGGESTIVE OF MALNUTRITION |
|---|---|

- Hair that is dull, brittle, dry, or falls out easily
- Swollen glands of the neck and cheeks
- Dry, rough, or spotty skin that may have a sandpaper feel
- Poor or delayed wound healing or sores
- Thin appearance with lack of subcutaneous fat
- Muscle wasting (decreased size and strength)
- Edema of the lower extremities
- Weakened hand grasp
- Depressed mood
- Abnormal heart rate, heart rhythm, or blood pressure
- Enlarged liver or spleen
- Loss of balance and coordination

## Clinical Data

Clinical data refer to physical signs and symptoms of malnutrition observed in the client. The problem with relying on physical appearance to reveal nutritional problems is that most signs cannot be considered diagnostic; rather, they must be viewed as suggestive of malnutrition because evaluation of "normal" versus "abnormal" findings is subjective, and the signs of malnutrition may be nonspecific. For instance, dull, dry hair may be related to severe protein deficiency or to overexposure to the sun. In addition, physical signs and symptoms of malnutrition can vary in intensity among population groups because of genetic and environmental differences. Lastly, physical findings occur only with overt malnutrition, not **subclinical** malnutrition. Physical signs and symptoms suggestive of malnutrition appear in Box 1.4.

**Subclinical:** asymptomatic.

## Dietary Data

Although the nurse may only be required to fill in a blank space next to the word "diet," simply asking the client "Are you on a diet?" will probably not give accurate or sufficient information to determine what the client eats. The client may interpret that leading question as "You should be on a diet. If you're a good patient, you'll tell me you follow a diet." A better question would be, "Do you avoid any particular foods?" or "Do you watch what you eat in any way?" Even the term "meal" may elicit a stereotypical mental picture. Questions to consider when asking a client about his or her usual intake appear in Box 1.5.

## Medical–Psychosocial History

A client's medical–psychosocial history may shed light on factors that influence intake, nutritional requirements, or nutrition counseling. Box 1.6 outlines criteria that may be considered.

**Medication.** Both prescription and over-the-counter drugs have the potential to affect and be affected by nutritional status. Sometimes drug–nutrient interactions are the intended actions of the drug. At other times, alterations in nutrient intake, metabolism, or excretion may be an unwanted side effect of drug therapy. Although well-nourished individuals on short-term drug therapy may easily withstand the negative effects of drug–nutrient interactions, malnourished clients and those on long-term drug regimens may experience

| BOX 1.5 | QUESTIONS TO CONSIDER ABOUT INTAKE |
|---------|-------------------------------------|

*How many meals and snacks do you eat in a 24-hour period?* This question helps to establish the pattern of eating and identifies unusual food habits such as pica, food faddism, eating disorders, and meal skipping.

*Do you have any food allergies or intolerances, and, if so, what are they?* The greater the number of foods restricted or eliminated in the diet, the greater the likelihood of nutritional deficiencies. This question may also shed light on the client's need for nutrition counseling. For instance, clients with hiatal hernia who are intolerant of citrus fruits and juices may benefit from counseling on how to ensure an adequate intake of vitamin C.

*What types of vitamin, mineral, herbal, or other supplements do you use and why?* A multivitamin, multimineral supplement that provides 100% or less of the Daily Value offers some protection against less than optimal food choices. Folic acid in supplements or fortified food is recommended for women of childbearing age; people older than 50 are encouraged to obtain vitamin $B_{12}$ from fortified foods or supplements. However, potential problems may arise from other types or amounts of supplements. For instance, large doses of vitamins A, $B_6$, and D have the potential to cause toxicity symptoms. Iron supplements may decrease zinc absorption and negatively impact zinc status over time.

*What concerns do you have about what or how you eat?* This question places the responsibility of healthy eating with the client, where it should be. A client who may benefit from nutrition intervention and counseling *in theory* may not be a candidate for such *in practice* depending on his or her level of interest and motivation. This question may also shed light on whether or not the client understands what he or she should be eating and if the client is willing to make changes in eating habits.

*For clients who are acutely ill, how has illness affected your choice or tolerance of food?* Sometimes food aversions or intolerances can shed light on what is going on with the client. For instance, someone who experiences abdominal pain that is relieved by eating may have a duodenal ulcer. Clients with little or no intake of food or liquids are at risk of dehydration and nutrient deficiencies.

*Who prepares the meals?* This person may need nutritional counseling.

*Do you have enough food to eat?* Be aware that pride and an unwillingness to admit inability to afford an adequate diet may prevent some clients and families from answering this question. For hospitalized clients, it may be more useful to ask the client to compare the size of the meals they are served in the hospital with the size of meals they normally eat.

*How much alcohol do you consume daily?* Risk begins at more than one drink daily for women and more than two drinks daily for men.

significant nutrient deficiencies and decreased tolerance to drug therapy. Clients at greatest risk for development of drug-induced nutrient deficiencies include those who

- Habitually consume fewer calories and nutrients than they need
- Have increased nutrient requirements including infants, adolescents, and pregnant and lactating women
- Are elderly
- Have chronic illnesses
- Take large numbers of drugs (five or more), whether prescription drugs, over-the-counter medications, or dietary supplements
- Are receiving long-term drug therapy
- Self-medicate
- Are substance abusers

---

| BOX 1.6 | MEDICAL–PSYCHOSOCIAL FACTORS THAT MAY INFLUENCE INTAKE, NUTRITIONAL REQUIREMENTS, OR NUTRITION COUNSELING |
|---|---|

*Medical factors*
- Acute status: current illness, hydration status, open wounds, dysphagia
- Chronic disease: cancer, cardiac disease, lung disease, diabetes, liver disease, GI disorders, renal disease, posttransplant

*Psychological factors*
- Depression
- Eating disorders
- Psychosis

*Social factors*
- Illiteracy
- Language barriers
- Limited knowledge of nutrition and food safety

- Altered or impaired intake related to culture
- Altered or impaired intake related to religion
- Lack of caregiver or social support system
- Social isolation
- Lack of or inadequate cooking arrangements
- Limited or low income
- Limited access to transportation to obtain food
- Advanced age (older than 80 years)
- Lack of or extreme physical activity
- Use of tobacco or recreational drugs
- Limited use or knowledge of community resources

## Nursing Diagnosis

A diagnosis is made after assessment data are interpreted. Nursing diagnoses in hospitals and long-term care facilities provide written documentation of the client's status and serve as a framework for the plan of care that follows. The diagnoses relate directly to nutrition when altered nutrition is the problem or indirectly when a change in intake will help to manage a nonnutritional problem. Box 1.7 lists nursing diagnoses with nutritional significance.

## Planning: Client Outcomes

Outcomes, or goals, should be measurable, attainable, specific, and client centered. How do you measure success against a vague goal of "gain weight by eating better"? Is "eating better" achieved by adding butter to foods to increase calories or by substituting 1% milk for

---

| BOX 1.7 | SELECTED NURSING DIAGNOSES WITH NUTRITIONAL SIGNIFICANCE |
|---|---|

**Obvious Diagnoses**
- Imbalanced nutrition: less than body requirements
- Imbalanced nutrition: more than body requirements
- Readiness for enhanced nutrition
- Risk for imbalanced nutrition: more than body requirements

**Less Obvious Diagnoses (Nutrition Interventions May Be Part of the Care Plan)**
- Acute pain
- Adult failure to thrive
- Chronic pain
- Constipation
- Deficient fluid volume

- Deficient knowledge (of nutrition/food)
- Diarrhea
- Excess fluid volume
- Fatigue
- Feeding self-care deficit
- Health-seeking behaviors (improved dietary intake)
- Impaired dentition
- Impaired oral mucous membrane
- Impaired skin integrity
- Impaired swallowing
- Ineffective health maintenance
- Ineffective infant eating pattern
- Nausea
- Noncompliance (with prescribed diet)
- Risk for aspiration
- Risk for constipation

whole milk because it is heart healthy? Is a 1-pound weight gain in 1 month acceptable or is 1 pound/week preferable? Is 1 pound/week attainable if the client has accelerated metabolism and catabolism caused by third-degree burns?

Client-centered outcomes place the focus on the client, not the health-care provider; they specify where the client is heading. Whenever possible, give the client the opportunity to actively participate in goal setting, even if the client's perception of need differs from yours. In matters that do not involve life or death, it is best to first address the client's concerns. Your primary consideration may be the patient's significant weight loss during the last 6 months of chemotherapy, whereas the patient's major concern may be fatigue. The two issues are undoubtedly related, but your effectiveness as a change agent is greater if you approach the problem from the client's perspective. Commitment to achieving the goal is greatly increased when the client "owns" the goal.

Keep in mind that the goal for all clients is to consume adequate calories and protein using foods they like and tolerate as appropriate. If possible, additional short-term goals may be set to alleviate symptoms or side effects of disease or treatments and to prevent complications or recurrences if appropriate. After short-term goals are met, attention can center on promoting healthy eating to reduce the risk of chronic diet-related diseases such as obesity, diabetes, hypertension, and atherosclerosis.

## Nursing Interventions

What can you or others do to effectively and efficiently help the client achieve his or her goals? Interventions may take the form of nutrition therapy and client teaching.

## Nutrition Therapy

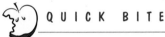 **QUICK BITE**

Estimating calorie requirements
A "rule-of-thumb" method of calculating calorie requirements:
Multiply weight in kg by
  30 cal/kg for most healthy adults
  25 cal/kg for elderly adults
  20–25 cal/kg for obese adults
Example: For an adult weighing 154 pounds:
  154 pounds ÷ 2.2 kg/pound = 70 kg
  70 kg × 30 cal/kg = 2100 cal/day

Throughout this book, the heading "Nutrition Therapy" is used in place of "Diet" because among clients *diet* is a four-letter word with negative connotations such as counting calories, deprivation, sacrifice, and misery. A diet is viewed as a short-term punishment to endure until a normal pattern of eating can resume. Clients respond better to terminology that is less emotionally charged. Terms such as *eating pattern, food intake, eating style,* or *the food you eat* may be used to keep the lines of communication open.

Nutrition therapy recommendations are usually general suggestions to increase/decrease, limit/avoid, reduce/encourage, or modify/maintain aspects of the diet because exact nutrient requirements are determined on an individual basis. Where more precise amounts of nutrients are specified, consider them as a starting point and monitor the client's response. Box 1.8 suggests ways the nurse can promote an adequate intake.

Nutrition theory does not always apply to practice. Factors such as the client's prognosis, outside support systems, level of intelligence and motivation, willingness to comply, emotional health, financial status,

**QUICK BITE**

Estimating protein requirements
  Healthy adults need 0.8 g protein/kg
Example: For an adult weighing 154 pounds:
  154 pounds ÷ 2.2 kg/pound = 70 kg
  70 kg × 0.8 g/kg = 56 g protein/day

| BOX 1.8 | WAYS TO PROMOTE AN ADEQUATE INTAKE |
| --- | --- |

- Reassure clients who are apprehensive about eating.
- Encourage a big breakfast if appetite deteriorates throughout the day.
- Advocate discontinuation of intravenous therapy as soon as feasible.
- Replace meals withheld for diagnostic tests.
- Promote congregate dining if appropriate.
- Question diet orders that appear inappropriate.
- Display a positive attitude when serving food or discussing nutrition.
- Order snacks and nutritional supplements.
- Request assistance with feeding or meal setup.
- Get the patient out of bed to eat if possible.
- Encourage good oral hygiene.
- Solicit information on food preferences.

| BOX 1.9 | WAYS TO FACILITATE CLIENT AND FAMILY TEACHING |
| --- | --- |

- Listen to the client's concerns and ideas.
- Encourage family involvement if appropriate.
- Reinforce the importance of obtaining adequate nutrition.
- Help the client to select appropriate foods.
- Counsel the client about drug–nutrient interactions.
- Avoid using the term "diet."
- Emphasize things "to do" instead of things "not to do."
- Keep the message simple.
- Review written handouts with the client.
- Advise the client to avoid foods that are not tolerated.

religious or ethnic background, and other medical conditions may cause the optimal diet to be impractical in either the clinical or the home setting. Generalizations do not apply to all individuals at all times. Also, comfort foods (e.g., chicken soup, mashed potatoes, ice cream) are valuable for their emotional benefits if not nutritional ones. Honor clients' requests for individual comfort foods whenever possible.

## Client Teaching

Compared with "well" clients, patients in a clinical setting may be more receptive to nutritional advice especially if they feel better by doing so or are fearful of a relapse or complications. But hospitalized patients are also prone to confusion about nutrition messages. The patient's ability to assimilate new information may be compromised by pain, medication, anxiety, or a distracting setting. Time spent with a dietitian or diet technician learning about a "diet" may be brief or interrupted, and the patient may not even know what questions to ask until long after the dietitian is gone. Box 1.9 suggests ways nurses can facilitate client and family teaching.

## Monitoring and Evaluation

In the "Nursing Process" sections of this textbook, monitoring and evaluation are grouped together, even though they are different in practice. In reality, monitoring precedes evaluation as a way to stay on top of progress or difficulties the client is experiencing. Box 1.10

| BOX 1.10 | **MONITORING SUGGESTIONS** |
|---|---|

- Observe intake whenever possible to judge the adequacy.
- Document appetite and take action when the client does not eat.
- Order supplements if intake is low or needs are high.
- Request a nutritional consult.
- Assess tolerance (i.e., absence of side effects).
- Monitor weight.
- Monitor progression of restrictive diets. Clients who are receiving nothing by mouth (NPO), who are restricted to a clear liquid diet, or who are receiving enteral or parenteral nutrition are at risk for nutritional problems.
- Monitor the client's grasp of the information and motivation to change.

offers general monitoring suggestions. Evaluation assesses whether client outcomes were achieved after the nursing care plan was given time to work. Given the limitations inherent in an abstract nursing care plan, monitoring and evaluation are combined in this textbook.

Ideally, the client's outcomes are achieved on a timely basis, and evaluation statements are client outcomes rewritten from "the client will" to "the client is." In reality, outcomes may be only partially met or not achieved at all; in those instances it is important to determine why the result was less than ideal. Were the outcomes realistic for this particular client? Were the interventions appropriate and consistently implemented? Evaluation includes deciding whether to continue, change, or abolish the plan.

Consider a male client admitted to the hospital for chronic diarrhea. During the 3 weeks before admission, the client experienced significant weight loss due to malabsorption secondary to diarrhea. Your goal is for the client to maintain his admission weight. Your interventions are to provide small meals of low-residue foods as ordered, to eliminate lactose because of the likelihood of intolerance, to increase protein and calories with appropriate nutrient-dense supplements, and to explain the nutrition therapy recommendations to the client to ease his concerns about eating. You find that the client's intake is poor because of lack of appetite and a fear that eating and drinking will promote diarrhea. You notify the dietitian, who counsels the client about low-residue foods, obtains likes and dislikes, and urges the client to think of the supplements as part of the medical treatment, not as a food eaten for taste or pleasure. You document intake and diligently encourage the client to eat and drink everything served. However, the client's weight continues to drop. You attribute this to his reluctance to eat and to the slow resolution of diarrhea due to inflammation. You determine that the goal is still realistic and appropriate but that the client is not willing or able to consume foods orally. You consult with the physician and dietitian about the client's refusal to eat and the plan changes from an oral diet to tube feeding.

## ▶ How Do You Respond?

**Should I save my menus from the hospital to help me plan meals at home?** This is not a bad idea if the in-house and discharge food plans are the same, but the menus should serve as a guide, not a gospel. Just because shrimp was never on the menu doesn't mean it is taboo. Likewise, if the client hated the orange juice served every morning, he or she shouldn't feel compelled to continue drinking it. By necessity, hospital menus are more rigid than at-home eating plans.

**Can you just tell me what to eat and I'll do it?** A black-and-white approach should be used only when absolutely necessary, such as for food allergies or for clients who insist on a rigid plan rather than the freedom to make choices. In most cases, flexible and individualized guidelines and recommendations will promote the greatest chance of compliance. Urge the client not to think of foods as "good" or "bad," but rather "more healthy" and "less healthy," except in situations of food allergy or intolerance. In most other cases, foods are negotiable.

## ▶ CASE STUDY

Steven is a 44-year-old male who is 5 ft 11 in tall and weighs 182 pounds. Over the last month he has lost approximately 10 pounds, which he blames on loss of appetite and fatigue. When he went to his family doctor with flu-like symptoms, a blood test revealed a very high white blood cell count, low platelets, and low hemoglobin. The doctor told him to proceed to the hospital for admission to rule out acute leukemia. Further lab tests are pending. His admitting orders include a regular diet. Steven does not have a significant medical history. He is married, has three children, and enjoys a successful career.

Calculate and evaluate Steven's weight according to the following standards:

- BMI
- IBW/percentage of IBW
- Percent weight change
- Based on Steven's weight and weight change, is he at nutritional risk?
- Does Steven's possible diagnosis place him at nutritional risk?
- What other criteria would help determine his level of risk?
- Using the shortcut method to determine his calorie needs, calculate his estimated calorie requirements. Calculate his recommended dietary allowance (RDA) for protein.
- If he is treated for leukemia, his protein need may increase to approximately 1.2 g protein/kg. How much would he then require?
- The hospital's diet manual says that, on average, a regular diet provides 2400 calories and 90 g of protein. Is it adequate to meet his needs?

## STUDY QUESTIONS

1. Nurses are in an ideal position to:
   a. Screen patients for risk of malnutrition
   b. Order therapeutic diets
   c. Conduct comprehensive nutrition assessments
   d. Calculate a patient's calorie and protein needs

2. The "ideal body weight" of a male who is 5 ft 10 in is:
   a. 150 pounds
   b. 155 pounds
   c. 160 pounds
   d. 166 pounds

3. Which of the following criteria would most likely be on a nutrition screen in the hospital?
   a. Prealbumin value
   b. Weight change
   c. Serum potassium value
   d. Cultural food preferences

4. Which of the following statements is accurate regarding physical signs and symptoms of malnutrition?
   a. "Physical signs of malnutrition appear before changes in weight or laboratory values occur."
   b. "Physical signs of malnutrition are suggestive, not definitive, for malnutrition."
   c. "Physical signs are easily identified as 'abnormal'."
   d. "All races and genders exhibit the same intensity of physical changes in response to malnutrition."

5. Your patient has a question about the cardiac diet the dietitian reviewed with him yesterday. What is the nurse's best response?
   a. "Ask your doctor when you go for your follow-up appointment."
   b. "What is the question? If I can't answer it, I will get the dietitian to come back to answer it."
   c. "Just do your best. The handout she gave you is simply a list of guidelines, not rigid instructions."
   d. "If I see the dietitian around, I will tell her you need to see her."

6. Which of the following statements is true regarding albumin?
   a. "Albumin is a reliable and sensitive indicator of protein status."
   b. "Albumin is not widely available because it is expensive."
   c. "Albumin has a short half-life, so it changes relatively quickly."
   d. "Low albumin is associated with increased length of hospital stay, complications, morbidity, and mortality because it reflects severity of illness."

## KEY CONCEPTS

- Nutrition is an integral part of nursing care. Like air, food is a basic human need.
- Nutrition screening is used to identify patients or clients who may be at risk of malnutrition. Screening tools are simple, quick, easy to use, and rely on available data.
- The Joint Commission stipulates that nutrition screens be performed within 24 hours to a health-care facility, but facilities are free to decide what criteria to include on a screen, what findings indicate risk, and who is to conduct the screen. Screens are often the responsibility of staff nurses because they can be completed during a history and physical examination upon admission.
- Patients who are identified to be a low or no nutritional risk are rescreened within a specified period of time to determine if their nutritional risk status has changed.
- Patients who are found to be a moderate to high nutritional risk at screening receive a comprehensive nutritional assessment by the dietitian that includes the steps of assessment, diagnosis, intervention, and monitoring and evaluation.
- Dietitians use information from the nursing history and physical to begin the assessment process. They may also obtain a nutritional history from the patient, calculate estimated protein and calorie needs, assess the adequacy and appropriateness of the diet order, and identify the patient's diagnostic code for malnutrition, if appropriate.
- Nurses can integrate nutrition into the nursing care process to develop care plans that address the individual's needs. Nurses are not expected to be dietitians, but rather use nutrition to provide quality nursing care.
- Accurate height and weight are essential for assessing risk and monitoring progress. They can be used to identify BMI, IBW, and percentage of ideal weight. Percentage of weight loss calculated to be significant or severe is also a risk.

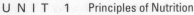

- There are no lab values that are specific and sensitive for malnutrition. Albumin is frequently used as a protein marker, but it is depleted by numerous nonnutritional factors. Prealbumin is a more sensitive indicator of protein status, but it is expensive and not routinely available.

- Clinical data are physical signs and symptoms of malnutrition. They are nonspecific, subjective, and develop slowly and should be considered suggestive, not diagnostic, of malnutrition.

- Dietary data can help determine if a nutrition problem is caused by intake or by illness or its treatments. The term *diet* inspires negative feelings in most people. Replace it with *eating pattern, eating style,* or *foods you normally eat* to avoid negative connotations.

- Medical–psychosocial history can reveal factors that influence intake, nutritional requirements, or nutrition counseling needs.

- Medications and nutritional supplements should be evaluated for their potential impact on nutrient intake, absorption, utilization, or excretion.

- Nursing diagnoses relate directly to nutrition when the client's intake of nutrients is too much or too little for body requirements. Many other nursing diagnoses, including constipation, impaired skin integrity, health-seeking behaviors, noncompliance, and risk for infection, relate indirectly to nutrition because nutrition contributes to the problem or solution.

- A nutrition priority for all clients is to obtain adequate calories and nutrients based on individual needs.

- Short-term nutrition goals are to attain or maintain adequate weight and nutritional status and (as appropriate) to avoid nutrition-related symptoms and complications of illness. Client-centered outcomes should be measurable, attainable, and specific.

- Intake recommendations are not always appropriate for all persons; what is recommended in theory may not work for an individual. Clients may revert to comfort foods during periods of illness or stress.

- Nurses can reinforce nutrition counseling done by the dietitian and initiate counseling for clients with low or mild risk.

- Use preprinted lists of "do's and don'ts" only if absolutely necessary such as in the case of food allergies. For most people, actual food choices should be considered in view of how much and how often they are eaten rather than as foods that "must" or "must not" be consumed.

## ANSWER KEY

1. **FALSE** The nurse is in an ideal position to provide nutrition information to patients and their families since he or she is the one with the greatest client contact.

2. **TRUE** Nutritional screening uses a small number of factors to identify patients or clients with malnutrition or at risk of malnutrition.

3. **FALSE** Hospitals and health-care facilities are free to decide what criteria they will use to identify risk for malnutrition and what defines risk. For instance, a hospital may use acute pancreatitis as a high-risk diagnosis, whereas another may not.

4. **FALSE** Changes in weight may be slow to occur. Weight changes are more reflective of chronic, not acute, changes in nutritional status.

5. **TRUE** A person can be malnourished without being underweight. Weight does not provide qualitative information about body composition.

6. **FALSE** Low serum albumin levels may be caused by problems other than protein malnutrition such as injury, infection, overhydration, and liver disease.

7. **TRUE** Weight loss is judged significant if there is a 5% loss over the course of 1 month.

8. **TRUE** People who take five or more prescription drugs, over-the-counter drugs, or dietary supplements are at increased risk for developing drug-induced nutrient deficiencies.

9. **TRUE** Determining what the patient normally eats can help diagnose the role of intake in the nutritional problem as primary, secondary, or insignificant.

10. **TRUE** Physical signs and symptoms of malnutrition develop only after other signs of malnutrition, such as laboratory and weight changes, are observed.

## WEBSITES

For Dietary Analysis and Intake Calculators, a variety of Dietary Assessment Tools, and Resource Information, go to "Dietary Assessment" under Topics A–Z at the Food and Nutrition Information Center at **www.nal.usda.gov/fnic.html**

## REFERENCES

American Dietetic Association Evidence Library. (2006). Nutrition Care Process. Available at www.adaevidencelibrary.com. Accessed on 3/11/08.

Charney, P., & Malone, A. (Ed.). (2004). *ADA Pocket Guide to Nutrition Assessment*. Chicago: American Dietetic Association.

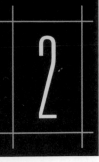

# 2

# Carbohydrates

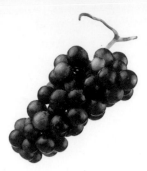

| TRUE | FALSE | | |
|------|-------|---|---|
| ☐ | ☐ | **1** | Starch is made from glucose molecules. |
| ☐ | ☐ | **2** | Sugar is higher in calories than starch. |
| ☐ | ☐ | **3** | The sugar in fruit is better for you than the sugar in candy. |
| ☐ | ☐ | **4** | Most commonly consumed American foods provide adequate fiber to enable people to meet the recommended intake. |
| ☐ | ☐ | **5** | Enriched wheat bread is nutritionally equivalent to whole wheat bread. |
| ☐ | ☐ | **6** | Soft drinks contribute more added sugars to the typical American diet than any other food or beverage. |
| ☐ | ☐ | **7** | Bread is just as likely as candy to cause cavities. |
| ☐ | ☐ | **8** | The sugar content on food labels refers only to added sugars, not those naturally present in the food. |
| ☐ | ☐ | **9** | Artificial sweeteners are dangerous for most people. |
| ☐ | ☐ | **10** | Sugar causes hyperactivity in kids. |

### UPON COMPLETION OF THIS CHAPTER, YOU WILL BE ABLE TO

- Classify the type(s) of carbohydrate found in various foods.
- Describe the functions of carbohydrates.
- Modify a menu to ensure that the adequate intake for fiber is provided.
- Calculate the calorie content of a food that contains only carbohydrates.
- Debate the usefulness of using glycemic load to make food choices.
- Suggest ways to limit sugar intake.
- Discuss the benefits and disadvantages of using sugar alternatives.

## ▶ CARBOHYDRATES

Sugar and starch come to mind when people hear the word "carbohydrates," but carbohydrates are so much more than just granulated sugar and bread. Foods containing carbohydrates can be empty calories, nutritional powerhouses, or something in-between. Globally, carbohydrates provide the majority of calories in almost all human diets.

This chapter describes what carbohydrates are, where they are found in the diet, and how they are handled in the body. Recommendations regarding intake and the role of carbohydrates in health are presented.

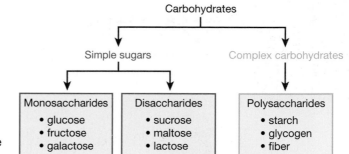

**FIGURE 2.1** Carbohydrate classifications.

## Carbohydrate Classifications

**Carbohydrates:** a class of energy-yielding nutrients that contain only carbon, hydrogen, and oxygen, hence the common abbreviation of CHO.

**Carbohydrates** are comprised of the elements carbon, hydrogen, and oxygen arranged into basic sugar molecules. They are classified as either **simple carbohydrates**, which contain only one or two sugar molecules, or **complex carbohydrates**, which are composed of many sugar molecules joined together (Fig. 2.1).

## Monosaccharides

**Simple Carbohydrates:** a classification of carbohydrates that includes monosaccharides and disaccharides; commonly referred to as sugars.

**Monosaccharide:** single (mono) molecules of sugar (saccharide), e.g., glucose, fructose, galactose.

**Monosaccharides,** the simplest of all sugars, are comprised of only one sugar molecule. The most common monosaccharides in foods are hexoses (six-carbon sugar molecules), namely glucose, fructose, and galactose. As basic units, these sugar molecules are absorbed "as is" without undergoing digestion.

**Glucose.** Glucose, also known as dextrose, is the sugar of greatest distinction: it circulates through the blood to provide energy for body cells; it is a component of all disaccharides and is virtually the sole constituent of complex carbohydrates; and it is the sugar the body converts all other digestible carbohydrates to. In foods, glucose is found in fruits, vegetables, honey, corn syrup, and cornstarch.

**Fructose.** Fructose ("fruit sugar") is found naturally in fruit and honey and is the sweetest of all natural sugars. High-fructose corn syrup (HFCS) is a commercially made liquid sweetener from the dextrose in cornstarch. It is composed of glucose and varying concentrations of fructose. Because HFCS is much sweeter than sucrose, less can be used to sweeten foods so the cost is less than using sugar. The beverage industry uses 90% of HFCS.

**Galactose.** Galactose does not occur in appreciable amounts in foods; it is significant only as it combines with glucose to form the disaccharide lactose.

## Disaccharides

**Disaccharide:** "double sugar" composed of two (di) monosaccharides, e.g., sucrose, maltose, lactose.

**Disaccharides** are composed of two linked monosaccharides, at least one of which is glucose. Disaccharides are split into their component monosaccharides before being absorbed. Sucrose, maltose, and lactose are disaccharides.

**Sucrose.** Sucrose, composed of glucose and fructose, is what is commonly called "sugar" or table sugar. It is produced when sucrose from sugarcane and sugar beets is refined and granulated. The differences among brown, white, confectioners, and turbinado sugars have to do with the degree of refining. Sucrose also occurs naturally in some fruits and vegetables.

**Maltose.** Maltose is composed of two glucose molecules joined together. Maltose is not found naturally in foods, but is added to some foods for flavoring (e.g., malted milk shakes) and to beer for coloring. Maltose occurs as an intermediate in starch digestion.

**Lactose.** Lactose ("milk sugar") is composed of glucose and galactose. It is the carbohydrate found naturally in milk and is used as an additive in many foods and drugs. Lactose enhances the absorption of calcium and promotes the growth of normal gastrointestinal (GI) flora that produce vitamin K. It is the least sweet of all sugars and the only animal source of sugar.

## Polysaccharides

**Polysaccharide:** carbohydrates consisting of many (poly) sugar molecules.

**Complex Carbohydrates:** a group name for starch, glycogen, and fiber; composed of long chains of glucose molecules.

**Starch:** the storage form of glucose in plants.

**Glycogen:** storage form of glucose in animals and humans.

**Insoluble Fiber:** nondigestible carbohydrates that do not dissolve in water.

**Soluble Fiber:** nondigestible carbohydrates that dissolve to a gummy, viscous texture.

**Dietary Fiber:** carbohydrates and lignin that are natural and intact components of plants that cannot be digested by human enzymes.

**Polysaccharides** are **complex carbohydrates** composed of hundreds to thousands of glucose molecules linked together. Despite being made of sugar, polysaccharides do not taste sweet because their molecules are too large to fit on the tongue's taste bud receptors that sense sweetness. Starch, glycogen, and fiber are types of polysaccharides.

**Starch.** Through the process of photosynthesis, plants synthesize glucose, which they use for energy. Glucose not used by the plant for immediate energy is stored in the form of **starch** in seeds, roots, or stems. Grains, such as wheat, rice, corn, barley, millet, sorghum, oats, and rye, are the world's major food crops and the foundation of all diets. Other sources of starch include potatoes, dried peas and beans, and other starchy vegetables (Fig. 2.2).

**Glycogen. Glycogen** is the animal (including human) version of starch; it is stored carbohydrate available for energy as needed. Humans have a limited supply of glycogen stored in the liver and muscles. Liver glycogen breaks down and releases glucose into the bloodstream between meals to maintain normal blood glucose levels and provide fuel for tissues. Muscles do not share their supply of glycogen but use it for their own energy needs. There is virtually no dietary source of glycogen because any glycogen stored in animal tissue is quickly converted to lactic acid at the time of slaughter. Miniscule amounts of glycogen are found in shellfish, such as scallops and oysters, which is why they taste slightly sweet compared to other fish.

**Fiber.** Although there is no universally accepted definition of fiber, it is generally considered a group name for polysaccharides that cannot be digested by human enzymes. Commonly referred to as "roughage," fiber is found only in plants as a component of plant cell walls.

Historically, fibers have been categorized as **insoluble** or **soluble** based on how readily they dissolve in water (Box 2.1). They differ in their physiologic effects in the body. Although sources of fiber are commonly labeled as either soluble or insoluble, almost all sources of fiber provide a blend of both types of fiber (Table 2.1).

The National Academy of Sciences recommends that the terms insoluble and soluble be phased out in favor of ascribing specific physiologic benefits to a particular fiber. **Dietary fiber**

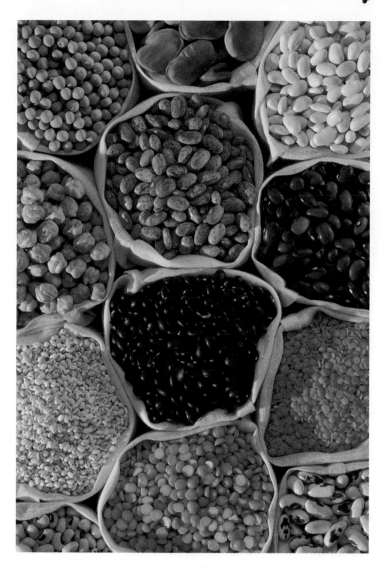

**FIGURE 2.2** Dried peas and beans are a good source of starch.

**Functional Fiber:** as proposed by the Food and Nutrition Board, functional fiber consists of extracted or isolated nondigestible carbohydrates that have beneficial physiological effects in humans.

**Total Fiber:** total fiber = dietary fiber + added fiber.

refers to intact and naturally occurring fiber found in plants; **functional fiber** refers to fiber that has been isolated or extracted from plants that has beneficial physiological effects in the body. The sum of dietary and functional fiber equals **total fiber.** The rationale for discontinuing soluble and insoluble fiber is that the amounts of soluble and insoluble fibers measured in a mixed diet are dependent on methods of analysis that are not able to exactly replicate human digestion.

It is commonly assumed that fiber does not provide any calories because it is not truly digested by human enzymes and may actually trap macronutrients eaten at the same time and prevent them from being absorbed. Yet most fibers, particularly soluble fibers, are fermented by bacteria in the colon to produce carbon dioxide, methane, hydrogen, and short-chain fatty acids which serve as a source of energy (calories) for the mucosal lining of the colon. For food labeling purposes in the United States, dietary fiber is assigned an energy value of 0 cal/g for insoluble fiber and 4 cal/g for soluble fiber (Lupton and Trumbo, 2006).

## BOX 2.1 TYPES, PHYSIOLOGICAL EFFECTS, AND SOURCES OF SOLUBLE AND INSOLUBLE FIBER

| Soluble Fiber (More Fermentable) | Insoluble Fiber (Less Fermentable) |
|---|---|
| **Types**<br>Pectin<br>Some hemicelluloses<br>Vegetable gums<br>Psyllium<br>Mucilages | **Types**<br>Cellulose<br>Many hemicelluloses<br>Lignans<br>Psyllium |
| **Mixed with water**<br>Dissolve to form a viscous gel | **Mixed with water**<br>Do not dissolve but act like a sponge in the intestine to soak up water |
| **Physiologic effects**<br>Slow gastric emptying time<br>Promote a feeling of fullness<br>Delay and blunt the rise in serum glucose after eating<br>Lower serum cholesterol, possibly by trapping cholesterol which increases cholesterol excretion | **Physiologic effects**<br>Increase stool bulk<br>Promote laxation<br>Prevent constipation |
| **Best Sources**<br>Dried peas and beans<br>Lentils<br>Oats<br>Certain fruits and vegetables | **Best Sources**<br>Whole wheat bread and cereals<br>Certain fruits and vegetables |

## TABLE 2.1 Fiber Content of Selected Foods

| Food Source | Soluble Fiber (g) | Insoluble Fiber (g) | Total Fiber (g) |
|---|---|---|---|
| **Grains** | | | |
| Barley, ½ cup cooked | 1 | 3 | 4 |
| Oatmeal, ½ cup cooked | 1 | 1 | 2 |
| Popcorn, popped, 3 cups | 0.1 | 1.9 | 2 |
| Puffed wheat cereal, 1 cup | 0.5 | 0.5 | 1.0 |
| Spaghetti, white, ½ cup | 0.4 | 0.5 | 0.9 |
| Spaghetti, whole wheat, ½ cup | 0.6 | 2.1 | 2.7 |
| White bread, 1 slice | 0.3 | 0.3 | 0.6 |
| Whole wheat, 1 slice | 0.3 | 1.2 | 1.5 |
| **Dried Peas and Beans (½ Cup Cooked)** | | | |
| Black beans | 2.4 | 3.7 | 6.1 |
| Black-eyed peas | 0.5 | 4.2 | 4.7 |
| Kidney beans, light red | 2 | 5.9 | 7.9 |
| Lima beans | 3.5 | 3 | 6.5 |
| Pinto beans | 1.4 | 4.7 | 6.1 |
| Lentils | 0.6 | 4.6 | 5.2 |

(table continues on page 23)

| TABLE 2.1 | **Fiber Content of Selected Foods** (continued) |

| Food Source | Soluble Fiber (g) | Insoluble Fiber (g) | Total Fiber (g) |
|---|---|---|---|
| **Fruit (1 Medium)** | | | |
| Apple | 1 | 3 | 4 |
| Bananas | 1 | 2 | 3 |
| Blackberries (½ cup) | 1 | 3 | 4 |
| Orange | 2 | 0–1 | 2–3 |
| Pears | 2 | 2 | 4 |
| Prunes (¼ cup) | 1.5 | 1.5 | 3 |
| **Vegetables (½ Cup Cooked)** | | | |
| Broccoli | 1 | 0.5 | 1.5 |
| Brussels sprouts | 3 | 1.5 | 4.5 |
| Carrots | 1 | 1.5 | 2.5 |
| Cauliflower | 0.4 | 0.6 | 1.0 |
| Corn, canned | 0.2 | 1.4 | 1.6 |
| Okra, frozen | 1 | 3.1 | 4.1 |
| Peas, frozen | 1.3 | 3.0 | 4.3 |

***Source:*** Soluble Fiber Tipsheet at www.nhlbi.nih.gov/chd/Tipsheets/solfiber.htm; and Fiber Content of Foods in Common Portions available at http://huhs.harvard.edu/assets/File/OurServices/Service_Nutrition_Fiber.pdf. Accessed on 10/5/07.

Although the exact energy value available to humans from the blend of fibers in food is unknown, current data indicate the value is between 1.5 cal/g and 2.5 cal/g (Institute of Medicine, 2005).

## Sources of Carbohydrates

Carbohydrates in food appear in the form of natural sugars, added sugars, starch, and fiber. Grains, Vegetables, Fruits, and Milk are the MyPyramid groups that provide the majority of carbohydrates (Fig. 2.3). Nuts and dried peas and beans from the Meat and Beans group provide significant starch and fiber, but they are generally consumed less often than the carbohydrate-free selections within this group. The Oils group is carbohydrate free. Table 2.2 estimates the grams of carbohydrate provided in the MyPyramid 2000 calorie food pattern.

### Grains

This group is synonymous with "carbs" and consists of grains (e.g., wheat, barley, oats, rye, corn, and rice) and products made with flours from grains (e.g., items made with wheat flour, such as bread, crackers, pasta, and tortillas). Grains are classified as "whole" or "refined" (Box 2.2).

**Whole Grains and Whole Grain Flours:** contain the entire grain, or seed, which includes the endosperm, bran, and germ.

**Whole grains** consist of the entire kernel of a grain, such as oatmeal, brown rice, whole wheat flour, and a whole kernel of corn (Fig. 2.4). They come in various forms, including cracked, ground, or milled into flour. Whole grains, regardless of the variety, are composed of three parts:

- The bran, or tough outer coating, which is an excellent source of insoluble fiber.
- The endosperm, the largest portion of the kernel, which supplies all of the grain's starch and is the basis of all flours.
- The germ (embryo), the smallest portion of the kernel that is rich in fat and thus makes whole wheat flour more susceptible to rancidity than refined flour.

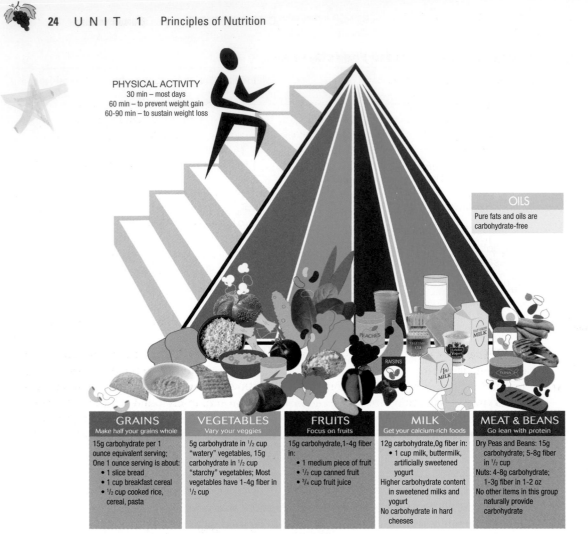

PHYSICAL ACTIVITY
30 min – most days
60 min – to prevent weight gain
60-90 min – to sustain weight loss

OILS
Pure fats and oils are
carbohydrate-free

| GRAINS Make half your grains whole | VEGETABLES Vary your veggies | FRUITS Focus on fruits | MILK Get your calcium-rich foods | MEAT & BEANS Go lean with protein |
|---|---|---|---|---|
| 15g carbohydrate per 1 ounce equivalent serving; One 1 ounce serving is about: <br>• 1 slice bread <br>• 1 cup breakfast cereal <br>• ½ cup cooked rice, cereal, pasta | 5g carbohydrate in ½ cup "watery" vegetables, 15g carbohydrate in ½ cup "starchy" vegetables; Most vegetables have 1-4g fiber in ½ cup | 15g carbohydrate,1-4g fiber in: <br>• 1 medium piece of fruit <br>• ½ cup canned fruit <br>• ¾ cup fruit juice | 12g carbohydrate,0g fiber in: <br>• 1 cup milk, buttermilk, artificially sweetened yogurt <br>Higher carbohydrate content in sweetened milks and yogurt <br>No carbohydrate in hard cheeses | Dry Peas and Beans: 15g carbohydrate; 5-8g fiber in ½ cup <br>Nuts: 4-8g carbohydrate; 1-3g fiber in 1-2 oz <br>No other items in this group naturally provide carbohydrate |

**FIGURE 2.3** Carbohydrate content of MyPyramid groups. (USDA, Center for Nutrition Policy and Promotion (2005). MyPyramid—Steps to Healthier You Food Guidance System. Available at www.MyPyramid.gov.)

---

**TABLE 2.2** **Carbohydrate Content of the MyPyramid 2000 Calorie Food Intake Pattern**

| Group | Amount Recommended in 2000 Calorie Diet* | CHO Content Per Unit of Measure† | Total CHO Content Per Group (g) |
|---|---|---|---|
| Grains | 6 oz equivalents | 15 g/equivalent | 90 |
| Vegetables | 2½ cups | 5 g/½ cup | 25 |
| Fruits | 2 cups | 15 g/½ cup | 60 |
| Milk | 3 cups | 12 g/cup | 36 |
| | | | Total carbohydrate‡: 211 g |

*United States Department of Agriculture, Center for Nutrition Policy and Promotion (2005). MyPyramid—Steps to Healthier You Food Guidance System. Available at www.MyPyramid.gov.

†Based on the American Diabetes Association, American Dietetic Association Choose your Foods: Exchange Lists for Diabetes, 2008.

‡Total carbohydrate does not account for any additional carbohydrate that may come from choosing nuts or dried peas and beans from the Meat group, or from added sugars in the discretionary calorie category.

BOX 2.2          **SOURCES OF WHOLE AND REFINED GRAINS**

| Generally Accepted Whole Grains | Refined Grains |
|---|---|
| Whole wheat grain, flour, bread, or cereals, such as wheat berries, bulgur (cracked wheat), whole wheat bread, whole wheat pasta, shredded wheat, Wheaties, whole wheat tortillas, whole wheat crackers | Enriched white or wheat flour, as found in white or wheat bread, white pasta, flour tortillas, pretzels, crackers |
| Whole oats, oatmeal, Cheerios | Cream of wheat, puffed wheat |
| Corn, popcorn | Oat flour |
| Brown rice, wild rice | Cornstarch, cornflakes, grits, hominy |
|  | White rice, Rice Krispies, Cream of rice, puffed rice |
| Whole grain barley | Pearl barley |
| Whole rye |  |
| Others: triticale, millet, quinoa, sorghum spelt, kamut, amaranth, teff Buckwheat |  |

**Refined Grains and Refined Flours:** consist of only the endosperm (middle part) of the grain and therefore do not contain the bran and germ portions.

**Enrichment:** adding back certain nutrients (to specific levels) that were lost during processing.

**Fortification:** adding nutrients that are not naturally present in the food or were present in insignificant amounts.

Bran cereals and wheat germ are not whole grains because they come from only one part of the whole.

**"Refined" grains** have most of the bran and germ removed. They are rich in starch, but lack the fiber, vitamins, trace minerals, fat, and phytochemicals found in whole grains (International Food Information Council (IFIC), 2007). The process of **enrichment** restores some B vitamins (thiamin, riboflavin, and niacin) and iron to levels found prior to processing. Other substances that are lost, such as other vitamins, other minerals, fiber, and phytochemicals, are not replaced by enrichment. Enriched grains are also required to be **fortified** with

**Endosperm**
Storage site
for starch; main
source of flour
*Provides:*
protein, starch,
small amounts
of vitamins,
and trace minerals

**Germ**
Embryo that
will sprout into
another plant
if fertilized
*Provides:*
B vitamins,
some protein,
healthy fat, vitamin E,
minerals, antioxidants,
and phytochemicals

**Bran**
Outer layer that protects rest of kernel
*Provides:*
fiber, antioxidants, B vitamin, iron, zinc,
copper, magnesium, and phytochemicals
from sunlight, pests, water, and disease

Refined grains:
• made only from endosperm
• are enriched with
  thiamin, riboflavin, niacin,
  and iron lost through processing
• are fortified with folic acid
• are inferior to whole
  grains in vitamin B6, protein,
  pantothenic acid, vitamin E,
  fiber, phytochemicals

**FIGURE 2.4** Whole wheat kernel. The components of the whole wheat kernel are the *bran,* the *germ,* and the *endosperm.*

folic acid, a mandate designed to reduce the risk of neural tube defects. Examples of refined grains include white flour, white bread, white rice, and refined cornmeal.

## Vegetables

Starch and some sugars provide the majority of calories in vegetables, but the content varies widely among individual vegetables. A ½ cup serving of "starchy" vegetables provides three times more carbohydrate than the same amount of "watery" vegetables. The average fiber content of vegetables is 2-3 g/serving.

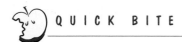

### Q U I C K   B I T E

| Examples of "starchy" vegetables | Examples of "watery" vegetables |
|---|---|
| Corn | Asparagus |
| Pinto beans | Bean sprouts |
| Lentils | Broccoli |
| Peas | Carrots |
| Potato | Green beans |
| Sweet potato | Greens |
| Winter squash (acorn, butternut) | Okra |
| Yam | Tomato |

## Fruits

### Q U I C K   B I T E

The effect of processing on fiber content

| | Fiber (g/serving) |
|---|---|
| Unpeeled fresh apple (1) | 3.0 |
| Peeled fresh apple (1) | 1.9 |
| Applesauce (½ cup) | 1.5 |
| Apple juice (¾ cup) | Negligible |

Generally, almost all of the calories in fruit come from sugar (mostly fructose), with small amounts of starch and minute quantities of protein providing negligible calories. The exceptions to this are avocado, olives, and coconut, which get the majority of their calories from fat. Generally a serving of fruit, defined as ¾ cup of juice, 1 piece of fresh fruit, ½ cup of canned fruit, or ¼ cup of dried fruit, provides 15 g of carbohydrate and approximately 2 g fiber. Because fiber is located in the skin of fruits, fresh whole fruits provide more fiber than do fresh peeled fruits, canned fruits, or fruit juices.

## Milk

### Q U I C K   B I T E

Carbohydrate content (both natural and added sugars) of various dairy foods

| | Carbohydrate (g) |
|---|---|
| Milk, 8 oz | 12 |
| Chocolate milk, 8 oz | 26.1 |
| Plain yogurt, 8 oz | 15.0 |
| Strawberry yogurt, 8 oz | 48.5 |
| Regular vanilla ice cream, ½ cup | 15.6 |
| Swiss cheese, 1 oz | 1.0 |

Although milk is considered a "protein," more of milk's calories come from carbohydrate than from protein. One cup of milk, regardless of the fat content, provides 12 g of carbohydrate in the form of lactose. Flavored milk and yogurt have added sugars, as do ice cream, ice milk, and frozen yogurt. With the exception of cottage cheese, which has about 6 g carbohydrate per cup, cheese is virtually lactose free because it is converted to lactic acid during production.

## Discretionary Calories

Sugar content of selected "extras"

|  | Sugar (g) |
|---|---|
| White sugar, 1 tsp | 4.0 |
| Brown sugar, 1 tsp | 4.5 |
| Jelly, 1 tsp | 4.5 |
| Gelatin, ½ cup | 19.0 |
| Cola drink, 12 oz | 40.0 |

Discretionary calories refer to "extras," either choices within food groups that are more calorically dense than the "ideal" choices or additional servings of food. Because it is a "catch-all" group, the carbohydrate content varies considerably, from none in items like butter and sausage to 100% of the calories in syrup, sweetened sodas, and hard candies.

# How the Body Handles Carbohydrates

## Digestion

Cooked starch begins to undergo digestion in the mouth by the action of salivary amylase, but the overall effect is small because food is not held in the mouth very long (Fig. 2.5). The stomach churns and mixes its contents, but its acid medium halts any residual effect of the swallowed amylase. Most carbohydrate digestion occurs in the small intestine, where pancreatic amylase reduces complex carbohydrates into shorter chains and disaccharides.

Disaccharidase enzymes (maltase, sucrase, and lactase) on the surface of the cells of the small intestine split maltose, sucrose, and lactose respectively into monosaccharides. Monosaccharides are the only form of carbohydrates the body is able to absorb intact and the form all other digestible carbohydrates must be reduced to before they can be absorbed. Normally 95% of starch is digested usually within 1 to 4 hours after eating.

## Absorption

Glucose, fructose, and galactose are absorbed through intestinal mucosa cells and travel to the liver via the portal vein. Small amounts of starch that have not been fully digested pass into the colon with fiber and are excreted in the stools. Fibers may impair the absorption of some minerals—namely calcium, zinc, and iron—by binding with them in the small intestine.

## Metabolism

Fructose and galactose are converted to glucose in the liver. The liver releases glucose into the bloodstream, where its level is held fairly constant by the action of hormones. A rise in blood glucose concentration after eating causes the pancreas to secrete insulin, which moves glucose out of the bloodstream and into the cells. Most cells take only as much glucose as they need for immediate energy needs; muscle and liver cells take extra glucose to store as glycogen. The release of insulin lowers blood glucose to normal levels.

**Postprandial:** following a meal.

In the **postprandial** state, as the body uses the energy from the last meal, the blood glucose concentration begins to drop. Even a slight fall in blood glucose stimulates the pancreas to release glucagon, which causes the liver to release glucose from its supply of glycogen. The result is that blood glucose levels increase to normal.

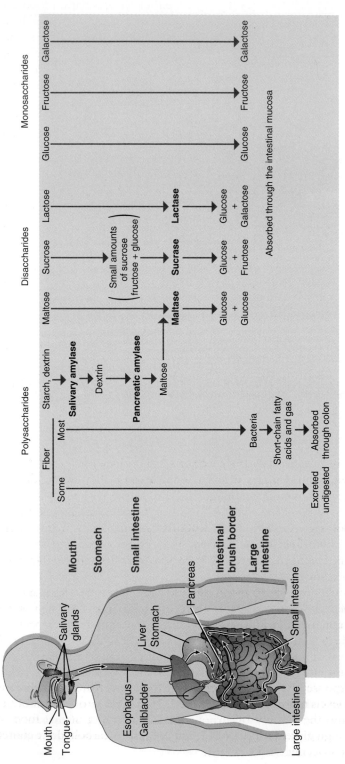

**FIGURE 2.5** Carbohydrate digestion. Dietary carbohydrates include the polysaccharides or complex carbohydrates (fiber, starch, and dextrin), the disaccharides (maltose, sucrose, and lactose), and the monosaccharides (glucose, fructose, and galactose). Digestion begins in the *mouth*, where food is chewed into pieces and salivary amylase begins the process of chemical digestion. The *stomach* churns and mixes the carbohydrate, but stomach acids halt residual action of the salivary amylase. The *small intestine* is the site of most carbohydrate digestion, and pancreatic amylase reduces complex carbohydrates into disaccharides. Disaccharide enzymes (maltase, sucrase, and lactase) on the surface of the small intestine cells split maltose, sucrose, and lactose into monosaccharides, thus completing the process of carbohydrate digestion. Fiber is not digested per se, but most is fermented by bacteria in the *large intestine* to yield gas, water, and short-chain fatty acids.

| TABLE 2.3 | Glycemic Index and Glycemic Load of Selected Foods | |
|---|---|---|
| Item | Glycemic Index (Glucose = 100) | Glycemic Load/Serving |
| White spaghetti | 58 | 28 |
| Baked potato | 85 | 26 |
| White bagel | 72 | 25 |
| Cornflakes | 92 | 24 |
| Long-grain white rice | 56 | 24 |
| Snickers Bar | 68 | 23 |
| Jelly beans | 78 | 22 |
| Macaroni | 45 | 22 |
| Sweet corn | 60 | 20 |
| Honey | 87 | 18 |
| Boiled sweet potato | 59 | 18 |
| Shredded wheat | 83 | 17 |
| Coca cola | 56 | 16 |
| Steamed brown rice | 50 | 16 |
| Pound cake | 54 | 15 |
| Unsweetened clear apple juice | 44 | 13 |
| Banana | 46 | 12 |
| White bread | 70 | 10 |
| Chickpeas | 33 | 10 |
| All-Bran cereal | 38 | 9 |
| Reduced-fat yogurt | 26 | 8 |
| Watermelon | 72 | 4 |
| Orange | 40 | 4 |
| Premium ice cream | 37 | 4 |
| Low-fat ice cream | 50 | 3 |
| Peanuts | 17 | 1 |

*Source:* Foster-Powell, K., Holt, S., and Brand-Miller, J. (2002). International table of glycemic index and glycemic load values: 2002. *The American Journal of Clinical Nutrition*; *76*(1), 50–56.

## Glycemic Response

**Glycemic Response:** the effect a food has on the blood glucose concentration; how quickly the glucose level rises, how high it goes, and how long it takes to return to normal.

**Glycemic Index:** a numeric measure of the glycemic response of 50g of a food sample; the higher the number, the higher the glycemic response.

**Glycemic Load:** a food's glycemic index multiplied by the amount of carbohydrate it contains to determine impact on blood glucose levels.

It was commonly believed that sugars produce a greater increase in blood glucose levels, or **glycemic response**, than complex carbohydrates because they are rapidly and completely absorbed. This proved to be too simplistic of an assumption, as illustrated by the lower glycemic index of cola (sugar) compared to that of baked potatoes (complex carbohydrate) (Table 2.3). A food's glycemic response is actually influenced by many variables including the amounts of fat, fiber, and acid in the food; the degree of processing, the method of preparation, the amount eaten, the degree of ripeness (for fruits and vegetables); and whether other foods eaten at the same time.

To assess a food's impact on blood glucose response more accurately, the concept of **glycemic index** was developed. A food's glycemic index is determined by comparing the impact on blood glucose after 50 g of a food sample is eaten to the impact of 50 g of pure glucose or white bread. For instance, a baked potato with a glycemic index of 76 elicits 76% of the blood glucose response as an equivalent amount of pure glucose.

Because the amount of carbohydrate contained in a typical portion of food also influences glycemic response, the concept of **glycemic load** was created to define a food's impact on blood glucose levels more accurately (Table 2.3). It takes into account both the glycemic index of a food and the amount of carbohydrate in a serving of that food. For example, watermelon has a high glycemic index of 72, but because its carbohydrate content is low (it is mostly water), the glycemic load is only 4.

In a practical sense, glycemic load is not a reliable tool for choosing a healthy diet and claims that a low glycemic index diet promotes significant weight loss or helps control appetite are unfounded. Soft drinks, candy, sugars, and high-fat foods may have low to moderate glycemic index but are not nutritious nor does eating them promote weight loss. And a food's actual impact on glucose levels is difficult to predict because of the many factors influencing glycemic load. Glycemic index may help people with diabetes fine-tune optimal meal planning (see Chapter 19) and athletes can use the glycemic index to choose optimal fuels for before, during, and after exercise (see Chapter 7).

## Functions of Carbohydrates

Glucose metabolism is a dynamic state of balance between burning glucose for energy (*catabolism*) and using glucose to build other compounds (*anabolism*). This process is a continuous response to the supply of glucose from food and the demand for glucose for energy needs.

### Glucose for Energy

The primary function of carbohydrates is to provide energy for cells. Glucose is burned more efficiently and more completely than either protein or fat, and it does not leave an end product that the body must excrete. Although muscles use a mixture of fat and glucose for energy, the brain is totally dependent on glucose for energy. All digestible carbohydrates provide 4 cal/g consumed.

As a primary source of energy, carbohydrates also spare protein and prevent ketosis.

### Protein Sparing

Although protein provides 4 cal/g just like carbohydrates, it has other specialized functions that only protein can perform, such as replenishing enzymes, hormones, antibodies, and blood cells. Consuming adequate carbohydrate to meet energy needs has the effect of "sparing protein" from being used for energy, leaving it available to do its special functions. An adequate carbohydrate intake is especially important whenever protein needs are increased such as for wound healing and during pregnancy and lactation.

### Preventing Ketosis

**Ketone Bodies:**
intermediate, acidic compounds formed from the incomplete breakdown of fat when adequate glucose is not available.

Fat normally supplies about half of the body's energy requirement. Yet glucose fragments are needed to efficiently and completely burn fat for energy. Without adequate glucose, fat oxidation prematurely stops at the intermediate step of **ketone body** formation. Although muscles and other tissues can use ketone bodies for energy, they are normally produced only in small quantities. An increased production of ketone bodies and their accumulation in the bloodstream causes nausea, fatigue, loss of appetite, and ketoacidosis. Dehydration and sodium depletion may follow as the body tries to excrete ketones in the urine.

### Using Glucose to Make Other Compounds

After energy needs are met, excess glucose can be converted to glycogen, be used to make nonessential amino acids and specific body compounds, or be converted to fat and stored.

**Glycogen.** The body's backup supply of glucose is liver glycogen. Liver and muscle cells pick up extra glucose molecules during times of plenty and join them together to form glycogen, which can quickly release glucose in time of need. Typically one-third of the body's glycogen reserve is in the liver and can be released into circulation for all body cells to use and two-thirds is in muscle, which is available only for use by muscles. Unlike fat, glycogen storage is limited and may provide only enough calories for about a half-day of moderate activity.

**Nonessential Amino Acids.** If an adequate supply of essential amino acids is available, the body can use them and glucose to make nonessential amino acids.

**Carbohydrate-Containing Compounds.** The body can convert glucose to other essential carbohydrates such as ribose, a component of ribonucleic acid (RNA) and deoxyribonucleic acid (DNA), keratin sulfate (in fingernails), and hyaluronic acid (found in the fluid that lubricates the joints and vitreous humor of the eyeball).

**Fat.** Any glucose remaining at this point—after energy needs are met, glycogen stores are saturated, and other specific compounds are made—is converted by liver cells to triglycerides and stored in the body's fat tissue. The body does this by combining acetate molecules to form fatty acids, which then are combined with glycerol to make triglycerides. Although it sounds easy for excess carbohydrates to be converted to fat, it is not a primary pathway; the body prefers to make body fat from dietary fat, not carbohydrates.

## Dietary Reference Intakes

### Total Carbohydrate

The Recommended Dietary Allowance (RDA) for carbohydrate is set at 130 g for both adults and children, based on the average *minimum* amount of glucose that is utilized to fuel the brain and assuming total calorie intake is adequate. Yet at this level total calorie needs are not met unless protein and fat intakes exceed levels considered healthy. A more useful guideline for determining appropriate carbohydrate intake is the Acceptable Macronutrient Distribution Range (AMDR); it suggests that carbohydrates provide 45% to 65% of total calories. As illustrated in Figure 2.6, the carbohydrate content using AMDR standards is

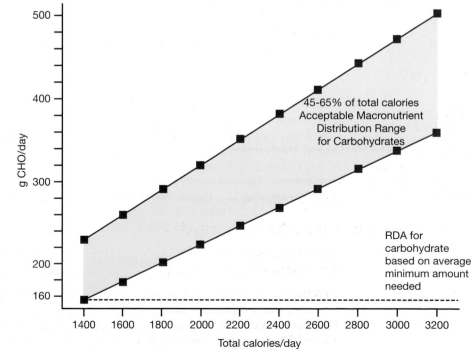

**FIGURE 2.6** Amount of total carbohydrates appropriate at various caloric levels based on the AMDR of 45% to 55% of total calories. The dotted line represents the RDA for carbohydrate based on average minimum amount needed.

45-65% of total calories Acceptable Macronutrient Distribution Range for Carbohydrates

RDA for carbohydrate based on average minimum amount needed

g CHO/day

Total calories/day

| TABLE 2.4 | Maximum Amount of Added Sugars Recommended Based on the Guideline of 25% of Total Calories or Less | |
| --- | --- | --- |
| Total Calories Consumed | Maximum Added Sugars (g/day) at 25% of Total Calories | Equivalent Amount of Sugar (tsp) |
| 1400 | 88 | 22 |
| 1600 | 100 | 25 |
| 1800 | 113 | 28 |
| 2000 | 125 | 31 |
| 2200 | 138 | 35 |
| 2400 | 150 | 38 |
| 2600 | 163 | 41 |
| 2800 | 175 | 44 |
| 3000 | 188 | 47 |
| 3200 | 200 | 50 |

significantly higher than the minimum of 130 g/day. According to National Health and Nutrition Examination Survey (NHANES) 2001–2002 data, the mean carbohydrate intake for men 19 and older was 316 g; for women in the same age category the mean intake was 232 g (Moshfegh, Goldman, & Cleveland, 2005). Table 2.2 estimates the carbohydrate content of a 2000 calorie MyPyramid meal pattern. A Tolerable Upper Intake Level (UL) has not been established for total carbohydrates.

## Fiber

An Adequate Intake (AI) for total fiber is set at 14 g/1000 calories or 25 g/day for women and 38 g/day for men. Fiber is not an essential nutrient that must be consumed through food in order to prevent a deficiency disease; the recommendation is based on intake levels that have been observed to protect against coronary heart disease. Mean fiber intake among American men and women over the age of 19 is 18 g and 14.3 g, respectively (Moshfegh et al., 2005), about half as much fiber as recommended. A tolerable upper intake level (UL) has not been established for fiber.

## Sugar

Although a UL has not been established for sugar, a maximal level of 25% of total calories or less from added sugars is recommended (Table 2.4). Diets containing added sugar at this level or higher are more likely to be inadequate in essential nutrients.

# ▶ CARBOHYDRATES IN HEALTH PROMOTION

Americans, on average, consume an appropriate percentage of their calories from carbohydrate but are urged to choose their carbohydrates wisely to promote health and avoid chronic disease. The 2005 *Dietary Guidelines for Americans* three key recommendations regarding carbohydrate intake appear in Box 2.3 and are discussed below (USHHS, USDA, 2005).

| BOX 2.3 | KEY RECOMMENDATIONS REGARDING CARBOHYDRATE INTAKE |
| --- | --- |

Choose fiber-rich fruits, vegetables, and whole grains often
Choose and prepare foods and beverages with little added sugars or caloric sweeteners
Reduce the incidence of dental caries by practicing good oral hygiene and consuming sugar- and starch-containing foods and beverages less frequently

## Concentrate on Fiber and Whole Grains

The most consistent benefit of consuming adequate fiber is to relieve or prevent constipation. Yet diets rich in whole grains provide fiber and a "whole package" of healthful components, such as essential fatty acids, antioxidants, vitamins, minerals, and phytochemicals, that are linked to a decreased risk of heart disease, cancer, diabetes, and obesity (International Food Information Council (IFIC), 2007).

Fruits, vegetables, dried peas and beans, and nuts provide fiber but are not likely to be consumed in amounts necessary to meet the AI for fiber. To consume an adequate amount of fiber, a consistent intake of whole grains is recommended. *The Dietary Guidelines* recommend that adults and children consume at least one-half of their grain servings, or a minimum of three servings per day, of whole grains. Not only are whole grains rich in fiber, they also offer a unique package of nutrients, phytochemicals, antioxidants, and other compounds that work together to promote health. For instance

- People who eat three or more servings of whole grains daily have a 20% to 30% lower risk of atherosclerotic cardiovascular disease (IFIC, 2007). Although the exact mechanism is unknown, various components of whole grains may synergistically work to influence cholesterol levels, blood pressure, blood clotting, and insulin sensitivity.
- Researchers at Tufts University found that people who eat three or more servings of whole grains daily, especially from high-fiber cereals, are less likely to develop insulin resistance and metabolic syndrome, common precursors of type 2 diabetes (McKeown et al., 2004). The American Diabetes Association's (ADA) guidelines for the primary prevention of diabetes recommend that half of grain consumption be in the form of whole grains (ADA, 2007).
- High fiber and whole grain intakes are associated with improved body weight management (Melanson et al., 2006). As part of the Nurses' Study, researchers concluded that women who consumed more whole grains consistently weigh less than their nonwhole grain eating counterparts (Liu et al., 2003). Whole grains may help to promote weight management because they are generally less calorically dense than refined foods; are high in bulk, which means they may take longer to consume; and prolong gastric emptying, delaying the return of hunger.

## Tips for Choosing Whole Grains

On average, Americans eat one serving per day of whole grains and over 30% of all Americans eat no whole grains at all (Malik & Hu, 2007). Factors contributing to the low intake of whole grains include consumers' inability to identify whole grains, a lack of awareness of their health benefits, the cost, taste, and unfamiliarity with how to prepare whole grains. Consumers need to understand that the recommendation to eat whole grains is qualified by the advice that whole grains *replace* refined grains, not that they are simply added to usual grain intake. Tips for eating more whole grains appear in Box 2.4.

## Limit Added Sugars

In foods, sugar adds flavor and interest. Few would question the value brown sugar adds to a bowl of hot oatmeal. Besides its sweet taste, sugar has important functions in baked goods. In yeast breads, sugar promotes fermentation by serving as food for the yeast. Sugar in cakes promotes tenderness and a smooth crumb texture. Cookies owe their crisp texture and light-brown color to sugar. In jams and jellies sugar inhibits the growth of mold; in candy it

| BOX 2.4 | **TIPS FOR INCREASING WHOLE GRAIN INTAKE** |

**Substitute:**
- whole wheat bread for white bread
- brown rice for white rice
- whole wheat pasta or pasta that is part whole wheat, part white flour for white pasta
- whole wheat pita for white pita
- whole wheat tortillas for flour tortillas
- whole grain or bran cereals for refined cereals
- half of the white flour in pancakes, waffles, muffins, quick breads, and cookies with whole wheat flour or oats
- whole wheat bread or cracker crumbs for white crumbs as a coating or breading for meat, fish, and poultry
- whole corn meal for refined corn meal in corn cakes, corn bread, and corn muffins

**Add:**
- barley, brown rice, or bulgur to soups, stews, bread stuffing, and casseroles
- a handful of oats or whole grain cereal to yogurt

**Snack on:**
- ready-to-eat whole grain cereal, such as shredded wheat or toasted oat cereal
- whole grain baked tortilla chips
- popcorn

influences texture. Sugar has many functional roles in foods including taste, physical properties, antimicrobial purposes, and chemical properties.

To some extent, sugar is inaccurately blamed for a variety of health problems. The idea that sugar causes hyperactivity in children has been around for decades, even though there is no supporting evidence, even among children who are reported to be sensitive to sugar. Similarly, type 2 diabetes is commonly blamed on a high-sugar diet, even though increasing intakes of sugar are not linked to increasing risk of diabetes. Type 2 diabetes is related to excess body weight, not from eating too much sugar.

Although sugar may not be the evil it is portrayed to be, limiting the intake of added sugar is a prudent idea. High added sugar foods are likely to be "empty calories": the higher the intake of "empty calories," the greater the risk that overall nutrient intake will be inadequate (if empty calorie foods displace more nutritious ones) or that calorie intake will be excessive (if empty calorie foods are added to the diet). Figure 2.7 illustrates the sources of added sugar in the typical American diet. Ways to limit added sugars appear in Box 2.5.

## Sugar Alternatives

**Nonnutritive Sweeteners:** synthetically made sweeteners that do not provide calories. Also known as artificial sweeteners.

One way to reduce sugar intake and not forsake sweetened foods is to consume sugar alternatives, such as sugar alcohols and **nonnutritive sweeteners**, in place of regular sugar.

**Sugar Alcohols.** Sugar alcohols (e.g., sorbitol, mannitol, xylitol) are natural sweeteners derived from monosaccharides. Sorbitol and mannitol are 50% to 70% as sweet as sucrose; xylitol has the same sweetness as sucrose. Although small amounts of sugar alcohols are found in some fruits and berries, most are commercially synthesized and used as alternatives to sugar. They are considered low-calorie sweeteners because they are incompletely absorbed, so their calorie value ranges from 1.6 to 3.0 cal/g. This slow and incomplete absorption causes them to produce a smaller effect on blood glucose levels and insulin secretion than sucrose does.

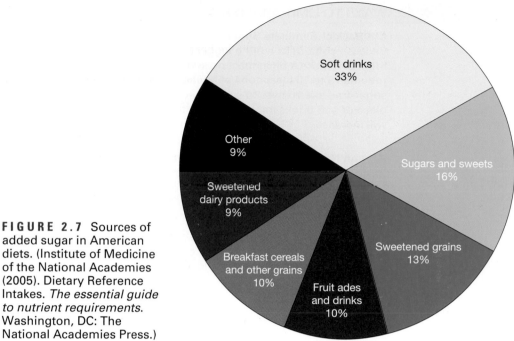

**FIGURE 2.7** Sources of added sugar in American diets. (Institute of Medicine of the National Academies (2005). Dietary Reference Intakes. *The essential guide to nutrient requirements*. Washington, DC: The National Academies Press.)

Sugar alcohols are approved for use in a variety of products, including candies, chewing gum, jams and jellies, baked goods, and frozen confections. Some people experience a laxative effect (abdominal gas, discomfort, osmotic diarrhea) after consuming sorbitol or mannitol. In small amounts and in products that stay in the mouth a long time, such as chewing gum and breath mints, sugar alcohols offer sweetness without promoting cavities.

**Nonnutritive Sweeteners.** Nonnutritive sweeteners are virtually calorie free and are hundreds to thousands of times sweeter than sugar. Sometimes combinations of nonnutritive sweeteners are used in a food to produce a synergistically sweeter taste, decrease the amount of sweetener needed, and minimize aftertaste. Because they do not raise blood glucose levels, nonnutritive sweeteners appeal to people with diabetes. The five nonnutritive sweeteners approved by the FDA for use in the United States are featured in Table 2.5.

**Risks and Benefits of Nonnutritive Sweeteners.** At first glance, nonnutritive sweeteners appear to answer Americans' passion for calorie-free sweetness. But do they really help people to manage their weight? Are they appropriate for diabetics? Are they safe for everyone, including pregnant women and children?

*Weight management.* Nonnutritive sweeteners are not a panacea for weight control. In theory, use of nonnutritive sweeteners in place of sugar can save 16 cal/tsp, or 160 calories in a 12-ounce can of cola. Eliminating one regularly sweetened soft drink per day for 22 days (160 calories × 22 days = 3520 calories) translates to a 1-pound loss (3500 calories equals 1 pound of body weight) without any other changes in eating or activity. This is because *all* calories in the regular soft drink have been eliminated. But foods whose calories come from a mixture of sugar, starch, protein, and fat still provide calories after sugar calories are reduced or eliminated. For instance, sugar-free cookies can provide as many or more calories than cookies sweetened with sugar. Many people falsely believe that low sugar means low calories and will overeat because they overestimate the calories saved by

| BOX 2.5 | **WAYS TO LIMIT ADDED SUGARS** |
|---|---|

### Cut Back or Eliminate Sugar-Sweetened Soft Drinks

Because soft drinks are the biggest source of added sugars in many diets, eliminating them can make a big impact on sugar intake. In fact, every 12-ounce can of soft drink provides 9 to 10 teaspoons of added sugar. Water, flavored water, and diet sodas are sugar-free alternatives to sweetened soft drinks. Using low-fat milk or 100% fruit juice in place of soft drinks may not impact total calorie intake, but vitamin and mineral intake will increase.

### Rely on Natural Sugars in Fruit to Satisfy a "Sweet Tooth"

Besides being less concentrated in sugars than candy, cookies, pastries, and cakes, fruits boost nutrient, phytochemical, and fiber intake.

### Cut Sugar in Home-Baked Products, If Possible

Although reducing the amount of sugar in some foods does not appreciably alter taste or other qualities, in others it can be disastrous. For instance, because sugar in jams and jellies inhibits the growth of mold, less sugar results in a product that supports mold growth.

### Read Labels

"Nutrition Facts" labels (see Chapter 9) list the amount of total carbohydrates and sugars per serving but they do not include sugar alcohols and do not distinguish between natural and added sugars. People concerned with limiting sugar who confine their focus to the grams of sugar per serving may inappropriately conclude that foods high in natural sugars, such as milk and fruit juice, should be avoided. When judging the value of a food high in sugar, it is important to look beyond sugar grams to the whole package. What other nutrients are provided and are they present in significant amounts? Are the sugars naturally present or are they added? The more added sugars on the ingredient label and the closer to the beginning of the list they appear, the higher the content of added sugar in that product. Look for these sources of sugar:

| | |
|---|---|
| Brown sugar | HFCS |
| Cane sugar | Honey |
| Confectioner's sugar | Invert sugar |
| Corn sweeteners | Lactose |
| Corn syrup | Malt |
| Crystallized cane sugar | Maltose |
| Dextrose | Molasses |
| Evaporated cane juice | Raw sugar |
| Fructose | Sucrose |
| Fruit juice concentrate | Turbinado sugar |
| Glucose | |

### Consider Using Sugar Alternatives Such As Sugar Alcohols or Nonnutritive Sweeteners

On the plus side, sugar alternatives are low in calories or calorie free; they do not produce a rise in blood glucose levels and do not promote tooth decay because they are not fermented by mouth bacteria. On the downside, the use of sugar alternatives does not guarantee lower calorie intake. Sugar free is not synonymous with calorie free (see section below on sugar alternatives).

| TABLE 2.5 | Nonnutritive Sweeteners Approved for Use in the United States |
| --- | --- |

| Sweetener | Sweetness (Sucrose = 1) | Taste Characteristics | Uses | Comments |
| --- | --- | --- | --- | --- |
| Saccharin (Sweet Twin™, Sweet 'n Low™) | 200–700 | Persistent aftertaste; bitter at high concentrations | Soft drinks, assorted foods, tabletop sweetener | Potential (weak) carcinogen; the FDA has officially withdrawn its proposed ban so warning labels no longer required |
| Aspartame (Nutrasweet™, Equal™, Spoonful™) | 180 | Similar to sucrose; no aftertaste | Tabletop sweeteners, dry beverage mixes, chewing gum, beverages, confections, fruit spreads, toppings, and fillings | Made from the amino acids aspartic acid and phenylalanine; people with PKU must avoid aspartame |
| Acesulfame K (Sunette™, Sweet One™) | 130–200 | Bitter aftertaste like saccharin | Tabletop sweeteners, dry beverage mixes, and chewing gum | Often mixed with other sweeteners to synergize the sweetness and minimize the aftertaste. Not digested; excreted unchanged in the urine |
| Sucralose (Splenda™) | 600 | Maintains flavor even at high temperatures | Soft drinks, baked goods, chewing gums, and tabletop sweeteners | Poorly absorbed; excreted unchanged in the feces |
| Neotame | 8000 | Clean, sugar-like taste; enhances flavors of other ingredients | Under review | Made from aspartic acid and phenylalanine but is not metabolized to phenylalanine so a warning label is not required. Has the potential to replace both sugar and HFCS |

*Source:* Brown, A. (2008). *Understanding food. Principles and preparation* (3rd ed.). Belmont, CA: Thomson Wadsworth.

replacing sugar. Ironically, the prevalence of obesity has increased significantly as the intake of nonnutritive sweeteners has increased.

*Diabetes mellitus.* Contrary to what was previously believed, regular sugar does not raise blood glucose levels more than complex carbohydrates do; a food's glycemic load is influenced by several factors, not just sugar content. The focus in management of blood glucose levels has shifted from avoiding simple sugars to maintaining a relatively consistent total carbohydrate intake with less emphasis on the source. For that reason, sweets can be included within the context of a nutritious, calorie-appropriate, carbohydrate-controlled diet. However, because most people with type 2 diabetes are overweight, substitution of calorie-free sweets for calorie-containing ones has the potential to improve blood glucose levels by promoting weight management. The full benefit of this is seen when "diet" carbonated beverages, jellies, syrups, and candies replace those containing sugar.

*Safety.* The FDA is responsible for approving the safety of all food additives, including artificial sweeteners. An **acceptable daily intake (ADI)** is established as a safety limit for each sweetener. For instance, the ADI of aspartame is 50 mg/kg of body weight; currently, aspartame users consume an average of just 3.0 mg/kg, or 6% of the safety limit.

**QUICK BITE**

The number of artificially sweetened soft drinks a 130-pound person can consume daily before meeting the ADI for each particular sweetener

| | |
|---|---|
| Saccharin | 1 |
| Aspartame | 24 |
| Acesulfame-K | 20 |

For most adults, nonnutritive sweeteners are safe when used within approved guidelines; for pregnant women, the issue is less straightforward. Some physicians recommend that women avoid all nonnutritive sweeteners during pregnancy; others suggest that they may be used in moderation. The position of the American Dietetic Association is that saccharin, aspartame, acesulfame-K, sucralose, and neotame are safe during pregnancy when consumed in amounts within ADI.

Saccharin has not been well studied in children, so caution is advised. Other nonnutritive sweeteners are relatively safe for children with the exception of aspartame for children with phenylketonuria (PKU). The qualifier *relatively* refers to the fact that any substance becomes toxic at some level, but average consumption of nonnutritive sweeteners among children is less than the ADI set for them. But even if they are relatively safe, are they really necessary? Regular sugar, which is the alternative to nonnutritive sweeteners, is not plagued with safety concerns and can fit within the context of a nutritious and balanced meal plan. One must look at the risk–benefit ratio to decide if use of nonnutritive sweeteners is appropriate for children.

## Take Steps to Avoid Dental Caries

Feeding on sugars and starches, bacteria residing in the mouth produce an acid that erodes tooth enamel. Although whole grain crackers and orange juice are more nutritious than caramels and soft drinks, their potential damage to teeth is the same. How often carbohydrates are consumed, what they are eaten with, and how long after eating brushing occurs may be more important than whether or not they are "sticky." Anticavity strategies include the following:

- Choose between-meal snacks that are healthy and teeth-friendly such as fresh vegetables, apples, cheese, and popcorn.
- Limit between-meal carbohydrate snacking including drinking soft drinks.
- Avoid high-sugar items that stay in the mouth for a long time such as hard candy, suckers, and cough drops.
- Brush promptly after eating.
- Chew gum sweetened with sugar alcohols (e.g., sorbitol, mannitol, and xylitol) or with nonnutritive sweeteners after eating. This may reduce the risk of cavities by stimulating production of saliva, which helps to rinse the teeth and neutralize plaque acids. Unlike sucrose and other nutritive sweeteners, sugar alcohols and artificial sweeteners are not fermented by bacteria in the mouth so they do not promote cavities.
- Use fluoridated toothpaste.

## ▶ How Do You Respond?

**Aren't carbohydrates fattening?** At 4 cal/g, carbohydrates are no more fattening than protein and are less than half as fattening as fat at 9 cal/g. Whether or not a food is "fattening" has more to do with frequency and total calories provided than whether the calories are in the form of carbohydrates, protein, or fat.

**Is whole "white" wheat bread as nutritious as whole wheat?** Whole "white" wheat flour is made from albino wheat that is white in color, not the characteristic bran color of whole wheat. Because it is a whole grain, it is nutritionally comparable to whole wheat. Many people not only prefer its lighter color, but also its milder flavor.

**"Light" or "diet" breads are high in fiber. Can I use them in place of whole grain breads?** So-called "light breads" usually have processed fiber from peas or other foods substituted for some starch; the result is a lower-calorie, higher-fiber bread that may help to prevent constipation but lacks the unique "package" of vitamins, minerals, and phyto-chemicals found in whole grains.

## ▶ Case Study

Amanda is convinced that white flour and white sugar cause her to overeat, resulting in an extra 30 pounds of weight she is carrying around. To control her impulse to overeat, she has decided to eliminate all foods made with white or whole wheat flour and white sugar from her diet. Her total calorie needs are estimated to be 2000 per day. Yesterday she ate the following:

| | |
|---|---|
| **Breakfast:** | 2 scrambled eggs and 2 sausage links |
| | 1 cup orange juice |
| | Lots of black coffee |
| **Snack:** | 2 ounces of cashews and a diet soda |
| **Lunch:** | tossed salad with 1 hard cooked egg, 3 ounces of sliced turkey, 2 ounces of sliced cheese, 3 tbsp of Italian dressing |
| | 1 can diet soda |
| | 1 cup of diet gelatin |
| **Snack:** | 2 ounces cheese curds and a diet soda |
| **Dinner:** | 6 ounces fried chicken |
| | 1 cup of French fries |
| | ½ cup corn |
| | ½ cup diet pudding with whipped cream |
| | 1 can diet soda |
| **Snack:** | 5 chicken wings with ¼ cup bleu cheese dressing |

- What foods did she eat yesterday that contained carbohydrates? Estimate how many grams of carbo-hydrate she ate. How does her in-take compare with the amount of total carbohydrate recommended for someone needing 2000 cal/day? How could she increase her carbo-hydrate intake within the restric-tions she has set for herself?
- What sources of fiber did she con-sume? Estimate how many grams of fiber she ate. How does her fiber intake compare with the amount of AI recommended for women? How could she increase her fiber intake within the restrictions she has set for herself?
- What would you tell her about her idea to forsake white and wheat flour and white sugar to manage her weight? What are the benefits and potential problems with her diet? What suggestions would you make about her intake?

1. The nurse knows her explanation of glycemic index was effective when the client says which of the following?
   a. "Choosing foods that have a low-glycemic index is an effective way to eat healthier."
   b. "Low-glycemic index foods promote weight loss because they do not stimulate the release of insulin."
   c. "Glycemic index may help me choose the best foods to eat before, during, and after training."
   d. "Glycemic index is a term to describe the amount of refined sugar in a food."

2. Which of the following recommendations would be most effective for someone wanting to eat more fiber?
   a. Replace white bread and refined cereals with whole grain breads and cereals.
   b. Eat raw vegetables in place of cooked vegetables.
   c. Use potatoes in place of white rice.
   d. Eat fruit for dessert in place of ice cream.

3. A client asks why sugar should be limited in the diet. Which of the following is the nurse's best response?
   a. "A high sugar intake increases the risk of heart disease and diabetes."
   b. "Foods high in sugar generally provide few nutrients other than calories and may make it hard to consume a diet that has enough of all the essential nutrients."
   c. "There is a direct correlation between sugar intake and the risk of obesity."
   d. "Sugar provides more calories per gram than starch, protein, or fat."

4. Which source of fiber may be the most effective in stimulating peristalsis and promoting laxation?
   a. Oatmeal
   b. Lentils
   c. Lettuce
   d. Whole wheat bread

5. The nurse knows her instructions about choosing dairy products that are lactose free have been effective when the client verbalizes she should consume more:
   a. Cottage cheese
   b. Skim milk
   c. Cheddar cheese
   d. Pudding

6. A client who has eaten too many dietetic candies sweetened with sorbitol may experience which of the following?
   a. Diarrhea
   b. Heartburn
   c. Vomiting
   d. Low-blood glucose

7. The client wants to eat fewer calories and lose weight by substituting regularly sweetened foods with those that are sweetened with sugar alternatives. Which of the following would be the most effective substitution?
   a. Sugar-free cookies for regular cookies.
   b. Sugar-free candy for regular candy.
   c. Sugar-free soda for regular soda.
   d. Sugar-free ice cream for regular ice cream.

8. A client is on a low-calorie diet that recommends she test her urine for ketones to tell how well she is adhering to the guidelines of the diet. What does the presence of ketones signify about her intake?
   a. It is too high in protein.
   b. It is too high in fat.
   c. It is too high in carbohydrates.
   d. It is too low in carbohydrates.

## KEY CONCEPTS

● Carbohydrates, which are found almost exclusively in plants, provide the major source of energy in almost all human diets.

● The two major groups are simple carbohydrates (monosaccharides and disaccharides) and complex carbohydrates (polysaccharides).

● Monosaccharides and disaccharides are composed of one or two sugar molecules respectively. They vary in sweetness.

● Polysaccharides, namely starch, glycogen, and fiber, are made up of many glucose molecules. They do not taste sweet because their molecules are too large to sit on taste buds in the mouth that perceive sweetness.

● Fiber, the undigestible part of plant cell walls, is commonly classified as either water-soluble or water-insoluble; each type has different physiologic effects.

● The most popular American foods do not represent rich sources of fiber. Whole grains, bran cereals, dried peas and beans, and unpeeled fruits and vegetables are the best sources of fiber.

● Carbohydrates are found in every MyPyramid group except Oils. Starches are most abundant in grains, vegetables, and the plant foods found in the meat and bean group; natural sugars occur in fruits and in the Milk group. Discretionary calorie items may provide sugar and/or starch, depending on the individual selection.

● The majority of carbohydrate digestion occurs in the small intestine, where disaccharides and starches are digested to monosaccharides. Monosaccharides are absorbed through intestinal mucosal cells and transported to the liver through the portal vein. In the liver, fructose and galactose are converted to glucose. The liver releases glucose into the bloodstream.

● The glycemic response is based on the glycemic index of a food and the carbohydrate content of that food. Because there are so many variables that influence the rise in blood glucose after eating, glycemic response is hard to predict in practice.

● The major function of carbohydrates is to provide energy, which includes sparing protein and preventing ketosis. Glucose can be converted to glycogen, used to make nonessential amino acids, used for specific body compounds, or converted to fat and stored in adipose tissue.

● The RDA for total carbohydrates is set as the minimum amount needed to fuel the brain but not as an amount adequate to satisfy typical energy needs. Most experts recommend that 45% to 65% of total calories come from carbohydrates and that added sugars be limited to less than 25% of total calories. Twenty-five to 38 g of fiber is recommended daily for adult women and men respectively.

● The 2005 *Dietary Guidelines* urges Americans to eat more fiber and whole grains, limit added sugars, and take steps to avoid dental caries.

● Whole grains appear to offer health benefits beyond the benefits of fiber. Whole grains may decrease the risk of heart disease, certain cancers, and type 2 diabetes. Whole grains also promote GI health and weight management.

● Sugars—as well as starches—promote dental decay by feeding bacteria in the mouth that produce an acid that damages tooth enamel. Sugar is also a source of empty calories. The higher the intake of empty calories, the greater the risk of an inadequate nutrient intake, an excessive calorie intake, or both.

● Sugar alcohols are considered to be low-calorie sweeteners because they are incompletely absorbed and, therefore, provide fewer calories per gram than regular sugar does. Because they do not promote dental decay, they are well suited for use in gum and breath mints that stay in the mouth a long time.

● Nonnutritive sweeteners provide negligible or no calories. Their use as food additives is regulated by the FDA, which sets safety limits known as ADI. The ADI, a level per kilogram of body weight, reflects an amount 100 times less than the maximum level at which no observed adverse effects have occurred in animal studies. Nonnutritive sweeteners have intense sweetening power, ranging from 180 to 8000 times sweeter than that of sucrose.

## ANSWER KEY

1. **TRUE** Starch, the storage form of carbohydrates in plants, is made from hundreds to thousands of glucose molecules.

2. **FALSE** All digestible carbohydrates—whether sugars or starch—provide 4 cal/g. Insoluble fiber does not provide calories because it is not digested; the mix of fiber in food may provide 1.5 to 2.5 cal/g.

3. **FALSE** The body cannot distinguish between the sugar in fruit and the sugar in candy. However, the *package* of nutrients in fruit (vitamins, minerals, fiber, phytochemicals) is better than the package of nutrients in candy (few to no other nutrients with the possible exception of fat).

4. **FALSE** The most commonly consumed American foods provide 1 to 3 g fiber/serving, which is why most Americans typically eat only about one-half the recommended intake of fiber.

5. **FALSE** Although enrichment returns certain B vitamins and iron lost through processing, other vitamins, minerals, phytochemicals, and fiber are not replaced so whole wheat bread is nutritionally superior to white or "wheat" bread. Enriched white bread offers the advantage of being fortified with folic acid.

6. **TRUE** Soft drinks contribute more added sugar to the average American diet than any other food or beverage.

7. **TRUE** All fermentable carbohydrates, whether sweet or not, promote dental decay by feeding bacteria in the mouth that damages tooth enamel.

8. **FALSE** Although "Nutrition Facts" labels do not distinguish between natural and added sugars, they do list the total sugar content per serving.

9. **FALSE** Alternative sweeteners approved for use in the United States are safe in amounts specified as the ADI. The exception is the use of aspartame by people who have PKU.

10. **FALSE** Sugar has not been proven to cause hyperactivity in children.

## WEBSITE

Learn about grains at **www.wholegrainscouncil.org**

# REFERENCES

American Diabetes Association. (2007). Nutrition recommendations and interventions for diabetes. A position statement of the American Diabetes Association. *Diabetes Care, 30* (Suppl. 1), S48–S65.

Brown, A. (2008). *Understanding food. Principles and preparation* (3rd ed.). Belmont, CA: Thomson Wadsworth.

Institute of Medicine of the National Academies (IOM). (2005). *Dietary Reference Intakes for energy, carbohydrates, fiber, fat, fatty acids, cholesterol, protein, and amino acids (macronutrients).* Washington, DC: National Academies Press.

International Food Information Council (IFIC). (2007). Whole grains fact sheet. Available at www.ific.org/publications/factsheets/wholegrainsfs.cfm. Accessed on 7/27/07.

*The American Journal of Clinical Nutrition, 84,* 1215–1223.

Kant, A., & Graubard, B. (2006). Secular trends in patterns of self-reported food consumption of adult Americans: NHANES 1971–1975 to NHANES 199–2002. *The American Journal of Clinical Nutrition, 84,* 1215–1223.

Liu, S., Willett, W., Manson, J., Hu, F., Rosner, B., & Colditz, G. (2003). Relation between changes in intakes of dietary fiber and grain products and changes in weight and development of obesity among middle-aged women. *The American Journal of Clinical Nutrition, 78,* 920–927.

Lupton, J., & Trumbo, P. (2006). Dietary fiber. In Shils, M., Shike, M., Ross, A., et al. (Eds.), *Modern Nutrition in Health and Disease* (10th ed.). Philadelphia: Lippincott Williams & Wilkins.

Malik, V., & Hu, F. (2007). Dietary prevention of atherosclerosis: Go with whole grains. *The American Journal of Clinical Nutrition, 85,* 1444–1445.

McKeown, N., Meigs, J. B., Liu, S., et al. (2004). Carbohydrate nutrition, insulin resistance, and the prevalence of the metabolic syndrome in the Framingham offspring cohort. *Diabetes Care, 27*(2), 538–546.

Moshfegh, A., Goldman, J., & Cleveland, L. (2005). What we eat in America, NHANES 2001–2002: Usual nutrient intakes from food compared to dietary reference intakes. US Department of Agriculture, Agricultural Research Service.

Melanson, K. J., Angelopoulos, T. J., Nguyen, V. T., et al. (2006). Consumption of whole-grain cereals during weight loss: Effects on dietary quality, dietary fiber, magnesium, vitamin B6, and obesity. *Journal of the American Dietetic Association, 106*(9), 1380–1388.

United State Department of Health and Human Services, United States Department of Agriculture. (2005). *Dietary Guidelines for Americans* (7th ed.). Available at www.health.gov/dietaryguidelines.

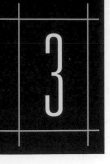

# 3

# Protein

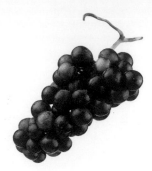

---

### UPON COMPLETION OF THIS CHAPTER, YOU WILL BE ABLE TO

- Discuss the functions of protein.
- Compare complete and incomplete proteins.
- Explain protein "sparing."
- Calculate an individual's protein requirement.
- Estimate the amount of protein in a sample meal plan.
- Give examples of conditions that increase a person's protein requirement.
- Select appropriate sources of nutrients that are most likely to be deficient in a vegetarian diet.
- Describe nitrogen balance and how it is determined.

---

## ▶ PROTEIN

In Greek, protein means "to take first place," and truly life could not exist without protein. Protein is a component of every living cell: plant, animal, and microorganism. In the adult, protein accounts for 20% of total weight. Dietary protein seems immune to the controversy over optimal intake that surrounds both carbohydrates and fat.

This chapter discusses the composition of protein, its functions, and how it is handled in the body. Sources, Dietary Reference Intakes, and the role of protein in health promotion are presented.

44

## Amino Acids

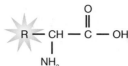

**FIGURE 3.1**
Generic amino acid structure.

Amino acids are the basic building blocks of all proteins and the end products of protein digestion. All amino acids have a carbon atom core with four bonding sites: one site holds a hydrogen atom, one an amino group ($NH_2$), and one an acid group (COOH) (Fig. 3.1). Attached to the fourth bonding site is a side group (R group), which contains the atoms that give each amino acid its own distinct identity. Some side groups contain sulfur, some are acidic, and some are basic. The differences in these side groups account for the differences in size, shape, and electrical charge among amino acids.

There are 20 common amino acids, 9 of which are classified as essential or indispensable because the body cannot make them so they must be supplied through the diet (Box 3.1). The remaining 11 amino acids are classified as nonessential or dispensable because cells can make them as needed through the process of transamination. Some dispensable amino acids may become indispensable when metabolic need is great and endogenous synthesis is not adequate. Note that the terms essential and nonessential refer to whether or not they must be supplied by the diet, not to their relative importance: all 20 amino acids must be available for the body to make proteins.

## Protein Structure

The types and amounts of amino acids and the unique sequence in which they are joined determine a protein's primary structure. Most proteins contain several dozen to several hundred amino acids: just as the 26 letters of the alphabet can be used to form an infinite number of words, so can amino acids be joined in different amounts, proportions, and sequences to form a great variety of proteins.

Proteins also vary in shape and may be straight, folded, coiled along one dimension, or a three-dimensional shape such as a sphere or globe. Larger proteins are created when two or more three-dimensional polypeptides combine. A protein's shape determines its function.

## Functions of Protein

Protein is the major structural and functional component of every living cell. Except for bile and urine, every tissue and fluid in the body contains some protein. In fact, the body may

---

**BOX 3.1**   **AMINO ACIDS**

| Essential (Indispensable) | Nonessential (Dispensable) | Conditionally* Essential (Indispensable) |
|---|---|---|
| Histidine | Alanine | Arginine |
| Isoleucine | Asparagine | Cysteine |
| Leucine | Aspartic acid | Glutamine |
| Lysine | Glutamic acid | Glycine |
| Methionine | Serine | Proline |
| Phenylalanine | | Tyrosine |
| Threonine | | |
| Tryptophan | | |
| Valine | | |

*Under most normal conditions, the body can synthesize adequate amounts of these amino acids. A dietary source is necessary only when metabolic demands exceed endogenous synthesis.

contain as many as 10,000 to 50,000 different proteins that vary in size, shape, and function. Amino acids or proteins are components of or involved in the following:

*Body structure and framework.* More than 40% of protein in the body is found in skeletal muscle and approximately 15% is found in each the skin and the blood. Proteins also form tendons, membranes, organs, and bones.

*Enzymes.* Enzymes are proteins that facilitate specific chemical reactions in the body without undergoing change themselves. Some enzymes (e.g., digestive enzymes) break down larger molecules into smaller ones; others (e.g., enzymes involved in protein synthesis in which amino acids are combined) combine molecules to form larger compounds.

*Other body secretions and fluids.* Neurotransmitters (e.g., serotonin, acetylcholine), antibodies, and some hormones (e.g., insulin, thyroxine, epinephrine) are made from amino acids as are breast milk, mucus, sperm, and histamine.

*Fluid balance.* Proteins help to regulate fluid balance because they attract water, which creates osmotic pressure. Circulating proteins, such as albumin, maintain the proper balance of fluid among the **intravascular**, **intracellular**, and **interstitial** compartments of the body. A symptom of low albumin is **edema**.

*Acid–base balance.* Because amino acids contain both an acid ($COOH$) and a base ($NH_2$), they can act as either acids or bases depending on the pH of the surrounding fluid. The ability to buffer or neutralize excess acids and bases enables proteins to maintain normal blood pH, which protects body proteins from being **denatured**.

*Transport molecules.* **Globular** proteins transport other substances through the blood. For instance, lipoproteins transport fats, cholesterol, and fat-soluble vitamins; hemoglobin transports oxygen; and albumin transports free fatty acids and many drugs.

*Other compounds.* Amino acids are components of numerous body compounds such as opsin, the light-sensitive visual pigment in the eye, and thrombin, a protein necessary for normal blood clotting.

*Some amino acids have specific functions within the body.* For instance, tryptophan is a precursor of the vitamin niacin and is also a component of serotonin. Tyrosine is the precursor of melanin, the pigment that colors hair and skin and is incorporated into thyroid hormone.

*Fueling the body.* Like carbohydrates, protein provides 4 cal/g. Although it is not the body's preferred fuel, protein is a source of energy when it is consumed in excess or when calorie intake from carbohydrates and fat is inadequate.

**Intravascular:** within blood vessels.

**Intracellular:** within cells.

**Interstitial:** between cells.

**Edema:** the swelling of body tissues secondary to the accumulation of excessive fluid.

**Denatured:** an irreversible process in which the structure of a protein is disrupted, leading to partial or complete loss of function.

**Globular:** spherical.

## How the Body Handles Protein

### Digestion

Chemical digestion of protein begins in the stomach, where hydrochloric acid denatures protein to make the peptide bonds more available to the actions of enzymes (Fig. 3.2). Hydrochloric acid also converts pepsinogen to the active enzyme pepsin, which begins the process of breaking down proteins into smaller polypeptides and some amino acids.

The majority of protein digestion occurs in the small intestine, where pancreatic proteases reduce polypeptides to shorter chains, tripeptides, dipeptides, and amino acids. The enzymes trypsin and chymotrypsin act to break peptide bonds between specific amino acids. Carboxypeptidase breaks off amino acids from the acid (carboxyl) end of polypeptides and dipeptides. Enzymes located on the surface of the cells that line the small intestine complete the digestion: aminopeptidase splits amino acids from the amino ends of short peptides and dipeptidase reduces dipeptides to amino acids. **Protein digestibility** is 90% to 99% for animal proteins, over 90% for soy and legumes, and 70% to 90% for other plant proteins.

**Protein Digestibility:** how well a protein is digested to make amino acids available for protein synthesis.

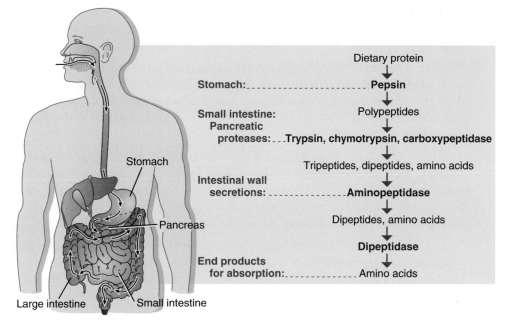

**FIGURE 3.2** Protein digestion. Chemical digestion of protein begins in the stomach. Hydrochloric acid converts pepsinogen to the active enzyme pepsin, which begins the process of breaking down proteins into small polypeptides and some amino acids. The majority of protein digestion occurs in the small intestine, where pancreatic proteases reduce polypeptides into shorter chains, tripeptides, dipeptides, and amino acids. Enzymes located on the surface of the cells that line the small intestine complete the digestion: aminopeptidase splits amino acids from the amino ends of short peptides, and dipeptidase reduces dipeptides to amino acids.

## Absorption

Amino acids, and sometimes a few dipeptides or larger peptides, are absorbed through the mucosa of the small intestine by active transport with the aid of vitamin $B_6$. Intestinal cells release amino acids into the bloodstream for transport to the liver via the portal vein.

## Metabolism

The liver acts as a clearinghouse for the amino acids it receives: it uses the amino acids it needs, releases those needed elsewhere, and handles the extra. For instance, the liver retains amino acids to make liver cells, nonessential amino acids, and plasma proteins such as heparin, prothrombin, and albumin; it regulates the release of amino acids into the bloodstream and removes excess amino acids from the circulation; it synthesizes specific enzymes to degrade excess amino acids; it removes the nitrogen from amino acids so that they can be burned for energy, and it converts certain amino acids to glucose if necessary; it forms urea from the nitrogenous wastes of protein when protein and calories are consumed in excess of need, the liver converts protein to fatty acids that form triglycerides for storage in adipose tissue.

**Protein Synthesis.** Protein synthesis is a complicated but efficient process that quickly assembles amino acids into proteins the body needs, such as proteins lost through normal wear and tear or those needed to support growth and development. Part of what makes every individual unique is the minute differences in body proteins, which are caused by variations in the sequencing of amino acids determined by genetics. Genetic codes created at conception hold the instructions for making all of the body's proteins. Cell function and life itself depend on the precise replication of these codes. Some important concepts related to protein synthesis are protein turnover, metabolic pool, and nitrogen balance.

*Protein Turnover.* Protein turnover is a continuous process that occurs within each cell as proteins are broken down from normal wear and tear and replenished. Body proteins vary in their rate of turnover. For example, red blood cells are replaced every 60 to 90 days, gastrointestinal cells are replaced every 2 to 3 days, and enzymes used in the digestion of food are continuously replenished.

*Metabolic Pool.* Although protein is not truly stored in the body as are glucose and fat, a supply of each amino acid exists in a metabolic pool of free amino acids within cells and circulating in blood. This pool consists of recycled amino acids from body proteins that have broken down and also amino acids from food. Because the pool accepts and donates amino acids as they become available or are needed, it is in a constant state of flux.

*Nitrogen Balance.* Nitrogen balance reflects the state of balance between protein breakdown and protein synthesis. It is determined by comparing nitrogen intake with nitrogen excretion over a specific period of time, usually 24 hours. To calculate nitrogen intake, protein intake is measured (in grams) over a 24-hour period and divided by 6.25 because protein is 16% nitrogen. The result represents total nitrogen intake for that 24-hour period. Nitrogen excretion is computed by analyzing a 24-hour urine sample for the amount (grams) of urinary urea nitrogen it contains and adding a coefficient of 4 to this number to account for the estimated daily nitrogen loss in feces, hair, nails, and skin. Subtracting grams of nitrogen excretion from grams of nitrogen intake will reveal the state of nitrogen balance, as illustrated in Box 3.2.

A neutral nitrogen balance, or state of equilibrium, exists when nitrogen intake equals nitrogen excretion, indicating protein synthesis is occurring at the same rate as protein breakdown. Healthy adults are in neutral nitrogen balance. When protein synthesis exceeds protein breakdown, as is the case during growth, pregnancy, or recovery from injury, nitrogen balance is positive. A negative nitrogen balance indicates that protein catabolism is occurring at a faster rate than protein synthesis, which occurs during starvation or the catabolic phase after injury.

---

**BOX 3.2**     **CALCULATING NITROGEN BALANCE**

Mary is a 25-year-old woman who was admitted to the hospital with multiple fractures and traumatic injuries from a car accident. A nutritional intake study indicated a 24-hour protein intake of 64 g. A 24-hour urinary urea nitrogen (UUN) collection result was 19.8 g.

1. Determine nitrogen intake by dividing protein intake by 6.25:

$$64 \div 6.25 = 10.24 \text{ g of nitrogen}$$

2. Determine total nitrogen output by adding a coefficient of 4 to the UUN:

$$19.8 + 4 = 23.8 \text{ g of nitrogen}$$

3. Calculate nitrogen balance by subtracting nitrogen output from nitrogen intake:

$$10.24 - 23.8 = -13.56 \text{ g in 24 hours}$$

4. Interpret the results.

A negative number indicates that protein breakdown is exceeding protein synthesis. Mary is in a catabolic state.

**Protein Catabolism for Energy.** Using protein for energy is a physiologic and economic waste because amino acids used for energy are not available to be used for protein synthesis, a function unique to amino acids. Normally the body uses very little protein for energy as long as intake and storage of carbohydrate and fat are adequate. If insufficient carbohydrate and fat are available for energy use (e.g., when calorie intake is inadequate), dietary and body proteins are sacrificed to provide amino acids that can be burned for energy. Over time, loss of lean body tissue occurs. Loss of 30% of body protein causes impaired breathing related to a decrease in muscle strength, altered immune function, altered organ function, and ultimately death (Shils et al., 2006). To "spare protein"—both dietary and body—from being burned for calories, an adequate supply of energy from carbohydrate and fat is needed.

## Sources of Protein

For most people, protein is synonymous with meat, but protein is also found in milk, grains, and vegetables (Fig. 3.3). As illustrated in Table 3.1, more than 40% of the protein in a MyPyramid 2000 calorie food pattern comes from the Meat and Beans group. Although a recommended serving size of meat may be 1–3 oz, restaurant portions may be much larger.

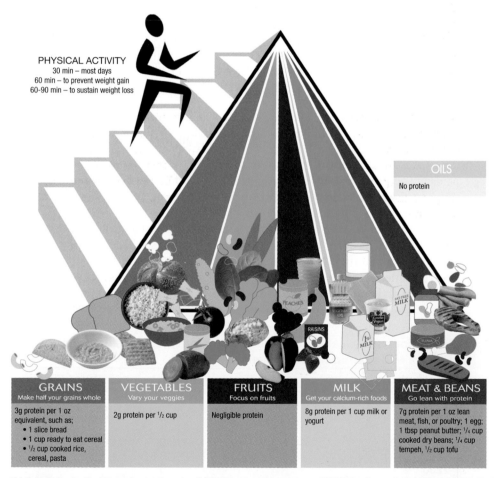

PHYSICAL ACTIVITY
30 min – most days
60 min – to prevent weight gain
60-90 min – to sustain weight loss

OILS
No protein

| GRAINS<br>Make half your grains whole | VEGETABLES<br>Vary your veggies | FRUITS<br>Focus on fruits | MILK<br>Get your calcium-rich foods | MEAT & BEANS<br>Go lean with protein |
|---|---|---|---|---|
| 3g protein per 1 oz equivalent, such as;<br>• 1 slice bread<br>• 1 cup ready to eat cereal<br>• ½ cup cooked rice, cereal, pasta | 2g protein per ½ cup | Negligible protein | 8g protein per 1 cup milk or yogurt | 7g protein per 1 oz lean meat, fish, or poultry; 1 egg; 1 tbsp peanut butter; ¼ cup cooked dry beans; ¼ cup tempeh, ½ cup tofu |

**F I G U R E  3.3** Protein content of MyPyramid groups. (USDA, Center for Nutrition Policy and Promotion (2005). MyPyramid—Steps to Healthier Food Guidance System. Available at www.MyPyramid.gov.)

| TABLE 3.1 | Protein Content of the MyPyramid 2000 Calorie Food Intake Pattern | | |
|---|---|---|---|
| Group | Amount Recommended in 2000 Calorie Diet | Protein Content Per Unit of Measure | Total Protein Content Per Group (g) |
| Grains | 6 oz equivalents | 3 g/equivalent | 18 |
| Vegetables | 2½ cups | 2 g/½ cup | 10 |
| Fruits | 2 cups | Negligible | 0 |
| Milk | 3 cups | 8 g/cup | 24 |
| Meat and Beans | 5.5 oz equivalents | 7 g/equivalent | 38.5 |
| | | Total protein*: | 90.5 |

*Total protein does not account for any additional protein in the discretionary calorie category.

Table 3.2 shows the MyPyramid recommendations for the Meat and Beans group at various calorie levels.

## Protein Quality

QUICK BITE

Comparison of meat portions
USDA official serving size of sirloin steak — 3 oz
Dinner house steak portion of sirloin steak — 7 oz
Steak house portion size of porterhouse steak — 20 oz

Dietary proteins differ in quality, based on their content of essential amino acids. For most Americans, protein quality is not important because the amounts of protein and calories consumed are more than adequate. But when protein needs are increased or protein intake is marginal, quality becomes a crucial concern. Terms that refer to protein quality are complete and incomplete.

**Complete and Incomplete Proteins.** Complete proteins provide all nine essential amino acids in adequate amounts and proportions needed by the body for protein synthesis. These high-quality proteins are generally from animal sources. Soy protein is the only plant source of complete protein.

Incomplete proteins also provide all the essential amino acids, but one or more are present in insufficient quantities to support protein synthesis. These amino acids are considered "limiting" in that they limit the process of protein synthesis. Different sources of incomplete proteins differ in their limiting amino acids. For instance, grains are typically low in lysine and isoleucine and legumes are low in methionine and cysteine. Two incomplete proteins that

| TABLE 3.2 | The Amount of Meat and Beans Group Equivalents Recommended at Various MyPyramid Calorie Levels |
|---|---|
| Total Daily Calories | Number of oz Equivalents Recommended |
| 1000 | 2 |
| 1200 | 3 |
| 1400 | 4 |
| 1600–1800 | 5 |
| 2000 | 5.5 |
| 2200 | 6 |
| 2400 | 6.5 |
| 2800–3200 | 7 |

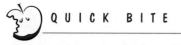

**QUICK BITE**

| Sources of complete/high-quality protein | Sources of incomplete/lower-quality protein |
|---|---|
| Meat | Grains |
| Poultry | Vegetables |
| Seafood | Dried peas and beans |
| Milk, yogurt, cheese | Nuts |
| Soybeans, soybean products | Gelatin |

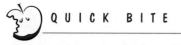

**QUICK BITE**

Examples of two complementary plant proteins
Black beans and rice
Bean tacos
Pea soup with toast
Lentil and rice curry
Falafel sandwich (ground chickpea patties on pita bread)
Peanut butter sandwich
Pasta e fagioli (pasta and white bean stew)

## Dietary Reference Intakes

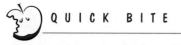

**QUICK BITE**

Examples of a plant protein complemented by a small amount of a complete protein
Bread pudding
Rice pudding
Corn pudding
Cereal and milk
Macaroni and cheese
Cheese fondue
French toast
Cheese sandwich
Vegetable quiche
Cheese enchilada
Bean burrito

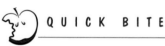

**QUICK BITE**

To calculate a healthy adult's RDA for protein
1. Divide weight in pounds by 2.2 to determine weight in kilograms
2. Multiply by 0.8 g/kg
3. Result is total grams protein/day

have different limiting amino acids are known as complementary proteins because together they form the equivalent of a complete protein. Likewise, small amounts of a complete protein combined with any incomplete protein are complementary. Eating complementary proteins at the same meal is not necessary as long as a variety of incomplete proteins are consumed over the course of a day and calorie intake is adequate.

The Recommended Dietary Allowance (RDA) for protein for healthy adults is 0.8 g/kg, derived from the absolute minimum requirement needed to maintain nitrogen balance plus an additional factor to account for individual variations and the mixed quality of proteins typically consumed. This figure also assumes calorie intake is adequate. For the reference adult male who weighs 154 pounds, this translates to 56 g protein/day; the reference female weighing 127 pounds needs 46 g/day. According to National Health and Nutrition Examination Survey (NHANES) 2001–2002 data, the mean intake for adult men and women aged 19 and older is 1.29 g/kg and 1.08 g/kg, respectively (Moshfegh et al., 2005).

The Acceptable Macronutrient Distribution Range (AMDR) for protein for adults is 10% to 35% of total calories. As illustrated in Figure 3.4, this is a wide range, with the upper end far greater than the median protein intake by American adult men of 71 to 101 g/day for various age groups during 1994–1996 and 1998, and 55 to

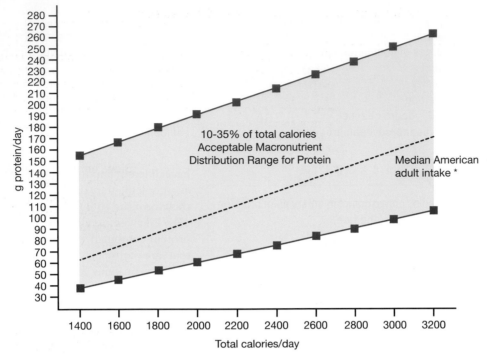

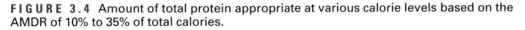

* median American adult intake of 15% of total calories

**FIGURE 3.4** Amount of total protein appropriate at various calorie levels based on the AMDR of 10% to 35% of total calories.

62 g/day for women (Institute of Medicine of the National Academies, 2005). For both men and women, protein provides approximately 15% of total calories consumed.

## When the RDA Doesn't Apply

The RDA is intended for healthy people only. Conditions that require tissue growth or repair increase a person's protein requirement (Box 3.3). Protein restriction is used for people with severe liver disease (because the liver metabolizes amino acids) and for those who are unable to adequately excrete nitrogenous wastes from protein metabolism due to impaired renal function.

---

### BOX 3.3 — CONDITIONS THAT INCREASE THE NEED FOR PROTEIN

*When calorie intake is inadequate and so protein is being used for energy*
- Very low calorie weight loss diets
- Starvation
- Protein–energy malnutrition

*When the body needs to heal itself*
- Hypermetabolic conditions such as burns, sepsis, major infection, and major trauma
- Skin breakdown
- Multiple fractures
- Hepatitis

*To replace excessive protein losses*
- Peritoneal dialysis
- Protein-losing renal diseases
- Malabsorption syndromes, such as protein-losing enteropathy and short bowel syndrome

*During periods of normal tissue growth*
- Pregnancy
- Lactation
- Infancy through adolescence

| TABLE 3.3 | Comparison Between Kwashiorkor and Marasmus |
|---|---|

| | Kwashiorkor | Marasmus |
|---|---|---|
| Cause | Acute, critical illness or infections that cause loss of appetite while increasing nutrient requirements and losses. Stressors in children in developing countries may be measles or gastroenteritis; in American adults, trauma or sepsis | Severe, prolonged starvation; may occur in children from chronic or recurring infections with marginal food intake; in adults from developed countries, may occur secondary to chronic illness |
| Onset | Rapid, acute; may develop in a matter of weeks | Slow, chronic; may take months or years to develop |
| Appearance | May look well nourished because of edema and enlarged liver | "Skin and bones" due to severe muscle loss with virtually no body fat |
| Weight Loss | Some | Severe |
| Other Clinical Symptoms That May Be Present | Poor appetite<br>Irritability<br>Patchy, scaly skin<br>Hair loss; loss of hair color; easy pluckability | Hunger |
| Mortality | High | Low, unless related to underlying disease |

*Source:* Shils, M., Shike, M., Ross, A., et al. (Eds.). (2006). *Modern nutrition in health and disease* (10th ed.). Philadelphia: Lippincott Williams & Wilkins.

## Protein Deficiency

**Kwashiorkor:** a type of protein–energy malnutrition caused by a deficiency of protein or from infections.

**Marasmus:** a type of protein–energy malnutrition caused from severe deficiency or impaired absorption of calories, protein, vitamins, and minerals.

Protein–energy malnutrition (PEM) occurs when protein, calories, or both are deficient in the diet. **Kwashiorkor** and **marasmus** are generally viewed as two distinctly different forms of PEM (Table 3.3), yet there is controversy as to whether kwashiorkor and marasmus simply represent the same disease at different stages. It may be that marasmus occurs when the body has adapted to starvation and kwashiorkor arises when adaptation fails due to illness.

Although PEM can affect people of any age, young children are the most common victims. Marasmus typically affects children between the ages of 1 to 4 years and kwashiorkor generally occurs in children less than 2 years of age. PEM is most prevalent in developing countries. Worldwide it is responsible for the deaths of about 6 million children annually.

In the United States, marasmus occurs secondary to chronic diseases, such as cancer, AIDS, and chronic pulmonary disease. It may also be seen among homeless people, elderly people living alone, fad dieters, adults who are addicted to drugs or alcohol, and people with eating disorders. Nutritional therapy is started slowly and advanced gradually to avoid life-threatening metabolic imbalances. In contrast, kwashiorkor results mainly from acute critical illnesses such as trauma, sepsis, and other illnesses seen in intensive care units (Shils et al., 2006). Aggressive nutritional support is used to restore metabolic balance as quickly as possible.

## Protein Excess

There are no proven risks from eating an excess of protein. Data are conflicting as to whether high-protein diets increase the risk of osteoporosis or renal stones. Although a UL has not been established, this does not mean there is no potential for adverse effects from a high protein intake from food or supplements (Institute of Medicine of the National Academies, 2005).

# ▶ PROTEIN IN HEALTH PROMOTION

Unlike carbohydrates and fat, protein intake, per se, is not addressed in the *Dietary Guidelines for Americans* (see Chapter 8). However, as a key recommendation regarding fat intake, Americans are urged to choose lean, low-fat, or fat-free selections of meat, poultry, dry beans, and milk or milk products. Table 3.4 lists very lean and lean options from the Meat and Beans group.

Many leading health organizations, including the World Cancer Research Fund and the American Cancer Society, recommend a plant-based diet. The American Heart Association and the Heart and Stroke Foundation of Canada recommend a balanced diet with an emphasis on grains, fruit, and vegetables. In a new report issued by the American Institute for Cancer Research, consumers are advised to eat no more than 18 ounces (cooked weight) per week of red meats, like beef, pork, and lamb, and to avoid processed meat such as ham, bacon, salami, hot dogs, and sausages based on evidence that red meat increases the risk of colorectal cancer (AICR, 2007).

| TABLE 3.4 | **Very Lean and Lean Choices from the Meat and Beans Group** | |
|---|---|---|
| **Item** | **Very Lean Choices (0–1 g fat/oz)** | **Lean Choices (3 g fat/oz)** |
| **Beef** | | Select or choice grades of trimmed round, sirloin, and flank steak; tenderloin; rib, chuck, and rump roast; T-bone, porterhouse, and cubed steak; ground round |
| **Pork** | | Fresh ham; canned, cured, or boiled ham; Canadian bacon; tenderloin, center loin chop |
| **Lamb** | | Roast, chop, or leg |
| **Veal** | | Lean chop, roast |
| **Poultry** | Skinless white meat chicken or turkey<br>Skinless Cornish hen | Skinless dark meat chicken or turkey<br>White meat with skin<br>Skinless domestic duck or goose |
| **Fish** | Cod, flounder, haddock, halibut, trout, smoked salmon, fresh or canned in water tuna | Smoked herring, oysters, fresh or canned salmon, catfish, sardines, tuna canned in oil |
| **Shellfish** | Clams, crab, lobster, scallops, shrimp, imitation shellfish | |
| **Game** | Skinless duck or pheasant, venison, buffalo, ostrich | Skinless goose, rabbit |
| **Cheese** | Fat-free or low-fat cottage cheese<br>Fat-free cheese | 4.5% cottage cheese<br>Grated parmesan<br>Cheese with 3 g of fat or less per ounce |
| **Processed meats** | Those with 1 g of fat or less per ounce, such as turkey ham | Those with 3 g of fat or less per ounce, such as turkey pastrami |
| **Other** | Egg whites, egg substitutes<br>Kidney<br>Sausage with 1 g of fat or less per ounce<br>Dried peas, beans, lentils (cooked) | Hot dogs with 3 g of fat or less per ounce<br>Liver, heart |

The health benefits of a plant-based diet may come from eating less of certain substances (such as saturated fat and cholesterol), eating more of others (such as fiber, antioxidants, and phytochemicals), or a combination of the two.

## Vegetarian Diets

Vegetarian eating patterns range from complete elimination of all animal products to simply avoiding red meat. Within each defined category of vegetarianism, individuals differ as to how strictly they adhere to their eating style. For instance, some vegans do not eat refried beans that contain lard because lard is an animal product, but other vegans do not avoid animal products so conscientiously. Flexitarians primarily follow a plant-based diet but occasionally allow themselves meat, fish, poultry, or dairy foods.

Vegetarians have lower incidences of obesity, cardiovascular disease, hypertension, type 2 diabetes, cancer, and dementia compared with nonvegetarians (American Dietetic Association (ADA), 2003). Vegetarians may also be at lower risk for renal disease, gallstones, and diverticular disease. However, vegetarian diets are not automatically healthier than nonvegetarian diets. Poorly planned vegetarian diets may lack certain essential nutrients, which endangers health. Also vegetarian diets can be excessive in fat and cholesterol if whole milk, whole-milk cheeses, eggs, and high-fat desserts are used extensively. Whether a vegetarian diet is healthy or detrimental to health depends on the actual food choices made over time. Tips for vegetarians appear in Box 3.4.

### Nutrients of Concern

Most vegetarian diets, even vegan ones, meet or exceed the RDA for protein despite containing less total protein and more lower-quality protein than nonvegetarian diets. Vegetarian sources of protein include dried peas and beans, nuts, nut butters, and soy products such as soy milk, tofu, tempeh, and veggie burgers (Fig. 3.5). A glossary of soy products is listed in Box 3.5.

---

**BOX 3.4**   **TIPS FOR FOLLOWING A VEGETARIAN DIET**

*Eat a variety of foods including whole grains, vegetables, fruits, dried peas and beans, nuts, seeds, and if desired, dairy products and eggs.* Consider meatless versions of familiar favorites, such as vegetable pizza, vegetable lasagna, vegetable stir-fry, vegetable lo mein, and vegetable kabobs.

*Experiment with meat substitutes made from vegetables.* For variety try soy sausage patties or links, veggie burgers, or soy hot dogs.

*Eat enough calories.* Adequate calories are necessary to avoid using amino acids for energy, which could lead to a shortage of amino acids for protein synthesis.

*Consume a rich source of vitamin C at every meal.* Eating a good source of vitamin C at every meal helps to maximize iron absorption from plants. Try orange and citrus fruits, tomatoes, kiwi, red and green peppers, broccoli, Brussels sprouts, cantaloupe, and strawberries.

*Include two servings daily of fats that supply omega-3 fats.* A serving is 1 teaspoon flaxseed oil, 1 tablespoon canola or soybean oil, 1 tablespoon ground flaxseed, or ¼ cup walnuts. Nuts and seeds may be used as substitutes from the Fat group.

*Don't go overboard on high-fat cheese as a meat substitute.* Full-fat cheese has more saturated fat and calories than many meats.

*Experiment with ethnic cuisines.* Many Asian, Middle Eastern, and Indian restaurants offer a variety of meatless dishes.

*Supplement nutrients that are lacking from food.* For vegans, this means vitamin $B_{12}$ (unless reliable fortified foods are consumed) and perhaps vitamin D. The adequacy of calcium, iron, and zinc intakes is evaluated on an individual basis.

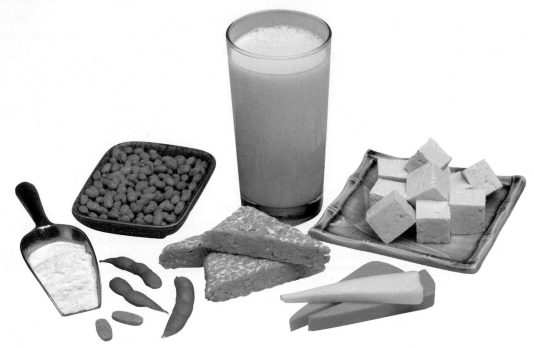

**FIGURE 3.5** A variety of soy products.

---

| BOX 3.5 | **GLOSSARY OF SOY PRODUCTS** |
|---------|------------------------------|

**Edamame:** parboiled fresh soybeans, usually in the pod, sold refrigerated or frozen
**Meat analogs:** imitation burgers, hot dogs, bacon, chicken fingers, etc. made from soy, not meat
**Miso:** fermented soybean paste
**Soy cheese:** cheese made from soy milk; can substitute for sour cream, cream cheese, or other cheese
**Soy milk:** the liquid from soaked, ground, strained soybeans. Available plain and in chocolate and vanilla flavors.
**Soy nuts:** whole soybeans that have been soaked in water then baked
**Soy nut butter:** crushed soy nuts blended with soy oil to resemble peanut butter
**Soy sprouts:** sprouted soybeans
**Tofu:** soybean curd
**Tempeh:** caked fermented soybeans
**Textured vegetable protein (TVP):** soy flour modified to resemble ground beef when rehydrated

---

Iron, zinc, calcium, vitamin D, and alpha-linolenic acid are nutrients of concern, not because they cannot be obtained in sufficient quantities from plants but because they may not be adequately consumed, depending on an individual's food choices. Vitamin $B_{12}$ is of concern because it does not occur naturally in plants. Table 3.5 lists vegetarian sources of these nutrients of concern.

## Is Vegetarianism for Everyone?

Vegetarianism is a personal choice, subject to personal interpretation. Although some view vegetarianism as a way of life, others prefer to simply opt for occasional meatless meals. Whatever the level of restriction, properly planned lacto-vegetarian, lacto-ovo vegetarian,

| TABLE 3.5 | **Sources of Nutrients of Concern in Vegan Diets** |

| Nutrient | Vegetarian Sources | Comments |
|---|---|---|
| Iron | Iron-fortified bread and cereals<br>Baked potato with skin<br>Kidney beans, black-eyed peas, and lentils<br>Cooked soybeans<br>Tofu<br>Veggie "meats"<br>Dried apricots, prunes, and raisins<br>Cooking in a cast iron pan, especially with acidic foods such as tomatoes | Because of the lower bioavailability of iron from plants, it is recommended that vegetarians consume 1.8 times the normal iron intake |
| Zinc | Whole grains, especially the bran and germ portions<br>White beans, kidney beans, chickpeas<br>Zinc-fortified cereals<br>Soybean products<br>Pumpkin seeds<br>Nuts | Zinc from plants is not absorbed as well as zinc from meats<br>Vegetarians are urged to meet or exceed the RDA for zinc |
| Calcium | Bok choy<br>Broccoli<br>Chinese/Napa cabbage<br>Collard greens<br>Kale<br>Okra<br>Turnip greens<br>Calcium-fortified orange juice<br>Tofu, soy milk<br>Calcium fortified breakfast cereals<br>Tortillas made from lime-processed corn | Spinach, beet greens, and Swiss chard are also high in calcium but their oxalate content interferes with calcium absorption<br>Calcium supplements are recommended for people who do not meet their calcium requirement through food |
| Vitamin D | Sunlight<br>Fortified milk<br>Fortified ready-to-eat cereals<br>Fortified soy milk<br>Fortified nondairy milk products | Supplements may be necessary depending on the quality of sunlight exposure and adequacy of food choices |
| Omega-3 Fatty Acids | Fortified foods, such as breakfast cereals and yogurt<br>Sources of alpha-linolenic acid are<br>Ground flaxseed and flaxseed oil<br>Walnuts and walnut oil<br>Canola oil<br>Soybean oil | Diets that exclude fish, eggs, and sea vegetables do not contain a direct source of omega-3 fatty acids<br>The body can convert small amounts of alpha-linolenic acid into one of the omega-3 fatty acids (DHA) |
| Vitamin B12 | Fortified soy milk, breakfast cereals, and veggie burgers | Seaweed, algae, spirulina, tempeh, miso, beer, and other fermented foods contain a form of vitamin $B_{12}$ that the body cannot use<br>Supplemental vitamin $B_{12}$ through food or pills is recommended for all people over the age of 50 regardless of the type of diet they consume because absorption decreases with age |

and vegan diets are nutritionally adequate during all phases of the life cycle including pregnancy and lactation. *Proper planning* means paying close attention to the nutrients of concern and using a vegetarian food guide for planning.

▶ HOW DO YOU RESPOND?

**Is ground turkey a low-fat alternative to ground beef?** Not necessarily. Ground turkey most likely contains skin, dark meat, and fat along with the breast, making it a higher fat product than 95% lean ground beef. Ground turkey breast and ground chicken breast are made only from white meat and are much lower in fat (0.5 g/3 oz cooked) than all varieties of ground beef (5.5–17 g fat/3 oz cooked).

**Isn't a high-protein diet better than a high-carbohydrate diet in promoting weight loss?** This may be true. A recent study showed that protein intake is a significant predictor of fat-free mass retention during calorie-restricted diets (Krieger et al., 2006). In fact, a daily protein intake of more than 1.05 g/kg was associated with greater muscle retention than was a protein intake closer to the RDA. In other words, protein eaters lost significantly more fat to muscle tissue than the carbohydrate eaters; obviously the loss of fat tissue is more desirable than the loss of muscle. Clients who choose to eat a high-protein diet in an attempt to lose weight should be reminded to choose low-fat sources of protein to keep calories under control.

**Does "vegetarian" on the label mean the product is also low fat?** No, vegetarian is not synonymous with low fat, particularly for items like vegetarian hot dogs, soy cheese, soy yogurt, and refried beans. Advise clients to read the "Nutrition Facts" label to determine if a vegetarian item is a good nutritional buy.

▶ CASE STUDY

For ethical reasons, Emily does not eat meat, eggs, or milk, although she is not so strict as to avoid baked goods that may contain milk or eggs. Over the last 6 months she has gained 15 pounds, although she actually expected to lose weight. She needs 2000 cal/day according to MyPyramid. A typical daily intake for her is as follows:

| | |
|---|---|
| **Breakfast:** | A smoothie made with soy milk, tofu, and fresh fruit |
| | A glazed doughnut |
| **Snack:** | Potato chips and soda |
| **Lunch:** | A peanut butter sandwich |
| | Soy yogurt |
| | Oatmeal cookies |
| | Soda |
| **Snack:** | A candy bar |
| **Dinner:** | Stir-fried vegetables over rice |
| | Bread with margarine |
| | A glass of soy milk |
| | Apple pie |
| **Snack:** | Buttered popcorn |

- What kind of vegetarian is Emily? What sources of protein is she consuming? Is she consuming enough protein? How does her daily intake compare to MyPyramid recommendations for a 2000-calorie diet? What suggestions would you make to her to improve the quality of her diet?
- Is Emily at risk of any nutrient deficiencies? If so, what would you recommend she do to ensure nutritional adequacy?
- What would you tell Emily about her weight gain? What foods would you recommend she eat less of if she wants to lose weight? What could she substitute for those foods?

1. What is the RDA for protein for a healthy adult who weighs 165 pounds?
   a. 60 grams
   b. 75 grams
   c. 100 grams
   d. 165 grams

2. The client asks what protein foods she can eat that are less expensive than meat. Which of the following foods would the nurse recommend she eat more of?
   a. Breads and cereals
   b. Dried peas and beans
   c. Fruit and vegetables
   d. Fish and shellfish

3. Which of the following sources of protein would be most appropriate on a low-fat diet?
   a. Eggs
   b. Ground chicken
   c. Boiled ham
   d. Turkey breast without skin

4. Which statement indicates the client understands vegetarian diets?
   a. "Vegetarians need to eat more calories than nonvegetarians in order to spare protein."
   b. "Vegetarian diets are always healthier than nonvegetarian diets."
   c. "Vegetarians usually do not consume enough protein."
   d. "Vegetarians may need to take supplements of iron, vitamin B12, and calcium."

5. A client who is in a positive nitrogen balance is most likely to be:
   a. A healthy adult
   b. Starving
   c. Pregnant
   d. Losing weight

6. An adult in the hospital has been diagnosed with marasmus. Which of the following would you expect?
   a. The client has experienced severe weight loss.
   b. The client denies hunger.
   c. The client has lost hair.
   d. The onset of the deficiency was rapid.

7. The nurse knows her instructions have been effective when the client verbalizes that a source of complete, high-quality protein is found in:
   a. Peanut butter
   b. Black-eyed peas
   c. Soy burgers
   d. Corn

8. A client says that she doesn't eat much meat. After teaching the client about serving sizes, the nurse determines that the teaching has been effective when the client states that an ounce of meat provides approximately the same amount of protein as which of the following?
   a. 8 ounces of milk
   b. 8 ounces of nuts
   c. ½ ounce of cheese
   d. 1 cup of black beans

- Protein is a component of every living cell. Protein in the body provides structure and framework. Amino acids are also components of enzymes, hormones, neurotransmitters, and antibodies. Proteins play a role in fluid balance and acid–base balance and are used to transport substances through the blood. Protein provides 4 cal/g of energy.

- Amino acids, which are composed of carbon, hydrogen, oxygen, and nitrogen atoms, are the building blocks of protein. Of the 20 common amino acids, 9 are considered essential because the body cannot make them. The remaining 11 amino acids are no less important but are considered nonessential because they can be made by the body if nitrogen is available. Some of these are considered conditionally essential under certain circumstances.

- Amino acids are joined in different amounts, proportions, and sequences to form the thousands of different proteins in the body.

- The small intestine is the principal site of protein digestion; amino acids and some dipeptides are absorbed through the portal bloodstream.

- In the body, amino acids are used to make proteins, nonessential amino acids, and other nitrogen-containing compounds. Some amino acids can be converted to glucose. Amino acids consumed in excess of need are burned for energy or converted to fat and stored.

- Healthy adults are in nitrogen balance, which means that protein synthesis is occurring at the same rate as protein breakdown. Nitrogen balance is determined by comparing the amount of nitrogen consumed with the amount of nitrogen excreted in urine, feces, hair, nails, and skin.

- Except for the Fruits and Oils, all MyPyramid groups provide protein in varying amounts.

- The quality of proteins varies. Complete proteins provide adequate amounts and proportions of all essential amino acids needed for protein synthesis. Animal proteins and soy protein are complete proteins. Incomplete proteins lack adequate amounts of one or more essential amino acids. Except for soy protein, all plants are sources of incomplete proteins. Gelatin is also an incomplete protein.

- The RDA for protein for adults is 0.8 g/kg of body weight. The AMDR for protein among adults is 10% to 35% of total calories. Most Americans consume more protein than they need.

- Pure vegans eat no animal products. Most American vegetarians are lacto-vegetarians or lacto-ovo vegetarians, whose diets include respectively milk products or milk products and eggs.

- Most vegetarian diets meet or exceed the RDA for protein and are nutritionally adequate across the life cycle. Pure vegans who do not have reliable sources of vitamin $B_{12}$ and vitamin D need supplements.

## ANSWER KEY

1. **TRUE** Most Americans consume more protein than they need.
2. **FALSE** Over the course of a day, if the food consumed is varied and contains sufficient calories, most vegetarian diets meet or exceed the RDA for protein.
3. **FALSE** Unlike glucose and fat, the body is not able to store excess amino acids for later use.
4. **TRUE** Soy protein is complete. It is a high biologic value protein and is comparable in quality to animal protein.
5. **FALSE** There are no proven risks to eating a high protein intake.

6. **FALSE** The quality of a protein is determined by the balance of essential amino acids provided.

7. **FALSE** Fruits generally provide negligible protein, and oils are protein free.

8. **FALSE** Healthy adults are in neutral nitrogen balance: protein synthesis is occurring at the same rate as protein breakdown.

9. **FALSE** Properly planned vegetarian diets are nutritionally adequate during all phases of pregnancy and lactation.

10. **TRUE** Due to lack of sufficient data, a UL has not been established for protein or any of the amino acids. However, the Institute of Medicine warns against using any single amino acid in amounts significantly higher than those found in food.

## WEBSITES FOR INFORMATION ABOUT GENERAL VEGETARIAN NUTRITION

Food and Nutrition Information Center, U.S. Department of Agriculture at **www.nal.usda.gov/fnic/etext/000059.html**
Vegan Health at **www.veganhealth.org**
The Vegan Society at **www.vegansociety.com**
Vegetarian Nutrition Dietetic Practice Group at **www.vegetariannutrition.net**
Vegetarian Resource Group at **www.vrg.org**
The Vegetarian Society of the United Kingdom at **www.vegsoc.org/health/**
Seventh-Day Adventist Dietetic Association at **www.sdada.org/health_tips.htm**
Soyfoods Association of North America at **www.soyfoods.org**
United Soybean Board at **www.soyconnection.com**

## REFERENCES

American Dietetic Association (ADA). (2003). Position of the American Dietetic Association and the Dietitians of Canada: Vegetarian diets. *Journal of the American Dietetic Association, 103*, 748–765.

American Institute of Cancer Research (AICR). (2007). Expert Report. Food, nutrition, physical activity and the prevalence of cancer: A global perspective. Available at www.dietandcancerreport.org. Accessed on 11/8/07.

Institute of Medicine of the National Academies (IOM). (2005). *Dietary Reference Intakes for energy, carbohydrates, fiber, fat, fatty acids, cholesterol, protein, and amino acids (macronutrients).* Washington, DC: National Academies Press.

Krieger, J., Sitren, H., Daniels, M., et al. (2006). Effects of variation in protein and carbohydrate intake on body mass and composition during energy restriction: A meta-regression. *American Journal of Clinical Nutrition, 83*, 260–274.

Moshfegh, A., Goldman, J., & Cleveland, L. (2005). *What we eat in America, NHANES 2001–2002: Usual nutrient intakes from food compared to dietary reference intakes.* US Department of Agriculture, Agricultural Research Service.

Shils, M., Shike, M., Ross, A., et al. (Eds.). (2006). *Modern nutrition in health and disease* (10th ed.). Philadelphia: Lippincott Williams & Wilkins.

# 4 Lipids

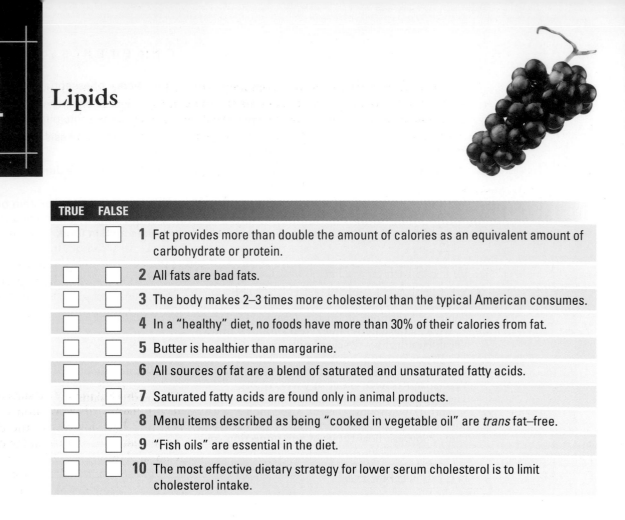

### UPON COMPLETION OF THIS CHAPTER, YOU WILL BE ABLE TO

- Compare saturated, monounsaturated, and polyunsaturated fatty acids.
- Propose ways to improve the type of fat present in a sample meal plan.
- Explain the functions of fat in the body.
- Discuss the digestion and absorption of fat.
- Give examples of foods that provide omega-3 fatty acids.
- Calculate the amount of calories from fat in various foods.
- Explain why there is not an RDA for total fat, trans fat, and saturated fat.

"Eat less fat" has long been a nutritional mantra. But decades of study have shown that the relationship between fat and chronic disease is far more complex than that simple advice implies. While an excess of calories from any source can lead to weight gain over time, switching to a low-fat diet does not guarantee weight loss. And although obesity increases the risk of certain cancers, the risk may come from an excess of calories, not specifically dietary fat. With heart disease and stroke, the type of fat may be more important than the amount of fat. The bottom line is that while all fats are calorically dense, some fats are "good" (unsaturated) and should be eaten in moderation and other fats are "bad" (saturated fat and trans fats) and should be limited.

**Lipids:** a group of water-insoluble, energy-yielding organic compounds composed of carbon, hydrogen, and oxygen atoms.

The three classes of **lipids**, commonly referred to as fat throughout the rest of this chapter and book, are triglycerides (fats and oils), phospholipids (e.g., lecithin), and sterols (e.g., cholesterol). This chapter describes fats, their dietary sources, and how they are handled in the body. The functions of fat are presented, as are recommendations regarding intake.

# ▶ TRIGLYCERIDES

**Triglycerides:** a class of lipids composed of a glycerol molecule as its backbone with three fatty acids attached.

Approximately 98% of the fat in foods is in the form of **triglycerides**. Chemically, triglycerides are made of the same elements as carbohydrates, namely carbon, hydrogen, and oxygen, but because there are proportionately more carbon and hydrogen atoms to oxygen atoms, they yield more calories per gram than carbohydrates. Structurally, triglycerides are composed of a three-carbon atom glycerol backbone with three fatty acids attached (Fig. 4.1). An individual triglyceride molecule may contain one, two, or three different types of fatty acids.

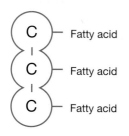

**FIGURE 4.1**
Generic triglyceride molecule.

## QUICK BITE

Fatty acids are commonly abbreviated by a C followed by the number of carbon atoms, a colon, and the number of double bonds.
Example: Stearic acid, an 18-carbon length fatty acid with no double bonds, is abbreviated as C18:0.

## QUICK BITE

The number of carbon atoms in fatty acids
Short chain: 2 to 4
Medium chain: 6 to 10
Long chain: 12 or more

## Fatty Acids

**Fatty acids** are basically chains of carbon atoms with hydrogen atoms attached (Fig. 4.2). At one end of the chain is a methyl group ($CH_3$) and at the other end is an acid group (COOH). Fatty acids vary in the length of their carbon chain and in the degree of unsaturation.

### Carbon Chain Length

Almost all fatty acids have an even number of carbon atoms in their chain, generally between 4 and 26 although both shorter and longer chains have been identified in

**Fatty Acids:** organic compounds composed of a chain of carbon atoms to which hydrogen atoms are attached. An acid group (COOH) is attached at one end and a methyl group ($CH_3$) at the other end.

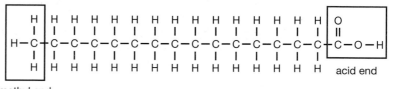

Palmitic acid: 16 carbon saturated fatty acid

**FIGURE 4.2** Fatty acid configurations.

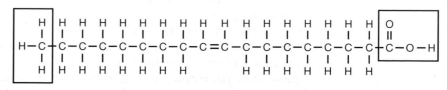

Oleic acid: 18 carbon n-9, monounsaturated fatty acid

certain body tissues. Long-chain fatty acids, predominate in meats, fish, and vegetables oils, are the most common length fatty acid in the diet. Smaller amounts of medium- and short-chain fatty acids are found primarily in dairy products.

## Degree of Saturation

**Saturated Fatty Acids:** fatty acids in which all the carbon atoms are bonded to as many hydrogen atoms as they can hold, so no double bonds exist between carbon atoms.

**Unsaturated Fatty Acids:** fatty acids that are not completely saturated with hydrogen atoms, so one or more double bonds form between the carbon atoms.

**Glycerol:** a three-carbon atom chain that serves as the backbone of triglycerides.

As dictated by nature, each carbon atom in a fatty acid chain must have four bonds connecting it to other atoms. When all the carbon atoms in a fatty acid have four single bonds each, the fatty acid is said to be **"saturated"** with hydrogen atoms. An **"unsaturated" fatty acid** does not have all the hydrogen atoms it can potentially hold; therefore, one or more double bonds form between carbon atoms in the chain. If one double bond exists between two carbon atoms, the fatty acid is monounsaturated; if there is more than one double bond between carbon atoms, the fatty acid is polyunsaturated.

Fatty acids can attach to **glycerol** molecules in various ratios and combinations to form a variety of triglycerides within a single food fat. The types and proportions of fatty acids present influence the sensory and functional properties of the food fat. For instance, butter tastes and acts differently from corn oil, which tastes and acts differently from lard.

All food fats contain a mixture of saturated, monounsaturated, and polyunsaturated fatty acids. When applied to sources of fat in the diet, "unsaturated" and "saturated" are not absolute terms used to describe the only types of fatty acids present; rather they are relative descriptions that indicate which kinds of fatty acids are present in the largest proportion (Fig. 4.3).

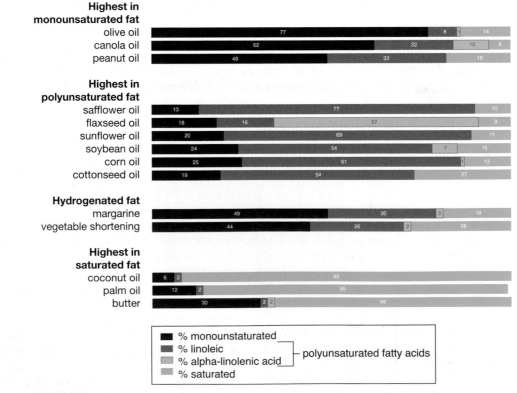

**FIGURE 4.3** Predominant types of fatty acids in selected fats and oils.

**Saturated Fats.** Saturated fats, because they are basically straight-line molecules, can pack tightly together and therefore tend to be solid at room temperature. Animal fats—the fat in meat, whole-milk dairy products, and egg yolks—are primarily saturated and provide approximately 60% of total saturated fat consumed in the typical American diet (American Dietetic Association (ADA), 2007). The only vegetable fats that are saturated are palm oil, palm kernel oil, and coconut oil.

Saturated fat is commonly known as a "bad" fat because it raises blood cholesterol levels. In general, as the intake of saturated fat increases, so does the level of total and **low-density lipoprotein (LDL) cholesterol** (Institute of Medicine of the National Academies, 2005). As total and LDL cholesterol levels rise, so does the risk of coronary heart disease. According to the *Dietary Guidelines for Americans*, reducing saturated fat intake is one of the most important changes needed in the typical American diet.

Saturated fat may also make the inner lining of arteries more prone to inflammation and the buildup of fatty plaques by interfering with the normal protective action of high-density lipoprotein (HDL) cholesterol (Nicholls et al., 2006). Although the effects may be temporary, frequent binges on high-saturated fat foods may be detrimental over time.

> **QUICK BITE**
>
> Most common saturated fatty acids in food
> | | |
> |---|---|
> | Myristic acid | C14:0 |
> | Palmitic acid | C16:0 |
> | Stearic acid | C18:0 |

**Low-Density Lipoprotein (LDL) Cholesterol:** the major class of atherogenic lipoproteins that carry cholesterol from the liver to the tissues.

**Unsaturated Fats.** Fatty acids with one more double bond in them are physically kinked and unable to pack together tightly thus they are liquid at room temperature. Monounsaturated fats are the predominate fat in olives, olive oil, canola oil, peanut oil, avocado, cashews, almonds, and most other nuts. Meat fat also contains moderate amounts of monounsaturated fats, providing approximately 60% of usual intake. Polyunsaturated fats are the predominate fat in corn, soybean, safflower, and cottonseeds oils, and also in fish. They are less ubiquitous than monounsaturated fats.

Unsaturated fats are commonly known as "good fats" because when they are eaten in place of saturated fats they lower LDL cholesterol and raise HDL cholesterol. When monounsaturated fats replace carbohydrates in the diet, improvements in triglyceride and HDL levels occur.

> **QUICK BITE**
>
> Common monounsaturated fatty acid
> | | |
> |---|---|
> | Palmitoleic acid | C16:1 |

*Position of the Double Bond.* Part of an unsaturated fatty acid's identity is determined by the location of the first or only double bond along the carbon chain. The most common method of identifying the bond is to count the number of carbon atoms from the methyl end, as denoted by the terms "$n$" or "omega." The location of the first double bond is significant because it determines the essentiality of a fatty acid: the body is unable to insert double bonds closer than $n$-9 when it makes fatty acids, so one $n$-6 fatty acid (linoleic acid) and one $n$-3 fatty acid (alpha-linolenic acid) are considered essential in the diet.

**Omega-6 ($n$-6) Fatty Acid:** an unsaturated fatty acid whose endmost double bond occurs six-carbon atoms from the methyl end of its carbon chain.

> **QUICK BITE**
>
> Common $n$-6 polyunsaturated fatty acids
> | | |
> |---|---|
> | Linoleic acid | C18:2 |
> | Arachidonic acid | C20:4 |

*Linoleic Acid.* Linoleic acid is the essential **$n$-6 fatty acid**. It is especially abundant in plant oils such as safflower, sunflower, corn, and soybean oils; poultry fat, nuts, and seeds are also sources. The body can make other $n$-6 fatty acids from linoleic acid, such as arachidonic acid. However, if a deficiency of linoleic acid develops, arachidonic acid becomes "conditionally essential" because the body is not able to make it without a supply of linoleic acid.

### Omega-3 Fatty Acid (*n*-3): an unsaturated fatty acid whose endmost double bond occurs three carbon atoms from the methyl end of its carbon chain.

### Fish Oils: a common term for the long-chain, polyunsaturated omega-3 fatty acids eicosapentaenoic acid (EPA) and docosahexaenoic acid (DHA) found in the fat of fish, primarily in cold-water fish.

### Rancidity: the chemical change that occurs when fats are oxidized, which causes an offensive taste and smell and the loss of fat-soluble vitamins A and E.

### Hydrogenation: a process of adding hydrogen atoms to unsaturated vegetable oils (usually corn, soybean, cottonseed, safflower, or canola oil), which reduces the number of double bonds; the number of saturated and monounsaturated bonds increases as the number of polyunsaturated bonds decreases.

### Cis Fats: unsaturated fatty acids whose hydrogen atoms occur on the same side of the double bond.

### Trans Fats: unsaturated fatty acids that have at least one double bond whose hydrogen atoms are on the opposite sides of the double bond; "trans" means across in Latin.

*Alpha-Linolenic Acid.* Alpha-linolenic acid is the essential ***n*-3 fatty acid** and the principal *n*-3 fatty acid in most Western diets. It is found in flaxseed, canola, soybean, and walnut oils; and in nuts, especially walnuts. To a limited extent, humans can convert alpha-linolenic acid to eicosapentaenoic acid (EPA) and docosahexaenoic acid (DHA) in the body. These two *n*-3 fatty acids are commonly referred to as **"fish oils"** because they are primarily found in fatty fish, especially salmon, anchovy, sardines, herring, lake trout, and mackerel.

**QUICK BITE**

Common *n*-3 polyunsaturated fatty acids
| | |
|---|---|
| Alpha-linolenic acid | C18:3 |
| Eicosapentaenoic acid | C20:5 |
| Docosahexaenoic acid | C22:6 |

*Stability of Fats.* The degree of unsaturation influences the stability of fats. Although all fats can become oxidized when exposed to light and oxygen over time, the greater the number of double bonds, the greater the susceptibility to rancidity. Therefore, polyunsaturated fats are most susceptible to **rancidity**, saturated fats are least susceptible, and monounsaturated fats are somewhere in-between.

To help extend the shelf life, food manufacturers may add antioxidants such as butylated hydroxyanisole (BHA) and butylated hydroxytoluene (BHT) to polyunsaturated fat-rich foods and oils. Another commercial method to make oils more stable is hydrogenation.

*Hydrogenation and Trans Fats.* **Hydrogenation** is a process that adds hydrogen atoms to heart-healthy polyunsaturated oils to saturate some of the double bonds so that the resulting product is less susceptible to rancidity and has improved function. Hydrogenation varies in degrees from "light" to "partial" according to the desired outcome. Lightly hydrogenated oils are more stable because they have fewer double bonds, but are still in liquid form. Partial hydrogenation results in a more solid (more saturated) product such as stick margarine and shortening, yet still maintains some unsaturated (double) bonds. Fully hydrogenated products are virtually completely saturated and do not contain trans fats (International Food Information Council, 2005).

Initially, hydrogenated fats appeared to be superior to both saturated and unsaturated fats, albeit for different reasons. Compared to the saturated fats in butter and lard, hydrogenated fats seemed more heart-healthy because they still provide some unsaturated fatty acids. And compared to liquid oils, products made with partially hydrogenated fats have a longer shelf life and better overall quality; hydrogenated fats make pie crusts flakier, French fries crispier, and frosting creamier. Seemingly a have-your-cake-and-eat-it-too type of product, partially hydrogenated fats permeated the food supply and quickly became a dietary staple in the 1970s.

However, the process of hydrogenation changes the placement of the hydrogen atoms around the remaining double bonds from the natural *cis* position to the rare *trans* position (Fig. 4.4). Only small amounts of **trans fats** occur naturally in some animal foods, such as milk and meat, and almost none appear naturally in plant oils. Most trans fat in a typical American diet comes from partially hydrogenated oils and foods made with partially hydrogenated oils, such as French fries, stick margarine, shortening, potato chips, baked goods, and crackers. In fact, most of these products contained more trans fat than saturated fat.

Over the last two decades, mounting evidence revealed that trans fats, like saturated fat, raise LDL cholesterol. Even worse, trans fats lower HDL cholesterol and have been shown to increase serum triglyceride levels as well as increase insulin resistance and raise biomarkers of inflammation (e.g., C-reactive protein, tumor necrosis factor receptors). It is now known that, ounce for ounce, trans fats are more unhealthy than saturated fats. However, because we consume so much less trans fat (an average of 2.6% of total calories among

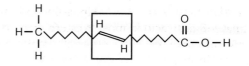

Trans-position: H on opposite sides of double bond

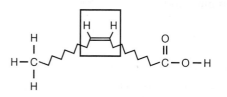

Cis-position: H on same side of double bond

**FIGURE 4.4** *Cis-* and *trans-*fatty acid configuration.

American adults) than saturated fat (an average of 11% to 12% of total calories), it is inaccurate to assume that cutting trans fat is a higher priority than reducing saturated fat intake.

In response to the clinical evidence that trans fats are "bad" and because of pressure from consumer groups, the FDA amended its nutrition labeling regulations to require trans fatty acids be declared on the "Nutrition Facts" label as of January 1, 2006. But beware: because amounts less than 0.5 g/serving can be rounded down to zero, the label can claim to have "zero trans fats" even if partially hydrogenated oils or shortenings appear on the ingredient list. And while 0.5 g trans fat per serving may sound insignificant, it can add up. For instance, most people will eat 3 cups of microwave popcorn at a time, which is actually 3 servings according to the label. At 0.5 g trans fat per serving, the total trans fat intake comes to 1.5 g. The American Heart Association recommends trans fat intake be less than 1% total calories, which translates to 2 g trans fat in a 2000-calorie diet. Only when the label says "no trans fats" is it actually free of trans fat.

Numerous cities around the United States, beginning with New York City, have banned the use of trans fats in restaurants and other foodservice establishments. The unhealthy image of trans fats has prompted food manufacturers to seek healthier alternatives and as a result, trans fat–free products are more commonplace on grocery store shelves. Likewise, many fast-food restaurants, hotel chains, cruise ship lines, and even the Disney theme parks have reformulated their recipes to virtually eliminate trans fats. In some items, such as French fries, partially hydrogenated fats (shortening) have been replaced with trans fat–free soybean oil. Ironically, in other products the choice of fat has come full circle and saturated fats are being used in place of partially hydrogenated fats. In the future, genetically engineered oils and new processing techniques will likely produce virtually trans fat–free customized oils as alternatives to hydrogenated fats (Tarrago-Trani et al., 2006).

## Functions of Triglycerides in the Body

The primary function of fat is to fuel the body. At rest, fat provides about 60% of the body's calorie needs. All fat, whether saturated or unsaturated, *cis-* or *trans-*, provides 9 cal/g, more than double the amount of calories as an equivalent amount of either carbohydrate or protein. Although fat is an important energy source, it cannot meet all of the body's energy needs because certain cells, such as brain cells and cells of the central nervous system, normally rely solely on glucose for energy.

Fat has other important functions in the body. Fat deposits insulate and cushion internal organs to protect them from mechanical injury. Fat under the skin helps to regulate body temperature by serving as a layer of insulation against the cold. And dietary fat facilitates the absorption of the fat-soluble vitamins A, D, E, and K when consumed at the same meal.

**Essential Fatty Acids:** fatty acids that cannot be synthesized in the body and so must be consumed through food.

The **essential fatty acids** have specific functions in the body. They play a role in maintaining healthy skin and promoting normal growth in children. As part of phospholipids, essential fatty acids are a component of cell membranes and are precursors of eicosanoids (e.g., prostaglandins, thromboxanes, and leukotrienes), a group of hormone-like substances that help regulate blood pressure, blood clotting, and other body functions. Although DHA is not an essential fatty acid, it is abundant in the structural lipids in the brain and in retinal membranes.

There is much interest in fish oils and the role they may play in preventing a variety of health problems, including heart disease, macular degeneration, cancer, and Alzheimer's disease. Unfortunately there have been few well designed, controlled studies testing their effectiveness. At this time, there is enough evidence to credit fish oils with decreasing the risk of heart disease through their impact on lipoproteins, triglycerides, and blood pressure (Balk et al., 2007). Overall results of clinical studies that looked at the role of $n$-3 fatty acids in asthma, cancer, dementia, neurological diseases, diabetes, inflammatory bowel disease, rheumatoid arthritis, kidney disease, lupus, eye health, and mental health are inconclusive or mixed (Balk et al., 2007). Also, there is a lack of convincing data that alpha-linolenic acid can substitute for fish oils to reduce the risk of heart disease, and a few studies showed that increased intakes of alpha-linolenic acid may increase the risk of advanced prostate cancer (Leitzmann et al., 2004). More quality human studies are needed to determine the role of $n$-3 fatty acids in maintaining health.

# ▶ OTHER LIPIDS

The other 2% of lipids in foods are phospholipids and sterols.

## Phospholipids

**Phospholipids:** a group of compound lipids that is similar to triglycerides in that they contain a glycerol molecule and two fatty acids. In place of the third fatty acid, phospholipids have a phosphate group and a molecule of choline or another nitrogen-containing compound.

**Emulsifier:** a stabilizing compound that helps to keep both parts of an emulsion (oil and water mixture) from separating.

Like triglycerides, **phospholipids** have a glycerol backbone with fatty acids attached. What makes them different from triglycerides is that a phosphate group replaces one of the fatty acids. Although phospholipids occur naturally in almost all foods, they make up a very small percentage of total fat intake.

Phospholipids are both fat-soluble (because of the fatty acids) and water-soluble (because of the phosphate group), a unique feature that enables them to act as **emulsifiers**. This role is played out in the body as they emulsify fats to keep them suspended in blood and other body fluids. As a component of all cell membranes, phospholipids not only provide structure but help to transport fat-soluble substances across cell membranes. Phospholipids are also precursors of prostaglandins.

Lecithin is the best-known phospholipid. Claims that it lowers blood cholesterol, improves memory, controls weight, and cures arthritis, hypertension, and gallbladder problems are unfounded. Studies show no benefit from taking supplements because lecithin is digested in the gastrointestinal tract into its component parts and is not absorbed intact to perform super functions. Lecithin is not even an essential nutrient because it is synthesized in the body. Many people who take lecithin supplements do not realize that they provide 9 cal/g, just like all other fats.

## Cholesterol

**Sterols:** one of three main classes of lipids that include cholesterol, bile acids, sex hormones, the adrenocortical hormones, and vitamin D.

Cholesterol is a **sterol**, a waxy substance whose carbon, hydrogen, and oxygen molecules are arranged in a ring. Cholesterol occurs in the tissues of all animals. It is found in all cell membranes and in myelin; brain and nerve cells are especially rich in cholesterol. The body synthesizes bile acids, steroid hormones, and vitamin D from cholesterol. Although cholesterol is made from acetyl-coenzyme A (acetyl-CoA), the body cannot break down cholesterol into CoA molecules to yield energy; so cholesterol does not provide calories.

### QUICK BITE

Cholesterol content of selected foods

| | Cholesterol (mg) | | Cholesterol (mg) |
|---|---|---|---|
| Beef brains, 3 oz | 1746 | Shrimp, 4 | 37 |
| Beef liver, 3 oz | 375 | Whole milk, 1 cup | 30 |
| Beef kidney, 3 oz | 329 | 2% milk, 1 cup | 15 |
| Egg yolk, 1 | 213 | Butter, 1 tbsp | 12 |
| Broiled lobster, 1 cup | 110 | Nonfat milk, 1 cup | 7 |
| Broiled steak, 4 oz | 71 | Egg whites | 0 |

Cholesterol is found exclusively in animals, with liver and egg yolks the richest sources. The cholesterol in food is just cholesterol; descriptions of "good" and "bad" cholesterol refer to the lipoprotein packages that move cholesterol through the blood (see Chapter 20). You cannot eat more "good" cholesterol, but you can make lifestyle changes, such as quitting smoking, exercising, and losing weight if overweight, that increase the amount of "good" cholesterol in the blood.

Because all body cells are capable of making enough cholesterol to meet their needs, cholesterol is not an essential nutrient. In fact, daily endogenous cholesterol synthesis is approximately two to three times more than average cholesterol intake (Harvard School of Public Health, 2007). When dietary cholesterol decreases, endogenous cholesterol production increases to maintain an adequate supply. The body makes cholesterol from acetyl-CoA, which can originate from carbohydrates, protein, fat, or alcohol. Thus eating an excess of calories, regardless of the source, can increase cholesterol synthesis.

Dietary cholesterol increases total and LDL cholesterol but the effect is lessened when saturated fat intake is low. Dietary cholesterol may have an independent effect on heart disease risk beyond its effect on serum cholesterol.

# ▶ HOW THE BODY HANDLES FAT

## Digestion

A minimal amount of chemical digestion of fat occurs in the mouth and stomach through the action of lingual lipase and gastric lipases, respectively (Fig. 4.5).

As fat enters the duodenum, it stimulates the release of the hormone cholecystokinin, which in turn stimulates the gallbladder to release bile. Bile, an emulsifier produced in the liver from bile salts, cholesterol, phospholipids, bilirubin, and electrolytes, prepares fat for digestion by suspending the hydrophobic molecules in the watery intestinal fluid. Emulsified fat particles have enlarged surface areas on which digestive enzymes can work.

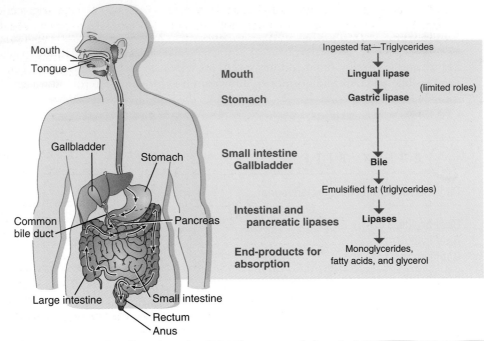

**FIGURE 4.5** Fat digestion. A minimal amount of chemical digestion of fat occurs in the mouth and stomach through the action of lingual lipase and gastric lipases, respectively. As fat enters the duodenum, it stimulates the release of the hormone cholecystokinin, which in turn stimulates the gallbladder to release bile. Bile prepares fat for digestion by suspending the hydrophobic molecules in the watery intestinal fluid. Most fat digestion occurs in the small intestine. Pancreatic lipase splits off one fatty acid at a time from the triglyceride molecule, working from the outside in until two free fatty acids and a monoglyceride remain. Usually the process stops at this point but sometimes digestion continues and the monoglyceride splits into a free fatty acid and glyceride molecule. The end products of digestion—mostly monoglycerides with free fatty acids and little glycerol—are absorbed into intestinal cells. It is normal for a small amount of fat (4 to 5 g) to escape digestion and be excreted in the feces.

**Monoglyceride:** a glyceride molecule with only one fatty acid attached.

Most fat digestion occurs in the small intestine. Pancreatic lipase, the most important and powerful lipase, splits off one fatty acid at a time from the triglyceride molecule, working from the outside in until two free fatty acids and a **monoglyceride** remain. Usually the process stops at this point but sometimes digestion continues and the monoglyceride splits into a free fatty acid and a glyceride molecule. The end products of digestion—mostly monoglycerides with free fatty acids and little glycerol—are absorbed into intestinal cells. It is normal for a small amount of fat (4 to 5 g) to escape digestion and be excreted in the feces.

The digestion of phospholipids is similar with the end products being two free fatty acids and a phospholipid fragment. Cholesterol does not undergo digestion; it is absorbed as is.

## Absorption

**Micelles:** fat particles encircled by bile salts to facilitate their diffusion into intestinal cells.

About 95% of consumed fat is absorbed, mostly in the duodenum and jejunum. Small fat particles, such as short- and medium-chain fatty acids and glycerol, are absorbed directly through the mucosal cells into capillaries. They bind with albumin and are transported to the liver via the portal vein.

The absorption of larger fat particles, namely monoglycerides and long-chain fatty acids, is more complex. Although they are insoluble in water, monoglycerides and long-chain fatty acids dissolve into **micelles**, which deliver fat to the intestinal cells. Once inside the intestinal

**Chylomicrons:** lipoproteins that transport absorbed lipids from intestinal cells through the lymph and eventually into the bloodstream.

cells, the monoglycerides and long-chain fatty acids combine to form triglycerides. The reformed triglycerides, along with phospholipids and cholesterol, become encased in protein to form **chylomicrons**. Chylomicrons distribute dietary lipids throughout the body.

Their job done, most of the released bile salts are reabsorbed in the terminal ileum, transported back to the liver, and recycled (enterohepatic circulation). Some bile salts become bound to fiber in the intestine and are excreted in the feces.

## Fat Catabolism

Whether from the most recent meal or from storage, triglycerides that are needed for energy are split into glycerol and fatty acids by lipoprotein lipase and are released into the bloodstream to be picked up by cells.

The catabolism of fatty acids increases when carbohydrate intake is inadequate (e.g., while on a very low-calorie diet) or unavailable (e.g., in the case of uncontrolled diabetes). Without adequate glucose, the breakdown of fatty acids is incomplete and ketones are formed. Eventually ketosis and acidosis may result.

Because fatty acids break down into two-carbon molecules, not three-carbon molecules, they cannot be reassembled to make glucose. Only the glycerol component of triglycerides can be used to make glucose, making fat an inefficient choice of fuel for glucose-dependent brain cells, nerve cells, and red blood cells. Fortunately, most body cells can use fatty acids for energy.

## Fat Anabolism

Most newly absorbed fatty acids recombine with glycerol to form triglycerides that end up stored in adipose tissue. Fat stored in adipose cells represents the body's largest and most efficient energy reserve; most other body cells are able to store only minute amounts of fat. Unlike glycogen, which can be stored only in limited amounts and is accompanied by water, adipose cells have a virtually limitless capacity to store fat and carry very little additional weight as intracellular water. While normal glycogen reserves may last for half a day of normal activity, fat reserves can last up to 2 months in people of normal weight. Each pound of body fat provides 3500 calories.

## ▶ FAT IN FOODS

Fat has many vital functions in food and serves to improve the overall palatability of the diet. For instance, it

- imparts its own flavor, from the mild taste of canola oil and corn oil to the distinctive tastes of peanut oil and olive oil;
- transfers heat to rapidly cook food, as in the case of frying;
- absorbs flavors and aromas of ingredients to improve overall taste;
- adds juiciness to meats;
- creates a creamy and smooth "mouth feel" in items such as ice cream, desserts, and cream soups;
- adds texture or body to many foods, such as flakiness, tenderness, elasticity, and viscosity (e.g., milk is watery and cheese is rubbery when fat is removed);
- imparts tenderness and moisture in baked goods, such as cookies, pies, and cakes, and delays staling;
- is insoluble in water, thus provides a unique flavor and texture to foods such as salad dressings.

The fat content in MyPyramid varies greatly among groups and between selections within each group (Fig. 4.6). It is recommended that people choose the lowest-fat selections from

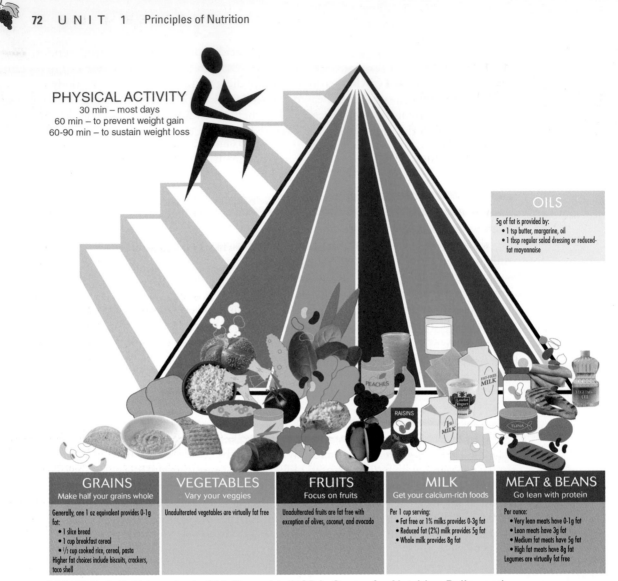

**PHYSICAL ACTIVITY**
30 min – most days
60 min – to prevent weight gain
60-90 min – to sustain weight loss

**OILS**

5g of fat is provided by:
- 1 tsp butter, margarine, oil
- 1 tbsp regular salad dressing or reduced-fat mayonnaise

| GRAINS | VEGETABLES | FRUITS | MILK | MEAT & BEANS |
|---|---|---|---|---|
| Make half your grains whole | Vary your veggies | Focus on fruits | Get your calcium-rich foods | Go lean with protein |
| Generally, one 1 oz equivalent provides 0-1g fat: • 1 slice bread • 1 cup breakfast cereal • ½ cup cooked rice, cereal, pasta Higher fat choices include biscuits, crackers, taco shell | Unadulterated vegetables are virtually fat free | Unadulterated fruits are fat free with exception of olives, coconut, and avocado | Per 1 cup serving: • Fat free or 1% milks provides 0-3g fat • Reduced fat (2%) milk provides 5g fat • Whole milk provides 8g fat | Per ounce: • Very lean meats have 0-1g fat • Lean meats have 3g fat • Medium fat meats have 5g fat • High fat meats have 8g fat Legumes are virtually fat free |

**FIGURE 4.6** Fat content of MyPyramid. (USDA, Center for Nutrition Policy and Promotion (2005). MyPyramid—Steps to Healthier You Food Guidance System. Available at www.MyPyramid.gov.)

each group. When higher-fat choices are made, the extra calories from the fat should be counted as part of a person's discretionary calories or oil allowance for the day. For instance, if a person chooses a Belgium waffle (made with added eggs and butter, providing 368 calories per waffle) instead of toast (considered fat free and about 80 calories per slice), the extra 288 calories in the waffle theoretically would be counted as discretionary calories. However, most discretionary calorie allowances are very small (between 150 and 300 discretionary calories per day, depending on total calorie needs), so the "budget" for higher-fat choices is limited.

Generally, three MyPyramid food groups provide little or no fat. Grains naturally contain very little fat, although some items within this group provide significant fat, such as granola cereals, crackers, biscuits, and waffles. Unadulterated vegetables contain little or no fat; vegetables that are fried, creamed, served with cheese, or mixed with mayonnaise provide significant fat. With the exception of avocado, coconut, and olives, fruits are naturally fat free. It is the other three groups—milk, meat and beans, and oils—that may provide significant fat.

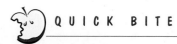 **Q U I C K   B I T E**

Added fats add up

|  | Fat (g) |  | Fat (g) |
|---|---|---|---|
| Boiled potato, ½ cup | trace | French fries, 10 | 8 |
| Mashed potatoes, ½ cup | 4.4 | Potato salad, ½ cup | 10.3 |
| Scalloped potatoes, ½ cup | 4.5 | Homemade hash browns, ½ cup | 10.8 |

**Q U I C K   B I T E**

| Grains with added fat | | The only fruits with natural fat | | |
|---|---|---|---|---|
| | g fat/serving | | Fat (g) | Saturated fat (g) |
| Apple cinnamon granola, 1 cup | 19 g | Avocado, 1 medium | 15 | 2.3 |
| Plain croissants, 1 | 17 g | Coconut, 2 tbsp shredded | 4.0 | 4.0 |
| Dry crispy chow mein noodles, 2 oz | 16 g | Coconut milk, 1 cup | 48.2 | 42.7 |
| Lemon poppy seed muffin, 1 | 13 g | Olives (green or ripe), 5 large | 3.0 | 0.5 |
| Cheese crackers, 1 oz | 7 g | | | |

## Milk

Because the fat content varies widely among Milk group selections, items within this group can be further classified into one of three subgroups: full-fat, reduced fat, and fat free. The fat in dairy products is predominately saturated and full-fat products have more cholesterol than in the lower-fat options.

Fat-free varieties of milk, yogurt, and cheese provide virtually no fat. The mid range is reserved for reduced-fat items—they have some of the fat and cholesterol removed yet retain some of the "mouthfeel" characteristic of whole milk. For this reason, reduced fat milk is suggested as a transition when switching from whole milk to fat-free milk.

## Meat and Beans

Similar to the Milk group, the amount of fat in items from the Meat and Beans group varies considerably. The American Diabetic Association's Exchange Lists for Meal Planning divides

**Q U I C K   B I T E**

Examples of meat and beans by fat content
*Very lean meats:* 0–1 g fat per ounce
 Skinless, white meat chicken and turkey
 Scallops, shrimp, and tuna canned in water
 Egg whites, egg substitutes
 Dried peas, beans, and lentils
*Lean meats:* 3 g fat per ounce
 Lean beef
 Salmon
 Lean pork

*Medium fat meats:* 5 g fat per ounce
 Ground beef
 Prime rib
 Fried fish
 Dark meat chicken
 Egg yolk
*High fat meats:* 8 g of fat per ounce
 Pork sausage
 Bologna
 Bacon
 Peanut butter

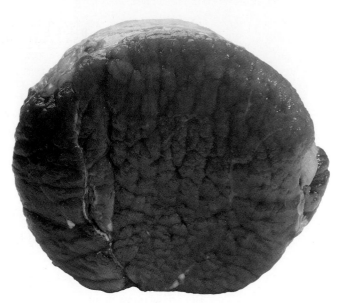

**FIGURE 4.7** A lean-only meat medallion trimmed of fat.

the Meat and Beans Group into four subgroups based on fat content. Details worth noting are as follows:

- The 1-ounce size cited in MyPyramid is simply a reference, not a serving size or a portion size. Typically, a *serving size* (the amount recommended for a meal) is 3 or 4 ounces and a *portion size* (the amount actually eaten at one time) may be much larger. For instance, fast-food triple cheeseburger contains approximately 9 ounces of meat.
- Fat added during cooking, such as frying or basting with fat, increases the overall fat content and counts as choices from the Oils group. It is recommended that meats be prepared by methods that do not add fat, such as baked, roasted, broiled, grilled, poached, or boiled.
- Untrimmed meats are higher in fat than lean-only portions (Fig. 4.7).
- "Red meats," namely beef, pork, and lamb, are higher in saturated fat than the "white meats" of poultry and seafood.
- White poultry meat is lower in fat than dark meat; removing poultry skin removes significant fat.
- Fat content varies among different cuts of meat. The leanest cuts are beef loin and round; veal and lamb from the loin or leg; and pork tenderloin or center loin chop.
- Beef grades can be used as a guide to fat content because grades are based largely on the amount of **marbling**. Beef graded "prime," sold mostly to restaurants, is the most heavily marbled grade and thus the fattiest. In retail stores, within any cut "choice" has more marbling and higher fat content than "select."
- Shellfish are very low in fat but have considerable cholesterol.
- Most wild game is very lean. The fat content in bison, venison, elk, ostrich, pheasant (without skin), rabbit, and squirrel ranges from 2 to 5 g per 3-ounce serving.
- Processed meats, such as sausage and hot dogs, may provide more fat calories than protein calories.
- Nuts have many healthy attributes; they contain plant protein, fiber, vitamin E, selenium, magnesium, zinc, phosphorus, potassium, in a low-saturated fat, cholesterol-free package. Their high fat content of 13 to 20 g/oz comes mostly from monounsaturated fats and polyunsaturated fats. Walnuts are a rich source of alpha-linolenic acid.

**Marbling:** fat deposited in the muscle of meat.

- Egg yolks have approximately 213 mg of cholesterol. The cholesterol content of typical cuts of beef, pork, lamb, and poultry is generally around 70 mg/3 oz. Veal averages slightly more at about 90 mg/3 oz. The exceptions are organ meats, which are very high in cholesterol. Egg whites, dried peas and beans, or nuts are cholesterol free.

## QUICK BITE

Oils and oil-rich food equivalents

| This much. . . | Is equivalent to this many teaspoons of oil. . . |
|---|---|
| 1 tbsp vegetable oil | 3 tsp |
| 1 tbsp soft margarine | 2½ tsp |
| 2 tbsp Italian dressing | 2 tsp |
| ½ medium avocado | 3 tsp |
| 2 tbsp peanut butter | 4 tsp |
| 1 oz nuts | 3–4 tsp |
| ½ oz sunflower seeds | 3 tsp |

## Oils

Oil allowances are small, usually 5 to 7 teaspoon/day for adults, depending on their total calorie needs. This group includes not only vegetable oils like canola, corn, and olive, but also oil-rich foods such as margarine and mayonnaise. Some other items on the oil list, such as avocado and nuts, are actually listed in other groups (fruit and meat and beans, respectively) but because the overwhelming majority of their calories comes from fat, their fat content is supposed to be counted as part of the oil allowance. For instance avocado is a fruit, yet 80% of its calories come from fat. Eating half of a medium avocado counts as a serving of fruit *and* as three teaspoons of oil, which is about half of a typical adult's daily oil allowance.

## ▶ DIETARY REFERENCE INTAKES

The issue of how much of each particular type of fat is needed, how much is optimal, and how much is too much is complex and in some cases controversial. Fats that the body can synthesize, namely saturated fatty acids, monounsaturated fatty acids, and cholesterol do not need to be consumed through food. Trans fats provide no known health benefits and so they are not essential. As such, neither an Adequate Intake (AI) nor Recommended Dietary Allowance (RDA) exists for any of these fats. The reference values that have been set are discussed later in the text.

### Total Fat

Neither an AI nor RDA is set for total fat due to insufficient data to define a level of total fat intake at which risk of deficiency or prevention of chronic disease occurs. An Acceptable Macronutrient Distribution Range (AMDR) is estimated to be 20% to 35% of total calories for adults (Fig. 4.8). Generally as total fat intake increases, the amount of saturated fat increases; therefore limiting total fat intake to 35% of total calories or less is prudent in order to limit saturated fat intake.

### Saturated and Trans Fat

The Additional Macronutrient Recommendation issued for both of these fats is that intake should be as low as possible within the context of a nutritionally adequate diet. Simply stated, neither of these fats need to be consumed in the diet, and both increase the risk of heart disease; therefore, their intake should be as low as possible without sacrificing nutritional adequacy. Because the risk of heart disease increases incrementally as saturated fat and trans fat intake increase, an upper limit (UL) could not be defined.

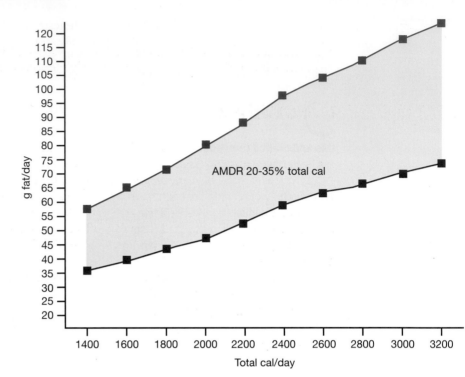

**FIGURE 4.8** Amount of total fat appropriate at various calorie levels based on AMDR of 20% to 35% of total calories.

| TABLE 4.1 | Dietary Reference Intakes for Essential Fatty Acids | | | |
|---|---|---|---|---|
| | **Acceptable Macronutrient Distribution Range** | | **Adequate Intake** | |
| | **Percent of Total Calories from Linoleic Acid (%)** | **Percent of Total Calories from Alpha-Linolenic Acid (%)** | **Linoleic Acid (g/day)** | **Alpha-Linolenic Acid (g/day)** |
| Adult men | 5–10 | 0.6–1.2 | 17 | 1.6 |
| Adult women | 5–10 | 0.6–1.2 | 12 | 1.1 |

## Essential Fatty Acids

Both an AMDR and AI have been set for the essential fatty acids linoleic acid and alpha-linolenic acid (Table 4.1). The AI values are based on the observed median intake in the United States, where fatty acid deficiencies do not exist in healthy people. AI should not be confused with RDA nor should they be assumed to be optimal levels of intake that confer the lowest risk of disease. There were insufficient data to set at UL for either of the essential fatty acids.

## Essential Fatty Acid Deficiency

Although the body cannot make essential fatty acids, it does store them, making deficiencies extremely rare in people eating a mixed diet. Those at risk for deficiency include infants and children consuming low-fat diets (their need for essential fatty acids is proportionately higher than that of adults), clients with anorexia nervosa, and people receiving lipid-free parenteral nutrition for long periods. People with fat malabsorption syndromes are also at risk. Symptoms of essential fatty acid deficiency include growth failure, reproductive failure, scaly dermatitis, and kidney and liver disorders.

## Cholesterol

Like saturated fat and trans fat, the Additional Macronutrient Recommendation issued for cholesterol is that intake be as low as possible while consuming a nutritionally adequate diet.

# ▶ FAT IN HEALTH PROMOTION

Over the last 30 years, fat has virtually been public health enemy number 1, blamed for causing heart disease, cancer, and obesity. For years, eating no more than 30% of total calories from fat was touted by various governmental and health agencies as the way to improve Americans' health. It now appears that the message to eat less fat was too simplistic because it ignored the different health effects produced by different types of fat. Multiple studies have shown that the type of fat in the diet can affect serum lipids more than the total amount of fat (Zarraga & Schwarz, 2006). Other study results about the role of fat in disease are summarized in Box 4.1.

Although the optimal amount of total fat is controversial, most leading health authorities recommend that Americans limit saturated fat and trans fat intake to less than 10% of total calories and cholesterol intake to 200 to 300 mg/day. The *2005 Dietary Guidelines for Americans* four key recommendations regarding fat intake appear in Box 4.2. Highlights are discussed in the following sections.

---

| BOX 4.1 | FAT AND DISEASE: WHAT'S THE CONNECTION? |
| --- | --- |

**Total Fat and Heart Disease**
Results from the large and long Women's Health Initiative Dietary Modification Trial (WHI DMT) showed that eating a low-fat diet for 8 years did not reduce the risk of coronary heart disease events or stroke (Howard, Van Horn, Hsia, et al., 2006) but critics argue that it is very difficult to actually achieve a low-fat intake and that study participants may not reduce fat intake enough to see positive results. Also, it may be that risk reduction takes longer to observe than the 8 year long WHI DMT.

**Type of Fat and Heart Disease**
Results from the Nurses' Health Study show that replacing only 30 calories (7 g) of carbohydrates every day with 30 calories (4 g) of trans fats nearly doubled the risk for heart disease (Willett et al., 1993). Saturated fat also increased the risk but not as much.

**Fat and Cancer**
The role of total fat in promoting cancer is controversial. Results from the WHI DMT showed that although a low–total fat diet did not prevent cancer, it did not rule out a potential modest benefit against breast cancer (Prentice et al., 2006). Evidence that certain types of fat promote cancer is suggestive, not conclusive and the impact of total fat is questionable.

**Fat and Weight**
Additional results from the WHI DMT show that women assigned to a low-fat diet did not lose, or gain, any more weight than women eating a "usual" diet (Howard, Manson, Stefanick, et al., 2006). In theory, cutting fat can cut calories and therefore promote weight loss; in practice low-fat diets are no more effective in promoting weight loss than are high-fat, low-carbohydrate diets. The key to managing weight is total calories, not the proportion of calories from carbohydrates, protein, or fat.

---

BOX 4.2 **2005 DIETARY GUIDELINES FOR AMERICANS: KEY RECOMMENDATIONS REGARDING FAT INTAKE**

- Consume less than 10% of calories from saturated fatty acids and less than 300 mg/day of cholesterol, and keep trans fatty acid consumption as low as possible.
- Keep total fat intake between 20% and 25% of calories, with most fats coming from sources of polyunsaturated and monounsaturated fatty acids, such as fish, nuts, and vegetable oils.
- When selecting and preparing meat, poultry, dry beans, and milk or milk products, make choices that are lean, low fat, or fat free.
- Limit intake of fats and oils high in saturated and/or trans fatty acids, and choose products low in such fats and oils.

## Eat Less Saturated Fat and Keep Trans Fat Consumption as Low as Possible

The recommendation to eat less saturated fat and trans fat is virtually universal among leading health agencies and generally the guideline is that combined saturated fat and trans fats contribute 10% or less of total calories. This translates to approximately 22 g/day in a 2000-calorie diet; about 27 g in a 2400-calorie diet.

To cut saturated fat intake, experts recommend limiting meat intake, especially red meat, and choosing lean varieties. Milk and dairy products should be reduced or nonfat. Hydrogenated fats and foods containing them should be avoided. Strategies for lowering total fat and "bad" fat as well as increasing "good" fat appear in Box 4.3.

## Limit Total Fat and Go for Unsaturated Fats

Americans, on average, currently consume approximately 34% of their total calories from fat, near the upper end of the AMDR. The most effective way to limit total and saturated fat and increase unsaturated fats may be with a plant-based diet rich in fruits and vegetables, whole grains, legumes, and nuts, with careful attention to the types and amounts of fat eaten in meats, fish, dairy products, oils, processed foods, and snacks.

---

BOX 4.3 **STRATEGIES FOR REDUCING AND MODIFYING FAT INTAKE**

**Eat Less Meat**

- Eat occasional meatless meals like bean burritos, meatless chilli, vegetable soup with salad, spaghetti with plain sauce.
- Limit meat to 5 oz/day, a recommended portion is size of a deck of cards or smaller.

**Eat Lean Meats**

- Eat meat, fish, and poultry that are baked, broiled, or roasted instead of fried.
- Remove the skin from chicken before eating.
- Choose "select" grades of beef, which have less marbling than "choice" grades.
- Trim all visible fat from meat.
- Choose ground beef that is at least 90% lean as indicated on the label.
- Choose beef cuts labeled "loin" or "round."
- Limit egg yolks to two per week.

BOX 4.3  **STRATEGIES FOR REDUCING AND MODIFYING FAT INTAKE** (continued)

### Substitute Low-Fat or Nonfat for Regular Varieties

- Use 1% or nonfat milk.
- Use low-fat or nonfat yogurt.
- Choose cheese with 3 g or less per serving.
- Try sherbet, reduced fat ice cream, nonfat ice cream, and yogurt.
- Try low-fat or nonfat salad dressing.
- Use nonstick spray in place of oil, margarine, or butter to sauté foods and "butter" pans.
- Use imitation butter spray to season vegetables and hot air popcorn.

### Limit Fat as a Flavoring

- Eat bread, rolls, muffins, or crackers without butter or margarine.
- Season with spice such as picante sauce, salsa, ginger, flavored vinegar, Italian spice blends.
- Eat potatoes and vegetables that are not fried.
- Instead of pouring dressing on salad, have it on the side; dip your fork into the dressing before spearing salad.
- Have desserts without cream or whipped cream toppings.

### Reduce Hydrogenated Fat Intake

- Use the soft margarine (liquid or tub) in place of butter or stick margarine. Look for margarine that is "trans fat–free," contains no more than 2 g saturated fat/tablespoon, and has liquid vegetable oil as the first ingredient.
- Look for processed foods made with unhydrogenated oil rather than hydrogenated or saturated fat.
- Avoid French fries, doughnuts, cookies, and crackers unless they are labeled fat free.
- Avoid fried fast foods that are made with hydrogenated shortenings and oils.

### Replace Fatty Foods With Fruit and Vegetables

- Eat fruit for dessert.
- Snack on raw vegetables or fresh fruit instead of snack chips.
- Double up on your usual portion of vegetables.

### Use "Good" Fats in Moderation

- Make canola or olive oil your oil of choice.
- Eat fatty fish twice a week.
- Eat nuts and nut butters that are rich in monounsaturated fats: walnuts, almonds, hazelnuts, pecans, pistachios, and pine nuts. Walnuts also contain alpha-linolenic acid. Cashews and macadamia nuts are higher in saturated fats.
- Sprinkle flaxseed (1–2 tablespoons/day) over cereal or yogurt or use as a fat substitute in many recipes: 3 tablespoons of ground flaxseed can replace 1 tablespoon fat or oil.

## Limit Cholesterol

Cholesterol intake becomes less important when saturated fat intake is low. Still because total and LDL cholesterol are positively related to the intake of saturated fat, trans fat, and cholesterol, the intake of these three lipids should be as low as possible within the context of a nutritionally AI (IOM, 2006). Eating less red meat, full-fat dairy products, and egg yolks significantly decreases cholesterol intake.

## What about "Fish Oils"?

Although the *Dietary Guidelines* do not include a recommendation about eating fatty fish, the American Heart Association suggests healthy people to eat at least two servings of fish per week, preferably fatty fish (American Heart Association, 2006). This recommendation is based on the assumption that 12 ounces of fatty fish per week averages out to approximately 500 mg/day of EPA and DHA, the amount recommended to reduce the risk of heart disease. The American Diabetes makes the same recommendation for the secondary prevention of diabetes (American Diabetes Association, 2007).

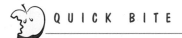

### QUICK BITE

The content of fish oils in selected foods

| Item (6 oz portion unless otherwise indicated) | Amount of DHA + EPA (mg) |
| --- | --- |
| Atlantic salmon, farmed | 3650 |
| Atlantic salmon, wild | 3130 |
| Rainbow trout, farmed | 1960 |
| Swordfish | 1390 |
| Flounder | 850 |
| Sole | 850 |
| Scallops | 620 |
| Yellow fish tuna, fresh | 560 |
| Catfish, wild | 400 |
| Lobster (3 oz) | 70 |
| Egg (1 large) | 20 |

*Source:* Liebman (2007). Omega medicine? Is fish oil good for what ails you? *Nutrition Action Health Letter, 34*(8), 1, 3–6.

For people who do not eat seafood, fish oil pills are an alternative source of omega-3 fats (Gebauer et al., 2006) but they have drawbacks (Box 4.4). A wide variety of products with added "omega-3s" or "DHA" are available, such as mayonnaise, margarine, eggs, cereal, milk, yogurt, and even puppy dog food. But beware: many products have alpha-linolenic acid added as the source of omega-3. While it is true that alpha-linolenic acid is an omega-3 fatty acid, it has not been shown to be protective against heart disease or any of the other

---

| BOX 4.4 | **POTENTIAL DRAWBACKS OF FISH OIL SUPPLEMENTS** |

- They prolong bleeding time. People taking anticoagulants and those with clotting abnormalities should be monitored while using fish oil supplements.
- Doses more than 3 g/day may suppress immune system function and may increase the risk of hemorrhagic stroke.
- Although most fish oil supplements do not contain vitamin A, those from shark and halibut liver oils contain high levels and they should not be used by pregnant women.
- Fish oils are susceptible to rancidity and should be stored in the refrigerator.

*Source:* Fragakis, A. and Thomson, C. (2007). The health professional's guide to popular dietary supplements (3rd ed.). Chicago, IL: The American Dietetic Association.

health problems that fish oils may benefit. Another downside is that some labels do not state how much omega-3s are contained in the product, which may be minimal. For instance, a 6-ounce container of yogurt "with DHA Omega-3" on the label has only 32 mg of DHA, the equivalent to the amount in ¾ teaspoon of salmon (Liebman, 2007).

## ▶ HOW DO YOU RESPOND?

**Is it true that not all saturated fatty acids raise cholesterol?** Strictly speaking, that is true. Specifically, stearic acid has a neutral effect on total, LDL, and HDL cholesterol (International Food Information Council, 2006). Animal fats are high in stearic acid—but they are also high in palmitic acid, which is atherogenic. Because fats in food contain mixtures of saturated fats, it is not practical to choose foods based on individual saturated fatty acid content. Therefore, the generalization to eat less saturated fat is appropriate, even though stearic acid has a neutral effect on cholesterol.

**What is flaxseed?** Flaxseed is derived from the flax plant, the same plant used to make linen. It is a nutritional powerhouse, providing essential fatty acids, fiber, and lignans. Specifically, 57% of its fat is from alpha-linolenic acid, the precursor of the omega-3 fats DHA and EPA. The fiber in flaxseed is predominately soluble, which helps to lower cholesterol levels and improves glucose levels in diabetics. Flaxseed contains 100 to 800 times more lignans than other grains; lignans, a group of plant estrogens, may help to reduce the risk of breast and prostate cancers. While flaxseed oil and flaxseed oil pills provide the benefits of alpha-linolenic acid, they lack the fiber found in the whole grain and the lignan content is variable. However, humans are unable to digest the tough outer coating so flaxseeds must be eaten ground, not whole. Because they are high in polyunsaturated fat, they are prone to rancidity. Ground flaxseed should be refrigerated and used within a few weeks.

**What is the best type of oil to buy?** Soy oil is often the oil of choice in restaurants and in many prepared grocery store items such as mayonnaise, salad dressings, spaghetti sauce, and cookies. In fact, soy oils account for more than 80% of all oil used in the United States, about half of which gets partially hydrogenated to make margarine or shortening. To balance that high intake of n-6 polyunsaturated fat, the best choice of oil to use at home may be canola because of its high content of monounsaturated fat and its n-3 fatty acid alpha-linolenic acid. However, consider flavor when appropriate. For instance, olive oil may be preferred for homemade salad dressing while canola oil is reliable for routine sautéing and baking.

**Why is the serving size of peanut butter on the meat list 2 tablespoons and on the oils list the size is 1 tablespoon?** Most people are probably unaware of the intricacies of the MyPyramid lists, particularly the double listing of some items and how they are to be "counted," especially when the serving sizes differ between lists. The reason for the discrepancies in the serving size lies with the nutrient of interest. On the meat list, 1-ounce equivalents are set based on protein content; each 1-ounce equivalent provides approximately 7 g of protein. Two tablespoons of peanut butter provide 7 g of protein. In contrast, oil allowances are listed in teaspoons of oil, which provide 5 g of fat. That same 2 tablespoons of peanut butter contains 16 g of fat—slightly more than the equivalent of 3 teaspoons of fat. The fat in 1 tablespoon of peanut butter is 8 g—closer but still more than the "standard" of 5 g of fat/equivalent. This point illustrates the imprecision of equivalents and estimating actual intake. Add to that the reality that people only estimate how much they actually eat, and the reliability of calculating a person's actual intake is questionable.

**Is it a good idea to substitute foods made with fat replacers for full-fat foods?** Although some foods can be made low fat by simply reducing the fat content (e.g., milk), others use fat replacers to simulate the functional properties of fat while reducing total fat, saturated fat, and calories. They are derived from carbohydrates, protein, or fat and thus their calorie content varies. Considering all the functional properties of fat in food, it is easy to understand that not all fat replacers are appropriate for all types of food. For instance, prune puree can substitute as fat in brownies by imparting moistness and some tenderness, but it cannot be used as a substitute for oil in frying French fries.

## QUICK BITE

Examples of fat replacers
*Home use:*
Lighter bake, made from prune puree, is used as a fat substitute in baking
*Commercial uses:*
Simplesse, made from the whey of milk or eggs, can only be used in uncooked products such as ice cream and cheese food

Olestra (brand name Olean) is not digested or absorbed so it is calorie free; found in salty snack foods and crackers

According to the American Dietetic Association (2005), "Fat replacers may offer a safe, feasible, and effective means to maintain the palatability of diets with controlled amounts of fat and/or energy." Whether they actually help Americans to eat less fat and fewer calories depends on whether they are used in addition to foods normally eaten or take the place of regular fat foods that would otherwise be eaten. Furthermore, diets low in fat are not guaranteed to be low in calories. For instance, even if the fat content of coffee cake is reduced, there are still considerable calories provided by starch and sugar. People who choose to use fat replacers should do so with the understanding that they are only one component of a total diet and as such they alone cannot transform an "unhealthy" diet into a healthy one.

**Aren't fatty fish contaminated and therefore not healthy?** The U.S. Food and Drug Administration and the Environmental Protection Agency advise pregnant women, women who could become pregnant, and young children not to eat shark, swordfish, king mackerel, or tilefish because of their mercury levels. They recommend that the intake of other fish and shellfish that are lower in mercury, such as shrimp, canned light tuna, salmon, pollack, and catfish, be limited to 12 oz/week and that the intake of albacore tuna be limited to 6 oz/week (USDHHS, EPA, 2004). Likewise, state and local advisories should be adhered to for locally caught fish. By adhering to the advisories, consumers should be able to reap the benefits of eating fish without increasing their exposure to environmental contaminants.

▶ CASE STUDY

Michael is a 40-year-old man who lost about 25 pounds 10 years ago by reducing his fat intake. He has slowly regained the weight and now wants to go back to a low-fat diet to manage his weight. He gives you a sample of his usual intake:

| | |
|---|---|
| **Breakfast:** | 3 cups of coffee with sugar and nondairy creamer |
| **On the way to work:** | A bagel with low-fat cream cheese and jelly |
| **Snack before lunch:** | Low-fat coffee cake; more coffee with sugar and nondairy creamer |
| **Lunch:** | Usually a burger, large order of French fries, and a diet soda from the fast-food restaurant near his office |
| **Snack before dinner:** | A glass of wine with cheese and crackers |
| **Dinner:** | Meat, potato, and vegetable; often double portions of meat
A salad with Italian dressing
Bread and butter
Sherbet for dessert |
| **Snack:** | A bowl of cornflakes with 2% milk and sugar |

- What foods and beverages did Michael eat that contain fat? What sources of saturated fat did he eat? What sources of unsaturated fat? What sources of omega-3 fats? What sources of cholesterol did he eat? What specific suggestions would you make for him to eat less fat and/or improve the type of fat he eats?
- What would you tell Michael about cutting fat intake to lose weight? What would you suggest he do to "eat healthier"?

STUDY QUESTIONS

1. The client asks if the cholesterol in shrimp is the "good" or "bad" type. Which of the following would be the nurse's best response?
   a. "All cholesterol is bad cholesterol."
   b. "Bad and good refer to how cholesterol is packaged for transport through the blood. The cholesterol in food is unpackaged and neither bad nor good."
   c. "Good cholesterol is found in plants; bad cholesterol is found in animal sources."
   d. "Shrimp has good cholesterol because it is low in saturated fat; foods high in cholesterol and saturated fat are a bad source of cholesterol."

2. When developing a teaching plan for a client who needs to limit saturated fat, which of the following foods would the nurse suggest the client limit?
   a. Seafood, and poultry.
   b. Full-fat dairy products and fried foods.
   c. Olive oil and canola oil.
   d. Red meat and full-fat dairy products.

3. What is the primary function of fat?
   a. To improve the flavor and taste of food.
   b. To provide energy.

c. To promote the absorption of fat-soluble vitamins.

      d. To facilitate carbohydrate metabolism.

**4.** The nurse knows her instructions have been effective when the client verbalizes the sources of trans fats are
    **a.** Red meat and full-fat dairy products.
    **b.** Commerical baked goods and stick margarine.
    **c.** Pretzels and nuts.
    **d.** Butter and lard.

**5.** A client asks why lowering saturated fat intake is necessary for lowering serum cholesterol levels. Which of the following is the nurse's best response?
    **a.** "Saturated fats raise the 'bad' cholesterol levels more than any other fat in the diet."
    **b.** "Sources of saturated fat also provide cholesterol and both should be limited to control blood cholesterol levels."
    **c.** "Saturated fat is high in calories and excess calories from any source increase the risk of high blood cholesterol levels."
    **d.** "Saturated fats make blood more likely to clot, increasing the risk of heart attack."

**6.** When teaching a client about "heart-healthy" types of fat, which of the following oils should the nurse recommend the client use?
    **a.** Vegetable and corn.
    **b.** Soybean and cottonseed.
    **c.** Olive and canola.
    **d.** Soybean and olive.

**7.** Which statement indicates the client understands about choosing low-fat foods from MyPyramid?
    **a.** "All items within a food group have approximately the same amount of fat."
    **b.** "You don't have to consciously select low-fat items because the discretionary calorie allowance will account for higher-fat choices."
    **c.** "It is best to eliminate as much fat from the diet as possible."
    **d.** "Within each food group, the foods lowest in fat should be chosen most often."

**8.** Which of the following are the best sources of omega-3 fatty acids?
    **a.** Salmon and trout.
    **b.** Flaxseed and walnuts.
    **c.** Olive and canola oils.
    **d.** Cod fish and haddock.

## KEY CONCEPTS

- Ninety-eight percent of lipids consumed in the diet are triglycerides, which are composed of one glyceride molecule and three fatty acids. Phospholipids and sterols are the other two types of dietary lipids.

- Saturation refers to the hydrogen atoms attached to the carbon atoms in the fatty acid chain. Saturated fatty acids do not have any double bonds between carbon atoms; each carbon is "saturated" with as much hydrogen as it can hold. Unsaturated fats have one (monounsaturated) or more than one (polyunsaturated) double bond between carbon atoms. When used to describe food fats, these terms are relative descriptions of the type of fatty acid present in the largest amount. All fats in foods contain a mixture of saturated, monounsaturated, and polyunsaturated fats.

- Generally, saturated fats are "bad" because they raise total and LDL cholesterol. Unsaturated fats are "good" because they lower total and LDL cholesterol when consumed in place of saturated fats.

● Trans fatty acids are produced through the process of hydrogenation. They are chemically unsaturated fats; however like saturated fat they raise total and LDL cholesterol. What is worse, they also lower HDL cholesterol, increase serum triglyceride levels, increase insulin resistance, and increase biomarkers of inflammation.

● Linoleic acid (*n*-6) and alpha-linolenic acid (*n*-3) are essential fatty acids because they cannot be made by the body. They are important constituents of cell membranes, are involved in eicosanoid synthesis, and they function to maintain healthy skin and promote normal growth. Deficiencies of essential fatty acids are nonexistent in healthy people.

● The major function of fat is to provide energy; 1 g of fat supplies 9 calories of energy. Fat also provides insulation, protects internal organs from mechanical damage, and promotes absorption of the fat-soluble vitamins.

● Fish oils lower the risk of heart disease by lowering serum lipids and triglycerides and by helping to regulate blood pressure. Although they may also be beneficial in preventing other health problems, the evidence is currently inconclusive or lacking.

● The best sources of *n*-3 fatty acids are fatty cold-water fish such as salmon, trout, herring, swordfish, sardines, and mackerel. Walnuts, soybeans, flaxseed, and canola oil are plant sources of the omega-3 fatty acid alpha-linolenic acid, but alpha-linolenic acid may not have the same cardio protective benefits as fish oils.

● Phospholipids are structural components of cell membranes that facilitate the transport of fat-soluble substances across cell membranes. They are widespread but appear in small amounts in the diet.

● Cholesterol, a sterol, is a constituent of all cell membranes and is used to make bile acids, steroid hormones, and vitamin D. Cholesterol is found in all foods of animal origin except egg whites. Most Americans eat about half as much cholesterol as the body makes each day.

● Fat digestion occurs mostly in the small intestine. Short- and medium-chain fatty acids and glycerol are absorbed through mucosal cells into capillaries leading to the portal vein. Larger fat molecules—namely cholesterol, phospholipids, and reformed triglycerides made from monoglycerides and long-chain fatty acids—are absorbed in chylomicrons and transported through the lymph system.

● Grains, fruits, and vegetables are generally low in fat, although certain preparation methods can add significant fat. Milk, meat and beans, and the oil food groups provide fat, with the type and quantity of fat varying considerably among items within each group.

● The AMDR for total fat is set at 20% to 35% of total calories. The intake of saturated fat, trans fat, and cholesterol should be as low as possible within the context of a nutritionally adequate diet. Most leading health authorities recommend that Americans limit saturated fat and trans fat intake to less than 10% of total calories and cholesterol intake to 200 to 300 mg/day.

● To achieve a more optimal fat intake, a plant-based diet rich in fruit, vegetables, whole grains is recommended with adequate amounts of fat-free dairy products and lean meats. Fats (e.g., margarine, salad dressings) should be trans fat–free and preferably made with canola oil. Two servings of fatty fish per week are suggested.

## ANSWER KEY

1. **TRUE** All fats, whether saturated or unsaturated, provide 9 cal/g compared to 4 cal/g from carbohydrates and protein.

2. **FALSE** "Good" fats, namely polyunsaturated and monounsaturated fats, may help to lower LDL cholesterol when used in place of saturated fat. Omega-3 fish oils are also "good": they lower triglyceride levels, decrease platelet aggregation, and may decrease inflammation in rheumatoid arthritis, Crohn's disease, and ulcerative colitis.

3. **TRUE** Endogenous cholesterol synthesis is generally two to three times higher than the average cholesterol intake in the United States.

4. **FALSE** The 30% guideline refers to the total diet, not individual foods. Over the course of the day, high-fat items (e.g., canola oil, peanut butter) are balanced by low-fat and fat-free items (nonfat milk, grains, vegetables, and fruit).

5. **FALSE** Even though some margarines contain more trans fats than butter, the combined amount of "bad" fat (saturated fat plus trans fat) is higher in butter than in margarine, even stick margarine. In addition, butter contains cholesterol; margarine generally does not.

6. **TRUE** All sources of fat are a blend of saturated, polyunsaturated, and monounsaturated fatty acids. The description of a fat as "saturated" means that there are more saturated fatty acids than polyunsaturated or monounsaturated fatty acids in that source, not that saturated fatty acids are the only fatty acids present.

7. **FALSE** Saturated fatty acids are found in varying proportions in all sources of fat. A fat labeled as "saturated" has saturated fatty acids providing the biggest percentage of fat in that item. Animal products (meat and full-fat dairy items) and coconut, palm kernel, and palm oils are considered saturated fats.

8. **FALSE** Vegetable oils are still vegetable oils, even when they are lightly or partially hydrogenated; therefore, the term "vegetable oil" is not synonymous with trans fat–free.

9. **FALSE** Fish oils are not essential in the diet because the body can convert alpha-linolenic acid to EPA and DHA, although only in limited quantities. Vegetarians do not appear to suffer adverse effects from eliminating fish from their diets.

10. **FALSE** Eating less saturated fat has a greater impact on lowering serum cholesterol than does simply limiting cholesterol intake.

## WEBSITES

American Heart Association at **www.americanheart.org**
American Oil Chemist's Society at **www.aocs.org**
Calorie Control Council's glossary of fat replacers at **www.caloriecontrol.org/frgloss.html**
Institute of Shortening and Edible Oils at **www.iseo.org**
International Food Information Council at **www.ific.org**
National Heart, Lung and Blood Institute at **www.nhlbi.nih.gov**

## REFERENCES

American Diabetes Association. (2007). Nutrition recommendations and interventions for diabetes. A position statement of the American Diabetes Association. *Diabetes Care, 30*(Suppl. 1), S48–S65.

American Dietetic Association. (2005). Position of the American Dietetic Association: Fat replacers. *Journal of the American Dietetic Association, 105*, 266–275.

American Dietetic Association. (2007). Position of the American Dietetic Association and Dietitians of Canada: Dietary fatty acids. *Journal of the American Dietetic Association, 107*, 1599–1611.

American Heart Association. (2006). *Our 2006 diet and lifestyle recommendations*. Available at www.americanheart.org/print_presenter.jhtml?identifier=851. Accessed on 10/19/07.

Balk, E. M., Horsley, T. A., Newberry, S. J., et al. (2007). A collaborative effort to apply the evidence-based review process to the field of nutrition: Challenges, benefits, and lessons learned. *American Journal of Clinical Nutrition, 85*, 1448–1456.

Gebauer, S. K., Psota, T. L., Harris, W. S., et al. (2006). n-3 fatty acid dietary recommendations and food sources to achieve essentiality and cardiovascular benefits. *American Journal of Clinical Nutrition, 83*(6 Suppl ), 1526S–1535S.

Harvard School of Public Health. (2007). Fats and cholesterol. Available at http://www.hsph.harvard.edu/nutritionsource/fats.html. Accessed on 04/26/07.

Howard, B. V., Manson, J. E., Stefanick, M. L., et al. (2006). Low-fat dietary pattern and weight change over 7 years: The Women's Health Initiative Dietary Modification Trial. *Journal of the American Medical Association, 295*, 39–49.

Howard, B. V., Van Horn, L., Hsia, J., et al. (2006). Low-fat dietary pattern and risk of cardiovascular disease: The Women's Health Initiative Randomized Controlled Dietary Modification Trial. *Journal of the American Medical Association, 295*, 655–666.

Institute of Medicine of the National Academies (IOM). (2005). *Dietary Reference Intakes for energy, carbohydrates, fiber, fat, fatty acids, cholesterol, protein, and amino acids (macronutrients).* Washington, DC: National Academies Press.

International Food Information Council. (2005). Translating the Facts about trans fat. Available at www.ific.org/foodinsight/2005/ma/transfatfi205.cfm. Accessed on 8/20/07.

International Food Information Council. (2006). Dietary fats and fat replacers. Available at www.ific.org/nutrition/fats/index.cfm. Accessed on 8/20/07.

Leitzmann, M. F., Stampfer, M. J., Michaud, D. S., et al. (2004). Dietary intake of *n*-3 and *n*-6 fatty acids and the risk of prostate cancer. *American Journal of Clinical Nutrition, 80*, 204–216.

Liebman, B. (2007). Omega medicine? Is fish oil good for what ails you? *Nutrition Action Health Letter, 34*(8), 1, 3–6.

Nicholls, S. J., Lundman, P., Harmer, J. A., et al. (2006). Consumption of saturated fat impairs the anti-inflammatory properties of high-density lipoproteins and endothelial function. *Journal of the American College of Cardiology, 48*(4), 715–720.

Prentice, R. L., Caan, B., Chlebowski, R. T., et al. (2006). Low-fat dietary pattern and risk of invasive breast cancer: The Women's Health Initiative Randomized Controlled Dietary Modification Trial. *Journal of the American Medical Association, 295*, 629–642.

Tarrago-Trani, M. T., Phillips, K. M., Lemar, L. E., et al. (2006). New and existing oils and fats used in products with reduced trans-fatty acid content. *Journal of the American Dietetic Association, 106*, 867–880.

USDHHS, EPA. (2004). What you need to know about Mercury in fish and shellfish. Available at www.cfsan.fda.gov/~dms/admehg3b.html. Accessed on 10/17/07.

Willett, W. C., Stampfer, M. J., Manson, J. E., et al. (1993). Intake of trans fatty acids and risk of coronary heart disease among women. *Lancet, 341*, 581–585.

Zarraga, I., & Schwarz, E. (2006). Impact of dietary patterns and interventions on cardiovascular health. *Circulation, 114*, 961–973.

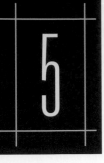

# 5 Vitamins

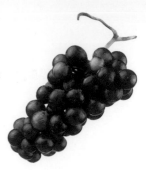

### UPON COMPLETION OF THIS CHAPTER, YOU WILL BE ABLE TO

- Compare and contrast fat- and water-soluble vitamins.
- Describe general functions and uses of vitamins.
- Judge when vitamin supplements may be necessary.
- Evaluate a vitamin supplement label.
- Give examples of food sources for individual vitamins.
- Identify characteristics to look for when choosing a vitamin supplement.

In 1913 thiamin was discovered as the first vitamin, the "vital amine" necessary to prevent the deficiency disease beriberi. Today, 13 vitamins have been identified as important for human nutrition; vitamin deficiency diseases are rare in the United States, and vitamin research focuses on whether consuming various vitamins above the minimum basic requirement can reduce the risk of heart disease, cancer, cataracts, cognitive decline in the elderly, and other chronic diseases.

This chapter describes vitamins and their uses. Generalizations about fat- and water-soluble vitamins are presented. Unique features of each vitamin are covered individually, and criteria for selecting a vitamin supplement are discussed.

# ▶ UNDERSTANDING VITAMINS

Vitamins are organic compounds made of carbon, hydrogen, oxygen, and sometimes nitrogen or other elements. They differ in their chemistry, biochemistry, function, and availability in foods. Vitamins facilitate biochemical reactions within cells to help regulate body processes such as growth and metabolism. They are essential to life. Unlike the organic compounds covered previously in this unit (carbohydrates, protein, and fat), vitamins

- Are individual molecules, not long chains of molecules linked together.
- Do not provide energy but are needed for the metabolism of energy.
- Are needed in microgram or milligram quantities, not gram quantities. Because they are needed in such small amounts, they are referred to as micronutrients (Fig. 5.1).

## Vitamins Are Chemically Defined

Vitamins are extremely complex chemical substances that differ widely in their structures. Because vitamins are defined chemically, the body cannot distinguish between natural vitamins extracted from food and synthetic vitamins produced in a laboratory. However, the absorption rates of natural and synthetic vitamins sometimes differ because of different chemical forms of the same vitamin (e.g., synthetic folic acid is better absorbed than natural folate in foods) or because the synthetic vitamins are "free," not "bound" to other components in food (e.g., synthetic vitamin $B_{12}$ is not bound to small peptides as natural vitamin $B_{12}$ is).

## Vitamins Are Susceptible to Destruction

**Oxidation:** a chemical reaction in which a substance combines with oxygen; the loss of electrons in an atom.

As organic substances, vitamins in food are susceptible to destruction and subsequent loss of function. Individual vitamins differ in their vulnerability to heat, light, **oxidation**, acid, and alkalis. For instance, thiamin is heat sensitive and is easily destroyed by high temperatures and long cooking times. Riboflavin is resistant to heat, acid, and oxidation but is quickly destroyed by light. That is why riboflavin-rich milk is sold in opaque, not transparent, containers. Baking soda (an alkali) added during cooking, a practice followed by some cooks to

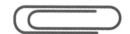

1 large paperclip weighs approximately 1 *gram*
**RDA** for protein for adult female who weighs 127 pounds is 46 g

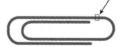

If you divide 1 large paperclip into 1000 equal portions, each piece weighs 1 *milligram*
**RDA** for thiamin for adult female is 1.1 mg

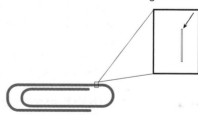

**FIGURE 5.1** Representative sizes of 1 g, 1 mg, and 1 mcg.

If you divide a 1 mg piece into 1000 equal portions, each piece weighs 1 *microgram*
**RDA** for vitamin $B_{12}$ for adult female is 2.4 μg

retain the color of beets and red cabbage, destroys thiamin. Fifty percent to 90% of folate in foods may be lost during preparation, processing, and storage. Vitamin C is destroyed by heat, air, and alkalis.

## Vitamins May Exist in More Than One Form

**Provitamins:** precursors of vitamins.

Many vitamins exist in more than one active form. Different forms perform different functions in the body. For instance, vitamin A exists as retinol (important for reproduction), retinal (needed for vision), and retinoic acid (acts as a hormone to regulate growth). Some vitamins have **provitamins**, an inactive form found in food that the body converts to the active form. Beta-carotene is a provitamin of vitamin A. Dietary Reference Intakes take into account the biologic activity of vitamins as they exist in different forms.

## Vitamins Are Essential

Vitamins are essential in the diet because, with a few exceptions, the body cannot make them. The body can make vitamin A, vitamin D, and niacin if the appropriate precursors are available. Microorganisms in the gastrointestinal (GI) tract synthesize vitamin K and vitamin B$_{12}$ but not in amounts sufficient to meet the body's needs.

## Some Vitamins Are Coenzymes

**Enzymes:** proteins produced by cells that catalyze chemical reactions within the body without undergoing change themselves.

**Coenzymes:** organic molecules that activate an enzyme.

Many **enzymes** cannot function without a **coenzyme**, and many coenzymes are vitamins. All B vitamins work as coenzymes to facilitate thousands of chemical conversions. For instance, thiamin, riboflavin, niacin, and biotin participate in enzymatic reactions that extract energy from glucose, amino acids, and fat. Folacin facilitates both amino acid metabolism and nucleic acid synthesis; without adequate folacin, protein synthesis and cell division are impaired. An adequate and continuous supply of B vitamins in every cell is vital for normal metabolism.

### QUICK BITE

Top 12 foods with the highest antioxidant contents per serving
Blackberries
Walnuts
Strawberries
Artichokes, prepared
Cranberries
Coffee
Raspberries
Pecans
Blueberries
Cloves, ground
Grape juice
Chocolate, baking, unsweetened

*Source:* Halvorsen, B. L., Carlsen, M. H., Phillips, K. M., Bøhn, S. K., Holte, K., Jacobs, D. R., Jr., et al. (2006). Content of redox-active compounds (eg, antioxidants) in foods consumed in the United States. *The American Journal of Clinical Nutrition, 84*, 95–135.

## Some Vitamins Are Antioxidants

**Free Radicals:** highly unstable, highly reactive molecular fragments with one or more unpaired electrons.

**Antioxidants:** substances that donate electrons to free radicals to prevent oxidation.

**Free radicals** are produced continuously in cells as they burn oxygen during normal metabolism. Ultraviolet radiation, air pollution, ozone, the metabolism of food, and smoking can also generate free radicals in the body. The problem with free radicals is that they oxidize body cells and DNA in their quest to gain an electron and become stable. These structurally and functionally damaged cells are believed to contribute to aging and various health problems such as cancer, heart disease, and cataracts. Polyunsaturated fatty acids (PUFAs) in cell membranes are particularly vulnerable to damage by free radicals.

**Antioxidants** protect body cells from being oxidized (destroyed) by free radicals by undergoing oxidation themselves, which renders free radicals harmless. Fruits, vegetables, and other plant-based food provide dozens, if not hundreds, of antioxidants. The major antioxidants are vitamin C, vitamin E, and beta-carotene. Each has a slightly different role, so one cannot completely substitute for another. For instance, water-soluble vitamin C works within cells to disable free radicals and fat-soluble vitamin E functions within fat tissue. Whether high doses of individual antioxidants offer the same health benefits as the package of substances found in food sources is an area of ongoing research.

## Some Vitamins Are Used As Food Additives

**Enrich:** to add nutrients back that were lost during processing, for example, white flour is enriched with B vitamins lost when the bran and germ layers are removed.

**Food Additive:** a substance added intentionally or unintentionally to food that affects its character.

Some foods have vitamins added to them simply to boost their nutritional content; examples include vitamin C–enriched fruit drinks, vitamin A and D fortified milk, and enriched flour and breads. Other foods have certain vitamins added to them to help preserve quality. For instance, vitamin C is added to frozen fish to help prevent rancidity and to luncheon meats to stabilize the red color. Vitamin E helps retard rancidity in vegetable oils, and beta-carotene adds color to margarine.

## Vitamins As Drugs

**Megadoses:** amounts at least 10 times greater than the RDA.

In **megadoses** vitamins function like drugs, not nutrients. Large doses of niacin are used to lower cholesterol, low-density lipoprotein (LDL) cholesterol, and triglycerides in people with hyperlipidemia who do not respond to diet and exercise. Tretinoin (retinoic acid, a form of vitamin A) is used as a topical treatment for acne vulgaris and orally for acute promyelocytic leukemia. Gram quantities of vitamin C promote healing in patients with impaired bone and wound healing.

## ▶ VITAMIN CLASSIFICATIONS BASED ON SOLUBILITY

Vitamins are classified according to their solubility. Vitamins A, D, E, and K are fat soluble. Vitamin C and the B vitamins (thiamin, riboflavin, niacin, folate, $B_6$, $B_{12}$, biotin, and pantothenic acid) are water soluble. Solubility determines vitamin absorption, transportation, storage, and excretion.

## Fat-Soluble Vitamins

Group characteristics of fat-soluble vitamins are summarized in Table 5.1. Table 5.2 highlights recommended intakes, sources, functions, deficiency symptoms, and toxicity symptoms of each fat-soluble vitamin. The complete table of Dietary Reference Intakes for vitamins appears in Appendix 2. Additional features of individual fat-soluble vitamins follow.

### Vitamin A

**Preformed Vitamin A:** the active form of vitamin A.

**Carotenoids:** a group name of retinol precursors found in plants.

In its preformed state, vitamin A exists as an alcohol (retinol), aldehyde (retinaldehyde), or acid (retinoic acid). **Preformed vitamin A** is found only in animal sources such as liver, whole milk, and fish. Low-fat milk, skim milk, margarine, and ready-to-eat cereals are fortified with vitamin A.

The term vitamin A also includes provitamin A **carotenoids**, natural plant pigments found in deep yellow and orange fruits and vegetables, and most dark green leafy vegetables. Although there are over 600 different carotenoids, only a few are considered precursors of retinol. Beta-carotene, lutein, and lycopene are among the most commonly

## TABLE 5.1 Group Characteristics of Fat-Soluble and Water-Soluble Vitamins

| Characteristic | Fat-Soluble Vitamins | Water-Soluble Vitamins |
|---|---|---|
| Sources | The fat and oil portion of foods | The watery portion of foods |
| Absorption | With fat encased in chylomicrons that enter the lymphatic system before circulating in the bloodstream | Directly into the bloodstream |
| Transportation through the blood | Attach to protein carriers because fat is not soluble in watery blood | Move freely through the watery environment of blood and within cells |
| Fat when consumed in excess of need | Are stored—primarily in the liver and adipose tissue | Are excreted in the urine, although some tissues may hold limited amounts of certain vitamins |
| Safety of consuming high intakes through supplements | Can be toxic. This applies primarily to vitamins A and D; large doses of vitamins E and K are considered relatively nontoxic | Are generally considered nontoxic, although side effects can occur from consuming very large doses of vitamin $B_6$ over a prolonged period |
| Frequency of intake | Generally do not have to be consumed daily because the body can retrieve them from storage as needed | Must be consumed daily because there is no reserve in storage |

## TABLE 5.2 Summary of Fat-Soluble Vitamins

| Vitamin and Sources | Functions | Deficiency/Toxicity Signs and Symptoms |
|---|---|---|
| **Vitamin A**<br>**Adult RDA:**<br>**Men: 900 micrograms**<br>**Women: 700 micrograms**<br>• Retinol: Liver, milk, butter, cheese, cream, egg yolk, fortified milk, margarine, and ready-to-eat cereals<br>• Beta-Carotene: Spinach, collard greens, kale, mango, broccoli, carrots, peaches, pumpkin, red peppers, sweet potatoes, winter squash, mango, watermelon, apricots, cantaloupe | The formation of visual purple, which enables the eye to adapt to dim light<br>Normal growth and development of bones and teeth<br>The formation and maintenance of mucosal epithelium to maintain healthy functioning of skin and membranes, hair, gums, and various glands<br>Important role in immune function | *Deficiency*<br>Slow recovery of vision after flashes of bright light at night is the first ocular symptom; can progress to xerophthalmia and blindness<br>Bone growth ceases; bone shape changes; enamel-forming cells in the teeth malfunction; teeth crack and tend to decay<br>Skin becomes dry, scaly, rough, and cracked; keratinization or hyperkeratosis develops; mucous membrane cells flatten and harden: eyes become dry (xerosis); irreversible drying and hardening of the cornea can result in blindness<br>Decreased saliva secretion → difficulty chewing, swallowing → anorexia<br>Decreased mucous secretion of the stomach and intestines → impaired digestion and absorption → diarrhea, increased excretion of nutrients<br>Impaired immune system functioning → increased susceptibility to respiratory, urinary tract, and vaginal infections increases |

(table continues on page 93)

| TABLE 5.2 | Summary of Fat-Soluble Vitamins (continued) | |
|---|---|---|
| **Vitamin and Sources** | **Functions** | **Deficiency/Toxicity Signs and Symptoms** |
| | | ***Toxicity***<br>Headaches, vomiting, double vision, hair loss, bone abnormalities, liver damage, which may be reversible or fatal<br>Can cause birth defects during pregnancy |
| **Vitamin D**<br>**Adult AI:**<br>**Up to age 51: 5 micrograms**<br>**51–70 years: 10 micrograms**<br>**Older than 70 years: 15 micrograms**<br>• Sunlight on the skin<br>• Cod liver oil, oysters, mackerel, most fish, egg yolks, fortified milk, some ready-to-eat cereals, and margarine | Maintains serum calcium concentrations by:<br>Stimulating GI absorption<br>Stimulating the release of calcium from the bones<br>Stimulating calcium absorption from the kidneys | ***Deficiency***<br>Rickets (in infants and children)<br>  Retarded bone growth<br>  Bone malformations (bowed legs)<br>  Enlargement of ends of long bones (knock-knees)<br>  Deformities of the ribs (bowed, with beads or knobs)<br>  Delayed closing of the fontanel → rapid enlargement of the head<br>  Decreased serum calcium and/or phosphorus<br>  Malformed teeth; decayed teeth<br>  Protrusion of the abdomen related to relaxation of the abdominal muscles<br>  Increased secretion of parathyroid hormone<br>Osteomalacia (in adults)<br>  Softening of the bones → deformities, pain, and easy fracture<br>  Decreased serum calcium and/or phosphorus, increased alkaline phosphatase<br>  Involuntary muscle twitching and spasms<br><br>***Toxicity***<br>Kidney stones, irreversible kidney damage, muscle and bone weakness, excessive bleeding, loss of appetite, headache, excessive thirst, calcification of soft tissues (blood vessels, kidneys, heart, lungs), death |
| **Vitamin E**<br>**Adult RDA: 15 mg**<br>• Vegetable oils, margarine, salad dressing, other foods made with vegetable oil, nuts, seeds, wheat germ, dark green vegetables, whole grains, fortified cereals | Acts as an antioxidant to protect vitamin A and PUFA from being destroyed<br>Protects cell membranes | ***Deficiency***<br>Increased RBC hemolysis<br>In infants, anemia, edema, and skin lesions<br><br>***Toxicity***<br>Relatively nontoxic<br>High doses enhance action of anticoagulant medications |
| **Vitamin K**<br>**Adult AI:**<br>**Men: 120 micrograms**<br>**Women: 90 micrograms**<br>• Bacterial synthesis<br>• Brussels sprouts, broccoli, cauliflower, Swiss chard, spinach, looseleaf lettuce, carrot, green beans, asparagus, eggs | Synthesis of blood clotting proteins and a bone protein that regulates blood calcium | ***Deficiency***<br>Hemorrhaging<br><br>***Toxicity***<br>No symptoms have been observed from excessive intake of vitamin K |

known carotenoids. Carotenoids account for about one-quarter to one-third of the usual intake of vitamin A.

Vitamin A is best known for its roles in normal vision, reproduction, growth, and immune system functioning. It is a relatively poor antioxidant. In contrast, beta-carotene is a major antioxidant in the body, prompting researchers to study whether it can prevent heart disease and cancer. Results of trials with beta-carotene supplements have varied from showing no effect on cancer incidence (Green, 1999; Greenberg, 1996; Lee et al., 1999) to a surprising increase in lung cancer incidence and deaths in smokers and male asbestos workers (The Alpha-Tocopherol, Beta Carotene Cancer Prevention Study Group, 1994; Omenn et al., 1996).

The body can store up to a year's supply of vitamin A, 90% of which is in the liver. Because deficiency symptoms do not develop until body stores are exhausted, it may take 1 to 2 years for them to appear. Although severe vitamin A deficiency is rare in the United States, a large percentage of adults may have suboptimal liver stores of vitamin A even though they are not clinically deficient. Worldwide, vitamin A deficiency is a major health problem and is the major cause of childhood blindness.

Only preformed vitamin A, the form found in animal foods, fortified foods, and supplements, is toxic in high doses. The risk of toxicity is much greater when supplements of vitamin A are consumed. Extremely high doses (at least 30,000 micrograms/day) consumed over months or years may cause central nervous system (CNS) changes; bone and skin changes; and liver abnormalities that range from reversible to fatal. At high doses during pregnancy, such as three to four times the recommended intake, vitamin A is teratogenic. Supplementation is not recommended during the first trimester of pregnancy unless there is specific evidence of vitamin A deficiency.

Beta-carotene is nontoxic because the body makes vitamin A from it only as needed and the conversion is not rapid enough to cause hypervitaminosis A. Instead, carotene is stored primarily in adipose tissue and may accumulate under the skin to the extent that it causes the skin color to turn yellowish-orange, a harmless condition known as hypercarotenemia. The upper limit (UL) for vitamin A does not apply to vitamin A derived from carotenoids.

## Vitamin D

Vitamin D is unique in that the body has the potential to make all the vitamin D it needs if exposure to sunlight is optimal and liver and kidney functions are normal. Cholecalciferol (vitamin $D_3$) is produced in the skin when it is exposed to ultraviolet B (UVB) rays in sunlight. Through a series of reactions involving the liver and kidneys, cholecalciferol is converted to 1,25-dihydroxyvitamin D [1,25(OH)D], the vitamin's active form.

Another distinctive feature of vitamin D is that it acts like a hormone because it is synthesized in one part of the body (skin) and stimulates functional activity elsewhere (e.g., GI tract, bones, kidneys) through vitamin D receptors. The primary function of vitamin D is to maintain normal blood concentrations of calcium and phosphorus by

- Stimulating calcium and phosphorus absorption from the GI tract.
- Mobilizing calcium and phosphorus from the bone as needed to maintain normal serum levels.
- Stimulating the kidneys to retain calcium and phosphorus.

In addition to its role in bone health, vitamin D is important for immune function, and low vitamin D status may increase the risk of various diseases, such as hypertension, certain cancers, multiple sclerosis, and type 1 diabetes (Holick, 2004; Lappe, 2007; Pittas et al., 2006; Giovanni, 2006; Giovanni et al., 2006; Mark & Carson, 2006).

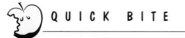

Factors that impair vitamin D synthesis
Dense clouds
Heavy smog
Clothing
Window glass
Sunscreen
Dark skin

It is possible to fulfill vitamin D requirement by taking a daily 15-minute walk in the sun under optimal conditions. However, significant rates of low vitamin D status are documented in studies of healthy adults and children in the United States and other countries (Egan, 2005; Tangpricha, 2002; Weng et al., 2007). Winter, living in northern latitudes, dark-skinned, and older age are associated with low vitamin D synthesis (Weng et al., 2007). During the winter months in northern latitudes, the angle of the sun is such that most UVB rays are absorbed by the earth's ozone layer, preventing most or all endogenous vitamin D synthesis. People living north of the line connecting San Francisco to Philadelphia are not likely to make adequate vitamin D. Elderly persons are particularly at risk for vitamin D deficiency because of various risk factors: inadequate intake, limited sun exposure, reduced skin thickness, impaired GI absorption, and impaired activation by the liver and kidneys. A dietary source is considered essential because few people meet optimal conditions.

Vitamin D occurs naturally in only a few foods: liver, fatty fish, and egg yolks. Fortified foods are important sources: all milks, most ready-to-eat cereals, and a few brands of orange juice, yogurt, margarine, and hot cereals are fortified.

Many experts believe the Adequate Intake (AI) for vitamin D is set too low and that, on average and without sun exposure, 20 to 25 micrograms (1000 IU) of vitamin D is needed daily (Vieth et al., 2007). Average current intake through food is approximately 2.5 micrograms/day (100 IU), maybe as high as 5 to 10 micrograms depending on the use of fortified foods (Vieth, 2006). Significant changes in sunlight exposure, the level of vitamin D fortification of foods, and/or the content of vitamin D in supplements would be necessary to achieve what experts consider a "healthy" vitamin D status (Vieth et al., 2007).

**IU:** International Units, the former unit of measure of vitamin D that has been replaced by micrograms of cholecalciferol, the active form of vitamin D.

**QUICK BITE**

| Vitamin D content of selected items | Micrograms of vitamin D |
|---|---|
| Cod-liver oil, 1 tbsp | 34 |
| Halibut, 3 oz | 17 |
| Catfish, 3 oz | 14 |
| Most multivitamin/ mineral supplements | 100 |
| Canned tuna, 1/4 cup | 3.25 |
| Milk, 1 cup | 2.45 |
| Minute maid calcium + vitamin D orange juice, 8 oz | 2.5 |
| Viactiv soft calcium chews, 1 chew | 2.5 |
| Egg, 1 | 0.65 |

Overt deficiency of vitamin D causes poor calcium absorption, leading to a calcium deficit in the blood that the body corrects by releasing calcium from bone. In children, the result is **rickets**, a condition characterized by abnormal bone shape and structure. Children at risk include breastfed infants who do not receive vitamin D supplements, toddlers given unfortified soy and rice beverages in place of milk, and children who replace milk with soft drinks. In adults, vitamin D deficiency can result in **osteomalacia**, a softening of the bones.

**Rickets:** vitamin D deficiency disease in children, most prominently characterized by bowed legs.

**Osteomalacia:** adult rickets characterized by inadequate bone mineralization due to the lack of vitamin D.

The current UL for vitamin D is set at 50 micrograms (2000 IU). A risk assessment by Hathcock et al. (2007) supports a UL of 250 micrograms/day (10,000 IU). Vitamin D is toxic only when it elevates serum calcium levels and this occurs only at extremely high intakes of vitamin D (e.g., 10,000 IU). Because the body destroys excess vitamin D produced from overexposure to the sun, there has never been a reported case of vitamin D toxicity from too much sun (Food and Nutrition Board, Institute of Medicine, 1997).

## Vitamin E

Vitamin E is a generic term that describes a group of at least eight naturally occurring compounds. Alpha-tocopherol is considered the most biologically active form of vitamin E, although other forms also have important roles in maintaining health. As a group, vitamin E functions as the primary fat-soluble antioxidant in the body, protecting PUFAs and other lipid molecules, such as LDL cholesterol, from oxidative damage. By doing so, it helps to maintain the integrity of PUFA-rich cell membranes; protects red blood cells against hemolysis; and protects vitamin A from oxidation. Vitamin E also has several important functions independent of its antioxidant activity, such as inhibiting cell proliferation, enhancing immune system functioning, improving vasodilation, inhibiting platelet aggregation, and suppressing tumor angiogenesis (Wright, 2006).

The need for vitamin E increases as the intake of PUFA increases. Fortunately, vitamin E and PUFA share many of the same food sources, particularly vegetable oils and products made from oil such as margarine, salad dressings, and other prepared foods. However, not all oils are rich in alpha-tocopherol, the active form of vitamin E. Soybean oil, the most commonly used oil in food processing, ranks low in alpha-tocopherol content.

### QUICK BITE

Oils containing active form of vitamin E (in descending order)
Wheat germ oil
Walnut oil
Sunflower oil
Cottonseed oil
Safflower oil
Palm oil
Canola oil
Sesame oil
Peanut oil
Olive oil
Corn oil
Soybean oil

It has been suggested that vitamin E, in doses higher than can be achieved by diet alone, may lower the risk for atherosclerosis, some types of cancer, cataracts, age-related macular degeneration, Parkinson's disease, and Alzheimer's disease. So far the results of clinical trials have been inconsistent. In fact, at doses above 400 IU/day, older, high-risk patients experienced an increased risk for death (Miller, 2005). A review of 19 clinical trials conducted between 1993 and 2004 found a lack of benefit from vitamin E supplements, especially at higher doses (IFIC, 2005). Clearly, more randomized clinical trials are needed to determine the safety and efficacy of using vitamin E supplements.

Vitamin E deficiency can occur in very specific instances. Premature infants who have not benefited from the transfer of vitamin E from mother to fetus in the last weeks of pregnancy are at risk for red blood cell hemolysis. The breaking of their red blood cell membranes is caused by oxidation; vitamin E corrects red blood cell hemolysis by preventing oxidation. Other cases of vitamin E deficiency are rare but may occur secondary to a genetic abnormality or malabsorption syndromes such as cystic fibrosis and short bowel syndrome. Vitamin E deficiency symptoms include peripheral neuropathy, ataxia, and ultimately death (Traber, 2006). Large amounts of vitamin E are relatively nontoxic but can interfere with vitamin K action (blood clotting) by decreasing platelet aggregation. Large doses may also potentiate the effects of blood-thinning drugs, increasing the risk of hemorrhage. The UL is 66 times higher than the Recommended Dietary Allowance (RDA).

## Vitamin K

Vitamin K occurs naturally in two forms: phylloquinone, found in plants, and menaquinones, which are synthesized in the intestinal tract by bacteria. Relatively, few foods contribute to the dietary phylloquinone intake of most people: collards, spinach, salad greens, broccoli, Brussels sprouts, and cabbage.

Vitamin K is a coenzyme essential for the synthesis of prothrombin and at least 6 of the other 13 proteins needed for normal blood clotting. Without adequate vitamin K, life is threatened: even a small wound can cause someone deficient in vitamin K to bleed to death. Vitamin K also activates at least three proteins involved in building and maintaining bone.

Newborns are prone to vitamin K deficiency because their sterile GI tracts cannot synthesize vitamin K and it may take weeks for bacteria to establish themselves in the newborn's intestines. To prevent hemorrhagic disease, a single water-soluble dose of vitamin K is given prophylactically at birth.

Clinically significant vitamin K deficiency is defined as vitamin K–responsive hypoprothrombinemia and is characterized by an increase in prothrombin time. Vitamin K deficiency does not occur from inadequate intake but may occur secondary to malabsorption syndromes or the use of certain medications that interfere with vitamin K metabolism or synthesis, such as anticoagulants and antibiotics. Anticoagulants, such as coumadin, interfere with hepatic synthesis of vitamin K–dependent clotting factors. People who take anticoagulants do not need to avoid vitamin K, but they should try to maintain a consistent intake so that the effect on coagulation time is as constant and as predictable as possible. Antibiotics kill the intestinal bacteria that synthesize vitamin K.

Due to the lack of data to estimate an average requirement, an AI, not an RDA, has been set. A UL has not been set because no adverse effects are associated with vitamin K intake from food or supplements.

## Water-Soluble Vitamins

Group characteristics of water-soluble vitamins are summarized in Table 5.1. Table 5.3 highlights sources, functions, deficiency symptoms, and toxicity symptoms of each water-soluble vitamin. The complete table of Dietary Reference Intakes for vitamins appears in Appendix 2. Additional features of individual water-soluble vitamins are summarized in the following sections.

## Thiamin

Thiamin (vitamin $B_1$) is a coenzyme in the metabolism of carbohydrates and branched-chain amino acids. In addition to its role in energy metabolism, thiamin is important in nervous system functioning.

In the United States and other developed countries, the use of enriched breads and cereals has virtually eliminated the thiamin deficiency disease known as beriberi. Today thiamin deficiency is usually seen only in alcoholics with limited food consumption because chronic alcohol abuse impairs thiamin intake, absorption, and metabolism. Edema occurs in wet beriberi; muscle wasting is prominent in dry beriberi. Cardiac and renal complications can be fatal.

No adverse effects have been noted from high intakes of thiamin from food or supplements, so a UL has not been set.

## Riboflavin

**Homocysteine:** an amino acid correlated with increased risk of heart disease.

**Methionine:** an essential amino acid.

Riboflavin (vitamin $B_2$) is an integral component of the coenzymes flavin adenine dinucleotide (FAD) and flavin mononucleotide (FMN) that function to release energy from nutrients in all body cells. Flavin coenzymes are also involved in the formation of some vitamins and their coenzymes and in the conversion of **homocysteine** to **methionine**. Riboflavin is unique among water-soluble vitamins in that milk and dairy products contribute the most riboflavin to the diet.

| TABLE 5.3 | Summary of Water-Soluble Vitamins | |
|---|---|---|
| **Vitamin and Sources** | **Functions** | **Deficiency/Toxicity Signs and Symptoms** |
| **Thiamin (Vitamin B$_1$)**<br>**Adult RDA**<br>**Men: 1.2 mg**<br>**Women: 1.1 mg**<br>• Whole grain and enriched breads and cereals, liver, nuts, wheat germ, pork, dried peas and beans | Coenzyme in energy metabolism<br>Promotes normal appetite and nervous system functioning | *Deficiency*<br>Beriberi<br>   Mental confusion, decrease in short-term memory<br>   Fatigue, apathy<br>   Peripheral paralysis<br>   Muscle weakness and wasting<br>   Painful calf muscles<br>   Anorexia, weight loss<br>   Edema<br>   Enlarged heart<br>   Sudden death from heart failure<br><br>*Toxicity*<br>No toxicity symptoms reported |
| **Riboflavin (Vitamin B$_2$)**<br>**Adult RDA**<br>**Men: 1.3 mg**<br>**Women: 1.1 mg**<br>• Milk and other dairy products; whole grain and enriched breads and cereals; liver, eggs, meat, spinach | Coenzyme in energy metabolism<br>Aids in the conversion of tryptophan into niacin | *Deficiency*<br>Dermatitis<br>Cheilosis<br>Glossitis<br>Photophobia<br>Reddening of the cornea<br><br>*Toxicity*<br>No toxicity symptoms reported |
| **Niacin (Vitamin B$_3$)**<br>**Adult RDA**<br>**Men: 16 mg**<br>**Women: 14 mg**<br>• All protein foods, whole grain and enriched breads and cereals | Coenzyme in energy metabolism<br>Promotes normal nervous system functioning | *Deficiency*<br>Pellagra: 4 D's<br>   Dermatitis (bilateral and symmetrical) and glossitis<br>   Diarrhea<br>   Dementia, irritability, mental confusion → psychosis<br>   Death, if untreated<br>*Toxicity* (from supplements/drugs)<br>Flushing, liver damage, gastric ulcers, low blood pressure, diarrhea, nausea, vomiting |
| **Vitamin B$_6$**<br>**Adult RDA**<br>**Men: 1.3–1.7 mg**<br>**Women: 1.3–1.5 mg**<br>• Meats, fish, poultry, fruits, green leafy vegetables, whole grains, nuts, dried peas and beans | Coenzyme in amino acid and fatty acid metabolism<br>Helps convert tryptophan to niacin<br>Helps produce insulin, hemoglobin, myelin sheaths, and antibodies | *Deficiency*<br>Dermatitis, cheilosis, glossitis, abnormal brain wave pattern, convulsions, and anemia<br><br>*Toxicity*<br>Depression, fatigue, irritability, headaches; sensory neuropathy characteristic |
| **Folate**<br>**Adult RDA: 400 micrograms**<br>• Liver, okra, spinach, asparagus, dried peas and beans, seeds, orange juice; breads, cereals, and other grains are fortified with folic acid | Coenzyme in DNA synthesis, therefore vital for new cell synthesis and the transmission of inherited characteristics | *Deficiency*<br>Glossitis, diarrhea, macrocytic anemia, depression, mental confusion, fainting, fatigue<br><br>*Toxicity*<br>Too much can mask B$_{12}$ deficiency |

*(table continues on page 99)*

| TABLE 5.3 | **Summary of Water-Soluble Vitamins** (continued) | | |
|---|---|---|
| **Vitamin and Sources** | **Functions** | **Deficiency/Toxicity Signs and Symptoms** |
| **Vitamin B$_{12}$**<br>**Adult RDA: 2.4 micrograms**<br>• Animal products: meat, fish, poultry, shellfish, milk, dairy products, eggs<br>• Some fortified foods | Coenzyme in the synthesis of new cells<br>Activates folate<br>Maintains nerve cells<br>Helps metabolize some fatty acids and amino acids | *Deficiency*<br>GI changes: glossitis, anorexia, indigestion, recurring diarrhea or constipation, and weight loss<br>Macrocytic anemia: pallor, dyspnea, weakness, fatigue, and palpitations<br>Neurologic changes: paresthesia of the hands and feet, decreased sense of position, poor muscle coordination, poor memory, irritability, depression, paranoia, delirium, and hallucinations<br><br>*Toxicity*<br>No toxicity symptoms reported |
| **Pantothenic Acid**<br>**Adult AI: 5 mg**<br>• Widespread in foods<br>• Meat, poultry, fish, whole-grain cereals, and dried peas and beans are among best sources | Part of coenzyme A used in energy metabolism | *Deficiency*<br>Rare; general failure of all body systems<br><br>*Toxicity*<br>No toxicity symptoms reported, although large doses may cause diarrhea |
| **Biotin**<br>**Adult AI: 30 micrograms**<br>• Widespread in foods<br>• Eggs, liver, milk, and dark green vegetables are among best choices<br>• Synthesized by GI flora | Coenzyme in energy metabolism, fatty acid synthesis, amino acid metabolism, and glycogen formation | *Deficiency*<br>Rare; anorexia, fatigue, depression, dry skin, heart abnormalities<br><br>*Toxicity*<br>No toxicity symptoms reported |
| **Vitamin C**<br>**Adult RDA**<br>**Men: 90 mg**<br>**Women: 75 mg**<br>• Citrus fruits and juices, red and green peppers, broccoli, cauliflower, Brussels sprouts, cantaloupe, kiwifruit, mustard greens, strawberries, tomatoes | Collagen synthesis<br>Antioxidant<br>Promotes iron absorption<br>Involved in the metabolism of certain amino acids<br>Thyroxin synthesis<br>Immune system functioning | *Deficiency*<br>Bleeding gums, pinpoint hemorrhages under the skin<br>Scurvy, characterized by<br>  Hemorrhaging<br>  Muscle degeneration<br>  Skin changes<br>  Delayed wound healing: reopening of old wounds<br>  Softening of the bones → malformations, pain, easy fractures<br>  Soft, loose teeth<br>  Anemia<br>  Increased susceptibility to infection<br>  Hysteria and depression<br><br>*Toxicity*<br>Diarrhea, mild GI upset |

Biochemical signs of an inadequate riboflavin status can appear after only a few days of a poor intake. The elderly and adolescents are at greatest risk for riboflavin deficiency. Riboflavin deficiency interferes with iron handling and contributes to anemia when iron intake is low. Other deficiency symptoms include sore throat, cheilosis, stomatitis, glossitis, and dermatitis, many of which may be related to the effect riboflavin deficiency has on the metabolism of folate and vitamin $B_6$. Certain diseases, such as cancer, heart disease, and diabetes, precipitate or exacerbate riboflavin deficiency.

## Niacin

Niacin (vitamin $B_3$) exists as nicotinic acid and nicotinamide. The body converts nicotinic acid to nicotinamide, which is the major form of niacin in the blood. All protein foods provide niacin, as do whole grain and enriched breads and fortified ready-to-eat cereals.

A unique feature of niacin is that the body can make it from the amino acid tryptophan: approximately 60 mg of tryptophan is used to synthesize 1 mg of niacin. Because of this additional source of niacin, niacin requirements are stated in **niacin equivalents (NEs)**. Median intake in the United States generously exceeds the RDA.

**Niacin Equivalents (NEs):** the amount of niacin available to the body including that made from tryptophan.

Niacin is part of the coenzymes nicotinamide adenine dinucleotide (NAD) and nicotinamide adenine dinucleotide phosphate (NADP), which are involved in energy transfer reactions in the metabolism of glucose, fat, and alcohol in all body cells. Reduced NADP is used in the synthesis of fatty acids, cholesterol, and steroid hormones.

Pellagra, the disorder caused by severe niacin deficiency, is rare in the United States and usually is seen only in alcoholics. However, pellagra is widespread in areas that rely on corn as a staple, such as parts of Africa and Asia, because corn is low in niacin and tryptophan. Before grain products were enriched with niacin in the early 20th century, pellagra was also common in the southern United States.

Niacin deficiency may be treated with niacin, or tryptophan, or both. Because a deficiency of niacin rarely occurs alone, treatment is most effective when other B-complex vitamins are also given, especially thiamin and riboflavin.

Large doses of niacin in the form of nicotinic acid (1 g to 6 g/day) are used therapeutically to lower total cholesterol and LDL cholesterol and raise high-density lipoprotein (HDL) cholesterol. Flushing is a common side effect caused by vasodilation. Large doses, which may cause liver damage and gout, should be used only with a doctor's supervision. The UL of 35 mg of NE does not apply for clinical applications using niacin as a drug.

## Vitamin $B_6$

Vitamin $B_6$ and pyridoxine are group names for six related compounds that include pyridoxine, pyridoxal, and pyridoxamine. All forms can be converted to the active form, pyridoxal phosphate, which is involved in more than 100 enzymatic reactions.

Vitamin $B_6$ plays a role in the synthesis, catabolism, and transport of amino acids and in the conversion of tryptophan to niacin. It is involved in the formation of heme for hemoglobin and in the synthesis of myelin sheaths and neurotransmitters. Vitamin $B_6$ helps to regulate blood glucose levels by assisting in the release of stored glucose from glycogen and is important in the maintenance of cellular immunity. Unlike other B vitamins, vitamin $B_6$ is stored extensively in muscle tissue.

Deficiencies of vitamin $B_6$, folic acid, and vitamin $B_{12}$ lead to an increase in blood homocysteine levels, a nonessential amino acid linked to an increased risk of vascular disease (McCully, 2007). Findings from both the HOPE2 trial (Lonn et al., 2006) and the NORVIT trial (Bønaa et al., 2006) showed that the combination of vitamin $B_6$, vitamin $B_{12}$, and folic acid lowers homocysteine levels in people with advanced vascular disease but has little effect on recurrent heart attack or stroke. Current trials are underway to determine whether lowering homocysteine with B vitamins plays a role in the primary prevention of cardiovascular disease. The American Heart Association recognizes that too much homocysteine is related to a higher risk of coronary heart disease and stroke, but acknowledges that evidence of benefit from lowering homocysteine levels is currently lacking (AHA, 2007).

Supplements of vitamin $B_6$ have been used for a variety of other conditions, although supportive evidence is lacking. Treating carpal tunnel syndrome with vitamin $B_6$ supplements is generally not supported by research (Goodyear-Smith & Arroll, 2004). Studies on the benefits of using vitamin $B_6$ in treating premenstrual syndrome (PMS) are equivocal, and most positive trials have been criticized for being poorly designed (Fragakis & Thomson, 2007). Likewise, well-designed studies are lacking on the use of vitamin $B_6$ supplement for autism and cognitive decline in the elderly.

High intakes of vitamin $B_6$ from food do not pose any danger. Long-term use of high-dose supplements (1000 to 4000 mg/day) is associated with neuropathy that is reversible with discontinuation (IOM, 2000).

Deficiencies of vitamin $B_6$ are uncommon but are usually accompanied by deficiencies of other B vitamins. Secondary deficiencies are related to alcohol abuse (the metabolism of alcohol promotes the destruction and excretion of vitamin $B_6$) and to other drug therapies such as isoniazid, the antituberculosis drug that acts as a vitamin $B_6$ antagonist.

## Folate

**Dietary Folate Equivalents (DFEs):** 1 DFE = 1 microgram of food folate = 0.6 micrograms of folic acid from fortified food or as a supplement consumed with food = 0.5 micrograms of a supplement taken on an empty stomach.

Folate is the generic term for this B vitamin that includes both synthetic folic acid found in vitamin supplements and fortified foods and naturally occurring folate in foods such as green leafy vegetables, dried peas and beans, seeds, liver, and orange juice. **Dietary folate equivalents (DFEs)**, used in establishing folate requirement, are based on the assumption that natural food folate is only half as available to the body as synthetic folic acid. A more recent study showed that bioavailability of food folate may be as high as 80% of synthetic folic acid (Winkels et al., 2007).

As part of the coenzymes tetrahydrofolate (THF) and dihydrofolate (DHF), folate's major function is in the synthesis of DNA. With the aid of vitamin $B_{12}$, folate is vital for synthesis of new cells and transmission of inherited characteristics. Folate is also involved in homocysteine metabolism.

Because folate is recycled through the intestinal tract (much like the enterohepatic circulation of bile), a healthy GI tract is essential to maintain folate balance. When GI integrity is impaired, as in malabsorption syndromes, failure to reabsorb folate quickly leads to folate deficiency. GI cells are particularly susceptible to folate deficiency because they are rapidly dividing cells that depend on folate for new cell synthesis. Without the formation of new cells, GI function declines and widespread malabsorption of nutrients occurs.

Folate deficiency impairs DNA synthesis and cell division and results in macrocytic anemia and other clinical symptoms. It is prevalent in all parts of the world. In developing countries, folate deficiency commonly is caused by parasitic infections that alter GI integrity. In the United States, alcoholics are at highest risk of folate deficiency because of alcohol's toxic effect on the GI tract. Groups at risk because of poor intake include the elderly, fad dieters, and people of low socioeconomic status. Because new tissue growth increases folate requirements, infants, adolescents, and pregnant women may have difficulty consuming adequate amounts.

Studies show that AI of folate before conception and during the first trimester of pregnancy reduces the risk of neural tube defects (e.g., spina bifida) in infants (Medical Research Council Vitamin Study Research Group, 1991). This discovery prompted the U.S. Public Health Service to recommend that all women of childbearing age who are capable of becoming pregnant consume 400 micrograms of synthetic folic acid from fortified food and/or supplements in addition to folate from a varied diet. Mandatory folic acid fortification of enriched bread and grain products began on January 1, 1998. However, this policy alone does not ensure adequate folate intake among women of childbearing age; supplements and wise food choices continue to be important.

The UL for folic acid is 1000 micrograms/day from fortified food or supplements, exclusive of food folate. Consistently high intakes of folate can mask vitamin $B_{12}$ deficiency, which can cause permanent neurologic damage if left untreated. Large doses may interfere with anticonvulsant therapy and precipitate convulsions in patients with epilepsy controlled by phenytoin.

## Vitamin $B_{12}$

Vitamin $B_{12}$ (cobalamin) has several interesting features. First, vitamin $B_{12}$ has an interdependent relationship with folate: each vitamin must have the other to be activated. Because it activates folate, vitamin $B_{12}$ is involved in DNA synthesis and maturation of red blood cells. Like folate, vitamin $B_{12}$ functions as a coenzyme in homocysteine metabolism. Unlike folate, vitamin $B_{12}$ has important roles in maintaining the myelin sheath around nerves. For this reason, large doses of folic acid can alleviate the anemia caused by vitamin $B_{12}$ deficiency (a function of both vitamins), but folic acid cannot halt the progressive neurologic impairments that only vitamin $B_{12}$ can treat. Nervous system damage may be irreversible without early treatment with vitamin $B_{12}$.

Vitamin $B_{12}$ also holds the distinction of being the only water-soluble vitamin that does not occur naturally in plants. Fermented soy products and algae may be enriched with vitamin $B_{12}$ but it is in an inactive, unavailable form. Some ready-to-eat cereals are fortified with vitamin $B_{12}$. All animal foods contain vitamin $B_{12}$.

Another unique feature of vitamin $B_{12}$ is that it requires an intrinsic factor, a glycoprotein secreted in the stomach, to be absorbed from the terminal ileum. But before it can bind to the intrinsic factor, vitamin $B_{12}$ must first be separated from the small peptides to which it is bound in food sources. Separation is accomplished by pepsin and gastric acid.

Vitamin $B_{12}$ deficiency symptoms may take 5 to 10 years or longer to develop because the liver can store relatively large amounts of $B_{12}$ and the body recycles $B_{12}$ by reabsorbing it.

Dietary deficiencies of vitamin $B_{12}$ are rare and are likely to occur only in strict vegans who consume no animal products and do not adequately supplement their diet. A more frequent cause of deficiency is the lack of intrinsic factor, which prevents absorption of vitamin $B_{12}$ regardless of intake; this condition is known as pernicious anemia. People with pernicious anemia, which can occur secondary to gastric surgery or gastric cancer, require parenteral injections of vitamin $B_{12}$. Most commonly, $B_{12}$ deficiency arises from inadequate gastric acid secretion, which prevents protein-bound vitamin $B_{12}$ in foods from being freed. Approximately 15% of adults older than 65 years of age may have this type of vitamin $B_{12}$ deficiency as a result of atrophic gastritis or from gastric resection, use of medications that suppress gastric acid secretion, or gastric infection with *Helicobacter pylori* (McCully, 2007). Because people with protein-bound vitamin $B_{12}$ deficiency are able to absorb synthetic (free) vitamin $B_{12}$, the National Academy of Sciences Institute of Medicine recommends that people over 50 obtain most of their requirement from fortified foods or supplements (Food and Nutrition Board, Institute of Medicine, 1998).

## Other B Vitamins

Pantothenic acid is part of CoA, the coenzyme involved in the formation of acetyl-CoA and in the TCA cycle. Pantothenic acid participates in more than 100 different metabolic reactions. It is widespread in the diet. The best sources of pantothenic acid are meat, fish, poultry, whole-grain cereals, and dried peas and beans.

As a coenzyme, biotin is involved in the TCA cycle, gluconeogenesis, fatty acid synthesis, and chemical reactions that add or remove carbon dioxide from other compounds. Biotin is widely distributed in nature and significant amounts are synthesized by GI flora, but it is not known how much is available for absorption. It is assumed that the average American diet provides adequate amounts of both pantothenic acid and biotin.

## Non-B Vitamins

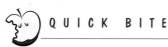

QUICK BITE

Substances often falsely promoted as
B vitamins
*Para*-aminobenzoic acid (PABA)
Bioflavonoids
Vitamin P
Hesperidin
Ubiquinone
Vitamin B$_{15}$
Vitamin B$_{17}$

Other substances, such as inositol, choline, and carnitine, are sometimes inaccurately referred to as B vitamins because they are coenzymes. Only choline has been assigned an AI value. Research is needed to determine if these substances are essential in the diet.

## Vitamin C

Vitamin C (ascorbic acid), most notably found in citrus fruits and juices, may be the most famous vitamin. Its long history dates back more than 250 years when it was determined that something in citrus fruits prevents scurvy, a disease that killed as many as two-thirds of sailors on long journeys. Years later, British sailors acquired the nickname "Limeys" because of Great Britain's policy to prevent scurvy by providing limes to all navy men. It wasn't until 1932 that the antiscurvy agent was identified as vitamin C. Since then, vitamin C has been touted as a cure for a variety of ills, including cancer, colds, and infertility.

Vitamin C prevents scurvy by promoting the formation of collagen, the most abundant protein in fibrous tissues such as connective tissue, cartilage, bone matrix, tooth dentin, skin, and tendon. Without adequate vitamin C, the integrity of collagen is compromised; muscles degenerate, weakened bones break, wounds fail to heal, teeth are lost, and infection occurs. Hemorrhaging begins as pinpoints under the skin and progresses to massive internal bleeding and death. Even though scurvy is deadly, it can be cured within a matter of days with moderate doses of vitamin C.

Vitamin C is a water-soluble antioxidant that protects vitamin A, vitamin E, PUFA, and iron from destruction. As an antioxidant, vitamin C is being studied for its ability to prevent heart disease, certain cancers, cataracts, and asthma. It is involved in many metabolic reactions including the promotion of iron absorption, the formation of some neurotransmitters, the synthesis of thyroxine, the metabolism of some amino acids, and normal immune system functioning.

The newest RDA for vitamin C represents an increase from the previous recommendation. Cigarette smokers are advised to increase their intake by 35 mg/day because smoking increases oxidative stress and metabolic turnover of vitamin C (Food and Nutrition Board, Institute of Medicine, 2000). The need for vitamin C also increases in response to other stresses such as fever, chronic illness, infection, and wound healing as well as from chronic use of certain medications such as aspirin, barbiturates, and oral contraceptives. There is no evidence that mental stress increases the need for vitamin C. Evidence consistently shows that intakes ≤ 300 mg/d are safe (Hathcock et al., 2005).

There is no clear and convincing evidence that large doses of vitamin C prevent colds, although it is possible that supplements may benefit those with low plasma vitamin C stores or those experiencing oxidative stress from intense physical exercise, such as ultramarathon runners (Peters et al., 1993). Efficacy is difficult to measure because it may be influenced by how much, how often, and how long supplements are used and by which outcome it is measured, such as frequency of colds, length of cold, and severity of symptoms (Fragakis & Thomson, 2007).

## Phytochemicals

**Phytochemicals:** plant chemicals that, though not essential for life, are thought to promote health.

**Phytochemicals** are literally plant ("phyto" in Greek) chemicals, a broad class of nonnutritive compounds that plants produce to protect themselves against viruses, bacteria, and fungi. In foods, phytochemicals impart color, taste, aroma, and other characteristics. When eaten in the "package" of fruit, vegetables, whole grains, or nuts, these chemicals work together with nutrients and fiber to promote health, such as by acting as antioxidants, detoxifying enzymes, stimulating the immune system, and regulating hormones, or by inactivating bacteria and viruses. Often their actions in the body are complementary and overlapping. Table 5.4 lists possible effects and sources of selected phytochemicals.

**TABLE 5.4** **Possible Effects and Sources of Selected Phytochemicals**

| Phytochemical (Name or Class) | Possible Effects | Sources |
| --- | --- | --- |
| Lycopene | Potent antioxidant that may reduce the risk of prostate cancer and heart disease | Red fruits and vegetables, such as tomatoes, tomato products, red grapefruit, red peppers, watermelon |
| Allyl sulfides | Boost levels of naturally occurring enzymes that may help to maintain healthy immune system | Garlic, onions, leeks, chives |
| Isoflavones (genistein and daidzein) | Antiestrogen activity, which may decrease the risk of estrogen-dependent cancers; may inhibit the formation of blood vessels that enable tumors to grow | Soybeans, soy flour, soy milk, tofu, other legumes |
| Ellagic acid | May reduce the risk of certain cancers and decrease cholesterol levels | Red grapes, strawberries, raspberries, blueberries, kiwifruit, currents |
| Limonene | Boosts levels of body enzymes that may destroy carcinogens | Oranges, grapefruit, tangerines, lemons, and limes |
| Polyphenols (catechins) | May help to prevent DNA damage by neutralizing free radicals | Onion, apple, tea, red wine, grapes, grape juice, strawberries, green tea, wine |
| Lignans | Act as a phytoestrogen; may reduce the risk of certain kinds of cancer | Flaxseed, whole grains |
| Phytic acid | May inhibit oxidative reactions in the colon that produce harmful free radicals | Whole wheat |
| Lutein | Acts as an antioxidant; may reduce the risk of heart disease, age-related eye diseases, and cancer | Kale, spinach, collard greens, kiwifruit, broccoli, Brussels sprouts, Swiss chard, romaine |
| Zeaxanthin | May help prevent macular degeneration and certain types of cancer | Corn, spinach, winter squash |
| Resveratrol | May reduce the risk of heart disease, cancer, and stroke | Red grapes, red grape juice, red wine |

Phytochemicals are an emerging area of nutrition research. At this time, researchers simply do not know all the components in plants, how they function, which ones are beneficial, which ones are potentially harmful, and the ideal combination and concentration of these chemicals to be able to create a pill to substitute for a varied diet rich in plants. More than likely it is the total package and balance of nutrients and nonnutritive substances that makes fruits and vegetables so healthy. Until science catches up to nature, the best advice is to eat a diet rich in plants. Variety is important because different plants supply different types and amounts of the thousands of phytochemicals that have already been identified.

## ▶ VITAMINS IN HEALTH PROMOTION

Unlike fats and carbohydrates, vitamins are not addressed by the *Dietary Guidelines for Americans* as a distinct topic. Under the heading of "Adequate Nutrients Within Calorie Needs," certain vitamins, namely vitamins A (as carotenoids), C, and E, are mentioned as being of concern for American adults based on dietary intake data or evidence of public health problems. Table 5.5 summarizes mean intake of vitamins for adult men and women compared to Dietary Reference Intakes.

A premise of the *Dietary Guidelines* is that nutrients should come primarily from food, not supplements (Fig. 5.2). MyPyramid and the DASH Eating Plan (Chapter 20) translate

| TABLE 5.5 | Comparison Between Usual Nutrient Intakes Among Adults and Dietary Reference Intakes* | | | |
|---|---|---|---|---|
| | **Men 19+ Years of Age** | | **Women 19+ Years of Age** | |
| **Vitamin** | **Mean Intake** | **Recommended Adult Intake** | **Mean Intake** | **Recommended Adult Intake** |
| Vitamin A (micrograms RAE) | 656 | 900 | 564 | 700 |
| Vitamin E (mg alpha-tocopherol) | 8.2 | 15 | 6.3 | 15 |
| Vitamin K (micrograms) | 88.9 | 120 | 95.6 | 90 |
| Thiamin (mg) | 1.89 | 1.2 | 1.37 | 1.1 |
| Riboflavin (mg) | 2.55 | 1.3 | 1.86 | 1.1 |
| Niacin (mg) | 27.0 | 16 | 18.7 | 14 |
| Vitamin $B_6$ (mg) | 2.23 | 1.3–1.7 | 1.53 | 1.3–1.5 |
| Folate (micrograms dietary folate equivalents) | 636 | 400 | 483 | 400 |
| Vitamin $B_{12}$ | 6.45 | 2.4 | 4.33 | 2.4 |
| Vitamin C (mg) | 105.2 | 90 | 83.6 | 75 |

*Dietary Reference Intakes are RDA for vitamins A, E, thiamin, riboflavin, niacin, vitamin $B_6$, folate, vitamin $B_{12}$, and vitamin C. Recommended intake is an AI for vitamin K.

Shaded areas represent nutrients whose mean intake falls below the recommended intake.

**Source:** Moshfegh, A., Goldman, J., & Cleveland, L. (2005). *What we eat in America, NHANES 2001–2002: Usual nutrient intakes from food compared to Dietary Reference Intakes.* US Department of Agriculture, Agricultural Research Service. Available at www.ars.usda.gov/SP2UserFiles/Place/12355000pdf.usualintaketables2001-2002.pdf. Accessed on 12/20/07.

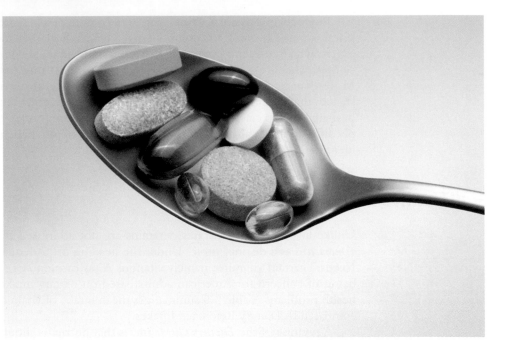

**FIGURE 5.2** Nutrients are best obtained from food, not pills.

the *Dietary Guidelines* into food plans aimed at ensuring nutrient adequacy. Generally, a food group approach rather than actual intake calculations is "good enough" to assess vitamin adequacy because

- Food composition data may be inaccurate (as in the case of vitamin E, which includes all types of E, not just the active form) or limited (e.g., biotin and pantothenic acid content of food is scarce).
- An individual's intake varies from day to day, so "usual" intake is hard to define.
- People tend to underreport their actual food intake.
- An individual's actual nutrient requirements are unknown; the RDAs are intended to meet the needs of 97% to 98% of all healthy people but not necessarily individuals.

Although all MyPyramid groups provide a mixture of vitamins in varying amounts (Fig. 5.3), the "vitamins of concern" are found almost exclusively in plants.

- Beta-carotene and vitamin C are found exclusively in fruits and vegetables. The amounts of fruits and vegetables recommended at various MyPyramid calorie levels appear in Table 5.6. According to food consumption data, less than 32% of adults consume fruits two or more times per day and approximately 27% eat vegetables three or more times per day (CDC, 2007). The variety of fruits and vegetables eaten is also limited, with apples, oranges, and bananas accounting for almost 50% of the fruit consumed in the United States. The most commonly eaten vegetables are potatoes and iceberg lettuce (Darmon et al., 2005). Tips for boosting fruit and vegetable intake appear in Box 5.1.
- Vitamin E is found mostly in vegetable oils, nuts, seeds, wheat germ, and green leafy vegetables. Some seafood, such as sardines, blue crab, and herring, also provide vitamin E. Although vitamin E is mentioned as a vitamin of concern, average intake among

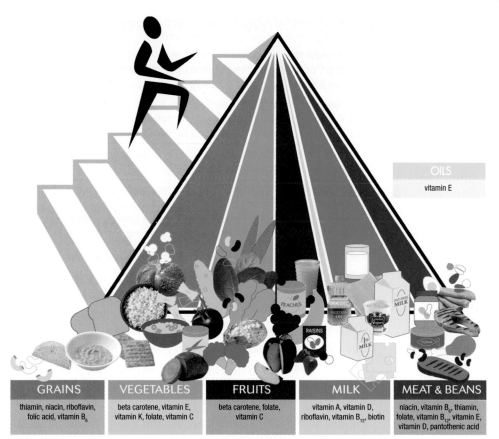

**FIGURE 5.3** Vitamins in MyPyramid food groups. (USDA, Center for Nutrition Policy and Promotion (2005). MyPyramid–Steps to Healthier Food Guidance System. Available at www.MyPyramid.gov.)

| TABLE 5.6 | Amounts of Fruits and Vegetables Recommended at Various MyPyramid Calorie Levels |

| Total Calorie Intake | Amount of Fruit Recommended/Day (in cups) | Amount of Vegetables Recommended/Day (in cups) |
|---|---|---|
| 1600 | 1.5 | 2 |
| 1800 | 1.5 | 2.5 |
| 2000 | 2 | 2.5 |
| 2200–2400 | 2 | 3 |
| 2600 | 2 | 3.5 |
| 2800 | 2.5 | 3.5 |
| 3000–3200 | 2.5 | 4 |

Americans may be underestimated because of (1) underreporting of total fat intake, (2) difficulty in estimating the amount of fat used in the food preparation (e.g., frying), and (3) vague ingredient lists that state "may contain one or more of the following oils" because vegetable oils differ in their vitamin E content. It is noteworthy that deficiency symptoms have never been reported in healthy people eating a low–vitamin E diet.

**BOX 5.1**     **TIPS FOR BOOSTING FRUIT AND VEGETABLE INTAKE**

- Eat at least five servings of fruits and vegetables every day. More is even better. Five servings of fruits and vegetables per day may provide more than 200 mg of vitamin C, far more than the RDA of 75 mg for adult women and 90 mg for adult men.

- Choose wholesome, nutrient-dense foods over refined or processed foods. For instance, fortified whole-grain cereal (e.g., total) is more nutritious than refined cereal (e.g., puffed wheat), and orange juice is more nutritious than orange drink.

- Concentrate on variety and color. Aim for at least one green, one orange, one red, one citrus, and one legume everyday.

- Make an effort to preserve the vitamin content of vegetables: store them in the refrigerator (except for onions, tomatoes, winter squash, and potatoes), prepare them with minimal peeling, and cook for as short a time as possible in as little water as necessary. Microwaving is a better option than boiling.

- Start at least one meal each day with a fresh salad.

- Eat raw vegetables or fresh fruits for snacks.

- Add vegetables to other foods such as zucchini to spaghetti sauce, grated carrots to meat loaf, and spinach to lasagna.

- Double the normal portion size of vegetables.

- Buy a new fruit or vegetable when you go grocery shopping.

- Eat occasional meatless entrees such as pasta primavera, vegetable stir fry, or black beans and rice.

- Order a vegetable when you eat out.

- Choose 100% fruit juice at breakfast and during the day instead of drinks, cocktails, ades, and/or carbonated beverages.

- Eat fruit for dessert.

- Make fruits and vegetables more visible. Leave a bowl of fruit on the center of your table. Keep fresh vegetables on the top shelf of the refrigerator in plain view.

## What About Supplements?

Multivitamin/multimineral supplements, used by about one-third of Americans, comprise the biggest share of the more than $23 billion spent on supplements annually in the United States (NIH State-of-the-Science Panel, 2007). More than half of American adults take some form of supplement based on the belief that it will make them feel better, give them more energy, improve their health, and prevent and treat disease (NIH State-of-the-Science Panel, 2007). Ironically, populations at greatest risk for nutritional inadequacy who may benefit from supplements are the least likely to use supplements.

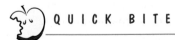 **QUICK BITE**

Demographics of multivitamin/multimineral users (Rock, 2007)
- Female
- Older age
- Higher level of education
- Engaged in regular physical activity
- Lower body mass index
- Non-Hispanic white

| BOX 5.2 | **KEY RECOMMENDATIONS FOR SPECIFIC POPULATION GROUPS** |

• *People over age 50. Consume vitamin $B_{12}$ in its crystalline form (i.e., fortified foods or supplements).*

Men and women over age 50 are urged to consume most of their RDA for vitamin $B_{12}$ via fortified cereals or supplements because they may not adequately absorb adequate $B_{12}$ from protein-bound food sources.

• *Women of childbearing age who may become pregnant. Eat foods high in heme-iron and/or consume iron-rich plant foods or iron-fortified foods with an enhancer of iron absorption, such as vitamin C–rich foods.*

Vitamin C enhances the absorption of iron from plant sources.

• *Women of childbearing age who may become pregnant and those in the first trimester of pregnancy. Consume adequate synthetic folic acid daily (from fortified foods or supplements) in addition to food forms of folate from a varied diet.*

Women capable of becoming pregnant are urged to obtain 400 micrograms of folic acid through supplements or fortified food in addition to natural folate obtained through a normal mixed diet. Notice the word "or." Women who consume folic acid–fortified cereal do not need a supplement; in fact, they may be at risk for an excessive folic acid intake if they consume both. Although fortified cereals only provide 400 micrograms of folic acid per serving, actual portion sizes eaten are usually much bigger.

• *Older adults, people with dark skin, and people exposed to insufficient ultraviolet band radiation (i.e., sunlight). Consume extra vitamin D from vitamin D–fortified foods and/or supplements.*

"Extra" is not defined.

*Source:* United States Department of Health and Human Services, United States Department of Agriculture. (2005). *Dietary Guidelines for Americans* (7th ed.). Available at www.cnpp.usda.gov/dietaryguidelines.htm

---

With few exceptions, healthy people who eat a variety of nutritious foods are able to obtain an adequate and balanced intake of vitamins, other essential nutrients, and healthy food components for which no recommendations have been made. Those exceptions are identified in the *Dietary Guidelines'* key recommendations for specific population groups (Box 5.2).

Other groups who many benefit from a multivitamin supplement include

• Dieters who consume less than 1200 calories. Even with optimal food choices, it may not be possible to consume adequate amounts of all nutrients on a low-calorie diet.
• Vegans, who eat no animal products, need supplemental $B_{12}$ because it is found naturally only in animal products. They may also need vitamin D if sunlight exposure is inadequate because the only plant sources of vitamin D are some fortified margarines and some fortified cereals.
• Finicky eaters and people who eliminate one or more food groups from their typical diet. For instance, someone who cannot tolerate citrus juices because of gastric reflux may not consistently obtain adequate vitamin C without the use of a vitamin supplement.
• The elderly, who may have an inadequate food intake related to a limited food budget, impaired chewing and swallowing, social isolation, physical limitations that make shopping

or cooking difficult, or a decreased sense of taste leading to poor appetite. In addition, their vitamin requirements may be elevated as a result of chronic disease or as a side effect of certain medications. Low-dose multivitamin and mineral supplements can help meet recommended intake levels in the elderly (ADA, 2005).

- Alcoholics, because alcohol alters vitamin intake, absorption, metabolism, and excretion. The nutrients most profoundly affected are thiamin, riboflavin, niacin, folic acid, and pantothenic acid.

## Can Supplements Be Used As Insurance Against Poor Food Choices?

While there is little scientific evidence to suggest that vitamin supplements can benefit the average person, there is also little evidence of harm from low-dose multivitamin or multivitamin and mineral supplements. Because vitamins work best together and in balanced proportions, a multivitamin that provides no more than 100% of the Daily Value (DV) is usually better than single-vitamin supplements that tend to provide doses much greater than the RDA. Remember that pills are not a substitute for healthy food: "supplement" means "add to," not "replace."

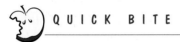

### QUICK BITE

Supplement labeling lingo

"High potency," at least to the FDA, means that at least ⅔ of the product's nutrients are provided at 100% of the DV. To most people, high potency means more than the DV.

"Advanced," "Complete," or "Maximum" formulas are not defined; manufacturers can use those terms as desired.

"Mature" or "50+" formulas usually have less iron and vitamin K. While seniors do need less iron, the need for vitamin K does not decrease with aging. In fact, vitamin K may help prevent hip fractures. However, people using anticoagulants should strive for a consistent vitamin K intake.

"Women's" formulas have 18 mg of iron, which is appropriate for premenopausal women. Postmenopausal women need around 8 mg, which is the same amount of iron as men need.

The FDA requires a standardized "Supplement Facts" label on all supplements (Fig. 5.4). Like the "Nutrition Facts" label, the supplement label is intended to provide consumers with better information. However, beware of label claims: because the FDA does not closely regulate the supplement industry, manufacturers' claims may be less than reliable and not defined. In fact, the term "multivitamin" does not have a standard regulatory definition (Yetley, 2007).

## A Word of Caution

Supplements taken to augment an intake that is already adequate are unnecessary; using supplements *and* fortified foods may be potentially dangerous—at least for vitamin A. In 2001, the Institute of Medicine lowered the RDA for vitamin A from 1000 to 900 micrograms retinol equivalent (RE) per day for men and from 800 to 700 micrograms/day for women. However, the Daily Reference Value used to calculate the percent DV on food

Cost is not an indication of quality. Large retail chains are high volume customers and can demand their own top-quality, private label supplements that are comparable to brand name varieties in quality and content.

For most people, a multivitamin that provides no more than 100% Daily Value for the 13 vitamins (and 8 minerals) for which there are established Daily Values. Note: Daily Values are the same as the 1968 USRDA and may not accurately reflect current DRI's.

USP on the label means the product passes tests for disintegration, dissolution, strength and purity. Does not ensure that the supplement is safe or beneficial to health.

Complete ingredient list must be stated.

Made to U.S. Pharmacopia (USP) quality, purity, and potency standards. Laboratory tested to dissolve within 60 minutes.

Ingredients: Cellulose, Ascorbic acid, cornstarch, dl-Alpha Tocophenyl acetate, Niacinamide, Stearic acid, Maltodextrin, Gelatin, d-Calcium Panthothenate, Pyridoxine hydrochloride, Sucrose, Riboflavin, Vitamin A acetate, Thiamine mononitrate, Lycopene, Folic Acid, Beta Carotene, dl-Alpha Tocopherol, Biotin, Cyanocobalamin, Ergocalciferol.

Serving size (and calories per serving, if any) must be stated.

## Supplement Facts

Serving Size 1 Tablet

| Each Tablet Contains | | % DV |
|---|---|---|
| Vitamin A | 3500 iu | 70% |
| 14% as beta carotene | | |
| Vitamin C | 90 mg | 150% |
| Vitamin D | 400 iu | 100% |
| Vitamin E | 45 iu | 150% |
| Vitamin K | 20 mcg | 25% |
| Thiamin (B$_1$) | 1.2 mg | 80% |
| Riboflavin (B$_2$) | 1.7 mg | 100% |
| Niacin (B$_3$) | 16 mg | 80% |
| Vitamin B$_6$ | 3 mg | 150% |
| Folic Acid | 400 mcg | 100% |
| Vitamin B$_{12}$ | 18 mcg | 300% |
| Biotin | 30 mcg | 10% |
| Pantothenic Acid | 5 mg | 50% |
| Lycopene | 0.6 mg | * |

* Daily Value not established

Median US intake of these B vitamins meets or exceeds recommendations; they aren't dangerous but probably aren't necessary.

Deficiencies of these vitamins almost never occur. They are not necessary.

Ingredients not proven to be important to health must appear at the bottom and be separated from established nutrients by a solid line.

dl-Alpha Tocopherol is the synthetic form of Vitamin E and is less well absorbed than natural Vitamin E labeled d-Alpha Tocopherol.

The amount of nutrient present and the % Daily Value must be listed.

FRESHNESS AND POTENCY GUARANTEED THROUGH JUN 2012

Beyond this date the ingredients may no longer meet standards of purity, strength, and/or quality.

Manufacturers are free to put in or leave out whatever nutrients they choose

For ingredients that do not have a Daily Value, an asterisk must be used to indicate there is no official recommendation for that substance.

**FIGURE 5.4** Sample supplement label.

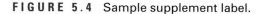

and supplement labels is 5000 IU (approximately 1500 micrograms RE), which is the 1968 RDA. This means that food and supplement labels *underreport* the percentage of vitamin A provided according to current recommendations. For instance, a vitamin supplement that supplies 100% of the DV, with all of it in the form of preformed vitamin A, is actually providing 1500 micrograms RE, not 700 or 900 micrograms as one would expect. With one vitamin supplement, the intake of vitamin A is above the recommended intake.

But that may be only half the problem. Because food manufacturers are free to decide which foods to **fortify** with vitamin A, which form of vitamin A to add, and at what level, the variety of foods fortified with preformed vitamin A is increasing. No longer limited to milk and some margarines, preformed vitamin A can now be found in cereals, cereal bars, energy bars, and even candy. Look how quickly the UL of 3000 micrograms/day is approached:

**Fortify:** to add nutrients that are not naturally found in the food, for example, milk is fortified with vitamin D and some breakfast cereals are fortified with vitamin $B_{12}$.

| Food Group | Micrograms of vitamin A |
|---|---|
| 1 vitamin supplement with 100% DV for vitamin A | 1500 |
| 1 meal replacement bar | 750 |
| 2 cups of milk | 300 |
| 1 cup of ready-to-eat cereal | 215 |
| Total | 2765 |

**Osteoporosis:** porous bones due to the loss of bone density.

While 2765 micrograms is small compared to the 30,000 micrograms/day for months associated with toxicity symptoms, **osteoporosis** and hip fracture are associated with preformed vitamin A intakes that are only twice the current RDA (Penniston & Tanumihardjo, 2006). Caution with using both fortified foods and a supplement is advised.

## ▶How Do You Respond?

**Is it better to take vitamin supplements with meals or between meals?** In general, it is better to take supplements with meals because food enhances the absorption of some vitamins.

**Should I choose vitamin-fortified foods over those that are not fortified?** For the most part, fortified foods are a good bet. Fortified milk and fortified cereals provide nutrients (vitamin D and iron respectively) that otherwise may not be consumed in adequate amounts by some people. On the other hand, a vitamin-fortified candy bar is still a candy bar. Be aware of slick marketing techniques that might lead you to believe that junk food with vitamins is healthy.

**I am under a lot of emotional stress. Should I take stress vitamins?** Although significant physical stress (e.g., thermal injury, trauma) increases the requirements for certain vitamins, mental stress does not. Misleading advertising is to blame for this widespread misconception.

## ▶ Case Study

Michael is a 22-year-old college student who lives off campus. Although he has a kitchen in his apartment, he has neither the time nor the interest in making his own food or stocking his own kitchen. All three of his daily meals come from fast food restaurants. A typical day's intake is as follows:

---

**Breakfast:** Two egg and bacon sandwiches on English muffins
Large coffee with creamer and sugar

**Lunch:** Two cheeseburgers with catsup
Large French fry
Soft drink
Cookies

**Dinner:** A foot-long submarine with cold cuts, cheese, mayonnaise, lettuce, tomato, onion, and pickles
Bag of potato chips
Soft drinks

**Snacks:** Chocolate bar
Chips and salsa
Popcorn

---

- What vitamins is Michael probably lacking in his diet? What vitamins is he probably getting enough of?
- Are there better choices he could make at fast food restaurants that would improve his vitamin intake?
- What suggestions would you make for keeping "quick" and "easy" food in his apartment that would improve his vitamin intake without being too much "bother"?
- How would you respond to this question from Michael: "Can I just take a multivitamin so I don't have to make changes in my eating habits?"

## STUDY QUESTIONS

1. When developing a teaching plan for a client who is on coumadin, which of the following foods would the nurse suggest the client consume a consistent intake of because of their vitamin K content?
   a. Liver, milk, and eggs
   b. Brussels sprouts, cauliflower, and spinach
   c. Fortified cereals, whole grains, and nuts
   d. Dried peas and beans, wheat germ, and seeds

2. A client asks if it is better to consume folic acid from fortified foods or from a vitamin pill. Which of the following is the nurse's best response?
   a. "It is better to consume folic acid through fortified foods because it will be better absorbed than through pill form."
   b. "It is better to consume folic acid through vitamin pills because it will be better absorbed than through fortified foods."
   c. "Fortified foods and vitamin pills have the same form of folic acid, so it does not matter which source you use because they are both well absorbed."
   d. "It is best to consume naturally rich sources of folic acid because that form is better absorbed than the folic acid in either fortified foods or vitamin pills."

3. Which population is at risk for combined deficiencies of thiamin, riboflavin, and niacin?
   a. Pregnant women
   b. Vegetarians
   c. Alcoholics
   d. Athletes

4. Which vitamin is given in large doses to facilitate wound and bone healing?
   a. Vitamin A
   b. Vitamin D
   c. Vitamin C
   d. Niacin

5. Which statement indicates that the client understands the instruction about using a vitamin supplement?
   a. "USP on the label guarantees safety and effectiveness."
   b. "Natural vitamins are always better for you than synthetic vitamins."
   c. "Vitamins are best absorbed on an empty stomach."
   d. "Taking a multivitamin cannot make up for poor food choices."

6. The client asks if taking supplements of beta-carotene will help reduce the risk of cancer. Which of the following would be the nurse's best response?
   a. "Supplements of beta-carotene may help reduce the risk of heart disease but not of cancer."
   b. "Supplements of beta-carotene have not been shown to lower the risk of cancer and may even promote cancer in certain people."
   c. "Although evidence is preliminary, taking beta-carotene supplements is safe and may prove to be effective against cancer in the future."
   d. "Natural supplements of beta-carotene are generally harmless; synthetic supplements of beta-carotene may increase cancer risk and should be avoided."

7. A client is diagnosed with pernicious anemia. What vitamin is he not absorbing?
   a. Folic acid
   b. Vitamin $B_6$
   c. Vitamin $B_{12}$
   d. Niacin

8. A client with hyperlipidemia is prescribed niacin. The client asks if he can just include more niacin-rich foods in his diet and forgo the need for niacin in pill form. Which of the following would be the nurse's best response?
   a. "The dose of niacin needed to treat hyperlipidemia is far more than can be consumed through eating a niacin-rich diet."
   b. "You can't get the therapeutic form of niacin through food."
   c. "Niacin from food is not as well absorbed as niacin from pills."
   d. "If you are able to consistently choose niacin-fortified foods in your diet, your doctor may allow you to forgo the pills and rely on dietary sources of niacin."

## KEY CONCEPTS

- Vitamins do not provide energy (calories) but they are needed for metabolism of energy. Most vitamins function as coenzymes to activate enzymes.
- The body needs vitamins in small amounts (microgram or milligram quantities). Vitamins are essential in the diet because they cannot be made by the body or they are synthesized in inadequate amounts.
- Fortification and enrichment have virtually eliminated vitamin deficiencies in healthy Americans.
- It is assumed that if a variety of nutritious foods are consumed, the diet's vitamin content will generally be adequate for most people.
- Vitamins are organic compounds that are soluble in either water or fat; their solubility determines how they are absorbed, transported through the blood, stored, and excreted.
- Vitamins A, D, E, and K are the fat-soluble vitamins. Because they are stored in liver and adipose tissue, they do not need to be consumed daily. Vitamins A and D are toxic when consumed in large quantities over a long period.
- The B-complex vitamins and vitamin C are water-soluble vitamins. Although some tissues are able to hold limited amounts of certain water-soluble vitamins, they are not generally stored in the body, so a daily intake is necessary. Because they are not stored, they are considered nontoxic; however, adverse side effects can occur from taking megadoses of certain water-soluble vitamins over a prolonged period.

● Phytochemicals are substances produced by plants to protect them from bacteria, viruses, and fungi. They add color, flavor, and aroma to foods. In the body, they impart important physiologic effects that may reduce the risk of chronic diseases.

● Not enough is known about phytochemicals to elevate them to the status of essential nutrients. Research is needed to determine which phytochemicals are protective, what quantity is optimal for health, and how they interact with other substances. Until then, the best advice is to eat a varied diet rich in fruits and vegetables.

● Antioxidant vitamins in foods are suspected of being beneficial, but high-dose supplements have not been proven to prevent disease and may disrupt nutrient balances. Long-term safety has not been established; some reports indicate that single-nutrient supplements may actually increase, not decrease, health risks.

● It is recommended that women who are capable of becoming pregnant consume 400 micrograms of folic acid through supplements or fortified food daily. People over the age of 50 are urged to consume most of their $B_{12}$ requirement from supplements or fortified food. Vegans need supplemental vitamin D, if exposure to sunshine is inadequate, and also supplemental vitamin $B_{12}$.

● Multivitamin supplements provide a limited safeguard when food choices are less than optimal. Other groups who may benefit from taking a daily multivitamin are the elderly, dieters, finicky eaters, and alcoholics.

● People who choose to take an all-purpose multivitamin should select one that provides 100% of the DV for vitamins with an established DV. The USP stamp ensures the quality, but not safety or benefits. High-cost supplements are not necessarily superior to lower-cost ones.

## ANSWER KEY

1. **FALSE** In theory, most healthy adults should be able to obtain all the nutrients they need by choosing a varied diet of nutrient-dense foods. Exceptions include (1) people over 50 who should consume synthetic vitamin $B_{12}$ from fortified food or supplements, (2) women who are capable of becoming pregnant need synthetic folic acid, and (3) anyone who obtains insufficient sunlight exposure needs supplemental vitamin D.

2. **FALSE** Vitamins are needed to release energy from carbohydrates, protein, and fat but are not a source of energy (calories).

3. **FALSE** Adverse side effects can occur from taking large doses of certain water-soluble vitamins over a long period of time. For instance, adverse effects can be seen from large doses of $B_6$ (neuropathy) and niacin (flushing).

4. **TRUE** Vitamins differ in their vulnerability to air, heat, light, acids, and alkalis. Proper food handling and storage, especially of fruits and vegetables, are needed to preserve vitamin content.

5. **FALSE** Cost and quality are not necessarily related.

6. **FALSE** "Natural" vitamins are not naturally better.

7. **TRUE** Under optimal conditions, such as exposing unprotected skin to the sun in the southern United States for several minutes, the body can make all the vitamin D it needs provided that kidney and liver functions are normal. However, sunscreen, smog, dark skin, clothing, and dense cloud cover hinder vitamin D synthesis.

8. **FALSE** Natural folate in foods is only half as available to the body as synthetic folic acid.

9. **FALSE** USP on a vitamin label means that the product passes tests that evaluate disintegration, dissolution, strength, and purity. It does not mean the product is safe. For instance, large doses of vitamin A are not safe but they may have USP on the label.

10. **FALSE** Because fat-soluble vitamins are stored, a daily intake is not considered essential. It is recommended that water-soluble vitamins be consumed daily because they are not stored in the body.

## WEBSITES

Produce for Better Health Foundation at **www.fruitsandveggiesmorematters.org**
Dietary Reference Intakes from the Institute of Medicine at **www.nap.edu**

## REFERENCES

American Dietetic Association. (2005). Position Paper of the American Dietetic Association: Nutrition across the spectrum of aging. *Journal of the American Dietetic Association, 105,* 616–633.

American Heart Association (AHA). (2007). *Homocysteine, folic acid and cardiovascular disease.* Available at www.americanheart.org/print_presenter.jhtml?identifier=4677. Accessed on 11/12/07.

Bønaa, K., Njølstad, I., Ueland, P., et al. (2006). Homocysteine lowering and cardiovascular events after acute myocardial infarction. *The New England Journal of Medicine, 354,* 1578–1588.

CDC. (2007). Fruit and vegetable consumption among adults—United States, 2005. *Morbidity and mortality weekly report,* March 16, 56(10), 213–217. Available at www.cdc.gov/mmwR/preview/mmwrhtml/mm5610a2.htm. Accessed on 11/12/07.

Darmon, N., Darmon, M., Maillot, M., et al. (2005). A nutrient density standard for vegetables and fruits: Nutrients per calorie and nutrients per unit cost. *Journal of the American Dietetic Association, 105,* 1881–1887.

Egan, K., Sosman, J., & Blot, W. (2005). Sunlight and reduced risk of cancer: Is the real story vitamin D? *Journal of the National Cancer Institute, 97,* 161–163.

Food and Nutrition Board, Institute of Medicine. (1997). *Dietary Reference Intakes for calcium, phosphorus, magnesium, vitamin D, and fluoride.* Washington, DC: National Academies Press.

Food and Nutrition Board, Institute of Medicine. (1998). *Dietary Reference Intakes for thiamin, riboflavin, niacin, vitamin $B_6$, folate, vitamin $B_{12}$, pantothenic acid, biotin, and choline.* Washington, DC: National Academies Press.

Food and Nutrition Board, Institute of Medicine (IOM). (2000). *Dietary Reference Intakes for vitamin C, vitamin E, selenium, and carotenoids.* Washington, DC: National Academies Press.

Food and Nutrition Board, Institute of Medicine. (2001). *Dietary Reference Intakes for vitamin A, vitamin K, arsenic, boron, chromium, copper, iodine, iron, manganese, molybdenum, nickel, silicon, vanadium, and zinc.* Washington, DC: National Academies Press.

Fragakis, A., & Thomson, C. (2007). *The health professional's guide to popular dietary supplements* (3rd ed.). Chicago: The American Dietetic Association.

Giovannucci, E. (2006). The epidemiology of vitamin D and colorectal cancer: Recent findings. *Current Opinion in Gastroenterology, 22,* 24–29.

Giovannucci, E., Liu, Y., Rimm, E., et al. (2006). Prospective study of predictors of vitamin D status and cancer incidence and mortality in men. *Journal of the National Cancer Institute, 98,* 451–459.

Goodyear-Smith, F., & Arroll, B. (2004). What can family physicians offer patients with carpal tunnel syndrome other than surgery? A systematic review of nonsurgical management. *Annals of Family Medicine, 2,* 267–273.

Green, A., Williams, G., Neale, R., et al. (1999). Daily sunscreen application and betacarotene supplementation in prevention of basal-cell and squamous-cell carcinomas of the skin: a randomized controlled trial. *Lancet, 354,* 723–729.

Halvorsen, B. L., Carlsen, M. H., Phillips, K. M., et al. (2006). Content of redox-active compounds (e.g., antioxidants) in foods consumed in the United States. *The American Journal of Clinical Nutrition, 84,* 95–135.

Hathcock, J. N., Azzi, A., Blumberg, J., et al. (2005). Vitamins E and C are safe across a broad range of intakes. *The American Journal of Clinical Nutrition, 81,* 736–745.

Hathcock, J. N., Shao, A., Vieth, R., et al. (2007). Risk assessment for vitamin D. *The American Journal of Clinical Nutrition, 85,* 6–18.

Holick, M. (2004). Vitamin D: Importance in the prevention of cancers, type 2 diabetes, heart disease, and osteoporosis. *The American Journal of Clinical Nutrition, 79,* 362–371.

International Food Information Council. (2005). The health effects of vitamin E: A case study in communicating emerging science. Available online at www.ific.org/foodinsight/2005/ja/vitaminefi405.cfm?renderforprint=1. Accessed on 9/17/07.

Lappe, J. M., Travers-Gustafson, D., Davies, K. M., et al. (2007). Vitamin D and calcium supplementation reduces cancer risk: Results of a randomized trial. *The American Journal of Clinical Nutrition, 85,* 1586–1591.

Lee, I., Cook, N., Manson, J., et al. (1999). Beta-carotene supplementation and incidence of cancer and cardiovascular disease: The Women's Health Study. *Journal of the National Cancer Institute, 91,* 2101–2106.

Lonn, E., Yusuf, S., Arnold, M. J., et al. (2006). Homocysteine lowering with folic acid and B vitamins in vascular disease. *The New England Journal of Medicine, 354,* 1567–1577.

Mark, B., & Carson, J. (2006). Vitamin D and autoimmune disease—Implications for practice from the multiple sclerosis literature. *Journal of the American Dietetic Association, 106,* 418–424.

McCully, L. (2007). Homocysteine, vitamins, and vascular disease prevention. *The American Journal of Clinical Nutrition, 86*(Suppl.), 1563S–1568S.

Medical Research Council Vitamin Study Research Group. (1991). Prevention of neural tube defects: Results of the Medical Research Council Vitamin Study. *Lancet, 338,* 131–137.

Miller, E. R. III, Pastor-Barriuso, R., Dalal, D., et al. (2005). Meta-analysis: high-dosage vitamin E supplementation may increase all-cause mortality. *Annals of Internal Medicine, 142,* 37–46.

Moshfegh, A., Goldman, J., & Cleveland, L. (2005). *What we eat in America, NHANES 2001–2002: Usual nutrient intakes from food compared to Dietary Reference Intakes.* US Department of Agriculture, Agricultural Research Service. Available at www.ars.usda.gov/SP2UserFiles/Place/12355000pdf.usualintaketables2001-2002.pdf. Accessed on 12/20/07.

National Institutes of Health State-of-the-Science Panel. (2007). National Institutes of Health State-of-the-Science Conference Statement: Multivitamin/mineral supplements and chronic disease prevention. *The American Journal of Clinical Nutrition, 85*(Suppl.), 257S–264S.

Omenn, G. S., Goodman, G. E., Thornquist, M. D., et al. (1996). Effects of a combination of beta carotene and vitamin A on lung cancer and cardiovascular disease. *The New England Journal of Medicine, 334,* 1150–1155.

Penniston, K., & Tanumihardjo, S. (2006). The acute and chronic toxic effects of vitamin A. *The American Journal of Clinical Nutrition, 83,* 191–201.

Peters, E. M., Goetzsche, J. M., Grobbelaar, B., et al. (1993). Vitamin C supplementation reduces the incidence of postrace symptoms of upper-respiratory-tract infection in ultramarathon runners. *The American Journal of Clinical Nutrition, 57,* 170–174.

Pittas, A. G., Dawson-Huges, B., Li, T., et al. (2006). Vitamin D and calcium intake in relation to type 2 diabetes in women. *Diabetes Care, 29,* 650–656.

Rock, C. (2007). Multivitamin-multimineral supplements: Who uses them? *The American Journal of Clinical Nutrition, 85*(Suppl.), 277S–279S.

Tangpricha, V., Pearce, E. N., Chen, T. C., et al. (2002). Vitamin D insufficiency among free-living healthy young adults. *The American Journal of Medicine, 112,* 659–662.

The Alpha-Tocopherol, Beta Carotene Cancer Prevention Study Group. (1994). The effect of vitamin D and beta carotene on the incidence of lung cancer and other cancers in small smokers. *The New England Journal of Medicine, 330,* 1029–1035.

United States Department of Health and Human Services, United States Department of Agriculture. (2005). *Dietary guidelines for Americans* (7th ed.). Available at www.cnpp.usda.gov/dietaryguidelines.htm

Vieth, R. (2006). Critique of the considerations for establishing tolerable upper intake levels for vitamin D: Critical need for revision upwards. *The Journal of Nutrition, 136,* 1117–1122.

Vieth, R., Bischoff-Ferrari, H., Boucher, B. J., et al. (2007). The urgent need to recommend an intake of vitamin D that is effective. *The American Journal of Clinical Nutrition, 85,* 649–650.

Weng, F. L., Shults, J., Leonard, M. B., et al. (2007). Risk factors for low serum 25-hydroxyvitamin D concentrations in otherwise healthy children and adolescents. *The American Journal of Clinical Nutrition, 86,* 150–158.

Winkels, R. M., Brouwer, I. A., Siebelink, E., et al. (2007). Bioavailability of food folates is 80% of that of folic acid. *The American Journal of Clinical Nutrition, 85,* 465–473.

Wright, M., Lawson, K., Weinstein, S., et al. (2006). Higher baseline serum concentrations of vitamin D are associated with lower total and cause-specific mortality in the Alpha-Tocopherol, Beta-Carotene Cancer Prevention Study. American Journal of Clinical Nutrition, 84, 1200–1207.

Yetley, E. (2007). Multivitamin and multimineral dietary supplements: Definitions, characterization, bioavailability, and drug interactions. *The American Journal of Clinical Nutrition, 85*(Suppl.), 269S–276S.

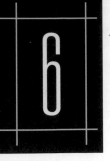

# 6 Water and Minerals

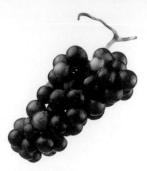

### UPON COMPLETION OF THIS CHAPTER, YOU WILL BE ABLE TO

- Calculate a person's fluid requirement.
- Evaluate the adequacy of fluid intake in a healthy adult.
- Give examples of mechanisms by which the body maintains mineral homeostasis.
- Identify sources of minerals.
- Predict potential consequences of mineral deficiencies or toxicities.
- Compare characteristics of minerals to those of vitamins.

## ▶ WATER

Water is fundamental to life. It is the single largest constituent of the human body, averaging 50% to 60% of the total body weight. It is the medium in which all biochemical reactions take place. Although most people can survive 6 weeks or longer without food, death occurs in a matter of days without water.

## Functions of Water

Water occupies essentially every space within and between body cells and is involved in virtually every body function. Water

- *Provides shape and structure to cells.* Approximately two-thirds of the body's water is located within cells (intracellular fluid). Muscle cells have a higher concentration of water (73%) than fat, which is only about 25% water. Men generally have more muscle mass than women have and, therefore, have a higher percentage of body water.
- *Regulates body temperature.* Because water absorbs heat slowly, the large amount of water contained in the body helps to maintain body temperature homeostasis despite fluctuations in environmental temperatures. Evaporation of water (sweat) from the skin cools the body.
- *Aids in the digestion and absorption of nutrients.* Approximately 7 to 9 L of water is secreted in the gastrointestinal tract daily to aid in digestion and absorption. Except for the approximately 100 mL of water excreted through the feces, all of the water contained in the gastrointestinal secretions (saliva, gastric secretions, bile, pancreatic secretions, and intestinal mucosal secretions) is reabsorbed in the ileum and colon.
- *Transports nutrients and oxygen to cells.* By moistening the air sacs in the lungs, water allows oxygen to dissolve and move into blood for distribution throughout the body. Approximately 92% of blood plasma is water.
- *Serves as a solvent for vitamins, minerals, glucose, and amino acids.* The solvating property of water is vital for health and survival.
- *Participates in metabolic reactions.* For instance, water is used in the synthesis of hormones and enzymes.
- *Eliminates waste products.* Water helps to excrete body wastes through urine, feces, and expirations.
- *Is a major component of mucus and other lubricating fluids.* Water reduces friction in joints where bones, ligaments, and tendons come in contact with each other and it cushions contacts between internal organs that slide over one another.

## Water Balance

Total body water is tightly regulated within ±0.2% of body weight. Normally, the sensation of thirst and the action of the hormone vasopressin control fluid balance on a day-to-day basis, a state where output and intake are approximately equal.

### Water Output

On average, adults lose approximately 1750 to 3000 mL of water daily (Table 6.1). Extreme environmental temperatures (very hot or very cold), high altitude, low humidity, and

---

**TABLE 6.1  Sources and Average Amounts of Daily Water Loss**

| Source of Water Loss | Average Amount Lost (mL/day) |
| --- | --- |
| Respiratory | 200–350 |
| Urinary | 1000–2000 |
| Fecal | 100–200 |
| Skin | 450 |
| Total | 1750–3000 |

*Source:* National Academy of Sciences, Institute of Medicine (2004). *Dietary Reference Intakes for water, potassium, sodium, chloride, and sulfate.* Washington, DC: National Academies Press.

strenuous exercise increase **insensible water losses** from respirations and the skin. Water evaporation from the skin is also increased by prolonged exposure to heated or recirculated air, such as during long airplane flights. **Sensible water losses** from urine and feces make up the remaining water loss. Because the body needs to excrete a minimum of 500 mL of urine daily to rid itself of metabolic wastes, the minimum daily total fluid output is approximately 1500 mL. To maintain water balance, intake should approximate output.

**Insensible Water Loss:** immeasurable losses.

**Sensible Water Loss:** measurable losses.

## Water Intake

Total water intake is comprised of water consumed in drinking water, other beverages, and solid foods.

**Drinking Water.** Drinking water, including both tap water and bottled water, accounts for 35% to 55% of total water consumed (PDRIEW, 2004). In 2007, bottled water was the seventh top consumer packaged good sold in U.S. retail stores, according to research on consumer trends by The Nielsen Company (Crowley, 2007). Nutritionally, tap water and bottled water are not significantly different, yet the cost of bottled water can be 10,000 times more expensive than that of tap water (Owen, 2006). The FDA has set standards of identity for bottled water products sold in the United States (Box 6.1). Soda water, tonic water, and club soda are carbonated soft drinks, not different varieties of water.

**Other Beverages.** Juice, carbonated beverages, coffee, tea, and milk account for 49% to 63% of total water consumed (PDRIEW, 2004). These beverages also currently provide 21% of total calories consumed by Americans older than 2 (Neilsen & Popkin, 2004). According to the Beverage Guidance Panel, a group formed to provide guidance on the nutritional

---

**BOX 6.1**     **STANDARDS OF IDENTITY FOR COMMON TYPES OF BOTTLED WATER**

- *Artesian water* originates from a well and is collected without mechanical pumping. The well must tap a confined aquifer, and the water level must stand at some height above the top of the aquifer. An aquifer is an underground layer of rock or sand with water.
- *Fluoridated water* has fluoride added within the limits established by the FDA.
- *Ground water* is from an underground source that is under pressure greater than or equal to atmospheric pressure.
- *Mineral water* contains at least 250 ppm total dissolved solids (minerals) that are naturally present, not added.
- *Purified water* is produced by distillation, deionization, reverse osmosis, or other suitable processes to remove minerals and other solids. It may also be referred to as "demineralized" water. Purified is not synonymous with "sterile."
- *Sparkling water* contains a "fizz" from carbon dioxide that was either present in the water when it emerged from its source or was present, removed in processing, and then replaced. Carbon dioxide levels cannot exceed the amount present in the original water. Seltzer, tonic water, and club soda are carbonated soft drinks that contain sugar and calories; they are not types of sparkling water.
- *Spring water* comes from an underground source that flows naturally to the surface. It must be collected at the spring or through a bored hole that taps the spring underground.
- *Sterile water* meets U.S. Pharmacopoeia (USP) requirements under "sterility tests."
- *Well water* is collected with a mechanical pump from an underground aquifer.

*Source:* National Science Foundation Consumer Information: Types and treatment of bottled water. Available at www.nsf.org/consumer/bottled_water/bw_types.asp?program+Bottledwat. Accessed on 12/5/07.

benefits and risks of various types of beverages, the current high intake of sweetened beverages contributes to an excess calorie intake and is a factor in the development of obesity (Popkin et al., 2006). Both portion sizes and the number of servings per day of sweetened beverages increased in national consumption surveys between 1977 and 1996 (Neilsen & Popkin, 2004). Although naturally calorie-free plain water could be used to completely satisfy fluid needs, other beverages have value in that they may provide nutrients, phytochemicals, and interest to the diet.

**Solid Foods.** Approximately 19% to 25% of total water intake comes from the water in food (PDRIEW, 2004). Fruits and vegetables are highest in water content, and fats and oils are lowest.

## Water Recommendations

### QUICK BITE

Percentage of water in selected foods

| | % water by weight |
|---|---|
| Lettuce | 95 |
| Watermelon | 92 |
| Broccoli | 91 |
| Milk | 89 |
| Carrot | 87 |
| Yogurt | 85 |
| Chicken | 65 |
| Whole wheat bread | 38 |
| Honey | 17 |
| Vegetable oil | 0 |

Water is an essential nutrient because the body cannot produce as much water as it needs. The DRI committee on fluid and electrolytes did not establish a Recommended Dietary Allowance (RDA) for water because of insufficient evidence linking a specific amount of water intake to health; actual requirements vary greatly among individuals (Weaver et al., 2006). The Adequate Intake (AI) for total water, which includes water from liquids and solids, is based on the median total water intake from U.S. food consumption survey data. For men aged 19 to older than 70 years, the AI is 3.7 L/day, which includes 3 L as drinking water and other beverages and the remainder coming from solid food. For women of the same age, the AI is 2.7 L, of which approximately 2.2 L comes from drinking water and beverages. Similar to AIs set for other nutrients, daily intakes below the AI may not be harmful to healthy people because normal hydration is maintained over a wide range of intakes. Intakes higher than the AI are recommended for rigorous activity in hot climates. Because the body cannot store water, it should be consumed throughout the day.

For healthy people, the universal, age-old advice has been to drink at least eight 8-ounce glasses of fluid daily, preferably in the form of water. Little scientific evidence supports this recommendation (Valtin, 2002). Food surveys show that many adults routinely consume less than the "8 × 8" recommendation without suffering any adverse effects because of the body's finely tuned osmoregulatory system that maintains fluid balance. For healthy adults, thirst is usually a reliable indicator of water need, and fluid intake is assumed to be adequate when the color of urine produced is pale yellow.

In some conditions and for some segments of the population, the sensation of thirst is blunted and may not be a reliable indicator of need. For the elderly and children, and during hot weather or strenuous exercise, drinking fluids should not be delayed until the sensation of thirst occurs because by then fluid loss is significant.

In clinical situations, actual water requirement is highly variable. Vomiting, diarrhea, fever, thermal injuries, uncontrolled diabetes, hemorrhage, and certain renal disorders increase water losses as does the use of drainage tubes. Fluid needs can be estimated by several methods (Table 6.2). Intake and output records are used to assess adequacy of intake.

| TABLE 6.2 | **Methods to Estimate Fluid Needs** | |
|---|---|---|
| **Method** | **Recommendation** | **Example (for a 70 kg person consuming 2000 cal/day)** |
| 1 | 30 mL/kg body weight | 70 kg × 30 mL/kg = 2100 mL/day |
| 2 | 1 mL/cal consumed | 1 mL/cal × 2000 cal/day = 2000 mL/day |
| 3 | 100 mL/kg for the first 10 kg, | 100 mL/kg for the first 10 kg = 1000 mL |
| | 50 mL/kg for the next 10 kg, | 50 mL/kg for the next 10 kg = 500 mL |
| | 15 mL/kg for each remaining kg of body weight | 15 mL/kg for the remaining 50 mg = 750 mL |
| | | Total 2250 mL/day |

**Source:** Bossingham, M., Carnell, N., & Campbell, W. (2005). Water balance, hydration status, and fat-free mass hydration in younger and older adults. *The American Journal of Clinical Nutrition, 81*, 1342–1350.

## Alterations in Intake

An inadequate intake of water can lead to dehydration, characterized by impaired mental function, impaired motor control, increased body temperature during exercise, increased resting heart rate when standing or lying down, and an increased risk of life-threatening heat stroke. A net water loss of as little as 1% of body weight increases plasma osmolality, and a loss of 20% can be life threatening (Bossingham et al., 2005).

A chronic high intake of water has not been shown to cause adverse effects in healthy people who consume a varied diet as long as intake approximates output (PDRIEW, 2004). An excessive water intake may cause hyponatremia, but it is rare in healthy people who consume a typical diet. People most at risk include infants, psychiatric patients with excessive thirst, women who have undergone surgery using a uterine distention medium, and athletes in endurance events who drink too much water, fail to replace lost sodium, or both. Symptoms of hyponatremia include lung congestion, muscle weakness, lethargy, and confusion. Hyponatremia can progress to convulsions and prolonged coma, and death can result.

## ▶ KEYS TO UNDERSTANDING MINERALS

Although minerals account for only about 4% of the body's total weight, they are found in all body fluids and tissues. Major minerals are present in the body in amounts greater than 5 g (the equivalent of 1 teaspoon). Calcium, phosphorus, magnesium, sulfur, sodium, potassium, and chloride are major minerals. Iron, iodine, zinc, selenium, copper, manganese, fluoride, chromium, and molybdenum are classified as trace minerals, or trace elements, because they are present in the body in amounts less than 5 g, not because they are less important than major minerals. Both groups are essential for life. As many as 30 other potentially harmful minerals are present in the body such as lead, gold, and mercury. Their presence appears to be related to environmental contamination.

## General Chemistry

**Inorganic:** not containing carbon or concerning living things.

Unlike the energy nutrients and vitamins, minerals are **inorganic** elements that originate from the earth's crust, not from plants or animals. Minerals do not undergo digestion nor are they broken down or rearranged during metabolism. Although they combine with other elements to form salts (e.g., sodium chloride) or with organic compounds (e.g., iron in hemoglobin), they always retain their chemical identities.

| TABLE 6.3 | General Functions of Minerals | |
|---|---|---|
| **Functions** | **Examples** | |
| Provide structure | Calcium, phosphorus, and magnesium provide structure to bones and teeth<br>Phosphorus, potassium, iron, and sulfur provide structure to soft tissues<br>Sulfur is a constituent of skin, hair, and nails | |
| Fluid Balance | Sodium, potassium, and chloride | |
| Acid–base balance | Sodium hydroxide and sodium bicarbonate are part of the carbonic acid–bicarbonate system that regulates blood pH<br>Phosphorus is involved in buffer systems that regulate kidney tubular fluids | |
| Nerve cell transmission and muscle contraction | Sodium and potassium are involved in transmission of nerve impulses<br>Calcium stimulates muscle contractions<br>Sodium, potassium, and magnesium stimulate muscle relaxation | |
| Vitamin, enzyme, and hormone activity | Cobalt is a component of vitamin $B_{12}$<br>Magnesium is a cofactor for hundreds of enzymes<br>Iodine is essential for the production of thyroxine<br>Chromium enhances the action of insulin | |

Unlike vitamins, minerals are not destroyed by light, air, heat, or acids during food preparation. In fact when food is completely burned, minerals are the ash that remains. Minerals are lost only when foods are soaked in water.

## General Functions

Minerals function to provide structure to body tissues and to regulate body processes such as fluid balance, acid–base balance, nerve cell transmission, muscle contraction, and vitamin, enzyme, and hormonal activities (Table 6.3).

## Mineral Balance

The body has several mechanisms by which it maintains mineral balance, depending on the mineral involved, such as

- *Releasing minerals from storage for redistribution.* Some minerals can be released from storage and redistributed as needed, which is what happens when calcium is released from bones to restore normal serum calcium levels.
- *Altering rate of absorption.* For example, normally only about 10% of the iron consumed is absorbed, but the rate increases to 50% when the body is deficient in iron.
- *Altering rate of excretion.* Virtually all of the sodium consumed in the diet is absorbed. The only way the body can rid itself of excess sodium is to increase urinary sodium excretion. For most people, the higher the intake of sodium, the greater the amount of sodium excreted in the urine. Excess potassium is also excreted in the urine.

## Mineral Toxicities

Minerals that are easily excreted, such as sodium and potassium, do not accumulate to toxic levels in the body under normal circumstances. Stored minerals can produce toxicity symptoms when intake is excessive, but excessive intake is not likely to occur from eating a balanced diet. Instead, mineral toxicity is related to excessive use of mineral supplements, environmental or industrial exposure, human errors in commercial food processing, or alterations in metabolism. For instance, more than a dozen Americans developed selenium toxicity after taking an improperly manufactured dietary supplement that contained 27.3 mg of selenium per tablet (500 times the RDA of 55 micrograms/day).

## Mineral Interactions

Mineral balance is significantly influenced by hundreds of interactions that occur among minerals and between minerals and other dietary components. For instance, caffeine promotes calcium excretion, whereas vitamin D and lactose promote its absorption. Mineral status must be viewed as a function of the total diet, not only from the standpoint of the quantity consumed.

## Sources of Minerals

Generally, unrefined or unprocessed foods have more minerals than refined foods. Trace mineral content varies with the content of soil from which the food originates. Within all food groups, processed foods are high in sodium and chloride. Drinking water contains varying amounts of calcium, magnesium, and other minerals; sodium is added to soften water. Fluoride may be a natural or added component of drinking water.

## ▶ MAJOR ELECTROLYTES

Sodium, chloride, and potassium are major minerals that are also major electrolytes in the body. Salient features for each electrolyte are presented in the following paragraphs. Table 6.4 details their recommended intakes, sources, functions, and signs and symptoms of deficiency and toxicity.

## Sodium

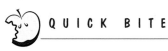

### QUICK BITE

**Examples of sodium additives**

To enhance flavor:
  Sodium chloride
  Monosodium glutamate (MSG)
  Soy sauce
  Teriyaki sauce
To preserve freshness:
  Brine
  Sodium benzoate
  Sodium nitrate or sodium nitrite
  Sodium propionate
  Sodium sulfite (for dried fruits)
As a leavening agent:
  Sodium bicarbonate (baking soda)
  Baking powder
As a stabilizer:
  Sodium citrate
  Disodium phosphate

By weight, salt (sodium chloride) is approximately 40% sodium; 1 teaspoon of salt (5 g) provides approximately 2300 mg of sodium. It is estimated that approximately 77% of the sodium consumed in the typical American diet comes from salt or sodium preservatives added to foods by food manufacturers. Only 12% of total sodium intake is from sodium that occurs naturally in foods such as milk, meat, poultry, vegetables, tap water, and bottled water (PDRIEW, 2004). Salt added during cooking or at the table accounts for the remaining sodium intake. Box 6.2 defines various types of salt. Wide variations in sodium intake exist between cultures and between individuals within a culture related to the amount of processed foods consumed.

As the major extracellular cation, sodium is largely responsible for regulating fluid balance. It also regulates cell permeability and the movement of fluid, electrolytes, glucose,

| TABLE 6.4 | Summary of Major Electrolytes |
|---|---|

| Electrolyte and Sources | Functions | Deficiency/Toxicity Signs and Symptoms |
|---|---|---|
| **Sodium (Na)**<br>Adult AI:<br>19–50 yr: 1.5 g<br>50–70 yr: 1.3 g<br>71+ yr: 1.2 g<br>Adult UL: 2.3 g<br>• Processed foods; canned meat, vegetables, soups; convenience foods; restaurant and fast foods | Fluid and electrolyte balance, acid–base balance, maintains muscle irritability, regulates cell membrane permeability and nerve impulse transmission | ***Deficiency***<br>Rare, except with chronic diarrhea or vomiting and certain renal disorders; nausea, dizziness, muscle cramps, apathy<br>***Toxicity***<br>Hypertension, edema |
| **Potassium (K)**<br>Adult AI: 4.7 g<br>No UL<br>• Canned tomato products, sweet potatoes, soy nuts, pistachios, prunes, clams, molasses, yogurt, tomato juice, prune juice, baked potatoes, cantaloupe, dried peas and beans, orange juice, bananas, peanuts, artichokes, fish, beef, lamb, avocados, apple juice, raisins, plantains, spinach, asparagus, kiwifruit, apricots | Fluid and electrolyte balance, acid–base balance, nerve impulse transmission, catalyst for many metabolic reactions, involved in skeletal and cardiac muscle activity | ***Deficiency***<br>Muscular weakness, paralysis, anorexia, confusion (occurs with dehydration)<br>***Toxicity (from supplements/drugs)***<br>Muscular weakness, vomiting |
| **Chloride (Cl)**<br>Adult AI: 19–50 yr: 2.3 g<br>50–70 yr: 2.0 g<br>71+ yr: 1.8 g<br>Adult UL: 3.6 g<br>• 1 tsp salt ≈ 3600 mg Cl<br>• Same sources as sodium | Fluid and electrolyte balance, acid–base balance, component of hydrochloric acid in stomach | ***Deficiency***<br>Rare, may occur secondary to chronic diarrhea or vomiting and certain renal disorders: muscle cramps, anorexia, apathy<br>***Toxicity***<br>Normally harmless; can cause vomiting |

insulin, and amino acids. Sodium is pivotal in acid–base balance, nerve transmission, and muscular irritability. Although sodium plays vital roles, under normal conditions the amount actually needed is very small, maybe even less than 200 mg/day.

Almost 98% of all sodium consumed is absorbed, yet humans are able to maintain homeostasis over a wide range of intakes, largely through urinary excretion. A salty meal causes a transitory increase in serum sodium, which triggers thirst. Drinking fluids dilutes the sodium in the blood to normal concentration, even though the volume of both sodium and fluid are increased. The increased volume stimulates the kidneys to excrete more sodium and fluid together to restore normal blood volume. Conversely, low blood volume or low extracellular sodium stimulates the hormone aldosterone to increase sodium reabsorption by the kidneys. In people who have minimal sweat losses, sodium intake and sodium excretion are approximately equal.

An AI for sodium is set at 1500 mg/day for young adults to ensure that the total diet provides adequate amounts of other essential nutrients and to compensate for sodium lost in sweat in unacclimatized people exposed to high temperatures or who become physically active. For men and women aged 50 to 70 years, the AI is 1300 mg, and after age 70 AI decreases to 1200 mg. An Upper Limit (UL) for adults is set at 2300 mg/day.

| BOX 6.2 | **TYPES OF SALT** |

*Table salt* is a fine-grained salt from salt mines that is refined until it is pure sodium chloride. It is mainly used in cooking and at the table and may or may not contain iodine. It often contains calcium silicate to keep it free flowing.

*Lite salt* is half regular salt (sodium chloride), half potassium chloride. It provides less sodium than table salt, but is not sodium free.

*Kosher salt* is a coarse-grain salt that does not contain any additives. It is used in the preparation of kosher meat according to Jewish dietary laws. Although the terms "kosher salt" and "sea salt" are often used interchangeably, kosher salt does not necessarily originate from the sea.

*Sea salt* may be fine or coarse grained. It has a slightly different taste than table salt due to its mineral content. Although it is often promoted as a healthier alternative to table salt, the sodium content is essentially the same. The advantage is that people may use less sea salt than table salt because of its more pronounced flavor. Examples include Mediterranean sea salt, Alaea (Hawaiian) sea salt, and Black salt—salts named after the originating sea.

*Pickling salt* is a fine-grained salt used for making pickles and sauerkraut. It does not contain additives or anticlumping agents.

*Specialty salts*, such as popcorn salt, come in various grains and textures and are intended for specific purposes. Generally, table salt can be substituted for these salts.

*Seasoned salt* is a blend of salt, herbs, and other seasoning ingredients. Examples include celery salt, onion salt, and garlic salt. The actual sodium content is lower than table salt because other ingredients dilute the concentration of sodium.

*Rock salt* is a nonedible salt of large crystals used to deice driveways and walkways. When combined with regular ice in home ice cream makers, it helps freeze homemade ice cream more quickly by absorbing heat.

**Source:** International Food Information Council. (2005). IFIC Review: Sodium in food and health. Available at www.ific.org/publications/reviews/sodiumir.cfm?renderforprint=1. Accessed on 12/4/07.

According to NHANES 2001–2002 data, estimated mean intake of sodium among adult men and women aged 31 to 50 years is 4252 and 3001 mg/day, respectively, and 100% of adult men and women exceed the AI of 1500 mg/day (Moshfegh et al., 2005). Figure 6.1 shows the relationship between the AI and UL for sodium and the sodium content of selected foods.

## Potassium

Most of the body's potassium is located in the cells as the major cation of the intracellular fluid. The remainder is in the extracellular fluid, where it works to maintain fluid balance, maintain acid–base balance, transmit nerve impulses, catalyze metabolic reactions, aid in carbohydrate metabolism and protein synthesis, and control skeletal muscle contractility.

In healthy people with normal kidney function, a high intake of potassium does not lead to an elevated serum potassium concentration because the hormone aldosterone promotes urinary potassium excretion to keep serum levels within normal range. Therefore, a UL has not been set. However, when potassium excretion is impaired, such as secondary to diabetes, chronic renal insufficiency, end-stage renal disease, severe heart failure, and adrenal insufficiency, high potassium intakes can lead to hyperkalemia and life-threatening cardiac arrhythmias.

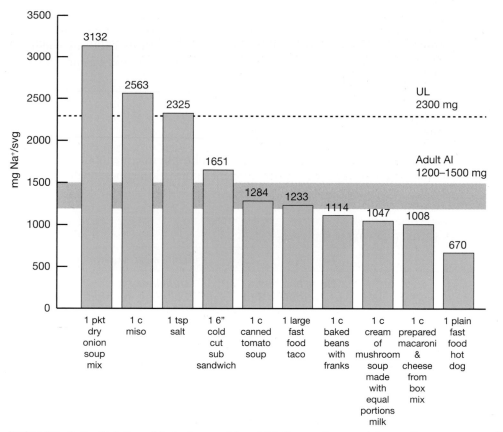

**FIGURE 6.1**   Relationship between AI and UL for sodium and the sodium content of selected foods.

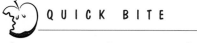

QUICK BITE

### Average potassium content by food group

*mg K/serving*

| | |
|---|---|
| Grains (except bran or whole wheat) | 35 mg/1 slice bread or ¾ cup most ready-to-eat cereals |
| Vegetables | 0–350 mg/½ cup of most |
| Fruit | 0–350 mg/½ cup or 1 small to medium piece fresh fruit |
| Milk | 370 mg/cup |
| Meat (not including dried peas and beans) | 100 mg/oz |
| Butter, margarine, oil | 10 mg/tsp |

## Chloride

Chloride is the major anion in the extracellular fluid, where it helps to maintain fluid and electrolyte balance in conjunction with sodium. Chloride is an essential component of hydrochloric acid in the stomach and, therefore, plays a role in digestion and acid–base balance. Its concentration in most cells is low.

Because almost all the chloride in the diet comes from salt (sodium chloride), the AI for chloride is set at a level equivalent (on a molar basis) to that of sodium. The AI for younger adults is 2.3 g/day, the equivalent to 3.8 g/day of salt or 1500-mg sodium. Sodium and chloride share dietary sources, conditions that cause them to become depleted in the body, and signs and symptoms of deficiency.

# ▶ MAJOR MINERALS

The remaining major minerals are calcium, phosphorus, magnesium, and sulfur. They are summarized in Table 6.5; additional salient information appears below.

### TABLE 6.5 Summary of Major Minerals

| Mineral and Sources | Functions | Deficiency/Toxicity Signs and Symptoms |
| --- | --- | --- |
| **Calcium (Ca)**<br>*Adult AI*<br>19–50 yr: 1000 mg<br>51+ yr: 1200 mg<br>Adult UL: 2.5 g/day<br>• Milk, yogurt, hard natural cheese, bok choy, broccoli, Chinese/Napa cabbage, collards, kale, okra, turnip greens, fortified breakfast cereal, fortified orange juice, dried peas and beans | Bone and teeth formation and maintenance, blood clotting, nerve transmission, muscle contraction and relaxation, cell membrane permeability, blood pressure | **Deficiency**<br>Children: impaired growth<br>Adults: osteoporosis<br>**Toxicity**<br>Constipation, increased risk of renal stone formation, impaired absorption of iron and other minerals |
| **Phosphorus (P)**<br>*Adult RDA*<br>Men and women: 700 mg<br>Adult UL:<br>To age 70: 4 g/day<br>70+ yr: 3 g/day<br>• All animal products (meat, poultry, eggs, milk), ready-to-eat cereal, dried peas and beans; bran and whole grains; raisins, prunes, dates | Bone and teeth formation and maintenance, acid–base balance, energy metabolism, cell membrane structure, regulation of hormone and coenzyme activity | **Deficiency**<br>Unknown<br>**Toxicity**<br>Low blood calcium |
| **Magnesium (Mg)**<br>*Adult RDA*<br>Men:<br>19–30 yr: 400 mg<br>31+ yr: 420 mg<br>Women:<br>19–30 yr: 310 mg<br>31+ yr: 320 mg<br>Adult UL: 350 mg/day from supplements only (does not include intake from food and water)<br>• Spinach, beet greens, okra, Brazil nuts, almonds, cashews, bran cereal, dried peas and beans, halibut, tuna, chocolate, cocoa | Bone formation, nerve transmission, smooth muscle relaxation, protein synthesis, CHO metabolism, enzyme activity | **Deficiency**<br>Weakness, confusion; growth failure in children<br>Severe deficiency: convulsions, hallucinations, tetany<br>**Toxicity**<br>No toxicity demonstrated from food<br>Supplemental Mg can cause diarrhea, nausea, and cramping<br>Excessive Mg from magnesium in Epsom salts causes diarrhea |
| **Sulfur (S)**<br>No recommended intake or UL<br>• All protein foods (meat, poultry, fish, eggs, milk, dried peas and beans, nuts) | Component of disulfide bridges in proteins; component of biotin, thiamin, and insulin | **Deficiency**<br>Unknown<br>**Toxicity**<br>In animals, excessive intake of sulfur-containing amino acids impairs growth |

# Calcium

Calcium is the most plentiful mineral in the body, making up about half of the body's total mineral content. Almost all of the body's calcium (99%) is found in bones and teeth, where it combines with phosphorus, magnesium, and other minerals to provide rigidity and structure. Bones serve as a large, dynamic reservoir of calcium that readily releases calcium when serum levels drop; this helps to maintain blood calcium levels within normal limits when calcium intake is inadequate.

The remaining 1% of calcium in the body is found in plasma and other body fluids, where it has important roles in blood clotting, nerve transmission, muscle contraction and relaxation, cell membrane permeability, and the activation of certain enzymes. Based on generally consistent evidence from several cohort studies, the American Institute of Cancer Research concludes that calcium probably protects against colorectal cancer (World Cancer Research Fund, 2007). In observational and experimental studies, the intakes of calcium or dairy products are associated with lower blood pressure (Zemel, 2001; Miller et al., 2000). Observational and clinical studies also indicate that calcium and dairy foods play a role in controlling body weight and obesity (Varenna et al., 2007).

Calcium balance—or, more accurately, calcium balance in the blood—is achieved through the action of vitamin D and hormones. When blood calcium levels fall, the parathyroid gland secretes parathormone (PTH), which promotes calcium reabsorption in the kidneys and stimulates the release of calcium from bones. Vitamin D has the same effects on the kidneys and bones and additionally increases the absorption of calcium from the gastrointestinal tract. Together, the actions of PTH and vitamin D restore low blood calcium levels to normal, even though bone calcium content may fall. A chronically low calcium intake compromises bone integrity without affecting blood calcium levels. When blood calcium levels are too high, the thyroid gland secretes calcitonin, which promotes the formation of new bone by taking excess calcium from the blood. A high calcium intake does not lead to hypercalcemia but rather maximizes bone density. Abnormal blood concentrations of calcium occur from alterations in the secretion of PTH.

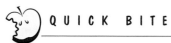

## QUICK BITE

### Absorption of Calcium

*Better-absorbed sources of calcium*

Milk, cheese, yogurt

Bok choy, broccoli, Chinese/Napa cabbage, collard greens, kale, okra, turnip greens

Fortified orange juice, fortified breakfast cereals, fortified soy milk

Calcium-set tofu, other soy foods

Sesame seeds, almonds, red and white beans, figs

*Not well-absorbed sources of calcium*

Spinach, beet greens, Swiss chard

Generally, three daily servings of milk, yogurt, or cheese plus nondairy sources of calcium are needed to ensure an adequate calcium intake. Milk is considered a "nearly perfect" source because it contains vitamin D and lactose that promote calcium absorption. People who are lactose intolerant can obtain calcium from yogurt, hard cheeses, and low-oxalate green vegetables such as broccoli, bok choy, collard greens, and kale (Fig. 6.2). Significant amounts of calcium can be found in calcium-fortified foods such as fruit juices, tomato juice, and ready-to-eat breakfast cereals.

An adequate calcium intake throughout the first three decades of life is needed to attain peak bone mass as determined by genetics. A dense bone mass offers protection against the inevitable net bone loss that occurs in all people after the age of about 35 years. Daily AI recommendations are set at 1300 mg for adolescents up to 18 years of age, 1000 mg between the ages of 19 and 50 years, and 1200 mg thereafter (IOM, 1997). Mean intake among American adults is 984 mg for men and 735 mg for women (Moshfegh et al., 2005). Only 25% of Americans meet their AI for calcium, and only 5% of women aged 51 to 70

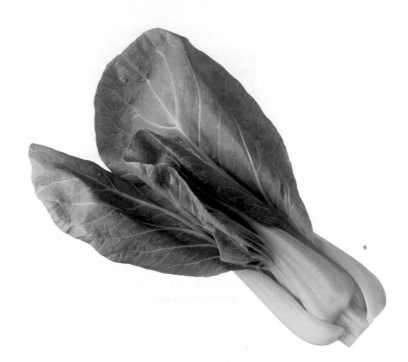

**FIGURE 6.2**
Baby bok choy; a
well-absorbed source
of calcium.

do so (Hunt & Johnson, 2007). However, a study by Hunt and Johnson showed that calcium balance is achievable at calcium intakes of 741 mg/day for people who consume typical amounts of sodium and protein; their data support an RDA of 1035 mg/day (Hunt & Johnson, 2007). Even though that amount is lower than the current AI, it is still a higher intake than most Americans typically consume. Supplements are an option for those who cannot meet their calcium need through food alone (Box 6.3).

## Phosphorus

After calcium, the most abundant mineral in the body is phosphorus. Approximately 85% of the body's phosphorus is combined with calcium in bones and teeth. The rest is distributed

---

**BOX 6.3**   **CALCIUM SUPPLEMENTS**

- Multivitamins contain much less calcium than calcium supplements.
- Calcium carbonate and calcium citrate are the preferred types of calcium supplements.
- Calcium from supplements is absorbed best in doses of 500 mg or less; spread tablets out over the course of the day.
- Calcium carbonate is the least expensive calcium supplement. It can cause constipation and is best absorbed when taken *with* food.
- Calcium citrate contains acids that promote calcium absorption, which is beneficial in elderly people who normally produce less stomach acid than younger adults. It is less likely to cause constipation than calcium carbonate and is better absorbed on an *empty stomach.*
- Look for supplements that contain vitamin D to maximize absorption.
- Take with milk because the lactose and vitamin D will promote calcium absorption.
- Avoid calcium supplements with dolomite, unrefined oyster shell, or bonemeal without a USP symbol. They may contain contaminants.
- Avoid taking calcium supplements at the same time as iron supplements.

in every body cell, where it performs various functions such as regulating acid–base balance (phosphoric acid and its salts), metabolizing energy (adenosine triphosphate), and providing structure to cell membranes (phospholipids). Phosphorus is an important component of RNA and DNA and is responsible for activating many enzymes and the B vitamins.

QUICK BITE

**What do phosphorus additives do?**
- Extend shelf life
- Improve taste, especially in soft drinks
- Prevent instant foods from clumping, such as instant coffee
- Keep fats from separating from liquids, such as in processed cheese, mayonnaise, and margarine
- Promote thickening and stability of instant foods, such as instant pudding and instant gravy
- Retain water in processed meat products, such as processed chicken nuggets
- Improve the texture of baked goods

Normally about 60% of natural phosphorus from food sources is absorbed, but absorption of phosphorus from food preservatives (e.g., phosphoric acid) is almost 100% (Bell et al., 1977). As with calcium, phosphorus absorption is enhanced by vitamin D and regulated by PTH. The major route of phosphorus excretion is in the urine.

Because phosphorus is pervasive in the food supply, dietary deficiencies of phosphorus do not occur. Animal proteins, dairy products, and legumes are rich natural sources of phosphorus; soft drinks contain phosphoric acid, and commercially prepared foods may contain significant sources of phosphate additives. Mean intake is estimated to be 1109 mg/day among adult women and 1552 mg/day among adult men, amounts significantly higher than the RDA of 700 mg (Moshfegh et al., 2005). However, most food databases do not count phosphorus derived from food additives, so the total amount of phosphorus consumed by the average person in the United States is unknown.

## Magnesium

Magnesium is the fourth most abundant mineral in the body; approximately 50% of the body's magnesium content is deposited in bone with calcium and phosphorus. The remaining magnesium is distributed in various soft tissues, muscles, and body fluids. Magnesium is a cofactor for more than 300 enzymes in the body, including those involved in energy metabolism, protein synthesis, and cell membrane transport. There is increasing interest in the role magnesium may play in preventing hypertension, and managing cardiovascular disease, and diabetes (Office of Dietary Supplements, 2005).

Mean magnesium intake among American adults is approximately 80% of the RDA. A low magnesium intake is related to the intake of refined grains over whole-grain breads and cereals because magnesium that is lost in the refining process is not added back through routine enrichment. However, food consumption data do not include the magnesium content of water, which is significant in water classified as "hard." Despite chronically low intakes, deficiency symptoms are rare and appear only in conjunction with certain diseases such as alcohol abuse, protein malnutrition, renal impairments, endocrine disorders, and prolonged vomiting or diarrhea.

## Sulfur

Sulfur does not function independently as a nutrient, but it is a component of biotin, thiamin, and the amino acids methionine and cysteine. The proteins in skin, hair, and nails are made more rigid by the presence of sulfur.

There is neither an RDA nor an AI for sulfur, and no deficiency symptoms are known. Although food and various sources of drinking water provide significant amounts of sulfur, the major source of inorganic sulfate for humans is body protein turnover of methionine and cysteine. The need for sulfur is met when the intake of sulfur amino acids is adequate. A sulfur deficiency is likely only when protein deficiency is severe.

# ▶ TRACE MINERALS

Although their presence in the body is small, their impact on health is significant. Each trace mineral has its own range over which the body can maintain homeostasis (Fig. 6.3). People who consume an adequate diet derive no further benefit from supplementing their intake with minerals and may induce a deficiency by upsetting the delicate balance that exists between minerals. Even though too little of a trace mineral can be just as deadly as too much, routine supplementation is not recommended. Factors that complicate the study of trace minerals are as follows:

- The high variability of trace mineral content of foods. The mineral content of the soil from which a food originates largely influences trace mineral content. For instance, grains, vegetables, and meat raised in South Dakota, Wyoming, New Mexico, and Utah are high in selenium, whereas foods grown in the southern states and from both coasts of the United States have much less selenium. Other factors that influence a food's trace mineral content are the quality of the water supply and food processing. Because of these factors, the trace mineral content listed in food composition tables may not represent the actual amount in a given sample.
- Food composition data are not available for all trace minerals. Food composition tables generally include data on the content of iron, zinc, manganese, selenium, and copper, but data on other trace minerals, such as iodine, chromium, and molybdenum, are not readily available.

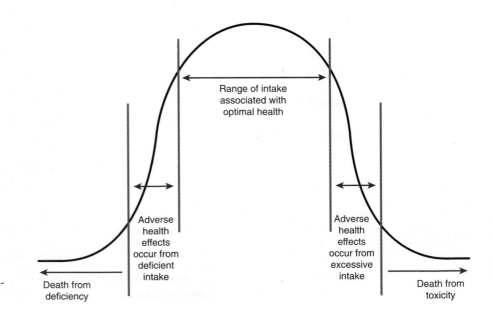

**FIGURE 6.3** Health effects seen over a range of trace mineral intakes.

- Bioavailability varies within the context of the total diet. Even when trace element intake can be estimated, the amount available to the body may be significantly less because the absorption and metabolism of individual trace elements is strongly influenced by mineral interactions and other dietary factors. An excess of one trace mineral may induce a deficiency of another. For instance, a high intake of zinc impairs copper absorption. Conversely, a deficiency of one trace mineral may potentiate toxic effects of another, as when iron deficiency increases vulnerability to lead poisoning.
- Reliable and valid indicators of trace element status (e.g., measured serum levels, results of balance studies, enzyme activity determinations) are not available for all trace minerals, so assessment of trace element status is not always possible.

Table 6.6 summarizes the sources, functions, recommended intakes, and signs and symptoms of deficiency and toxicity of trace minerals that have either an RDA or AI. Additional salient features are presented in the following sections.

## Iron

Approximately two-thirds of the body's 3 to 5 g of iron is contained in the heme portion of hemoglobin. Iron is also found in transferrin, the transport carrier of iron, and in enzyme systems that are active in energy metabolism. Ferritin, the storage form of iron, is located in the liver, bone marrow, and spleen.

Iron in foods exists in two forms: heme iron, found in meat, fish, and poultry, and non-heme iron, found in plants such as grains, vegetables, legumes, and nuts. The majority of iron in the diet is nonheme iron.

Normally the overall rate of iron absorption, which includes both heme and nonheme iron, is only 10% to 15% of total intake. In times of need such as during growth, pregnancy,

| TABLE 6.6 | Summary of Trace Minerals | |
|---|---|---|
| **Mineral and Sources** | **Functions** | **Deficiency/Toxicity Signs and Symptoms** |
| **Iron (Fe)**<br>**Adult RDA**<br>Men: 8 mg<br>Women:<br>    19–50 yr: 18 mg<br>    51+ yr: 8 mg<br>Adult UL: 45 mg<br>• Beef liver, red meats, fish, poultry, clams, tofu, oysters, lentils, dried peas and beans, fortified cereals, bread, dried fruit | Oxygen transport via hemoglobin and myoglobin; constituent of enzyme systems | **Deficiency**<br>Impaired immune function, decreased work capacity, apathy, lethargy, fatigue, itchy skin, pale nail beds and eye membranes, impaired wound healing, intolerance to cold temperatures<br>**Toxicity**<br>Increased risk of infections, apathy, fatigue, lethargy, joint disease, hair loss, organ damage, enlarged liver, amenorrhea, impotence<br>Accidental poisoning in children causes death |
| **Zinc (Zn)**<br>**Adult RDA**<br>Men: 11 mg<br>Women: 8 mg<br>Adult UL: 40 mg<br>• Oysters, red meat, poultry, dried peas and beans, fortified breakfast cereals, yogurt, cashews, pecans, milk | Tissue growth and wound healing, sexual maturation and reproduction; constituent of many enzymes in energy and nucleic acid metabolism; immune function; vitamin A transport, taste perception | **Deficiency**<br>Growth retardation, hair loss, diarrhea, delayed sexual maturation and impotence, eye and skin lesions, anorexia, delayed wound healing, taste abnormality, mental lethargy<br>**Toxicity**<br>Anemia, elevated LDL, lowered HDL, diarrhea, vomiting, impaired calcium absorption, fever, renal failure, muscle pain, dizziness, reproductive failure |

*(table continues on page 134)*

| TABLE 6.6 | Summary of Trace Minerals (continued) | |
|---|---|---|
| **Mineral and Sources** | **Functions** | **Deficiency/Toxicity Signs and Symptoms** |
| **Iodine**<br>*Adult RDA*<br>150 micrograms<br>Adult UL: 1100 micrograms<br>• Iodized salt, seafood, bread, dairy products | Component of thyroid hormones that regulate growth, development, and metabolic rate | *Deficiency*<br>Goiter, weight gain, lethargy<br>During pregnancy may cause severe and irreversible mental and physical retardation (cretinism)<br>*Toxicity*<br>Enlarged thyroid gland, decreased thyroid activity |
| **Selenium (Se)**<br>*Adult RDA*<br>Men and women: 55 micrograms<br>Adult UL: 400 micrograms /day<br>• Brazil nuts, tuna, beef, cod, turkey, egg, cottage cheese, rice, enriched and whole-wheat bread | Component of antioxidant enzymes, immune system functioning, thyroid gland activity | *Deficiency*<br>Enlarged heart, poor heart function, impaired thyroid activity<br>*Toxicity*<br>Rare; nausea, vomiting, abdominal pain, diarrhea, hair and nail changes, nerve damage, fatigue |
| **Copper (Cu)**<br>*Adult RDA:* 900 micrograms<br>Adult UL: 10,000 micrograms<br>• Organ meats, seafood, nuts, seeds, whole grains, cocoa products, drinking water | Used in the production of hemoglobin; component of several enzymes; used in energy metabolism | *Deficiency*<br>Rare; anemia, bone abnormalities<br>*Toxicity*<br>Vomiting, diarrhea, liver damage |
| **Manganese (Mn)**<br>*Adult AI*<br>Men: 2.3 mg<br>Women: 1.8 mg<br>Adult UL: 11 mg<br>• Widely distributed in foods. Best sources are whole grains, oat bran, tea, pineapple, spinach, dried peas and beans | Component of enzymes involved in the metabolism of carbohydrates, protein, and fat, and in bone formation | *Deficiency*<br>Rare<br>*Toxicity*<br>Rare; nervous system disorders |
| **Fluoride (Fl)**<br>*Adult AI*<br>Men: 4 mg<br>Women: 3 mg<br>Adult UL: 10 mg<br>• Fluoridated water, water that naturally contains fluoride, tea, seafood | Formation and maintenance of tooth enamel, promotes resistance to dental decay, role in bone formation and integrity | *Deficiency*<br>Susceptibility to dental decay, may increase risk of osteoporosis<br>*Toxicity*<br>Fluorosis (mottling of teeth), nausea, vomiting, diarrhea, chest pain, itching |
| **Chromium (Cr)**<br>*Adult AI*<br>Men:<br>19–50 yr: 35 micrograms<br>51+ yr: 30 micrograms<br>Women<br>51+ yr: 30 micrograms<br>19–50 yr: 25 micrograms<br>Adult UL:<br>Undetermined<br>• Broccoli, grape juice, whole grains, red wine | Cofactor for insulin | *Deficiency*<br>Insulin resistance, impaired glucose tolerance<br>*Toxicity*<br>Dietary toxicity unknown<br>Occupational exposure to chromium dust damages skin and kidneys |
| **Molybdenum (Mo)**<br>*Adult RDA:* 45 micrograms<br>Adult UL: 2000 micrograms<br>• Milk, legumes, bread, grains | Component of many enzymes; works with riboflavin to incorporate iron into hemoglobin | *Deficiency*<br>Unknown<br>*Toxicity*<br>Occupational exposure to molybdenum dust causes gout-like symptoms |

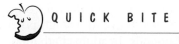

**QUICK BITE**

**Nonheme iron absorption**

Nonheme iron absorption is *enhanced* when consumed at the same time as:

Vitamin C-rich foods, such as orange juice or tomato products

Heme iron, found in meat, fish, and poultry

Nonheme iron absorption is *impaired* when consumed at the same time as:

Coffee

Tea

Calcium

Phytates found in dried peas and beans, rice, and grains

Oxalates found in spinach, chard, berries, chocolate

or iron deficiency, iron is absorbed more efficiently to boost the overall absorption rate to as high as 50%.

The bioavailability of heme and nonheme iron differs greatly. The rate of heme iron absorption is normally about 15% and is influenced only by need, not by dietary factors. In contrast, nonheme iron absorption is enhanced or inhibited by numerous dietary factors. Only 1% to 7% of nonheme iron is absorbed from plant foods when they are consumed as a single food. That rate increases when nonheme iron is consumed with an absorption enhancer. For instance, consuming 50 mg of vitamin C with a meal, which is the amount of vitamin C found in one small orange, can increase nonheme iron absorption three to six times above normal. Conversely, tea, an absorption inhibitor, can reduce iron absorption in a meal by 60%.

Based on average absorption rates and to compensate for daily (and monthly) iron losses, the RDA for iron is set at 8 mg for men and postmenopausal women and 18 mg for premenopausal women. Iron requirements increase during growth and in response to heavy or chronic blood loss related to menstruation, surgery, injury, gastrointestinal bleeding, or aspirin abuse. Iron recommendations for vegetarians are 1.8 times higher than that for nonvegetarians because of the lower bioavailability of iron from a vegetarian diet (IOM, 2001). Most adult men and postmenopausal women consume adequate amounts of iron. Women of childbearing age, pregnant women, and breastfeeding women generally do not consume the recommended amounts of iron.

**Microcytic:** small blood cells.

**Hypochromic:** pale red blood cells related to the decrease in hemoglobin pigment.

**Pica:** ingestion of nonfood substances such as dirt, clay, or laundry starch.

Iron deficiency anemia, a **microcytic, hypochromic** anemia, occurs when total iron stores become depleted, leading to a decrease in hemoglobin. The World Health Organization considers iron deficiency the most common and widespread nutritional disorder in the world, affecting more than 30% of the world's population (WHO, 2008). In the United States, about 10% of the population is iron deficient. Because the typical American diet provides only 6 to 7 mg of iron per 1000 calories, many menstruating women simply do not consume enough calories to satisfy their iron requirement. Other groups most likely to be deficient from an inadequate iron intake are older infants and toddlers, adolescent girls, and pregnant women. Some people with iron deficiency anemia practice **pica**, which impairs iron absorption. Because symptoms of iron deficiency are similar to iron overload, namely apathy, lethargy, and fatigue, iron supplements should not be taken on the basis of symptoms alone.

Because very little iron is excreted from the body, the potential for toxicity is moderate to high. Although repeated blood transfusions, rare metabolic disorders, and megadoses of supplemental iron can cause iron overload, the most frequent cause is hemochromatosis, one of the most common genetic disorders in the United States. The absorption of excessive amounts of iron leads to iron accumulation in body tissues, especially the liver, heart, brain, joints, and pancreas. Left untreated, excess iron can cause heart disease, cancer, cirrhosis, diabetes, and arthritis. Phlebotomies are used to reduce body iron. Given the prevalence of iron enrichment and iron fortification in the U.S. food supply, a low-iron diet is not recommended, nor could it be realistically achieved.

Acute iron toxicity, caused by the overdose of medicinal iron, is the leading cause of accidental poisoning in small children. As few as five to six high-potency tablets can provide enough iron to kill a child weighing 22 pounds. In adults, high intakes of iron supplements can cause constipation, nausea, vomiting, and diarrhea, especially when the supplements are taken on an empty stomach.

## Zinc

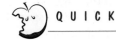

**QUICK BITE**

100% DV for zinc can be met with six medium battered and fried oysters

The small amount of zinc contained in the body (about 2 g) is found in almost all cells and is especially concentrated in the eyes, bones, muscles, and prostate gland. Zinc in tissues is not available to maintain serum levels when intake is inadequate, so a regular and sufficient intake is necessary.

Zinc is a component of DNA and RNA and is part of more than 100 enzymes involved in growth, metabolism, sexual maturation and reproduction, and the senses of taste and smell. Zinc plays important roles in immune system functioning and wound healing. Mean intake among American adults exceeds the RDA for zinc.

There is no single laboratory test that adequately measures zinc status, so zinc deficiency is not readily diagnosed. Risk factors for zinc deficiency include poor calorie intake, alcoholism, and malabsorption syndromes such as celiac disease, Crohn's disease, and short bowel syndrome. Vegetarians are also at increased risk because zinc is only half as well absorbed from plants as it is from animal sources. Although overt zinc deficiency is not common in the United States, the effects of marginal intakes are poorly understood.

## Iodine

Iodine is found in the muscles, the thyroid gland, the skin, the skeleton, endocrine tissues, and the bloodstream. It is an essential component of thyroxine ($T_4$) and triiodothyronine ($T_3$), the thyroid hormones responsible for regulating metabolic rate, body temperature, reproduction, growth, the synthesis of blood cells, and nerve and muscle function.

The iodine content of most food sources is low. In the United States, approximately 50% of the population uses iodized salt, making it the biggest source of iodine in the American diet. Seafood is naturally high in iodine. Milk has become a significant source of iodine in part because of the use of iodine chemicals to sanitize and disinfect udders, milking machines, and milk tanks. Processed foods may also contain higher amounts of iodine because of the addition of iodized salt or additives containing iodine.

Although the average American adult consumes more than the RDA for iodine, most countries have some degree of iodine deficiency, which may lead to goiter, hypothyroidism, or growth and developmental defects. The effect of **goitrogens** on iodine balance is clinically insignificant except when iodine deficiency exists.

**Goitrogens:** thyroid antagonists found in cruciferous vegetables (e.g., cabbage, cauliflower, broccoli), soybeans, and sweet potatoes.

## Selenium

**QUICK BITE**

One ounce of Brazil nuts provides 544 micrograms of selenium—enough to meet the DV for almost 8 days

Selenium is a component of a group of enzymes, called glutathione peroxidases, that function as antioxidants to disarm free radicals produced during normal oxygen metabolism. Selenium is also

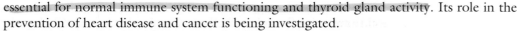

essential for normal immune system functioning and thyroid gland activity. Its role in the prevention of heart disease and cancer is being investigated.

Although areas of the country with selenium-poor soil produce selenium-poor foods, mass transportation mitigates the effect on total selenium intake (IOM, 2000). Also because selenium is associated with protein, some meats and seafood provide selenium. The average American adult consumes adequate amounts of selenium.

Selenium deficiency is rare in the United States. It is most likely to occur secondary to severe gastrointestinal problems, such as Crohn's disease, or from surgical removal of part of the stomach. People with acute severe illness who develop inflammation and widespread infection often have low blood levels of selenium.

## Copper

Copper is distributed in muscles, liver, brain, bones, kidneys, and blood. Copper is a component of several enzymes involved in hemoglobin synthesis, collagen formation, wound healing, and maintenance of nerve fibers. Copper also helps cells to use iron and plays a role in energy metabolism.

Americans typically consume adequate amounts of copper. Excess zinc intake has the potential to induce copper deficiency by impairing its absorption, but copper deficiency is rare. Supplements, not food, may cause copper toxicity, as do some genetic disorders such as Wilson's disease.

## Manganese

Mean manganese intake among American adults is well above the AI, and dietary deficiencies have not been noted. Manganese toxicity is a well-known occupational hazard for miners who inhale manganese dust over a prolonged period of time, leading to central nervous system abnormalities with symptoms similar to those of Parkinson's disease. There is some evidence to suggest that high manganese intake from drinking water, which may be more bioavailable than manganese from food, also produces neuromotor deficits similar to Parkinson's disease. The UL for adults is set at 11 mg/day, approximately four times the usual intake.

## Fluoride

**Cariogenic:** cavity promoting.

Fluoride promotes the mineralization of developing tooth enamel prior to tooth eruption and the remineralization of surface enamel in erupted teeth. It concentrates in plaque and saliva to inhibit the process by which **cariogenic** bacteria metabolize carbohydrates to produce acids that cause tooth decay. Fluoridation of municipal water in the second half of the 20th century is credited with a major decline in the prevalence and severity of dental caries in the U.S. population.

Fluoridation of municipal water is endorsed by the National Institute of Dental Health, the American Dietetic Association, the American Medical Association, the National Cancer Institute, and the Centers for Disease Control and Prevention (CDC). According to the CDC, 67% of Americans had access to optimally fluoridated water in 2004. National health goals are to increase fluoridation to 75% or more of the U.S. population served by municipal water systems (Carmona, 2004). It is estimated that for every $1 spent on fluoridation, $38 or more is saved in treatment costs. For both children and adults, fluoridation is the most effective public health measure to prevent tooth decay and improve oral health over a lifetime (Carmona, 2004).

Children under the age of 8 are susceptible to mottled tooth enamel if they ingest several times more fluoride than the recommended amount during the time of tooth enamel formation. The swallowing of fluoridated toothpaste is to blame.

## Chromium

Chromium enhances the action of the hormone insulin to help regulate blood glucose levels. A deficiency of chromium is characterized by high blood glucose and impaired insulin response.

Even though chromium is widespread in foods, many foods provide less than 1 to 2 micrograms per serving. Because existing databases lack information on chromium, few food intake studies utilizing few laboratories are available to estimate usual intake. However, it appears that average intake is adequate. Unrefined foods are higher in chromium than processed foods.

## Molybdenum

Molybdenum plays a role in red blood cell synthesis and is a component of several enzymes. Average American intake falls within the recommended range. Dietary deficiencies and toxicities are unknown.

## Other Trace Elements

Although definitive evidence is lacking, future research may reveal that other trace elements are essential for human nutrition. However, evidence is difficult to obtain, and quantifying human need is even more formidable. In addition, as with all trace minerals, the potential for toxicity exists. Consider the following:

- Nickel, silicon, vanadium, and boron have been demonstrated to have beneficial health effects in some animals and may someday be classified as essential for humans.
- Cobalt is an essential component of vitamin $B_{12}$, but it is not an essential nutrient and does not have an RDA.
- It is possible that minute amounts of cadmium, lithium, tin, and even arsenic are also essential to human life.

# ▶ WATER AND MINERALS IN HEALTH PROMOTION

## Water

The 2005 Dietary Guidelines for Americans recommends that thirst be the guide to consuming adequate fluid and does not suggest specific amounts or types of beverages to satisfy fluid need. Specific fluids are mentioned within the context of other topics based on their nutritional makeup, not their fluid content. For instance, three daily servings (equivalent to three cups) of milk and milk products are recommended to meet calcium need, not as part of fluid needs. For healthy people, hydration is unconsciously maintained with ad lib access to water.

## Sodium and Potassium

Americans, on average, consume more than twice the AI for sodium and roughly half the AI for potassium. The 2005 Dietary Guidelines for Americans key recommendations regarding sodium and potassium intake appear in Box 6.4.

**2005 DIETARY GUIDELINES FOR AMERICANS**

Key recommendations regarding sodium and potassium are as follows:

• Consume less than 2300 mg (~ 1 teaspoon of salt) of sodium per day.
• Choose and prepare foods with little salt. At the same time, consume potassium-rich foods, such as fruits and vegetables.

Key recommendations for specific population groups are as follows:

• *Individuals with hypertension, blacks, and middle-aged and older adults* aim to consume no more than 1500 mg of sodium per day, and meet the potassium recommendation (4700 mg/day) with food.

## Less Sodium

A high sodium intake is believed to contribute to increased blood pressure, which is a risk factor for coronary heart disease, stroke, congestive heart failure, and renal diseases. Generally, blood pressure increases progressively and continuously over the continuum of sodium intake without an obvious threshold. Certain groups are more "salt sensitive" and so have greater responses to changes in sodium intake, namely people with hypertension, older people, and African Americans; they are encouraged to reduce sodium intake to not more than 1500 mg/day. The DASH (Dietary Approaches to Stop Hypertension) study showed that the DASH diet (rich in potassium, calcium, magnesium, fiber, and protein) combined with a reduced sodium intake lowers blood pressure in hypertensive and normotensive people (NIH, 2001). Tips for reducing sodium intake appear in Box 6.5.

**TIPS FOR LOWERING SODIUM INTAKE**

• Avoid or limit convenience foods, such as boxed mixes, frozen dinners, and canned foods.
• Eat home-cooked meals more often.
• Eat more fresh or frozen vegetables.
• Compare labels to choose brands or varieties with the lowest amount of sodium.
• Use fresh veggies in place of pickles.
• Substitute low-sodium tuna and roasted chicken for deli meats.
• Replace sausages and hot dogs with fresh meats such as rotisserie chicken.
• Use cheese sparingly.
• Choose nut butters with no sodium added.
• Cook rice and pasta without salt.
• Switch to pasta sauce without added salt or combine equal parts of no-salt-added tomato sauce with bottled pasta sauce.
• Choose cereals with no added salt, such as shredded wheat, puffed whole-grain cereal, and unsalted oatmeal.
• Use lower salt condiments, such as salt-free ketchup, Worcestershire sauce, vinegar, and low-sodium mayonnaise.
• Substitute homemade vinegar and oil dressing for bottled varieties.
• If you use canned vegetables, drain away liquid and rinse thoroughly.
• Limit salty snacks.
• Instead of salt, season food with spices, herbs, lemon, vinegar, or salt-free seasonings.

| BOX 6.6 | DESCRIPTORS OF SODIUM CONTENT |
| --- | --- |
| **If the label says . . .** | **One serving contains. . .** |
| Sodium free | <5 mg |
| Very low sodium | <35 mg |
| Low sodium | <140 mg |
| Reduced or less sodium | At least 25% less sodium compared with a standard serving size of the traditional food |
| Light in sodium | 50% less sodium than the traditional food (restricted to >40 calories per serving or >3 g fat per serving) |
| Salt free | <5 mg |
| Unsalted or no added salt | No salt added during processing (this does not necessarily mean the food is sodium free) |

Because the Daily Value (DV) for sodium used on food labels predates the latest AI and UL set for sodium, those values do not reliably reflect a food's contribution to recommended (lower) sodium intake levels. The Daily Reference Value for sodium used on the "Nutrition Facts" label is 2400 mg, which exceeds the current UL set at 2300 mg. A food that supplies 50% of the DV for sodium in a serving actually provides 1200 mg, which is 100% the current AI for adults aged 71 and older. Until the DV figure is updated, %DV is best used to compare the sodium content of similar products, not to estimate intake with the goal of consuming the AI. Descriptive terms on food labels do have legally defined meanings and can assist in food selection (Box 6.6).

## More Potassium

The AI for potassium is set at 4.7 g/day for all adults, a level believed necessary to maintain lower blood pressure levels, lessen the adverse effects of high sodium intake on blood pressure, reduce the risk of kidney stones, and possibly reduce bone loss. Indeed, moderate potassium deficiency, which typically occurs without hypokalemia, is characterized by increased blood pressure, increased salt sensitivity, an increased risk of kidney stones, and increased bone turnover (IOM, 2004). An inadequate potassium intake may also increase the risk of cardiovascular disease, particularly stroke.

Typically, American women consume only half the AI for potassium and men consume approximately two-thirds (Moshfegh et al., 2005). The Dietary Guidelines urges Americans to consume more potassium as part of a comprehensive lifestyle change designed to prevent or delay the onset of high blood pressure or to lower existing hypertension. Food sources are recommended over supplements, and fruits and vegetables are preferred because potassium is better absorbed from them than from meat, milk, and cereal products. Because African Americans have relatively low potassium intakes and a high prevalence of salt sensitivity and hypertension, a higher potassium intake may be even more beneficial for this population group. Figure 6.4 illustrates how food processing generally lowers potassium content and raises sodium content.

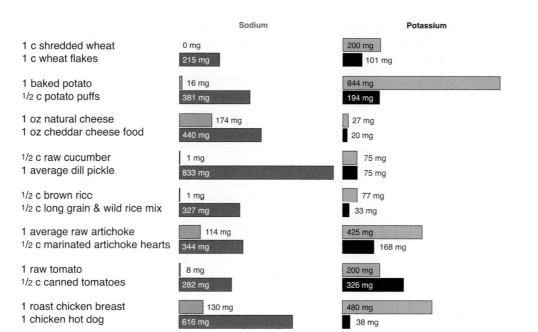

|  | Sodium | Potassium |
|---|---|---|
| 1 c shredded wheat | 0 mg | 200 mg |
| 1 c wheat flakes | 215 mg | 101 mg |
| 1 baked potato | 16 mg | 844 mg |
| 1/2 c potato puffs | 381 mg | 194 mg |
| 1 oz natural cheese | 174 mg | 27 mg |
| 1 oz cheddar cheese food | 440 mg | 20 mg |
| 1/2 c raw cucumber | 1 mg | 75 mg |
| 1 average dill pickle | 833 mg | 75 mg |
| 1/2 c brown rice | 1 mg | 77 mg |
| 1/2 c long grain & wild rice mix | 327 mg | 33 mg |
| 1 average raw artichoke | 114 mg | 425 mg |
| 1/2 c marinated artichoke hearts | 344 mg | 168 mg |
| 1 raw tomato | 8 mg | 200 mg |
| 1/2 c canned tomatoes | 282 mg | 326 mg |
| 1 roast chicken breast | 130 mg | 480 mg |
| 1 chicken hot dog | 616 mg | 38 mg |

**FIGURE 6.4**   Effect of food processing on the sodium content of selected foods.

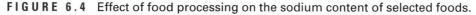

## ▶ How Do You Respond?

**Do zinc lozenges cure the common cold?** The effectiveness of zinc lozenges in reducing the severity or duration of the common cold is controversial. Although some studies indicate that zinc lozenges decrease the duration of common colds, others have found that cold symptoms get no better with zinc lozenges than with a placebo (Office of Dietary Supplements, 2002). Until more studies are done, it is not unreasonable or unsafe to use zinc lozenges to *treat* a cold. However, long-term use to *prevent* colds is not recommended because regular consumption of too much zinc can impair the immune system and lower the concentration of high-density lipoprotein ("good") cholesterol.

**Does chlorine in drinking water cause cancer?** When organic matter is present in water, chlorine reacts with it to form a by-product called trihalomethane (THM). If THM forms, it is in such small quantities that it is not a cancer risk. The benefits of chlorine in preventing outbreaks of cholera, hepatitis, and other diseases far outweigh the negligible effects of THM.

**What are chelated minerals?** A chelated mineral is surrounded by an amino acid to protect it from other food components such as oxalates and phytates that can bind to the mineral and prevent it from being absorbed. Chelated minerals are probably not worth the added expense: chelated calcium is absorbed 5% to 10% better than ordinary calcium but costs about five times more.

## ▶ Case Study

Bill is a 45-year-old bachelor who eats a grab-and-go breakfast, all of his lunches out, and has take-out or "something easy" for dinner. Bill's doctor is concerned that his blood pressure is progressively rising with every office visit and has advised him to "cut out the salt" to lower his sodium intake. Bill rarely uses salt from a saltshaker and is unsure what else he can do to lower his sodium intake. A typical day's intake is as follows:

| **Breakfast:** | Black coffee<br>2 jelly doughnuts |
| --- | --- |
| **Midmorning snack:** | Black coffee<br>Cookies |
| **Lunch:** | 2 fast-food tacos with tortilla chips and salsa or a 6-in. cold cut submarine with potato chips<br>Cola |
| **Midafternoon snack:** | Candy bar |
| **Dinner:** | If take-out, then Chinese food or pizza<br>If "something easy," then boxed macaroni and cheese with a couple of hot dogs, canned soup with a cold cut sandwich, or frozen TV dinners |
| **Dessert:** | Instant pudding or ice cream or candy bars |
| **Evening snacks:** | Cereal with milk or potato chips and dip |

- What foods did Bill eat yesterday that were high in sodium? What foods were relatively low in sodium? What would be better choices for him when eating out? How could he lower his sodium intake while still relying on "something easy" when he prepares food at home?
- Knowing that potassium may help blunt the effect of a high sodium intake on blood pressure, what foods would you recommend he add to his diet that would increase his potassium intake?
- In overweight people, weight loss helps lower high blood pressure. Bill is "a little heavy." What changes/substitutions would help him lose weight?

## STUDY QUESTIONS

1. The client asks if bottled water is better than tap water. Which of the following would be the nurse's best response?
   a. "Bottled water is safer than tap water because it has impurities removed."
   b. "Bottled water is not nutritionally superior to tap water."
   c. "The chlorine in tap water may increase the risk of cancer."
   d. "Bottled water is better than tap water because it is higher in minerals."

2. When developing a teaching plan for a client who is lactose intolerant, which of the following foods would the nurse suggest as sources of calcium the client could tolerate?
   a. Cheddar cheese, bok choy, broccoli
   b. Spinach, beet greens, skim milk
   c. Poultry, meat, eggs
   d. Whole grains, nuts, and cocoa

3. The nurse knows her instructions about reading labels for sodium information have been effective when the client verbalizes:
   a. "Foods labeled as "no salt added" are sodium free."
   b. "The %DV on the "Nutrition Facts" labels is based on the current adult AI of 1500 mg Na."

c. "The best way to use the "Nutrition Facts" label is to compare the sodium content or %DV of one brand or variety of a food to another."

d. "Spaghetti sauce labeled "reduced sodium" has less sodium in it than spaghetti sauce labeled as "light in sodium.""

4. Which of the following recommendations would be most effective at increasing potassium intake?
   a. Choose enriched grains in place of whole grains.
   b. Eat more fruits and vegetables.
   c. Eat more seafood and poultry in place of red meat.
   d. Because there are few good dietary sources of potassium, it is best obtained by taking potassium supplements.

5. A client asks why eating less sodium is important for healthy people. The nurse's best response is:
   a. "Low-sodium diets tend to be low in fat and therefore may reduce the risk of heart disease."
   b. "Low-sodium diets are only effective at preventing high blood pressure, not lowering existing high blood pressure, so the time to implement a low-sodium diet is when you are healthy."
   c. "Blood pressure tends to go up as sodium intake rises—without an obvious threshold; lowering sodium regardless of how much you consume may help prevent or delay high blood pressure."
   d. "Low-sodium diets are inherently low in calories and help people lose weight, which can help prevent a variety of chronic diseases."

6. Which of the following recommendations would be most effective at helping a client maximize iron absorption?
   a. Drink orange juice when you eat iron-fortified breakfast cereal.
   b. Avoid drinking coffee when you eat red meat.
   c. Drink milk with all meals.
   d. Eat dried peas and beans in place of red meat.

7. A client says he never adds salt to any foods that his wife serves so he believes he is consuming a low-sodium diet. Which of the following is the nurse's best response?
   a. "If you don't add salt to any of your foods, you are probably eating a low-sodium diet. Continue with that strategy."
   b. "Even though you aren't adding salt to food at the table, your wife is probably salting food as she cooks. She should stop doing that."
   c. "Lots of foods are naturally high in sodium, such as milk and meat; in addition to not using a saltshaker you must also limit foods that are naturally high in sodium."
   d. "The major source of sodium is processed and convenience foods; limiting their intake makes the biggest impact on overall sodium intake."

8. What should you tell the client about taking calcium supplements?
   a. "Calcium supplements are essentially all equal in quality and amount, so focus on price when deciding which brand to buy."
   b. "Look for a supplement that supplies the AI for calcium because many contain much smaller doses."
   c. "Calcium from supplements is best absorbed in doses of 500 mg or less, so spread tablets out over the day."
   d. "Taking iron supplements with calcium supplements will help maximize absorption."

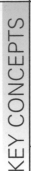

## KEY CONCEPTS

- Because water is involved in almost every body function, is not stored, and is excreted daily, it is more vital to life than food.

- Under normal conditions, water intake equals water output to maintain water balance. In most healthy people, thirst is a reliable indicator of need.

- The body's need for water is influenced by many variables, including activity, climate, and health. A general guideline is to consume 1.0 mL of fluid per calorie consumed, with a minimum of 1500 mL/day.

- Minerals are inorganic substances that cannot be broken down and rearranged in the body.

- Mineral toxicities are not likely to occur from diet alone. They are most often related to excessive use of mineral supplements, environmental exposure, or alterations in metabolism.

- Depending on the mineral involved, the body can maintain mineral balance by altering the rate of absorption, altering the rate of excretion, or releasing minerals from storage when needed.

- The absorption of many minerals is influenced by mineral–mineral interactions. Too much of one mineral may promote a deficiency of another mineral.

- Sodium, potassium, and chloride are electrolytes because they carry electrical charges when they are dissolved in solution.

- Macrominerals are needed in relatively large amounts and are found in the body in quantities greater than 5 g. Trace minerals are needed in very small amounts and are found in the body in amounts less than 5 g.

- As much as 75% of sodium consumed in the average American diet is from processed food. Virtually all Americans consume more than the UL for sodium.

- The potassium content of the diet tends to decrease as the sodium content increases, largely because high-sodium processed foods tend to be low in potassium.

- Many American adults consume less than the AI for calcium, placing them at risk of osteoporosis and possibly hypertension. Milk and yogurt are the richest sources of calcium, and their vitamin D and lactose content promote its absorption.

- Phosphorus is pervasive in foods and is also widely used in food additives to extend shelf life, enhance flavor, or improve quality characteristics. Americans consume more than they need.

- Although most Americans consume less than the RDA for magnesium, overt deficiency symptoms are rare and occur only secondary to certain diseases such as protein malnutrition and alcoholism.

- Trace minerals are not less important than major minerals; "trace" refers to the small amount normally found and needed in the body.

- The typical American diet supplies only 6 to 7 mg of iron per 1000 calories, so menstruating females typically do not eat enough calories to meet their RDA of 18 mg. Iron deficiency anemia is one of the most common nutritional deficiencies in the world.

- Americans generally consume adequate amounts of zinc. A regular intake is necessary because zinc in tissues cannot be released to maintain normal blood levels.

- Iodized salt is the biggest source of iodine in the U.S. diet, and Americans typically consume more than the RDA for iodine.

- Selenium is a component of substances that act as antioxidants. It is being studied for its potential to decrease the risk of cancer and heart disease.

- Fluoridated water has dramatically reduced the prevalence and severity of cavities in the U.S. population. Bottled water may not be fluoridated.

- Americans are urged to reduce their intake of sodium because of its potential role in the development of hypertension. The UL established for sodium is lower than the DV used on the "Nutrition Facts" label.

- A high potassium intake may blunt the effect of a high sodium intake and may also decrease the risk of kidney stones, help prevent bone loss, and reduce the risk of stroke. Americans are urged to increase their potassium intake by eating more fruits and vegetables. Meat, fish, whole grains, and dried peas and beans are also sources of potassium, but it is less well absorbed in them than the potassium in fruits and vegetables.

## ANSWER KEY

1. **FALSE** Although many healthy people do not consume the eight 8-ounce glasses of fluid recommended daily, the body is able to maintain homeostasis over a wide range of intakes.

2. **FALSE** Although the body rids itself of some excess minerals such as sodium and potassium through urinary excretion, homeostasis of other minerals is achieved by adjusting the rate of mineral absorption (e.g., iron, calcium).

3. **FALSE** Calcium is the most plentiful mineral in the body. For most Americans, sodium is the most abundant mineral in the diet.

4. **TRUE** An increase in sodium intake is associated with an increase in blood pressure. In addition, the dose-dependent rise in blood pressure is progressive, continuous, and appears to occur throughout the continuum of sodium intake without an obvious threshold.

5. **FALSE** Bottled water may taste better than tap water to some people but it usually lacks fluoride, the trace element that protects against dental decay.

6. **TRUE** Foods high in sodium tend to be low in potassium (e.g., processed foods like frozen entrees), and foods high in potassium tend to be low in sodium (e.g., fresh vegetables and whole grains).

7. **FALSE** The "major" and "trace" descriptions refer to the relative quantity of the mineral found in the body, not to their importance in maintaining health.

8. **TRUE** For most people, thirst is a reliable indicator of fluid needs. Exceptions are the elderly, children, and during hot weather or strenuous exercise.

9. **TRUE** Trace mineral balance is a function of not just the quantity of the element consumed, but also the presence of other trace minerals and dietary factors. For instance, nonheme iron absorption is impaired by tea but enhanced by orange juice.

10. **FALSE** A chronically low intake of calcium compromises the density and strength of bones but does not lead to hypocalcemia. Serum levels of calcium are maintained within normal range, regardless of calcium intake at the expense of calcium in bones.

## WEBSITES

Iron Overload Diseases Association at **www.ironoverload.org**
National Dairy Council at **www.nationaldairycouncil.org**
National Academy of Sciences, Institute of Medicine for Reference Dietary Intakes at **www.nap.edu**
Facts about dietary supplements (including mineral supplements) from the National Institutes of Health at **http://dietary-supplements.info.nih.gov**
Nutrient sources at USDA National Nutrient Database for Standard Reference, Release 20. Available at **www.ars.usda.gov/Main/docs.htm?docid=15869.**

# REFERENCES

Bell, R., Draper, J., Tzeng, D., et al. (1977). Physiological responses of human adult to foods containing phosphate additives. *The Journal of Nutrition, 107*, 45–50.

Bossingham, M., Carnell, N., & Campbell, W. (2005). Water balance, hydration status, and fat-free mass hydration in younger and older adults. *The American Journal of Clinical Nutrition, 81*, 1342–1350.

Carmona, R. (2004). *Surgeon General's statement on community water fluoridation.* Available at www.cdc.gov/fluoridation/fact_sheets/sg04.htm. Accessed on 1/2/08.

Crowley, L. (2007). *Sodas and cereal most popular food items in 2007.* Available at http://www.foodnavigator-usa.com/Financial-Industry/Sodas-and-cereal-most-popular-food-items-in-2007. Accessed on 12/13/07.

Hunt, C., & Johnson, L. (2007). Calcium requirements: New estimations for men and women by cross-sectional statistical analyses of calcium balance data from metabolic studies. *The American Journal of Clinical Nutrition, 86*, 1054–1063.

International Food Information Council. (2005). *Sodium in Food and Health.* Available at www.ific.org/publications/reviews/sodiumir.cfm?renderforprint=1. Accessed on 12/4/07.

Miller, G., DiRienzo, D., Reusser, M., et al. (2000). Benefits of dairy product consumption on blood pressure in humans: A summary of the biomedical literature. *Journal of the American College of Nutrition, 19*, 127S–164S.

Moshfegh, A., Goldman, J., & Cleveland, L. (2005). *What we eat in American, NHANES 2001–2002: Usual Nutrient Intakes from Food Compared to Dietary Reference Intakes.* US Department of Agriculture, Agricultural Research Service. Available at http://www.ars.usda.gov/SP2UserFiles/Place/12355000/pdf/usualintaketables2001-02.pdf. Accessed on 12/20/07.

National Academy of Sciences, Institute of Medicine. (1997). *Dietary Reference Intakes for calcium, phosphorus, magnesium, vitamin D, and fluoride.* Washington, DC: National Academy Press.

National Academy of Sciences, Institute of Medicine. (2000). *Dietary Reference Intakes for vitamin C, vitamin E, selenium, and carotenoids.* Washington, DC: National Academy Press.

National Academy of Sciences, Institute of Medicine (IOM). (2001). *Dietary Reference Intakes for vitamin A, vitamin K, arsenic, boron, chromium, copper, iodine, iron, manganese, molybdenum, nickel, silicon, vanadium, and zinc.* Washington, DC: National Academy Press.

National Academy of Sciences, Institute of Medicine (IOM). (2004). *Dietary Reference Intakes for water, potassium, sodium, chloride, and sulfate.* Available at http://www.nap.edu/openbook.php?isbn=0309091691. Accessed on 2/23/04.

National Science Foundation. *Types and treatment of bottled water.* (2004). Available at www.nsf.org/consumer/bottled_water/bw_types.asp?program=BottledWat. Accessed on 12/5/07.

Neilsen, S., & Popkin, B. (2004). Changes in beverage intake between 1977 and 2001. *American Journal of Preventive Medicine, 27*, 205–210.

Office of Dietary Supplements, National Institutes of Health. (2005). *Magnesium.* Available at http://ods.od.nih.gov/factsheets/magnesium.asp. Accessed on 1/3/08.

Office of Dietary Supplements, National Institutes of Health. (2002). *Facts about dietary supplements: Zinc.* Available at http://ods.od.nih.gov/factsheets/cc/zinc.html. Accessed on 1/3/08.

Owen, J. (2006). Bottled water isn't healthier than tap, report reveals. Available at http://news.nationalgeographic.com/news/2006/02/0224_060224_bottled_water.html. Accessed on 12/5/07.

Panel on Dietary Reference Intakes for Electrolytes and Water (PDRIEW), Standing Committee on the Scientific Evaluation of Dietary Reference Intakes, Food and Nutrition Board, Institute of Medicine. (2004). *Dietary Reference Intakes: Water, potassium, chloride, and sulfate.* Washington, DC: National Academies Press.

Popkin, B., Armstrong, L., Bray, G., et al. (2006). A new proposed guidance system for beverage consumption in the United States. *The American Journal of Clinical Nutrition, 83*, 529–542.

Valtin, H. (2002). "Drink at least eight glasses of water a day." Really? Is there scientific evidence for "8 × 8"? *American Journal of Physiology. Regulatory, Integrative and Comparative Physiology, 283*, R993–R1004.

Varenna, M., Binelli, L., Casari, S., et al. (2007). Effects of dietary calcium intake on body weight and prevalence of osteoporosis in early postmenopausal women. *The American Journal of Clinical Nutrition, 86*, 639–644.

Weaver, C., Lupton, J., King, J., et al. (2006). Dietary guidelines vs beverage guidance system. *The American Journal of Clinical Nutrition, 84,* 1245–1246.

World Cancer Research Fund/American Institute for Cancer Research. (2007). *Food, nutrition, physical activity, and the prevention of cancer: A global perspective.* Washington DC: AICR.

World Health Organization. (2008). Micronutrient deficiencies. Available at www.who.int/nutrition/topics/ida/en/print.html. Accessed on 1/3/08.

Zemel, M. (2001). Calcium modulation of hypertension and obesity: Mechanisms and implications. *Journal of the American College of Nutrition, 20,* 428S–435S.

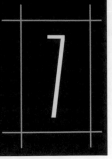

# 7 Energy Balance

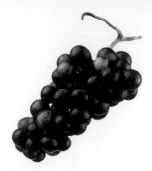

| TRUE | FALSE | |
|:---:|:---:|---|
| ☐ | ☐ | **1** A food that is high in "energy" is high in calories. |
| ☐ | ☐ | **2** A pound of body fat is equivalent to 3500 calories. |
| ☐ | ☐ | **3** People shaped like "apples" are at greater health risk than people shaped like "pears." |
| ☐ | ☐ | **4** Starvation diets can lower metabolic rate. |
| ☐ | ☐ | **5** Thirty minutes a day of moderate-intensity exercise is recommended to manage weight and prevent weight gain in adulthood. |
| ☐ | ☐ | **6** The majority of calories expended daily by most Americans are on basal needs. |
| ☐ | ☐ | **7** Building muscle speeds metabolic rate. |
| ☐ | ☐ | **8** To reap health benefits, you must participate in continuous activity for at least 30 minutes. |
| ☐ | ☐ | **9** The best exercise is the one the individual sticks with. |
| ☐ | ☐ | **10** An effective strategy for limiting calorie intake is to limit food and beverages high in added sugar and fat. |

### UPON COMPLETION OF THIS CHAPTER, YOU WILL BE ABLE TO

- Estimate an individual's total calorie requirements.
- Determine an individual's BMI.
- Evaluate weight status based on BMI.
- Assess a person's waist circumference.
- Give examples of the healthiest ways to reduce calorie intake.
- Evaluate a person's usual activity level based on Dietary Guidelines recommendations.

**Calorie:** unit by which energy is measured; the amount of heat needed to raise the temperature of 1 kg of water by 1°C. Technically, calorie is actually kilocalorie or kcal.

Technically, a **calorie** is the amount of energy required to raise the temperature of 1 kg of water by 1°C. In nutrition, calories are the measure of the amount of energy in a food or used by the body to fuel activity. Energy balance is a function of calorie intake versus calorie output (Fig. 7.1).

This chapter addresses the dynamics of energy balance and how total calorie requirements are estimated. Methods to determine healthy body weight and standards for evaluating body weight are presented. Energy in health promotion focuses on the Dietary Guidelines for Americans (DGA) recommendations for weight management and physical activity (PA).

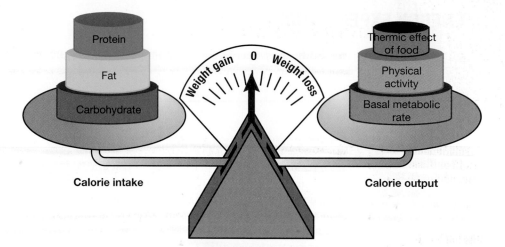

**FIGURE 7.1** Energy balance: calorie intake versus calorie output.

# ► ENERGY INTAKE

Calories come from carbohydrates, protein, fat, and alcohol. The total number of calories in a food or diet can be estimated by multiplying total grams of these nutrients by the appropriate calories per gram, namely 4 cal/g for carbohydrates and protein, 9 cal/g for fat, and 7 cal/g for alcohol.

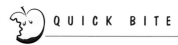 QUICK BITE

Calories by food groups according to Exchange Lists for Diabetes*

| Food Group | Average Calories/ Serving |
| --- | --- |
| Starch/grains | 80 |
| Fruits | 60 |
| Milk | |
|   Skim or 1% | 100 |
|   2% | 120 |
|   Whole | 160 |
| Nonstarchy vegetables | 25 |
| Meat and beans | |
|   Plant-based protein | Varies |
|   Lean | 45 |
|   Medium fat | 75 |
|   High fat | 100 |
| Fat/oils | 45 |

***Source:*** American Diabetes Association, American Dietetic Association. (2008). *Choose your foods: Exchange lists for diabetes.* Alexandria, VA: The American Diabetes Association.

In practice, "counting calories" is an imprecise and painstaking process dependent upon knowing accurate portion sizes of all foods consumed and the exact nutritional composition of each item, neither of which conditions are easily met. Even when all food consumed is measured, the nutrient values available in food composition references represent *average* not *actual* nutrition content based on analysis of a number of food samples.

A less accurate but easier way to estimate calorie intake is to estimate or count the number of servings from each food group a person consumes; multiply the number of servings by the average amount of calories in a serving; then add the calories from each group to get an approximation of the total calories consumed. Be aware that representative foods within each of the Exchange Lists for Diabetics food groups are generally free of added fat or sugar. For instance, items like onion rings, brownies, and sugar-sweetened cereals are not part of those food groups. As with "counting calories," the accuracy of "counting servings" is dependent upon the quality of foods consumed and accuracy of portion size estimation.

## ▶ ENERGY EXPENDITURE

The body uses energy for involuntary activities and purposeful PA. The total of these expenditures represent the number of calories a person uses in a day.

## Basal Metabolism

**Basal Metabolic Rate (BMR) or Basal Energy Expenditure (BEE):** the minimum caloric requirement to sustain life in a resting individual.

**Resting Energy Expenditure (REE):** basal energy needs that do not adhere to the criterion of a 12-hour fast and, therefore, include the energy spent on digesting, absorbing, and metabolizing food.

Basal metabolism is the caloric cost of staying alive or the amount of calories required to fuel the involuntary activities of the body at rest after a 12-hour fast. These involuntary activities include maintaining body temperature and muscle tone, producing and releasing secretions, propelling the gastrointestinal (GI) tract, inflating the lungs, and beating the heart. For most people, the **Basal Metabolic Rate (BMR)** accounts for approximately 60% of total calories expended. The less active a person is, the greater the proportion of calories used for **Basal Energy Expenditure (BEE)**. The terms "BEE" and **Resting Energy Expenditure (REE)** are often used interchangeably.

One rule-of-thumb guideline for estimating BMR is to multiply healthy weight (in pounds) by 10 for women and 11 for men. For example, a 130-pound woman expends approximately 1300 cal/day on BMR (130 lb × 10 cal/lb = 1300 cal). When actual weight exceeds healthy weight, an "adjusted" weight of halfway between healthy and actual can be used. For instance, if healthy weight is 130 but actual weight is 170, 150 pounds would be the "adjusted" weight for estimating basal calories. Methods used to determine BMR and total calorie requirements in the clinical setting are covered in Chapter 16.

A drawback of using a "rule-of-thumb" method for determining BMR is that it is based only on weight; it does not account for other variables that affect metabolic rate, such as body composition. Lean tissue (muscle mass) contributes to a higher metabolic rate than fat tissue. Therefore, people with more muscle mass have higher metabolic rates than do people with proportionately more fat tissue. This explains why men, who have a greater proportion of muscle, have higher metabolic rates than women, who have a greater proportion of fat. Conversely, the loss of lean tissue that usually occurs with aging beginning sometime around age 30 is one reason why calorie requirements decrease as people get older. However, the loss of lean tissue can be limited in severity by healthy eating and exercise (Rivlin, 2007). Other factors that affect BMR appear in Table 7.1.

## Physical Activity

PA, or voluntary muscular activity, accounts for approximately 30% of total calories used, although it may be as low as 20% in sedentary people and as high as 50% in people who are very active. The actual amount of energy expended on PA depends on the intensity and duration of the activity and the weight of the person performing the activity (Table 7.2). The more intense and longer the activity, the greater the amount of calories burned. Heavier people, who have more weight to move, use more energy than lighter people to perform the same activity.

Although it is possible to get a reasonable estimate of total calories expended in a day by keeping a thorough record of all activity for a 24-hour period, it is a tedious process. An easier rule-of-thumb method for estimating daily calories expended on PA is to calculate the percentage increase above BMR on the basis of estimated intensity of usual daily activities.

TABLE 7.1          **Factors That Influence BMR**

| Variables | Effect on Metabolism |
| --- | --- |
| Age | Loss of lean body mass with age lowers BMR |
| Growth | The formation of new tissue, as seen in children and during pregnancy, increases BMR |
| Stresses | Stresses, such as infection and many diseases, raise BMR |
| Thyroid hormones: tetraiodothyronine (thyroxine, or $T_4$) and triiodothyronine ($T_3$) | An oversecretion of thyroid hormones (hyperthyroidism) speeds up BMR; undersecretion of thyroid hormones (hypothyroidism) lowers BMR. The change may be as great as 50% |
| Fever | BMR increases 7% for each degree Fahrenheit above 98.6 |
| Height | When considering two people of the same gender who weigh the same, the taller one has a higher BMR than the shorter one because of a larger surface area |
| Extreme environmental temperatures | Very hot and very cold environmental temperatures increase the BMR because the body expends more energy to regulate its own temperature |
| Starvation, fasting, and malnutrition | Part of the decline in BMR that occurs with these conditions is attributed to the loss of lean body tissue. Hormonal changes may contribute to the decrease in metabolic rate |
| Weight loss from calorie deficits | With smaller body mass, less energy is required to fuel metabolism |
| Smoking | Nicotine increases BMR |
| Caffeine | Increases BMR |
| Certain drugs, such as barbiturates, narcotics, and muscle relaxants | Decrease BMR |
| Sleep, paralysis | Decrease BMR |

TABLE 7.2          **Calories/Hour Expended in Common Physical Activities**

| Moderate Physical Activity | Approximate Calories/Hour for a 154-lb Person* |
| --- | --- |
| Hiking | 370 |
| Light gardening/yard work | 330 |
| Dancing | 330 |
| Golf (walking and carrying clubs) | 330 |
| Bicycling (<10 mph) | 290 |
| Walking (3.5 mph) | 280 |
| Weight lifting (general light workout) | 220 |
| Stretching | 180 |

| Vigorous Physical Activity | Approximate Calories/Hour for a 154-lb Person* |
| --- | --- |
| Running/jogging (5 mph) | 590 |
| Bicycling (>10 mph) | 590 |
| Swimming (slow freestyle laps) | 510 |
| Aerobics | 480 |
| Walking (4.5 mph) | 460 |
| Heavy yard work (chopping wood) | 440 |
| Weight lifting (vigorous effort) | 440 |
| Basketball (vigorous) | 440 |

Some examples of PAs commonly engaged in and the average amount of calories a 154-pound individual will expend by engaging in each activity for 1 hour. The expenditure value encompasses both resting metabolic rate calories and activity expenditure. Some of the activities can constitute either moderate- or vigorous-intensity PA depending on the rate at which they are carried out (for walking and bicycling).

*Calories burned per hour will be higher for persons who weigh more than 154 lb (70 kg) and lower for persons who weigh less.

Adapted from the 2005 DCAC Report.

**Source:** USDHHS, USDA. *Dietary Guidelines for Americans 2005.* Available at www.health.gov/dietaryguidelines

| BOX 7.1 | **ESTIMATING TOTAL CALORIE EXPENDITURE\*** |
|---------|---------------------------------------------|

**1. Estimate basal metabolic rate**

Multiply your healthy weight (in pounds) by 10 for women or 11 for men. If you are overweight, multiply by the average weight within your healthy weight range (see Chapter 14).

_____ (weight in pounds) × _____ = _____ calories for BMR

**2. Estimate total calories according to usual activity level**

Choose the category that describes your usual activities and then multiply BMR by the appropriate percentage.

| Usual Activity Most Days of the Week | BMR Used (%) |
|---|---|
| Sedentary: mostly sitting, driving, sleeping, standing, reading, typing, and other low-intensity activities | 20 |
| Light activity: light exercise such as walking not more than 2 hours/day | 30 |
| Moderate activity: moderate exercise such as heavy housework, gardening, and very little sitting | 40 |
| High activity: active in physical sports or a labor-intensive occupation such as construction work | 50 |

**3. Add BMR calories and PA calories to determine total calories per day**

_____ calories for BMR + _____ calories spent on activity = _____ total daily calories expended daily

**Thermic Effect of Food:** an estimation of the amount of energy required to digest, absorb, transport, metabolize, and store nutrients.

\*The **thermic effect of food** is another category of energy expenditure that represents the "cost" of processing food. In a normal mixed diet, it is estimated to be about 10% of the total calorie intake. For instance, people who consume 1800 cal/day use about 180 calories to process their food. The actual thermic effect of food varies with the composition of food eaten, the frequency of eating, and the size of meals consumed. Although it represents an actual and legitimate use of calories, the thermic effect of food in practice is usually disregarded when calorie requirements are estimated because it constitutes such a small amount of energy and is imprecisely estimated.

## Estimating Total Calorie Requirements

Box 7.1 illustrates how daily needs are estimated using BMR and activity level. Other more complex mathematical formulas are available for estimating total calorie requirements in healthy people, such as the one put forth by the DRI Committee (estimated energy requirements or EERs) based on age, weight, height, and PA, with defined PA factors for men and women based on intensity of activity (NAS, IOM, 2005). A quicker and easier reference is the MyPyramid calorie level table based on gender, age, and activity (Table 7.3).

## ▶ CALORIES IN VERSUS CALORIES OUT

The state of energy balance is the relationship between the amount of calories consumed and the amount of calories expended. As illustrated in Figure 7.2, when calorie intake and output are approximately the same, body weight is stable.

| TABLE 7.3 | MyPyramid Food Intake Pattern Calorie Levels | | | | | | |
|---|---|---|---|---|---|---|---|
| **Age** | **Activity Level for Males** | | | **Age** | **Activity Level for Females** | | |
| | Sedentary* | Mod. Active* | Active* | | Sedentary* | Mod. Active* | Active* |
| 2 | 1000 | 1000 | 1000 | 2 | 1000 | 1000 | 1000 |
| 3 | 1000 | 1400 | 1400 | 3 | 1000 | 1200 | 1400 |
| 4 | 1200 | 1400 | 1600 | 4 | 1200 | 1400 | 1400 |
| 5 | 1200 | 1400 | 1600 | 5 | 1200 | 1400 | 1600 |
| 6 | 1400 | 1600 | 1800 | 6 | 1200 | 1400 | 1600 |
| 7 | 1400 | 1600 | 1800 | 7 | 1200 | 1600 | 1800 |
| 8 | 1400 | 1600 | 2000 | 8 | 1400 | 1600 | 1800 |
| 9 | 1600 | 1800 | 2000 | 9 | 1400 | 1600 | 1800 |
| 10 | 1600 | 1800 | 2200 | 10 | 1400 | 1800 | 2000 |
| 11 | 1800 | 2000 | 2200 | 11 | 1600 | 1800 | 2000 |
| 12 | 1800 | 2200 | 2400 | 12 | 1600 | 2000 | 2200 |
| 13 | 2000 | 2200 | 2600 | 13 | 1600 | 2000 | 2200 |
| 14 | 2000 | 2400 | 2800 | 14 | 1800 | 2000 | 2400 |
| 15 | 2200 | 2600 | 3000 | 15 | 1800 | 2000 | 2400 |
| 16 | 2400 | 2800 | 3200 | 16 | 1800 | 2000 | 2400 |
| 17 | 2400 | 2800 | 3200 | 17 | 1800 | 2000 | 2400 |
| 18 | 2400 | 2800 | 3200 | 18 | 1800 | 2000 | 2400 |
| 19–20 | 2600 | 2800 | 3000 | 19–20 | 2000 | 2200 | 2400 |
| 21–25 | 2400 | 2800 | 3000 | 21–25 | 2000 | 2200 | 2400 |
| 26–30 | 2400 | 2600 | 3000 | 26–30 | 1800 | 2000 | 2400 |
| 31–35 | 2400 | 2600 | 3000 | 31–35 | 1800 | 2000 | 2200 |
| 36–40 | 2400 | 2600 | 2800 | 36–40 | 1800 | 2000 | 2200 |
| 41–45 | 2200 | 2600 | 2800 | 41–45 | 1800 | 2000 | 2200 |
| 46–50 | 2200 | 2400 | 2800 | 46–50 | 1800 | 2000 | 2200 |
| 51–55 | 2200 | 2400 | 2800 | 51–55 | 1600 | 1800 | 2200 |
| 56–60 | 2200 | 2400 | 2600 | 56–60 | 1600 | 1800 | 2200 |
| 61–65 | 2000 | 2400 | 2600 | 61–65 | 1600 | 1800 | 2000 |
| 66–70 | 2000 | 2200 | 2600 | 66–70 | 1600 | 1800 | 2000 |
| 71–75 | 2000 | 2200 | 2600 | 71–75 | 1600 | 1800 | 2000 |
| 76 and up | 2000 | 2200 | 2400 | 76 and up | 1600 | 1800 | 2000 |

MyPyramid assigns individuals to a calorie level based on their sex, age, and activity level.
The above chart identifies the calorie levels for males and females by age and activity level.
Calorie levels are provided for each year of childhood, from 2 to 18 years, and for adults in 5-year increments.
*Calorie levels are based on the Estimated Energy Requirements (EER) and activity levels from the Institute of Medicine Dietary Reference Intakes Macronutrients Report, 2002.
Sedentary = less than 30 minutes a day of moderate PA in addition to daily activities.
Mod. Active = at least 30 minutes up to 60 minutes a day of moderate PA in addition to daily activities.
Active = 60 or more minutes a day of moderate PA in addition to daily activities.
*Source:* United Sates Department of Agriculture.

A "positive" energy balance occurs when calorie intake exceeds calorie output, whether the imbalance is caused by overeating, low activity, or both (Fig. 7.3). Over time, the calories consumed in excess of need contribute to weight gain. Because a pound of body fat is equivalent to 3500 calories, an "extra" 500 cal/day for a whole week can result in a 1-pound weight gain. Conversely, a "negative" calorie balance occurs when calorie output exceeds intake, whether the imbalance is from decreasing calorie intake, increasing PA, or (preferably) both (Fig. 7.4).

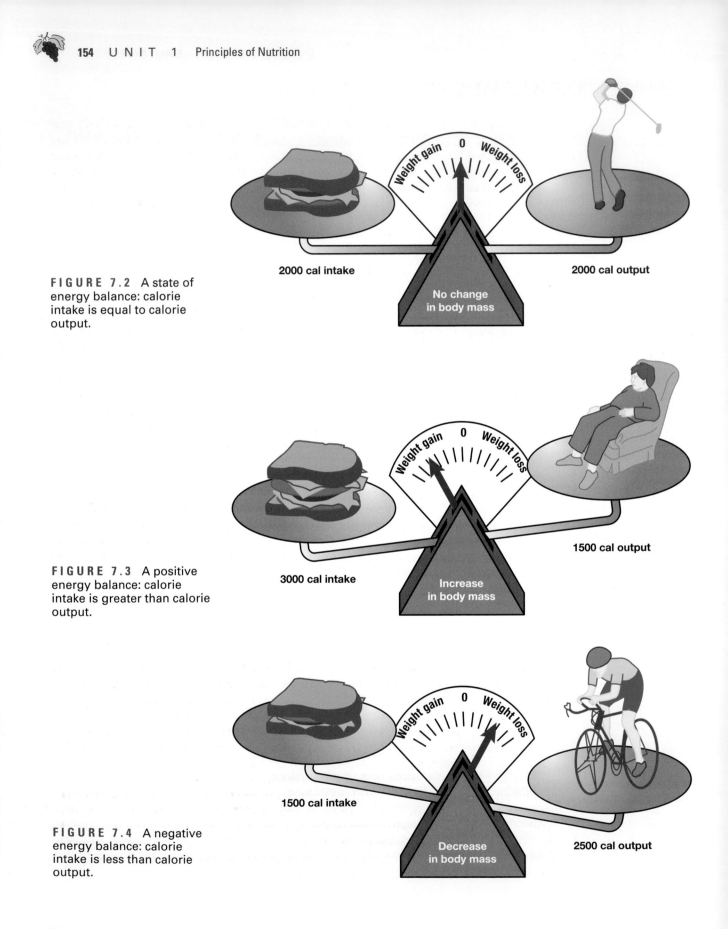

**FIGURE 7.2** A state of energy balance: calorie intake is equal to calorie output.

2000 cal intake

Weight gain | 0 | Weight loss

No change in body mass

2000 cal output

**FIGURE 7.3** A positive energy balance: calorie intake is greater than calorie output.

3000 cal intake

Weight gain | 0 | Weight loss

Increase in body mass

1500 cal output

**FIGURE 7.4** A negative energy balance: calorie intake is less than calorie output.

1500 cal intake

Weight gain | 0 | Weight loss

Decrease in body mass

2500 cal output

## ▶ WHAT IS "NORMAL" WEIGHT?

From a health perspective, "normal" or "desirable" weight is that which is statistically correlated to good health. But the relationship between body weight and good health is more complicated than simply the number on the scale. The amount of body *fat* a person has and where a person's weight is distributed also influence health risks, as does the presence of certain diseases or conditions (comorbidities). The three criteria used for assessing overweight and obesity are body mass index (BMI), waist circumference, and existing health problems.

## Body Mass Index

**Skinfold Measurements:** a measure of body fat and its distribution obtained by a pincer caliper at various body sites, such as the triceps, iliac crest, abdomen, and chest.

**Bioelectrical Impedance:** a computerized system that uses a small alternating current to determine percentage body fat; the amount of water in the body (fat-free tissue) impedes the electric flow, which can be translated into percentage body fat.

In the clinical setting, BMI has replaced traditional weight–height calculations that were used to determine "ideal" or "desirable" body weight. After a review of the evidence-based literature, the U.S. Preventive Services Task Force concluded that BMI is reliable and valid for identifying adults at increased risk for mortality and morbidity due to overweight and obesity (McTigue et al., 2003). BMI is recommended because it provides an estimate of body fat and is related to risk of disease (Kushner & Blatner, 2005).

The formula to calculate BMI is weight in kilogram divided by height in meters squared or weight in pounds divided by height in inches squared multiplied by 703. Nomograms and tables are available to eliminate complicated mathematical calculations (Table 7.4). After obtaining height and weight, the table can be used to determine BMI; the step that follows is to classify BMI according to standards (Table 7.5). Because the relationship between increasing weight and risk of disease is continuous, the BMI levels that define overweight and obesity are somewhat arbitrary.

Using BMI to evaluate body weight is nonthreatening and noninvasive to clients and requires minimal equipment and skill. The drawback is that it does not take body composition into account. A lean athlete may have well-developed muscle mass and little fat tissue, yet if his BMI is high, he would fall under the designation of overweight or obese. Conversely, an elderly person may have a normal BMI and be deemed "healthy" despite a high amount of body fat masked by a low percentage of muscle mass. **Skinfold measurements** and **bioelectrical impedance** can assess body composition, but neither technique is widely used.

## Waist Circumference

The location of excess body fat may be a more important and reliable indicator of disease risk than the degree of total body fatness. Storing a disproportionate amount of total body fat in the abdomen increases risks for type 2 diabetes, dyslipidemia, hypertension, and cardiovascular disease. Generally, men and postmenopausal women tend to store excess fat in the upper body, particularly in the abdominal area, whereas premenopausal women tend to store excess fat in the lower body, particularly in the hips and thighs. Regardless of gender, people with a high distribution of abdominal fat (i.e., "apples") have a greater relative health risk than people with excess fat in the hips and thighs (i.e., "pears") (Fig. 7.5).

Abdominal fat is clinically defined as a waist circumference greater than or equal to 40 in. in men and greater than or equal to 35 in. in women (USDA, USDHHS, 2005). As illustrated in Table 7.5, people with a large waist circumference are at higher cardiovascular risk than people with normal waist sizes within healthy, overweight, and obesity class I categories. In people with a BMI of 35 or higher, waist measurement is unnecessary because health risk is already considered "very high" based on BMI alone.

| TABLE 7.4 | Body Mass Index | | | | | | | | | | | | | | | |
|---|---|---|---|---|---|---|---|---|---|---|---|---|---|---|---|---|
| | Normal | | | | | | Overweight | | | | | | Obese | | | |
| BMI | 19 | 20 | 21 | 22 | 23 | 24 | 25 | 26 | 27 | 28 | 29 | 30 | 31 | 32 | 33 | 34 | 35 |
| Height (inches) | Body Weight (pounds) | | | | | | | | | | | | | | | |
| 58 | 91 | 96 | 100 | 105 | 110 | 115 | 119 | 124 | 129 | 134 | 138 | 143 | 148 | 153 | 158 | 162 | 167 |
| 59 | 94 | 99 | 104 | 109 | 114 | 119 | 124 | 128 | 133 | 138 | 143 | 148 | 153 | 158 | 163 | 168 | 173 |
| 60 | 97 | 102 | 107 | 112 | 118 | 123 | 128 | 133 | 138 | 143 | 148 | 153 | 158 | 163 | 168 | 174 | 179 |
| 61 | 100 | 106 | 111 | 116 | 122 | 127 | 132 | 137 | 143 | 148 | 153 | 158 | 164 | 169 | 174 | 180 | 185 |
| 62 | 104 | 109 | 115 | 120 | 126 | 131 | 136 | 142 | 147 | 153 | 158 | 164 | 169 | 175 | 180 | 186 | 191 |
| 63 | 107 | 113 | 118 | 124 | 130 | 135 | 141 | 146 | 152 | 158 | 163 | 169 | 175 | 180 | 186 | 191 | 197 |
| 64 | 110 | 116 | 122 | 128 | 134 | 140 | 145 | 151 | 157 | 163 | 169 | 174 | 180 | 186 | 192 | 197 | 204 |
| 65 | 114 | 120 | 126 | 132 | 138 | 144 | 150 | 156 | 162 | 168 | 174 | 180 | 186 | 192 | 198 | 204 | 210 |
| 66 | 118 | 124 | 130 | 136 | 142 | 148 | 155 | 161 | 167 | 173 | 179 | 186 | 192 | 198 | 204 | 210 | 216 |
| 67 | 121 | 127 | 134 | 140 | 146 | 153 | 159 | 166 | 172 | 178 | 185 | 191 | 198 | 204 | 211 | 217 | 223 |
| 68 | 125 | 131 | 138 | 144 | 151 | 158 | 164 | 171 | 177 | 184 | 190 | 197 | 203 | 210 | 216 | 223 | 230 |
| 69 | 128 | 135 | 142 | 149 | 155 | 162 | 169 | 176 | 182 | 189 | 196 | 203 | 209 | 216 | 223 | 230 | 236 |
| 70 | 132 | 139 | 146 | 153 | 160 | 167 | 174 | 181 | 188 | 195 | 202 | 209 | 216 | 222 | 229 | 236 | 243 |
| 71 | 136 | 143 | 150 | 157 | 165 | 172 | 179 | 186 | 193 | 200 | 208 | 215 | 222 | 229 | 236 | 243 | 250 |
| 72 | 140 | 147 | 154 | 162 | 169 | 177 | 184 | 191 | 199 | 206 | 213 | 221 | 228 | 235 | 242 | 250 | 258 |
| 73 | 144 | 151 | 159 | 166 | 174 | 182 | 189 | 197 | 204 | 212 | 219 | 227 | 235 | 242 | 250 | 257 | 265 |
| 74 | 148 | 155 | 163 | 171 | 179 | 186 | 194 | 202 | 210 | 218 | 225 | 233 | 241 | 249 | 256 | 264 | 272 |
| 75 | 152 | 160 | 168 | 176 | 184 | 192 | 200 | 208 | 216 | 224 | 232 | 240 | 248 | 256 | 264 | 272 | 279 |
| 76 | 156 | 164 | 172 | 180 | 189 | 197 | 205 | 213 | 221 | 230 | 238 | 246 | 254 | 263 | 271 | 279 | 287 |

**Source:** Adapted from U.S. Department of Health and Human Services. (1998). *Clinical guidelines on the identification, evaluation, and treatment of overweight and obesity in adults: The evidence report.* Rockville, MD: Author.

| TABLE 7.5 | Weight Classifications and Disease Risk Based on BMI and Waist Circumference | | |
|---|---|---|---|

| | | Disease risk (for type 2 diabetes, hypertension, and CVD) compared to normal weight and waist circumference | |
|---|---|---|---|
| Assessment | BMI | ≤40 in. for men ≤35 in. for women | >40 in. for men >35 in. for women |
| Underweight | <18.5 | — | — |
| Normal (healthy) weight* | 18.5–24.9 | — | — |
| Overweight | 25.0–29.9 | Increased | High |
| Obesity class I | 30.0–34.9 | High | Very high |
| Obesity class II | 35.0–39.9 | Very high | Very high |
| Obesity class III (extreme obesity) | ≥40.0 | Extremely high | Extremely high |

*Increased waist circumference may also indicate increased risk in people whose weight is normal.

**Source:** Adapted from National Institutes of Health, National Heart, Lunch and Blood Institute. (1998). *Clinical guidelines on the identification, evaluation, and treatment of overweight and obesity in adults.* USDHHS, Bethesda, MD, Public Health Service.

| Extreme Obesity | | | | | | | | | | | | | | | | | | |
|---|---|---|---|---|---|---|---|---|---|---|---|---|---|---|---|---|---|---|
| 36 | 37 | 38 | 39 | 40 | 41 | 42 | 43 | 44 | 45 | 46 | 47 | 48 | 49 | 50 | 51 | 52 | 53 | 54 |

**Height (inches)** — **Body Weight (pounds)**

| 36 | 37 | 38 | 39 | 40 | 41 | 42 | 43 | 44 | 45 | 46 | 47 | 48 | 49 | 50 | 51 | 52 | 53 | 54 |
|---|---|---|---|---|---|---|---|---|---|---|---|---|---|---|---|---|---|---|
| 172 | 177 | 181 | 186 | 191 | 196 | 201 | 205 | 210 | 215 | 220 | 224 | 229 | 234 | 239 | 244 | 248 | 253 | 258 |
| 178 | 183 | 188 | 193 | 198 | 203 | 208 | 212 | 217 | 222 | 227 | 232 | 237 | 242 | 247 | 252 | 257 | 262 | 267 |
| 184 | 189 | 194 | 199 | 204 | 209 | 215 | 220 | 225 | 230 | 235 | 240 | 245 | 250 | 255 | 261 | 266 | 271 | 276 |
| 190 | 195 | 201 | 206 | 211 | 217 | 222 | 227 | 232 | 238 | 243 | 248 | 254 | 259 | 264 | 269 | 275 | 280 | 285 |
| 196 | 202 | 207 | 213 | 218 | 224 | 229 | 235 | 240 | 246 | 251 | 256 | 262 | 267 | 273 | 278 | 284 | 289 | 295 |
| 203 | 208 | 214 | 220 | 225 | 231 | 237 | 242 | 248 | 254 | 259 | 265 | 270 | 278 | 282 | 287 | 293 | 299 | 304 |
| 209 | 215 | 221 | 227 | 232 | 238 | 244 | 250 | 256 | 262 | 267 | 273 | 279 | 285 | 291 | 296 | 302 | 308 | 314 |
| 216 | 222 | 228 | 234 | 240 | 246 | 252 | 258 | 264 | 270 | 276 | 282 | 288 | 294 | 300 | 306 | 312 | 318 | 324 |
| 223 | 229 | 235 | 241 | 247 | 253 | 260 | 266 | 272 | 278 | 284 | 291 | 297 | 303 | 309 | 315 | 322 | 328 | 334 |
| 230 | 236 | 242 | 249 | 255 | 261 | 268 | 274 | 280 | 287 | 293 | 299 | 306 | 312 | 319 | 325 | 331 | 338 | 344 |
| 236 | 243 | 249 | 256 | 262 | 269 | 276 | 282 | 289 | 295 | 302 | 308 | 315 | 322 | 328 | 335 | 341 | 348 | 354 |
| 243 | 250 | 257 | 263 | 270 | 277 | 284 | 291 | 297 | 304 | 311 | 318 | 324 | 331 | 338 | 345 | 351 | 358 | 365 |
| 250 | 257 | 264 | 271 | 278 | 285 | 292 | 299 | 306 | 313 | 320 | 327 | 334 | 341 | 348 | 355 | 362 | 369 | 376 |
| 257 | 265 | 272 | 279 | 286 | 293 | 301 | 308 | 315 | 322 | 329 | 338 | 343 | 351 | 358 | 365 | 372 | 379 | 386 |
| 265 | 272 | 279 | 287 | 294 | 302 | 309 | 316 | 324 | 331 | 338 | 346 | 353 | 361 | 368 | 375 | 383 | 390 | 397 |
| 272 | 280 | 288 | 295 | 302 | 310 | 318 | 325 | 333 | 340 | 348 | 355 | 363 | 371 | 378 | 386 | 393 | 401 | 408 |
| 280 | 287 | 295 | 303 | 311 | 319 | 326 | 334 | 342 | 350 | 358 | 365 | 373 | 381 | 389 | 396 | 404 | 412 | 420 |
| 287 | 295 | 303 | 311 | 319 | 327 | 335 | 343 | 351 | 359 | 367 | 375 | 383 | 391 | 399 | 407 | 415 | 423 | 431 |
| 295 | 304 | 312 | 320 | 328 | 336 | 344 | 353 | 361 | 369 | 377 | 385 | 394 | 402 | 410 | 418 | 426 | 435 | 443 |

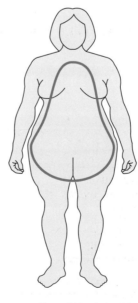
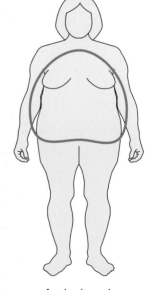

**FIGURE 7.5** Pear shape versus apple shape.

Pear shaped          Apple shaped

| BOX 7.2 | **ASSESSMENT OF RISK FOR DISEASE COMPLICATIONS AND MORTALITY BASED ON COMORBIDITIES** |

People with the following conditions are at *very high risk* related to overweight and obesity:

- Established coronary heart disease
- Other atherosclerotic diseases, such as peripheral arterial disease, abdominal aortic aneurysm, or symptomatic carotid artery disease
- Type 2 diabetes
- Sleep apnea

Three or more of the following risk factors place people at *high risk:*

- Cigarette smoking
- Hypertension
- High concentration of low-density lipoprotein (LDL) cholesterol
- Low concentration of high-density lipoprotein (HDL) cholesterol
- Impaired fasting glucose
- Family history of premature heart disease
- Age (45 years or older for men, 55 years or older or postmenopausal for women)

Incremental risk above the preceding risks occurs from

- Physical inactivity
- High serum triglyceride levels

## Existing Health Problems

The presence of existing health problems impacts a person's absolute risk related to weight (Box 7.2). Generally, the number and severity of comorbid conditions increases with increasing levels of obesity.

## ▶ ENERGY BALANCE IN HEALTH PROMOTION

Although estimates vary, approximately 66% of the adult American population is overweight or obese (CDC, 2007), and the prevalence of obesity has doubled in the past two decades (USDA, USDHHS, 2005). Overweight and obesity are a public health concern because excess body fat increases the risk of premature death, type 2 diabetes, hypertension, dyslipidemia, cardiovascular disease, stroke, gallbladder disease, respiratory disorders, gout, osteoarthritis, and certain kinds of cancer (USDA, USDHHS, 2005).

As a wellness issue, preventing or reducing overweight is achieved by adopting a lifestyle approach that includes healthier food choices, increasing PA, and behavior modification. Key recommendations for weight management and PA—intended for "healthy" Americans—appear in Box 7.3. As a clinical issue, the management of overweight and obesity, including therapeutic diet approaches, is presented in Chapter 14.

**QUICK BITE**

Lifestyle tips to manage weight
- Think "healthy choices" not diet
- Eat only to satisfy hunger, not to relieve boredom or anxiety
- Eat out wisely
- Shop smart—and never when hungry
- Eat breakfast everyday
- Choose healthy foods to snack on
- Monitor your weight
- Limit TV watching—a passive activity that may spur mindless munching

| BOX 7.3 | **2005 DIETARY GUIDELINES FOR AMERICANS RECOMMENDATIONS REGARDING WEIGHT MANAGEMENT AND PHYSICAL ACTIVITY** |
|---------|---|

**Weight Management**
Key recommendations:

- To maintain body weight in a healthy range, balance calories from foods and vegetables with calories expended.
- To prevent gradual weight gain over time, make small decreases in food and beverage calories and increase PA.

**Physical Activity**
Key recommendations:

- Engage in regular PA and reduce sedentary activities to promote health, psychological well-being, and a healthy body weight.
  - To reduce the risk of chronic disease in adulthood: engage in at least 30 minutes of moderate-intensity PA, above usual activity, at work or home on most days of the week.
  - For most people, greater health benefits can be obtained by engaging in PA of more vigorous intensity or longer duration.
  - To help manage body weight and prevent gradual, unhealthy body weight gain in adulthood: engage in approximately 60 minutes of moderate- to vigorous-intensity activity on most days of the week while not exceeding caloric intake requirements.
  - To sustain weight loss in adulthood: participate in at least 60 to 90 minutes of daily moderate-intensity PA while not exceeding caloric intake requirements. Some people may need to consult with a health care provider before participating in this level of activity.
- Achieve physical fitness by including cardiovascular condition, stretching exercises for flexibility, and resistance exercises or calisthenics for muscle strength and endurance.

## Healthier Choices

Making healthier choices to lower calorie intake encompasses a two-pronged approach: eating less of certain items, eating more of others. Foods to limit include those that are high in fat and added sugars, such as regular soft drinks, most desserts, fried foods, full-fat dairy products, high-fat meat, and most fast foods. Items to emphasize are nutrient-dense, minimally processed, high-fiber foods, such as fruits, vegetables, whole grains, legumes, and lean protein. MyPyramid recommendations for replacing foods high in added sugar and/or fat appear in Box 7.4.

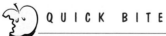 QUICK BITE

A closer look at reduced-fat cookies shows they are not a calorie bargain

|  | Serving size | Fat (g) | Calories |
|---|---|---|---|
| Chips Ahoy! Chocolate Chip | 3 | 8 | 160 |
| Chips Ahoy! Reduced fat | 3 | 5 | 140 |
| Fig Newtons | 2 | 3 | 110 |
| Fat-Free Fig Newtons | 2 | 0 | 90 |
| Oatmeal Raisin | 1 | 4 | 110 |
| Fat-Free Oatmeal Raisin | 1 | 0 | 105 |
| Raspberry-Filled Cookies | 1 | 4 | 100 |
| Raspberry Oatmeal Fat-Free Cookies | 1 | 4 | 110 |

| BOX 7.4 | STEPS TO A HEALTHIER WEIGHT |

**Making Nutrient-Dense Food Choices**

Here are some foods that contain extra calories from solid fats and added sugars and some "smarter" replacements. Choices on the right side are more nutrient dense—lower in solid fats and added sugars. Try these new ideas instead of your usual choices. This guide gives sample ideas—it is not a complete list. Use the "Nutrition Facts" label to help identify more alternatives.

| Instead of. . . | Replace with. . . |
| --- | --- |
| **Milk Group** | |
| Sweetened fruit yogurt | Plain fat-free yogurt with fresh fruit |
| Whole milk | Low-fat or fat-free milk |
| Natural or processed cheese | Low-fat or reduced-fat cheese |
| **Meat Group** | |
| Beef (chuck, rib, brisket) | Beef (loin, round), fat trimmed off |
| Chicken with skin | Chicken without skin |
| Lunch meats (such as bologna) | Low-fat lunch meats (95%–97% fat free) |
| Hot dogs (regular) | Hot dogs (lower fat) |
| Bacon or sausage | Canadian bacon or lean ham |
| Refried beans | Cooked or canned kidney or pinto beans |
| **Grain Group** | |
| Granola | Reduced-fat granola |
| Sweetened cereals | Unsweetened cereals with cut-up fruit |
| Pasta with cheese sauce | Pasta with vegetables (primavera) |
| Pasta with white sauce (alfredo) | Pasta with red sauce (marinara) |
| Croissants or pastries | Toast or bread (try whole grain types) |
| **Fruit Group** | |
| Apple or berry pie | Fresh apple or berries |
| Sweetened applesauce | Unsweetened applesauce |
| Canned fruit packed in syrup | Canned fruit packed in juice or "lite" syrup |
| **Vegetable Group** | |
| Deep-fried French fries | Oven-baked "French fries" |
| Baked potato with cheese sauce | Baked potato with salsa |
| Fried vegetables | Steamed or roasted vegetables |
| **Solid Fats** | |
| Cream cheese | Light or fat-free cream cheese |
| Sour cream | Plain low-fat or fat-free yogurt |
| Regular margarine or butter | Light-spread margarines, diet margarine |
| **Added Sugars** | |
| Sugar-sweetened soft drinks | Seltzer mixed with 100% fruit juice |
| Sweetened tea or drinks | Unsweetened tea or water |
| Syrup on pancakes or French toast | Unsweetened applesauce or berries as a topping |
| Candy, cookies, cake, or pastry | Fresh or dried fruit |
| Sugar in recipes | Experiment with reducing amount and adding spices (cinnamon, nutmeg, etc.) |

*Source:* MyPyramid.gov. United States Department of Agriculture.

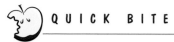 Q U I C K  B I T E

| Compare the calories in sugar-free varieties to their original counterparts | | | |
|---|---|---|---|
| | *Calories* | | *Calories* |
| Archway Chocolate Chip Cookie, 1 | | Nature's Own Bread, 1 slice | |
| Original | 130 | Original | 50 |
| Sugar free | 110 | Sugar free | 50 |
| Peanut butter, 2 tbsp | | Mrs. Smith Frozen Pies, 1/8 pie | |
| Original | 190 | Original | 340 |
| Sugar free | 190 | Sugar free | 350 |

Note that the emphasis is on healthy and wholesome choices, not commercially pre-pared "junk" foods that have been modified to be "fat free" or "sugar free." Those labels may give the impression that the food is also "calorie free," but that is not necessarily true. Fat-free milk is a good choice because milk is fundamentally healthy food made healthier by the elimination of fat. In contrast, fat-free cookies are still cookies—"treats" made with sugar and refined flour—not an inherently healthy food. In both cases, these fat-free foods still contain calories from protein and carbohydrates.

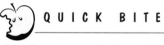 Q U I C K  B I T E

| Calorie content of selected alcoholicbeverages | | | |
|---|---|---|---|
| *Alcoholic Beverages* | *Calories* | *Alcoholic Beverages* | *Calories* |
| 12 oz regular beer | 144 | 1.5 oz 80 proof distilled spirits | |
| 12 light beer | 108 | (e.g., gin, rum, vodka, whiskey) | 96 |
| 5 oz white wine | 100 | 1.5 oz coffee liqueur | 308 |
| 5 oz red wine | 105 | 1 (4.5 oz) pina colada | 245 |
| 3 oz sweet dessert wine | 141 | 1 whiskey sour | |
| | | (2 oz mix + 1.5 oz whiskey) | 158 |

*Source:* USDHHS, USDA. *Dietary Guidelines for Americans.* Available at www.health.gov/dietaryguidelines/default.htm

Reducing alcohol intake is another way to consume fewer calories. Alcohol generally provides few essential nutrients and is considered a source of "empty calories." Although moderate alcohol consumption (1 drink/day for women, 2 drinks/day for men) may have beneficial health effects, its calorie content can be significant. Heavy alcohol consumption increases the risk of liver cirrhosis, hypertension, cancers of the upper GI tract, injury, vio-lence, and death (USHHS, 2005).

## Portion Control

Portion sizes have grown over the last 20 years. The number of "large-sized" food pack-ages sold in grocery stores increased 10-fold between 1970 and 2000 (Young & Nestle, 2003). Jumbo-sized portions in restaurants are consistently 250% larger than the regular portion (Wansink & Ittersum, 2007). The average dinner plate used in the home has in-creased by 36% since 1960 (Wansink, 2006). Over time, the effects of larger portion sizes distort peoples' perception of how much food is "normal" or necessary to create a feeling of fullness and alter their ability to monitor how much food they have consumed, resulting

**QUICK BITE**

Portion Distortion
Look at how portion sizes have grown over the last 20 years

| | 20 Years Ago | Today |
|---|---|---|
| Blueberry muffin | 1.5 oz | 5 oz |
| | 210 calories | 500 calories |
| Bagel | 3 in. diameter | 6 in. diameter |
| | 140 calories | 350 calories |
| Soda | 6.5 oz | 20 oz |
| | 85 calories | 250 calories |
| French fries | 2.4 oz | 6.9 oz |
| | 210 calories | 610 calories |
| Spaghetti with meatballs | 1 cup pasta with sauce and 3 meatballs | 2 cup pasta with sauce and 3 large meatballs |
| | 500 calories | 1025 calories |

*Source:* USDHHS, NHLBI, NIH. *Portion distortion.* Available at hp2010.nhlbihin.net/portion/index.htm. Accessed on 1/15/08.

in an increase in the amount of food consumed in a single eating occasion (Wansink & Ittersum, 2007). "Portion distortion" appears to be a widespread problem not linked to income, education, hunger, or body weight (Wansink & Ittersum, 2007).

According to Wansink and Ittersum, telling people to remind themselves not to overeat is not the answer; changing the environment that led to large portion sizes is easier. In other words, food should be less accessible, less visible, and proportioned in smaller quantities. Tips for changing the environment to control portion sizes appear in Box 7.5.

## Physical Activity

Despite the proven benefits of regular exercise, most Americans are not getting enough. Only 30% of American adults engage in regular leisure-time PA, and 39% of adults do not engage in any leisure-time PA (CDC, NCHS, 2006) (Fig. 7.6). A sedentary lifestyle increases the risk of overweight, obesity, coronary artery disease, hypertension, type 2 diabetes, osteoporosis, and certain types of cancer, and helps manage mild to moderate depression and anxiety (USDHHS, 2005).

The benefits of increasing activity are dose dependent and occur along a continuum (Fig. 7.7). A minimum of 30 min/day of moderate-intensity activity above usual activity is recommended to reduce the risk of chronic disease in adulthood. For bigger benefits, such as managing weight and preventing gradual weight gain, 60 minutes of moderate- to

---

**BOX 7.5**      **TIPS FOR CHANGING THE ENVIRONMENT TO CONTROL PORTION SIZES**

- Buy smaller packages of food at the grocery store.
- Buy prepackaged, portion-controlled items, such as "100-calorie" packages.
- Keep food out of sight.
- Order smaller portions at restaurants.
- Fill a "doggie bag" *before* beginning to eat.
- Use smaller dinner plates, bowls, glasses, and utensils.

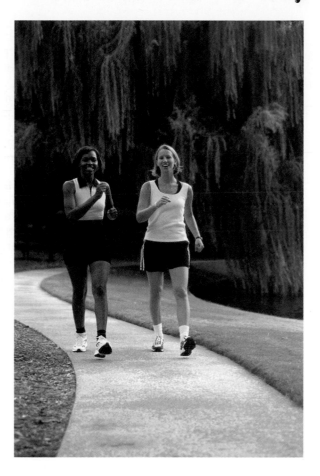

**FIGURE 7.6** Women power walking. Enlisting the support of a "buddy" helps sustain motivation.

**FIGURE 7.7** The benefits of increasing activity along a continuum of duration, frequency, and intensity.

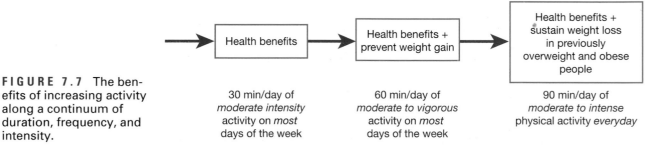

vigorous-intensity activity on most days of the week is recommended. This translates to approximately 2100 calories of activity per week (Tate et al., 2007). Tips for increasing activity appear in Box 7.6.

In addition to regular aerobic exercises, other types of exercise are also recommended. Stretching exercises are important for flexibility, and resistance exercises are vital for muscle strength and endurance. Resistance exercises build muscle, raising the metabolic rate and increasing the likelihood of weight loss and body fat loss. Changes in body composition—more muscle, less fat—are positive outcomes of strength training exercises that are not reflected on the scale, as is improved bone density and decreased risk of osteoporosis.

| BOX 7.6 | **TIPS FOR INCREASING ACTIVITY** |
|---|---|

- **Find something enjoyable.** The best chance of success comes from choosing activities that are enjoyable to the individual. The best activity or exercise is one that is done, not just contemplated.
- **Use the buddy system.** Committing to an exercise program or increased PA with a friend makes the activity less of a chore and helps to sustain motivation.
- **Spread activity over the entire day if desired.** This recommendation is particularly important for people who "don't have time to exercise." Many people find it easier to fit three 10-minute activity periods into a busy lifestyle than to find 30 uninterrupted minutes to dedicate to activity.
- **Start slowly and gradually increase activity.** For people who have been inactive, it is prudent to start with only a few minutes of daily activity, such as walking, and gradually increase the frequency, duration, and then intensity. People with existing health problems such as diabetes, heart disease, and hypertension should consult a physician before beginning a PA program, as should all men older than 40 and all women older than 50 years.
- **Move more.** Just moving more can make a cumulative difference in activity. Take the stairs instead of the elevator, park at the far end of the parking lot, walk around while talking on the portable phone, walk instead of driving short distances, play golf without a golf cart or caddy, fidget.
- **Keep an activity log.** Just as people tend to underestimate the amount of food they eat, people usually overestimate the amount of PA they perform. Documenting the type and duration of activity can help to track progress.

## ▶ How Do You Respond?

**Do calories eaten at night promote weight gain?** What determines whether or not calories are stored as fat is not when they are eaten but in what quantity. Food eaten in the evening is not more calorically dense than it is during the day, but mindless snacking in the evening, if it causes calorie intake to exceed calorie expenditure, can lead to weight gain over time.

**Which diet is best for losing weight—a low-carb diet or a low-fat diet?** *Any diet that creates a calorie deficit leads to weight loss over time.* What ultimately determines weight loss is the amount of calories consumed compared to the amount of calories expended, not what macronutrient the calories are from. In other words, if a 1500-calorie intake will promote weight loss, it does not matter if these calories come from French fries and cola or carrots and kidney beans. From a health standpoint, the recommended distribution of calories is 45 to 55% carbohydrate, 15 to 35% protein, and 20 to 35% fat (NAS, IOM, 2005).

## ▶ Case Study

Tonya is 5 ft. 3 in. tall, weighs 151 pounds, and is 38 years old. Her waist circumference is 37 in. As a receptionist for a law firm and mother of two socially active children, her life is busy but sedentary. She simply does not have the time or energy to stay with an exercise program after working all day and caring for her children. She would like to lose about 20 pounds but knows "dieting" doesn't work for her—all the diets she has tried in the past have left her hungry and feeling deprived. Losing weight has taken on greater importance since her doctor told her that both her blood pressure and glucose are at "borderline" high levels.

- What is her BMI? Assess her weight based on BMI. Based on her BMI and waist circumference, what is her level of disease risk?
- Estimate her total calorie requirements using the "rule-of-thumb" method of calculating BMR and adding calories for a sedentary lifestyle. How does it compare to the level of calories recommended in Table 7.3 for a woman of her age and sedentary lifestyle? Which calorie level do you think is most accurate? Why?
- How many calories would she need to eat to lose 1 pound of weight per week if her activity level stays the same? Two pounds per week? Is a 2-pound weight loss per week a reasonable goal?
- She likes to walk and is willing to try to walk for an hour during her lunch break. According to Table 7.2, approximately how many calories would she expend at a 3.5 mph pace? If she was able to walk an hour every day, how many calories would she need to cut out of her usual intake to produce a 1-pound weight loss/week?
- To help her avoid feeling hungry while eating fewer calories, what foods would you recommend she consume more of? She knows she should drink fewer soft drinks. What advice would you give her to help her do that?

## STUDY QUESTIONS

1. A client who wants to prevent further weight gain should be encouraged to exercise:
   a. At moderate intensity for 30 minutes/day on most days of the week
   b. At moderate intensity for 30 minutes/day everyday of the week
   c. At moderate to vigorous intensity for 60 minutes/day on most days of the week
   d. At moderate to vigorous intensity for 90 minutes/day everyday

2. The nurse knows her instructions about portion control have been effective when the client verbalizes she will:
   a. Prepare a doggie bag after she feels she is full enough while eating out
   b. Use a smaller dinner plate
   c. Be careful not to overfill her cereal bowl when she serves herself from the large, family-sized box
   d. Remind herself not to overeat

3. A client asks how she can speed up her metabolism. The best response is
   a. "You can't. Metabolic rate is genetically determined."
   b. "Ask your doctor to check your thyroid hormone levels. Taking thyroid hormone will stimulate metabolism."
   c. "Include resistance training in your exercise program because adding muscle tissue will increase metabolic rate."
   d. "Eat fewer calories because that will stimulate metabolic rate."

4. How much weight will a person lose in a week if he eats 500 fewer calories/day than he needs and increases his exercise expenditure by 500 calories/day?
   a. 1 pound/week
   b. 2 pounds/week
   c. 3 pounds/week
   d. There isn't enough information provided to estimate weekly weight loss

5. A client is wondering whether to go on a low-fat diet or a low-carb diet to lose weight. What should you tell her?
   a. "Lowering fat intake causes a great calorie deficit than lowering carbohydrate intake because fat has more calories/gram than carbohydrates do."
   b. "A low-carb diet is easier to achieve and more filling than a low-fat diet. I would try that if I were you."

c. "For weight loss, it doesn't matter if you lower fat or lower carbohydrates; what is necessary is to consume fewer calories than you expend."
    d. "The best approach is to eat a diet that is low in both carbohydrates and fat. That means concentrate on eating a diet high in fat-free protein."

**6.** Waist circumference is an indicator of
    a. Percentage of body fat
    b. Abdominal fat content
    c. The ratio of body fat to muscle mass
    d. Body mass index

**7.** Which of the following substitutions results in a healthier choice?
    a. Beef loin instead of beef rib
    b. Refried beans instead of cooked or canned pinto beans
    c. Natural cheese instead of low-fat cheese
    d. Baked potato with cheese sauce instead of baked potato with salsa

**8.** A BMI of 26 is classified as:
    a. Normal
    b. Overweight
    c. Class I obesity
    d. Class II obesity

## KEY CONCEPTS

- Calories are a measure of energy. The body obtains calories from carbohydrates, protein, fat, and alcohol.

- Basal metabolism refers to the calories used to conduct the involuntary activities of the body, such as beating the heart and inflating the lungs. For most Americans, basal metabolism accounts for approximately 60% of total daily calories used.

- The sum of calories spent on basal metabolism and PA represent a person's total calorie expenditure.

- The thermic effect of food is the cost of digesting, absorbing, and metabolizing food. At about 10% of total calories consumed, it is a small part of total energy requirements and is usually not factored into the total energy equation.

- MyPyramid calorie levels are based on gender, age, and activity. Sedentary women need approximately 1600 to 2000 cal/day, and sedentary men 2000 to 2600 cal/day.

- Normal weight is defined as weight for height that is statistically correlated to good health. BMI, waist circumference, and existing health conditions are used to assess risk related to overweight and obesity.

- BMI may be the best method of evaluating weight status, but it does not account for how weight is distributed. Overweight is defined as a BMI of 25 to 29.9; obesity is defined as a BMI of 30 or higher.

- Waist circumference is a tool to assess for abdominal fatness. "Apples" (people with upper-body obesity) have more health risks than "pears" (people with lower-body obesity).

- The Dietary Guidelines urge Americans to maintain body weight in a healthy range and to balance calories from foods and beverages with calories expended. Regular PA is recommended.

- Healthy food choices involve eating less of items that are high in added sugar and fat and more of unprocessed, high-fiber foods like fruits, vegetables, whole grains, and lean protein.

● Portion sizes have grown over the last two decades, and people often overestimate how much food they really need. Portion control is facilitated by eating less at restaurants, using smaller dinner plates, and buying prepackaged, portion-controlled foods.

● The vast majority of Americans do not get the recommended amount of PA. The benefits of PA are dose dependent and range from decreased risk of chronic disease to weight loss and maintenance.

● Exercise leads to modest weight loss if calories are not also restricted. In the long term, exercise promotes weight loss by promoting fat loss and preventing loss of muscle, which contributes to metabolic rate.

## ANSWER KEY

1. **TRUE** Calorie is a unit of measure pertaining to energy in foods. Thus a food that is high in "energy" is high in calories.

2. **TRUE** One pound of body fat is equivalent to 3500 calories. To lose 1 pound of weight per week, a daily deficit of 500 calories for 7 days is necessary, whether from eating less, doing more, or both.

3. **TRUE** People of either gender with a high distribution of abdominal fat ("apples") have a greater health risk than people with excess fat in the hips and thighs ("pears").

4. **TRUE** Starvation diets (e.g., fasting) may cause less loss of body fat than low-calorie diets because the body seeks to lower its metabolic rate to sustain life when food is not available. It does so by breaking down muscle.

5. **FALSE** To manage weight and prevent weight gain in adulthood, 60 min/day of moderate- to vigorous-intensity activity is recommended on most days of the week, while not exceeding calorie intake requirements.

6. **TRUE** On average, basal metabolism accounts for 60 of total calories expended in a day. Active people use a smaller percentage of total calories on BMR.

7. **TRUE** Building muscle speeds metabolic rate because lean tissue is metabolically active compared with fat tissue, which is relatively inert and requires few calories to exist.

8. **FALSE** Activity does not need to be sustained for any given duration to provide health benefits. Snippets of activity accumulated over the entire day can provide the same health benefits as one exercise session of the same total length of time.

9. **TRUE** The best exercise is one the individual sticks with. Exercise prescriptions are not one-size-fits-all.

10. **TRUE** These items tend to be calorie dense, not nutrient dense, providing few nutrients for the amount of calories they contain. Limiting alcohol is another strategy for limiting calorie intake.

## WEBSITES

American College of Sports Medicine at **www.acsm.org**
American Council on Exercise at **www.acefitness.org**
Calculate your own BMR at **www.room42.com/nutrition/basal.shtml**
National Institute of Diabetes and Digestive and Kidney Diseases, Physical Activity and Weight
    Control at **www.niddk.nih.gov/health/nutrit/pubs/physact.htm**
President's Council on Physical Fitness and Sports at **www.fitness.gov**

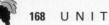 

# REFERENCES

American Diabetes Association, American Dietetic Association. (2008). *Choose your foods: Exchange lists for diabetes.* Alexandria, VA: The American Diabetes Association.

Center for Disease Control, National Center for Health Statistics. (2007). Overweight. Available as sss.cdc.gov/nchs/fastats/overwt.htm.

Kushner, R., & Blatner, D. (2005). Risk assessment of the overweight and obese patient. *Journal of the American Dietetic Association, 105,* S53–S62.

McTigue, K., Harris, R., Hemphill, B., et al. (2003). Screening and interventions for obesity in adults: Summary of the evidence for the US Preventive Services Task Force. *Annals of Internal Medicine, 139,* 933–949.

National Academy of Sciences Institute of Medicine (NAS, IOM). (2005). *Dietary Reference Intakes for energy, carbohydrate, fiber, fat, fatty acids, cholesterol, protein, and amino acids.* Washington, DC: The National Academies Press.

National Heart, Lung, and Blood Institute Expert Panel on the Identification, Evaluation, and Treatment of Overweight and Obesity in Adults. (1998). *Executive summary of the clinical guidelines on the identification, evaluation, and treatment of overweight and obesity in adults.* Rockville, MD.

Rivlin, R. (2007). Keeping the young-elderly health: Is it too late to improve our health through nutrition? *The American Journal of Clinical Nutrition, 86*(Suppl), 1572S–1576S.

Tate, D., Jeffery, R., Sherwood, N., et al. (2007). Long-term weight losses associated with prescription of higher physical activity goals. Are higher levels of physical activity protective against weight regain? *The American Journal of Clinical Nutrition, 85,* 954–959.

U.S. Department of Agriculture (USDA), U.S. Department of Health & Human Services (USDHHS). Dietary Guidelines for Americans. (2005). Accessed at www.health.gov/dietaryguidelines/default.htm.

Wansink, B. (2006). *Mindless eating: Why we eat more than we think.* New York: Bantam Dell.

Wansink, B., & Ittersum, K. (2007). Portion size me: Downsizing our consumption norms. *Journal of the American Dietetic Association, 107,* 1103–1106.

Young, L., & Nestle, M. (2003). Expanding portion sizes in the US marketplace: Implications for nutritional counseling. *Journal of the American Dietetic Association, 103,* 231–234.

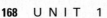 

# REFERENCES

American Diabetes Association, American Dietetic Association. (2008). *Choose your foods: Exchange lists for diabetes.* Alexandria, VA: The American Diabetes Association.

Center for Disease Control, National Center for Health Statistics. (2007). Overweight. Available as sss.cdc.gov/nchs/fastats/overwt.htm.

Kushner, R., & Blatner, D. (2005). Risk assessment of the overweight and obese patient. *Journal of the American Dietetic Association, 105,* S53–S62.

McTigue, K., Harris, R., Hemphill, B., et al. (2003). Screening and interventions for obesity in adults: Summary of the evidence for the US Preventive Services Task Force. *Annals of Internal Medicine, 139,* 933–949.

National Academy of Sciences Institute of Medicine (NAS, IOM). (2005). *Dietary Reference Intakes for energy, carbohydrate, fiber, fat, fatty acids, cholesterol, protein, and amino acids.* Washington, DC: The National Academies Press.

National Heart, Lung, and Blood Institute Expert Panel on the Identification, Evaluation, and Treatment of Overweight and Obesity in Adults. (1998). *Executive summary of the clinical guidelines on the identification, evaluation, and treatment of overweight and obesity in adults.* Rockville, MD.

Rivlin, R. (2007). Keeping the young-elderly health: Is it too late to improve our health through nutrition? *The American Journal of Clinical Nutrition, 86*(Suppl), 1572S–1576S.

Tate, D., Jeffery, R., Sherwood, N., et al. (2007). Long-term weight losses associated with prescription of higher physical activity goals. Are higher levels of physical activity protective against weight regain? *The American Journal of Clinical Nutrition, 85,* 954–959.

U.S. Department of Agriculture (USDA), U.S. Department of Health & Human Services (USDHHS). Dietary Guidelines for Americans. (2005). Accessed at www.health.gov/dietaryguidelines/default.htm.

Wansink, B. (2006). *Mindless eating: Why we eat more than we think.* New York: Bantam Dell.

Wansink, B., & Ittersum, K. (2007). Portion size me: Downsizing our consumption norms. *Journal of the American Dietetic Association, 107,* 1103–1106.

Young, L., & Nestle, M. (2003). Expanding portion sizes in the US marketplace: Implications for nutritional counseling. *Journal of the American Dietetic Association, 103,* 231–234.

- Portion sizes have grown over the last two decades, and people often overestimate how much food they really need. Portion control is facilitated by eating less at restaurants, using smaller dinner plates, and buying prepackaged, portion-controlled foods.

- The vast majority of Americans do not get the recommended amount of PA. The benefits of PA are dose dependent and range from decreased risk of chronic disease to weight loss and maintenance.

- Exercise leads to modest weight loss if calories are not also restricted. In the long term, exercise promotes weight loss by promoting fat loss and preventing loss of muscle, which contributes to metabolic rate.

## ANSWER KEY

1. **TRUE** Calorie is a unit of measure pertaining to energy in foods. Thus a food that is high in "energy" is high in calories.

2. **TRUE** One pound of body fat is equivalent to 3500 calories. To lose 1 pound of weight per week, a daily deficit of 500 calories for 7 days is necessary, whether from eating less, doing more, or both.

3. **TRUE** People of either gender with a high distribution of abdominal fat ("apples") have a greater health risk than people with excess fat in the hips and thighs ("pears").

4. **TRUE** Starvation diets (e.g., fasting) may cause less loss of body fat than low-calorie diets because the body seeks to lower its metabolic rate to sustain life when food is not available. It does so by breaking down muscle.

5. **FALSE** To manage weight and prevent weight gain in adulthood, 60 min/day of moderate- to vigorous-intensity activity is recommended on most days of the week, while not exceeding calorie intake requirements.

6. **TRUE** On average, basal metabolism accounts for 60 of total calories expended in a day. Active people use a smaller percentage of total calories on BMR.

7. **TRUE** Building muscle speeds metabolic rate because lean tissue is metabolically active compared with fat tissue, which is relatively inert and requires few calories to exist.

8. **FALSE** Activity does not need to be sustained for any given duration to provide health benefits. Snippets of activity accumulated over the entire day can provide the same health benefits as one exercise session of the same total length of time.

9. **TRUE** The best exercise is one the individual sticks with. Exercise prescriptions are not one-size-fits-all.

10. **TRUE** These items tend to be calorie dense, not nutrient dense, providing few nutrients for the amount of calories they contain. Limiting alcohol is another strategy for limiting calorie intake.

## WEBSITES

American College of Sports Medicine at **www.acsm.org**
American Council on Exercise at **www.acefitness.org**
Calculate your own BMR at **www.room42.com/nutrition/basal.shtml**
National Institute of Diabetes and Digestive and Kidney Diseases, Physical Activity and Weight
    Control at **www.niddk.nih.gov/health/nutrit/pubs/physact.htm**
President's Council on Physical Fitness and Sports at **www.fitness.gov**

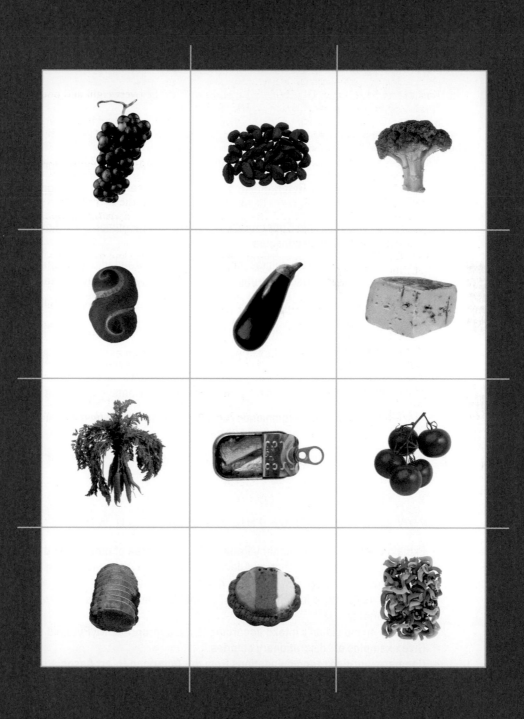

UNIT TWO

Nutrition in Health Promotion

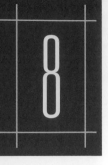

# 8  Guidelines for Healthy Eating

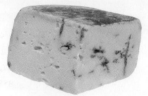

### UPON COMPLETION OF THIS CHAPTER, YOU WILL BE ABLE TO

- Explain the objectives of Healthy People 2010 in the area of nutrition and overweight.
- Compare Recommended Dietary Allowance (RDA) and Adequate Intake (AI).
- Summarize the *Dietary Guidelines for Americans*.
- Design a day's intake for your own MyPyramid that illustrates variety, moderation, and proportionality.
- Evaluate an individual's intake according to the appropriate MyPyramid plan.
- Give examples of "discretionary calories."
- Compare nutrition recommendations from the American Heart Association, the American Cancer Society, and the American Institute for Cancer Research.

## ▶ HOW TO CHOOSE A "HEALTHY DIET"

A healthy diet provides enough of all essential nutrients to avoid deficiencies but not excessive amounts that may increase the risk of nutrient toxicities or chronic diseases. Today, nutrient deficiency diseases are rare in the United States except among the poor, elderly, alcoholics, fad dieters, and hospitalized patients. Conversely, four of the ten leading causes of death in the United States are associated with dietary excesses, namely, heart disease, cancer, stroke, and diabetes. Many other health problems, such as obesity, hypertension, and hypercholesterolemia, are related, at least in part, to dietary excesses. A healthy diet has the potential to alleviate the high economic and personal costs of morbidity and mortality associated with these diseases (Krebs-Smith & Kris-Etherton, 2007; Kennedy, 2006).

This chapter focuses on what constitutes an "optimal" intake to promote health and prevent disease. Professional and consumer tools for choosing an optimal diet are presented, including the **Dietary Reference Intakes (DRIs)**, Dietary Guidelines for Americans, MyPyramid, and diet recommendations from leading health agencies.

> **QUICK BITE**
>
> The 10 leading causes of death in the United States in 2004 (in descending order)
>
> 1. Heart disease
> 2. Cancer
> 3. Stroke
> 4. Chronic obstructive pulmonary disease
> 5. Accidents
> 6. Diabetes
> 7. Alzheimer's disease
> 8. Influenza and pneumonia
> 9. Kidney disease
> 10. Septicemia
>
> *Source:* Miniño, A., Heron, M., & Smith, B. (2006). Deaths: Preliminary data for 2004. *National Vital Statistics Reports, 54*(19), June 28, 2006. Available at www.cdc.gov.

**Dietary Reference Intakes:** a set of four nutrient-based reference values used to plan and evaluate diets.

## Healthy People 2010

In January 2000, the Department of Health and Human Services introduced a 10-year national health promotion program called Healthy People 2010 (Centers for Disease Control and Prevention, National Center for Health Statistics, 2007). Its overall goals are to increase quality and years of healthy life and eliminate health disparities among Americans. Twenty-eight focus areas, ranging from cancer and diabetes to substance abuse and immunizations, outline areas of public health concern. From these, 467 specific, measurable objectives serve as the basis for monitoring and measuring improvements in the nation's health over the 10-year period from 2000 to 2010. Box 8.1 summarizes the objectives in the area of nutrition and overweight.

## Primarily Professional

**Recommended Dietary Allowances (RDAs):** the average daily dietary intake level sufficient to meet the nutrient requirement of 97% to 98% of healthy individuals in a particular life stage and gender group.

Historically, the **Recommended Dietary Allowances (RDAs)** in the United States and the Recommended Nutrient Intakes in Canada established recommended levels of nutrients set at a level to protect people from nutrient deficiency diseases. The old RDAs have been replaced with a new set of standards, the DRIs, that incorporate an expanded focus of reducing the risk of chronic diseases associated with dietary excesses.

### Dietary Reference Intakes

In the early 1990s, Canadian scientists and the Food and Nutrition Board of the Institute of Medicine embarked on a comprehensive, multiyear project to update and expand nutrient intake recommendations. The outcome has been a series of eight in-depth reports featuring a new set of references called DRIs that cover vitamins, minerals, the energy nutrients, cholesterol, fiber, electrolytes, and water.

The DRIs is a group name that includes four separate reference values that are based on the concepts of probability and risk: updated RDAs, estimated average requirement (EAR), adequate intake (AI), and the tolerable upper intake level (UL) (Otten, Hellwig, Meyers (Eds.), 2006).

---

**BOX 8.1**      **HEALTHY PEOPLE 2010—SUMMARY OF NUTRITION AND OVERWEIGHT OBJECTIVES**

**Goal: Promote Health and Reduce Chronic Disease Associated with Diet and Weight**

**Weight Status and Growth**
- Increase proportion of adults who are at healthy weight
- Reduce obesity among adults
- Reduce overweight or obesity among children and adolescents
- Reduce growth retardation among low-income children

**Food and Nutrient Consumption**
- Increase fruit intake
- Increase vegetable intake
- Increase grain intake with at least 3 servings from whole grains
- Decrease saturated fat intake to <10% of total calories
- Decrease total fat intake to <30% of total calories
- Decrease sodium intake to <2400 mg/day
- Meet dietary recommendations for calcium

**Iron Deficiency and Anemia**
- Decrease iron deficiency in young children and in women of childbearing age
- Decrease anemia in low-income pregnant women
- Decrease iron deficiency in pregnant women

**Schools, Worksites, and Nutrition Counseling**
- Increase the positive impact of meals and snacks at school
- Increase worksites that promote nutrition education and weight management
- Increase nutrition counseling for medical conditions

**Food Security**
- Increase food security to reduce hunger

*Source:* http://www.healthypeople.gov/Document/HTML/Volume2/19Nutrition.htm#_Toc490383121

---

Each of these reference values has a specific purpose and represents a different level of intake (Fig. 8.1). Each reference value is viewed as an average daily intake over time, at least 1 week for most nutrients. Summary tables of the DRIs appear in Appendices 1 and 2. Additional reference values include Acceptable Macronutrient Distribution Ranges (AMDRs) and an Estimated Energy Requirement (EER).

**QUICK BITE**

Nutrients with RDAs for people older than 1 year

- Carbohydrates
- Protein
- Vitamin A
- Vitamin C
- Vitamin E
- Thiamin
- Riboflavin
- Niacin
- Vitamin $B_6$
- Folate
- Vitamin $B_{12}$
- Copper
- Iodine
- Iron
- Magnesium
- Molybdenum
- Phosphorus
- Zinc

**Recommended Dietary Allowances.** The RDAs represent the average daily recommended intake to meet the nutrient requirements of 97% to 98% of healthy individuals by life stage and gender. The recommendations are based on specific criteria indicators for estimating requirements such as plasma and serum nutrient concentrations and are set high enough to account for daily variations in intake. When estimating the nutritional needs of people with health disorders, health professionals use the RDAs as a starting point and adjust them according to the individual's need.

**Estimated Average Requirement (EAR):** the nutrient intake estimated to meet the requirement of half of the healthy individuals in a particular life stage and gender group.

**Estimated Average Requirement.** The **EAR** is the amount of a nutrient that is estimated to meet the requirement of half of healthy people in a lifestyle or gender group. "Average" actually means *median*. By definition, the EAR exceeds the requirements of half of the group and falls below the requirements of the other half. The EAR is not based solely on the prevention of nutrient deficiencies but includes consideration for reducing the risk of chronic disease and takes into account the bioavailability of the nutrient, that is, how its absorption is impacted by other food components. EAR values are used to determine RDA values.

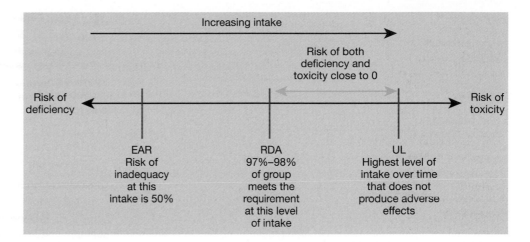

**FIGURE 8.1**
Representation of DRI along a continuum of intake.

**Adequate Intake.** An AI is set when an RDA cannot be determined due to lack of sufficient data on requirements. It is a recommended average daily intake level thought to meet or exceed the needs of virtually all members of a life stage or gender group based on observed or experimentally determined estimates of nutrient intake by groups of healthy people. The primary purpose of the AI is as a goal for the nutrient intake of individuals. This is similar to the use of the RDA except that the RDA is expected to meet the needs of almost all healthy people, while in the case of an AI, it is not known what percentage of people are covered.

**Adequate Intake (AI):** an intake level thought to meet or exceed the requirement of almost all members of a life stage and gender group. An AI is set when there are insufficient data to define an RDA.

**Tolerable Upper Intake Level (UL):** the highest average daily intake level of a nutrient likely to pose no danger to most individuals in the group.

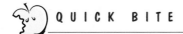

**QUICK BITE**

Nutrients with an AI for people older than 1 year
- Water
- Fiber
- Linoleic acid
- Alpha-linolenic acid
- Vitamin D
- Vitamin K
- Pantothenic acid
- Biotin
- Choline
- Calcium
- Chromium
- Fluoride
- Manganese
- Potassium
- Sodium
- Chloride

**Tolerable Upper Intake Level.** The UL is the highest level of average daily nutrient intake that is likely to pose no risk of adverse health effects to almost all individuals in the general population. It is not intended to be a recommended level of intake; there is no benefit in consuming amounts greater than the RDA or AI. Not all nutrients have an established UL.

**QUICK BITE**

Nutrients with Tolerable Upper Intake Levels for people older than 1 year
- Vitamin A
- Vitamin C
- Vitamin D
- Vitamin E
- Niacin
- Vitamin B$_6$
- Folate
- Choline
- Boron
- Calcium
- Copper
- Fluoride
- Iodine
- Iron
- Magnesium
- Manganese
- Molybdenum
- Nickel
- Phosphorus
- Selenium
- Zinc
- Sodium
- Chloride

**Acceptable Macronutrient Distribution Ranges (AMDRs):** an intake range as a percentage of total calories for energy nutrients.

**Estimated Energy Requirements (EERs):** level of calorie intake estimated to maintain weight in normal-weight individuals based on age, gender, height, weight, and activity.

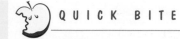

## QUICK BITE

The Acceptable Macronutrient Distribution Ranges for adults are

| | Total calories consumed (%) |
|---|---|
| Carbohydrate | 45–65 |
| Protein | 10–35 |
| Fat | 20–35 |
| Linoleic acid (n-6) | 5–10 |
| Alpha-linolenic (n-3) | 0.6–1.2 |

**Source:** Dietary Reference Intakes for energy, carbohydrate, fiber, fat, fatty acids, cholesterol, protein, and amino acids (2002). This report may be accessed via www.nap.edu.

**Acceptable Macronutrient Distribution Ranges.** The AMDRs are broad ranges for each energy nutrient, expressed as a percentage of total calories consumed, that is, associated with reduced risk of chronic disease while providing AIs of essential nutrients. Over time, intakes above or below this range may increase the risk of chronic disease or deficiency, respectively.

**Estimated Energy Requirements.** Similar to the EAR, the EERs are defined as the dietary energy intake predicted to maintain energy balance in healthy, normal weight individuals of a defined age, gender, weight, height, and level of physical activity consistent with good health. Exceeding the EER may produce weight gain. See Chapter 7 for more on determining energy needs.

## How Are the DRIs Used?

DRIs are used by scientists and nutritionists who work in research or academic settings and by dietitians who plan menus for specific populations such as elderly feeding programs, schools, prisons, hospitals, nursing homes, and military feeding programs. They are also used to assess the adequacy of an individual's intake by comparing estimated intake with estimated requirements. Keep in mind that obtaining a reliable estimate of a person's actual intake is difficult due to reporting errors, flaws in estimating portion sizes, and day-to-day variation in food intake. Unless a person has participated in a nutrient requirement study, it is impossible to quantify exact nutrient requirements for an individual. Because consumers eat food and not nutrients, the DRIs are not suited to teaching people how to make healthy choices.

## Conveying the Concept of a Healthy Diet to Consumers

The most prominent tools to assist Americans in making wise food choices are the Dietary Guidelines for Americans and its companion tool, MyPyramid. Numerous health agencies, including the American Heart Association, the American Cancer Society, and the American Institute of Cancer Research, have also issued dietary recommendations to help Americans choose diets aimed at reducing the risk of chronic diseases.

## Dietary Guidelines for Americans

The Dietary Guidelines for Americans, published jointly every 5 years by the U.S. Department of Health and Human Services and the U.S. Department of Agriculture, serves as the federal policy on nutrition, dictating how education, communication, and food assistance programs are conducted by the government. The most recent edition, published in 2005, generated, for the first time, *evidence-based* recommendations on diet and physical activity to promote health and decrease the risk of chronic diet-related diseases such as hypertension, diabetes, abnormal blood lipid levels, overweight, and obesity (United States Department of Health and Human Services, United States Department of Agriculture, 2005).

The Dietary Guidelines cover nine major messages with 23 key recommendations (Box 8.2). Eighteen additional recommendations are made for specific population groups.

BOX 8.2   **DIETARY GUIDELINES FOR AMERICANS, 2005**

**Key Recommendations for the General Population**

*Adequate Nutrients Within Calorie Needs*
- Consume a variety of nutrient-dense foods and beverages within and among the basic food groups while choosing foods that limit the intake of saturated and *trans* fats, cholesterol, added sugars, salt, and alcohol.
- Meet recommended intakes within energy needs by adopting a balanced eating pattern, such as the U.S. Department of Agriculture (USDA) MyPyramid or the Dietary Approaches to Stop Hypertension (DASH) Eating Plan.

*Weight Management*
- To maintain body weight in a healthy range, balance calories from foods and beverages with calories expended.
- To prevent gradual weight gain over time, make small decreases in food and beverage calories, and increase physical activity.

*Physical Activity*
- To promote health, psychological well-being, and a healthy body weight, engage in regular physical activity and reduce sedentary activities.
- To reduce the risk of chronic disease in adulthood, engage in at least 30 minutes of moderate-intensity physical activity, above usual activity, at work or home on most days of the week.
- To obtain greater health benefits, engage in physical activity of more vigorous intensity or longer duration.
- To help manage body weight and prevent gradual, unhealthy body weight gain in adulthood, engage in approximately 60 minutes of moderate- to vigorous-intensity activity on most days of the week while not exceeding caloric intake requirements.
- To sustain weight loss in adulthood, participate in at least 60 to 90 minutes of daily moderate-intensity physical activity while not exceeding caloric intake requirements. Some people may need to consult with a health-care provider before participating in this level of activity.
- To achieve physical fitness, include cardiovascular conditioning, stretching exercises for flexibility, exercises to increase muscle strength and endurance, and include resistance exercises or calisthenics.

*Food Groups to Encourage*
- Consume sufficient amount of fruits and vegetables while staying within energy needs. Two cups of fruit and 2½ cups of vegetables per day are recommended for a reference 2000-calorie intake, with higher or lower amounts depending on the calorie level.
- Choose a variety of fruits and vegetables each day. In particular, select from all five vegetable subgroups (dark green, orange, legumes, starchy vegetables, and other vegetables) several times a week.
- Consume 3 or more ounce-equivalents of whole-grain products per day, with the rest of the recommended grains coming from enriched or whole-grain products. In general, at least half the grains should come from whole grains.
- Consume 3 cups per day of fat-free or low-fat milk or equivalent milk products.

*Fats*
- Consume less than 10% of calories from saturated fatty acids and less than 300 mg/day of cholesterol, and keep *trans* fatty acid consumption as low as possible.

*(box continues on page 176)*

BOX 8.2      DIETARY GUIDELINES FOR AMERICANS, 2005 (continued)

- Keep total fat intake between 20% and 35% of calories, with most fats coming from sources of polyunsaturated and monounsaturated fatty acids, such as fish, nuts, and vegetable oils.
- When selecting and preparing meat, poultry, dry beans, and milk or milk products, make choices that are lean, low fat, or fat free.
- Limit intake of fats and oils high in saturated and/or *trans* fatty acids and choose products low in such fats and oils.

### Carbohydrates

- Choose fiber-rich fruits, vegetables, and whole grains often.
- Choose and prepare foods and beverages with little added sugars or caloric sweeteners, such as amounts suggested by the USDA MyPyramid and the DASH Eating Plan.
- Reduce the incidence of dental caries by practicing good oral hygiene.
- Consume sugar- and starch-containing foods and beverages less frequently.

### Sodium and Potassium

- Consume less than 2300 mg (approximately 1 teaspoon of salt) of sodium per day.
- Choose and prepare foods with little salt. At the same time, consume potassium-rich foods such as fruits and vegetables.

### Alcoholic Beverages

- Those who choose to drink alcoholic beverages should do so sensibly and in moderation—defined as the consumption of up to one drink per day for women and up to two drinks per day for men.
- Alcoholic beverages should not be consumed by some individuals, including those who cannot restrict their alcohol intake, women of childbearing age who may become pregnant, pregnant and lactating women, children and adolescents, individuals taking medications that can interact with alcohol, and those with specific medical conditions.
- Alcoholic beverages should be avoided by individuals engaging in activities that require attention, skill, or coordination, such as driving or operating machinery.

### Food Safety

To avoid microbial food borne illness:

- Clean hands, food contact surfaces, and fruits and vegetables. Meat and poultry should not be washed or rinsed.
- Separate raw, cooked, and ready-to-eat foods while shopping, preparing, or storing foods.
- Cook foods to a safe temperature to kill microorganisms.
- Chill (refrigerate) perishable food promptly and defrost foods properly.
- Avoid raw (unpasteurized) milk or any products made from unpasteurized milk, raw or partially cooked eggs or foods containing raw eggs, raw or undercooked meat and poultry, unpasteurized juices, and raw sprouts.

**Note:** The Dietary Guidelines for Americans 2005 contain additional recommendations for specific populations. The full document is available at www.healthierus.gov/dietaryguidelines. (U.S. Department of Health and Human Services and U.S. Department of Agriculture.)

The guidelines are intended to represent a pattern of eating for Americans older than 2 years and should ideally be implemented as a whole. The major themes are to eat fewer calories, be more physically active, and make wiser food choices.

## MyPyramid

In early 2005, MyPyramid was launched as the newest generation of the food guide that features a new graphic and an interactive online guidance system (United States Department of

Agriculture, Center for Nutrition Policy and Promotion, 2005). MyPyramid serves as the vehicle by which the Dietary Guidelines for Americans are translated into food and activity choices for healthy individuals older than 2 years. At its foundation rests the philosophy that nutrient needs, to the greatest extent possible, should be met through food not supplements. It is a total diet approach designed to cover all aspects of the diet, from calories and fat to particular types of vegetable subgroups and whole grains. Its basic messages are as follows:

- Eat more fruit, vegetables, and whole grains. Weekly totals of a variety of specific vegetable categories are recommended.
- Eat less saturated fat, trans fat, and cholesterol.
- Limit sweets and salt.
- Use alcohol in moderation, if at all.
- Balance calorie intake with calorie expenditure.
- Be physically active most days of the week.

The MyPyramid graphic has rainbow-colored, vertical groups and a three-dimensional shape that depicts physical activity on the side (Fig. 8.2). It is designed to convey the concepts of

**Activity**
Activity is represented by the steps and the person climbing them, a reminder of the importance of daily physical activity.

**Personalization**
Personalization is shown by the person on the steps, the slogan, and the URL. Find the kinds and amounts of food to eat each day at MyPyramid.gov.

**Gradual Improvement**
Gradual improvement is encouraged by the slogan. It suggests that individuals can benefit from taking small steps to improve their diet and lifestyle each day.

**Moderation**
Moderation is represented by the narrowing of each food group from bottom to top. The wider base stands for foods with little or no solid fats or added sugars. These should be selected more often. The narrower top area stands for foods containing more added sugars and solid fats. The more active you are, the more of these foods can fit into your diet.

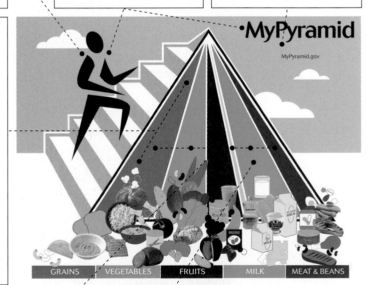

**Variety**
Variety is symbolized by the 6 color bands representing the 5 food groups of the pyramid and oils. This illustrates that foods from all groups are needed each day for good health.

**Proportionality**
Proportionality is shown by the different widths of the food group bands. The widths suggest how much food a person should choose from each group. The widths are just a general guide, not exact proportions. Check the Web site for how much is right for you.

**FIGURE 8.2**
MyPyramid. (USDA, Center for Nutrition Policy and Promotion (2005). MyPyramid— Steps to Healthier You Food Guidance System. Available at www.MyPyramid.gov.)

| TABLE 8.1 | | **Food Intake Patterns at Various MyPyramid Calorie Levels** | | | | | | | | | | |
|---|---|---|---|---|---|---|---|---|---|---|---|---|
| **Group** | **1000** | **1200** | **1400** | **1600** | **1800** | **2000** | **2200** | **2400** | **2600** | **2800** | **3000** | **3200** |
| Grains (oz-eq) | 3 | 4 | 5 | 5 | 6 | 6 | 7 | 8 | 9 | 10 | 10 | 10 |
| Vegetables (in cups) | 1 | 1.5 | 1.5 | 2 | 2.5 | 2.5 | 3 | 3 | 3.5 | 3.5 | 4 | 4 |
| Fruits (in cup/s) | 1 | 1 | 1.5 | 1.5 | 1.5 | 2 | 2 | 2 | 2 | 2.5 | 2.5 | 2.5 |
| Milk (in cup/s) | 2 | 2 | 2 | 3 | 3 | 3 | 3 | 3 | 3 | 3 | 3 | 3 |
| Meat and Beans (oz-eq) | 2 | 3 | 4 | 5 | 5 | 5.5 | 6 | 6.5 | 6.5 | 7 | 7 | 7 |
| Oils (tsp) | 3 | 4 | 4 | 5 | 5 | 6 | 6 | 7 | 8 | 8 | 10 | 11 |
| Discretionary calorie allowance* | 165 | 171 | 171 | 132 | 195 | 267 | 290 | 362 | 410 | 426 | 512 | 648 |

eq = equivalent
*The following are considered 1 oz Grain equivalent:*
1 slice of bread
1 cup of ready-to-eat cereal
¹/₂ cup cooked rice, pasta, or cooked cereal

*1 oz Meat and Beans equivalent is:*
1 oz of lean meat, poultry, or fish
1 egg
1 tbsp peanut butter
¹/₄ cup cooked dry beans
¹/₂ ounce nuts or seeds

*Discretionary Calorie Allowance is the remaining amount of calories in a food intake pattern after accounting for the calories needed for all for all food groups, using forms of foods that are fat free or low fat and with no added sugars.
***Source:*** www.myPyramid.gov

variety, moderation, proportionality, gradual improvement, personalization, and physical activity. Rather than the previous one-size-fits-all model designed for the "average" American, MyPyramid actually represents 12 individualized pyramids, each one representing a different calorie level ranging from 1000 to 3200 calories in increments of 200 calories (Table 8.1). This customization of calorie levels reflects not only the broad range of calorie needs across the population but also the increasing attention paid to obesity as a major health problem.

### QUICK BITE

A comparison between 1-oz grain equivalent servings and a typical American portion

| | *Amount that qualifies as 1-oz grain equivalent* | *Common portion* |
|---|---|---|
| Bread | 1 slice | 2 slices |
| Pancakes | 1 (4½-in. diameter) | 3 (4½-in. diameter) |
| Popcorn | 3 cups, popped | 12 cups, popped |
| Rice or pasta | ½ cup cooked | 1 cup cooked |
| Tortillas | 1 small (6 in.) | 1 large (12 in.) |

***Source:*** www.MyPyramid.gov

Visitors to the website www.MyPyramid.gov enter their age, gender, and usual activity level (height and weight are optional) to see the MyPyramid plan most appropriate for their estimated calorie needs. Figure 8.3 illustrates the format used to convey basic MyPyramid plan recommendations. The pdf version of a MyPyramid plan features the pyramid graphic, recommended daily amounts from each group, and additional basic information, as illustrated in the 2000-calorie MyPyramid food pattern in Figure 8.4.

## MyPyramid Plan

Eat these amounts from each food group daily. This plan is a _____ calorie food pattern. It is based on average needs for someone like you. (A __ year old _____ , __ feet __ inches tall, pounds, physically active _____ **minutes** a day.) Your calorie needs may be more or less than the average, so check your weight regularly. If you see unwanted weight gain or loss, adjust the amount you are eating.

| ▶ Grains¹ | _ ounces | tips |
| ▶ Vegetables² | ____ cups | tips |
| ▶ Fruits | ____ cups | tips |
| ▶ Milk | ____ cups | tips |
| ▶ Meat & Beans | ____ ounces | tips |

Click the food groups above to learn more.

**¹ Make Half Your Grains Whole**

Aim for at least _ ounces of whole grains a day ●

**² Vary Your Veggies**

Aim for this much every week:

Dark Green Vegetables = _ cups weekly
Orange Vegetables = _ cups weekly
Dry Beans & Peas = _ cups weekly
Starchy Vegetables = _ cups weekly
Other Vegetables = ____ cups weekly

**Oils & Discretionary Calories**

Aim for _ teaspoons of oils a day

Limit your extras (extra fats & sugars) to __ Calories

**Physical Activity**

Physical activity is also important for health. Adults should get at least 30 minutes of moderate level activity most days. Longer or more vigorous activity can provide greater health benefits. Click here to find out if you should talk with a health care provider before starting or increasing physical activity. Click here for more information about physical activity and health.

Recommended amounts are listed in ounces or cups to eliminate confusion over "serving" or "portion" sizes

"Tips" give suggestions for selections within each group

Specifies minimum amount of whole grains to be eaten

Amounts of each vegetable subgroup are specified to ensure variety and adequacy

Oils and "extras" are separately listed from the food groups and at the end of the food recommendations, signifying less of a prominent position in the diet

Physical activity was not previously addressed in other food group nutrition teaching tools

**FIGURE 8.3**
Format of MyPyramid. (USDA, Center for Nutrition Policy and Promotion (2005). MyPyramid—Steps to Healthier You Food Guidance System. Available at www.MyPyramid.gov.)

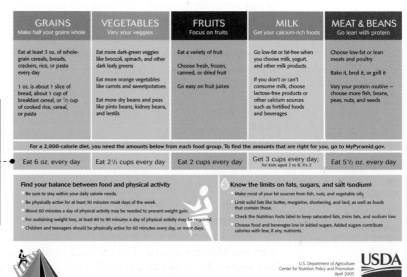

**FIGURE 8.4**
PDF version of MyPyramid's 2000 calorie eating plan. (USDA, Center for Nutrition Policy and Promotion (2005). MyPyramid—Steps to Healthier You Food Guidance System. Available at www.MyPyramid.gov.)

These amounts vary with total calories; all other information is consistent in all 12 pyramids.

**Clearing Up Controversy.** Despite the enormous amount of information available to consumers on the website www.MyPyramid.gov, putting knowledge into practice is difficult as evidenced by the lack of widespread improvements in the typical American diet (International Food Information Council, 2006). General concepts of healthy eating are familiar to consumers, but misunderstandings about servings and food group placement are common (Britten, Haven, & Davis, 2006). Specifically, consumers may need clarification on the appropriate calorie level, the concept of discretionary calories and how they are appropriated, the importance of serving sizes, and how the concept of variety should be applied.

*Appropriate Calorie Level.* The specific MyPyramid calorie level recommended for an individual is actually an estimate of how many calories a person of similar age and average height and weight needs to maintain an appropriate weight, not an exact individual requirement. If an individual's actual weight is more or less than "appropriate weight," weight change may occur as a result of following MyPyramid recommendations. MyPyramid makes a disclaimer that weight should be monitored to determine whether adjustments to calorie intake need to be made.

**Calorie-Dense Foods:** generally thought of as foods that provide significant calories with little nutritional value, such as fats, sweets, and alcohol.

**Empty-Calorie Foods:** subjectively defined by what they are not—not fruit, vegetables, dairy, meat, or bread.

*Discretionary Calories.* Discretionary calories allow consumers to incorporate small amounts of **calorie-dense** or **"empty-calorie" foods** into their eating plan and still meet nutrient needs without exceeding total calorie constraints. Discretionary calorie allowances can be quite low, allowing for only small amounts of alcohol or calorie-dense items *if* the bulk of the day's food choices are of nutrient-dense foods (American Dietetic Association, 2007).

While it may be obvious that discretionary calories can be used to allow for "extras" to the meal plan, such as a glass of wine or can of cola, consumers may not realize that discretionary calories may be "eaten up" by choosing foods within the existing plan that are high in fat or added sugar. At each calorie level, the recommendations for the amount of food to consume are based on the **"healthiest"** choices within each group, such as the very leanest cuts of meat trimmed of all visible fat. If less-than-optimal food choices are made, such as choosing whole milk instead of fat-free milk, the difference in calories is considered discretionary calories. Selecting the healthiest choices from each food group is vital for achieving appropriate calorie and nutrient recommendations (Gao et al., 2006).

**Healthiest Foods:** subjectively defined as foods that provide the most nutrients with the least amount of extraneous calories from fat or sugar.

*Serving Sizes.* Just as the quality of foods chosen influences total calorie intake, so does the quantity of foods eaten. Americans from all walks of life appear to have an inflated perception of what a "normal" serving size is and of how much food we actually need to eat to be full (Wansink & Ittersum, 2007). Because people tend to eat more when served more, the large size of many restaurant meals and the ability to "supersize" a regular meal for only pennies more may contribute to the risk of overeating. Even at-home dinnerware has grown, with the surface area of the average dinner plate now 36% bigger than it was in 1960 (Wansink, 2006). The result is more food consumed during meals and snacks. Using common objects is an excellent way to convey the concept of normal **serving sizes**, but the most effective way to downsize **portion sizes** may be to change a person's environment. That means buying smaller packages from the grocery store, ordering smaller portions out, and using smaller dinnerware at home.

**Serving Size:** the amount of food "officially" recommended.

**Portion Size:** the amount of food usually consumed.

### QUICK BITE

Serving sizes/common items

| This amount . . . . | Looks like . . . . |
|---|---|
| 3 oz of meat | a deck of cards |
| 2 tbsp of peanut butter | a ping-pong ball |
| 1 oz of cheese | 4 dice |
| ½ cup of nuts | a level adult handful |
| ½ cup cooked pasta, rice, or cereal | a scoop of ice cream |
| 1 medium-sized piece of fruit | a baseball |

*Variety.* Following a varied diet helps ensure that the more than 40 known essential nutrients are consumed in adequate amounts, based on the rationale that some nutrients, such as iron, calcium, vitamin C, and vitamin A, are concentrated in a few foods. For instance, choosing a variety of vegetables, such as carrots, broccoli, tomatoes, and garbanzo beans helps ensure adequate nutrient intake because each has a different nutrient profile. Conversely, choosing a variety of refined grains (e.g., white bread, white pasta, hamburger bun) does little to ensure nutritional adequacy, because although they are each different foods, their nutrient profile is remarkably similar. A study by McCrory et al. found that increased variety within food groups is associated with higher calorie intake and greater body fatness (McCrory et al., 1999).

## Guidelines and Graphics in Other Countries

MyPyramid is a pervasive icon in the United States, yet because of cultural differences in communicating symbolism and other cultural norms, the pyramid shape is not necessarily superior or even appropriate for food guides in other countries. A circle or dinner plate with each section depicting relative proportion to the total diet is used by many countries, including the United Kingdom (Fig. 8.5), Germany, and Mexico. Korea and China use a pagoda shape and Canada uses a rainbow shape (Fig. 8.6). Despite the differences in the shape of the graphics, the core recommendations are consistently similar: eat plenty of grains, vegetables, and fruit; limit fat, saturated fat, and sugars; eat a variety of foods; eat to balance intake with activity.

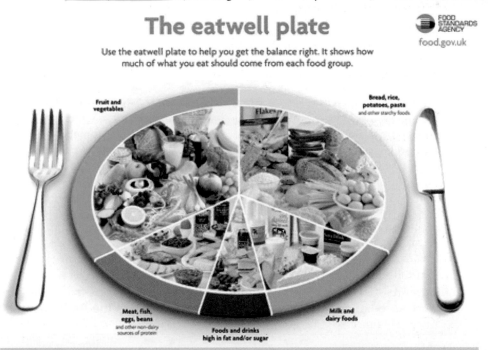

**FIGURE 8.5**
Great Britain's food guide: The Balance of Good Health Food Standards Agency (UK).

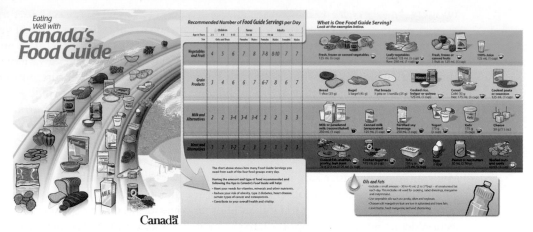

**FIGURE 8.6**
Canada's Food Guide to Healthy Eating. (© Her Majesty the Queen in Right of Canada, represented by the Minister of Healthy Canada, 2007.)

## Recommendations From Health Agencies

Many health agencies publish guidelines or recommendations for healthy eating such as the American Heart Association, the American Cancer Society, and the American Institute of Cancer Research (Table 8.2). The recommendations are similar to each other and to the Dietary Guidelines for Americans.

**The New American Plate.** The New American Plate is a campaign by the American Institute of Cancer Research to teach Americans how to implement their diet guidelines using a dinner plate as a visual aid (Fig. 8.7). It is based on recommendations stemming from a comprehensive landmark report entitled *Food Nutrition and the Prevention of Cancer: A Global Perspective* that was based on more then 4500 research studies from around the world. The report estimates that around one-third of all cancers could be prevented by changes in intake and activity. The guidelines are illustrated by a plate of food that is two-thirds or more covered with plants (fruits, vegetables, whole grains, and dried peas and beans) and one-third or less devoted to animal protein (fish, poultry, meat, low-fat dairy products). Additional recommendations regarding physical activity and weight management are offered.

| TABLE 8.2 | Comparison of Nutrition and Lifestyle Recommendations from the American Heart Association, the American Cancer Society, and the American Institute for Cancer Research | | |
|---|---|---|---|
| Criteria | Our 2006 Diet and Lifestyle Recommendations by the American Heart Association* | Choices for Good Health: American Cancer Society Guidelines for Nutrition and Physical Activity for Cancer Prevention† | AICR Diet and Health Guidelines for Cancer Prevention by the American Institute for Cancer Research‡ |
| Weight/ Calorie Balance | Use up at least as many calories as you take in. | Maintain healthy weight throughout life.<br>• Balance caloric intake with physical activity.<br>• Avoid excessive weight gain throughout the life cycle.<br>• Achieve and maintain a healthy weight if currently overweight or obese. | Be as lean as possible without becoming underweight. |

*(table continues on page 183)*

| | Our 2006 Diet and Lifestyle Recommendations by the American Heart Association* | Choices for Good Health: American Cancer Society Guidelines for Nutrition and Physical Activity for Cancer Prevention[†] | AICR Diet and Health Guidelines for Cancer Prevention by the American Institute for Cancer Research[‡] |
|---|---|---|---|
| **Criteria** | | | |
| Physical Activity | Aim for at least 30 minutes of moderate physical activity on most days of the week or—best of all—at least 30 minutes every day. | Adopt a physically active lifestyle.<br>• Adults: get at least 30 minutes or more of moderate to vigorous physical activity, above usual activities, on 5 or more days of the week; 45–60 minutes of intentional activity on 5 or more days per week is preferred. | Be physically active for at least 30 minutes each day. |
| Food | Eat a variety of nutritious foods from all the food groups.<br>• Eating a variety of fruits and vegetables may help you control your weight and your blood pressure.<br><br>• Unrefined whole-grain foods contain fiber that can help lower your blood cholesterol and help you feel full, which may help you manage your weight.<br>• Eat fish at least twice a week. | Eat a variety of healthy foods, with an emphasis on plant sources.<br>• Choose foods and beverages in amounts that help you achieve and maintain a healthy weight.<br>• Eat 5 or more servings of a variety of vegetables and fruits each day.<br>• Choose whole grains in preference to processed (refined) grains. | Eat more of a variety of vegetables, fruits, whole grains, and legumes such as beans.<br>Don't use supplements to protect against cancer.<br><br>Limit consumption of red meats (such as beef, pork, and lamb) and avoid processed meats.<br>Limit consumption of energy-dense foods (particularly processed foods high in added sugar, or low in fiber, or high in fat).<br>Avoid sugary drinks.<br>Limit consumption of salty foods and foods processed with salt (sodium). |
| | Eat less of the nutrient-poor foods.<br>• Choose lean meats and poultry without skin and prepare them without added saturated and trans fat.<br>• Select fat-free, 1%, and low-fat dairy products.<br>• Cut back on foods containing partially hydrogenated vegetable oils to reduce trans fat in your diet.<br>• Cut back on foods high in dietary cholesterol. Aim to eat < 300 mg of cholesterol each day.<br>• Cut back on beverages and foods with added sugars.<br>Choose and prepare foods with little or no salt. Aim to eat < 2300 mg of sodium/day. | • Limit consumption of processed and red meats. | |
| Alcohol | If you drink alcohol, drink in moderation. That means one drink/day if you're a woman and 2 drinks/day if you're a man. | If you drink alcoholic beverages, limit consumption.<br>Drink no more than 1 drink/day for women or 2/day for men. | If consumed at all, limit alcoholic drinks to 2 for men and 1 for women a day. |
| Tobacco | Don't smoke tobacco—and stay away from tobacco smoke. | | Do not use, smoke, or chew tobacco. |

*Sources:* *American Heart Association (2006). Our 2006 diet and lifestyle recommendations. Available at www.americanheart.org/pring_presenter.jhtml?identifier+851. Accessed on 7/4/07.

[†]American Cancer Society (2006). The complete guide—Nutrition and physical activity. Available at www.cancer.org. Accessed on 7/9/07.

[‡]World Cancer Research Fund, American Institute for Cancer Research. *Food, nutrition, physical activity, and the prevention of cancer: A global perspective.* Washington DC: AICR, 2007.

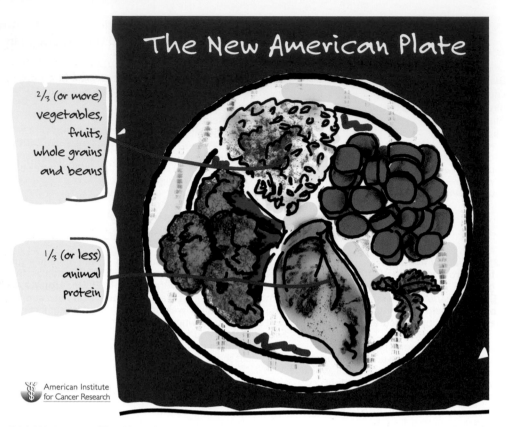

**FIGURE 8.7** The New American Plate. (Permission granted by American Institute for Cancer Research.)

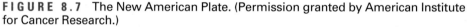

## ▶ HOW DO YOU RESPOND?

**Which foods are "good"? Which foods are "bad"?** Instead of thinking as individual foods as good or bad, consider how a food fits within the context of the total intake. For instance, broccoli is among the best plant foods available, yet if someone ate only broccoli all day long, it would not be "good" because it does not supply adequate amounts of all essential nutrients for health. What matters is how often a particular food is eaten, what size the portion is, *why* a particular food is eaten (e.g., by choice or from mindless eating), and overall calorie balance. If most of a person's intake is of healthful foods, small amounts of less-than-healthful choices can fit into the diet without wreaking great havoc as long as total calorie intake is appropriate. The keys to fitting in less-than-healthful foods are to eat them *infrequently, in small amounts, and by conscious decision.*

**How can I eat healthy if I don't like whole-wheat bread?** Just as there are no good or bad foods, there is not one particular food you must eat to be healthy, nor is there one particular food you must never eat to be healthy. Instead of whole-wheat bread, consider whole-wheat bagels or tortillas made with whole-wheat flour for sandwiches and wraps. "Low-calorie" breads are another alternative; although they lack the phytochemicals, vitamins, and minerals of whole-wheat bread, they do provide generous amounts of fiber added in place of some starch. Besides whole-wheat bread, other sources of insoluble fiber include bran and whole-grain cereals and dried peas and beans.

▶ CASE STUDY

Andrew wants to eat healthier and went online to learn about MyPyramid. He came away overwhelmed at all the information and was turned off by reading about ounces and cups—concepts that are unfamiliar to him. He is clearly interested in changing his food habits, but is stuck on the idea that that isn't possible unless he weighs and measures his food. He is wondering if eating healthier is worth the trouble.

- How would you encourage him to approach the goal of eating healthier? What information would you gather about his usual intake? His willingness to change? How would you use MyPyramid to help him make better choices without overwhelming him?

- Would Andrew be a candidate for using the plate method? What additional suggestions would you make to help him effectively use this tool?

- Andrew's doctor told him he is not meeting his RDA for vitamin C based on what Andrew told him about his eating habits. Andrew is worried that he will develop scurvy. Can you assume that he is at risk for scurvy if he isn't consuming the RDA for vitamin C? Why may the doctor's assessment be flawed? How can you determine if Andrew isn't consuming enough vitamin C? What would you tell Andrew to calm his fears?

## STUDY QUESTIONS

1. The greatest percentage of calories in the diet should come from:
   a. Carbohydrates
   b. Protein
   c. Fat
   d. Either carbohydrate or protein

2. The Dietary Guidelines for Americans recommends most fats in the diet come from foods such as:
   a. Dried peas and beans
   b. Beef, pork, and chicken
   c. Fish, nuts, and vegetable oils
   d. Margarine, eggs, and low fat milk

3. "Moderate" alcohol consumption is:
   a. 3 to 4 drinks/week for women, 6 to 8 drinks/week for men
   b. Up to 1 drink/day for both men and women
   c. Up to 1 drink/day for women, up to 2 drinks/day for men
   d. Up to 2 drinks/day for women, up to 3 drinks/day for men

4. The nurse knows her instructions about grain equivalents have been understood when the client verbalizes that one grain equivalent is equal to:
   a. 1 slice of bread
   b. 2 cups ready-to-eat cereal
   c. 1 cup cooked pasta
   d. 1 cup cooked rice

5. A client states that there is no way he can eat all the vegetables recommended in his MyPyramid plan. Which of the following would be the nurse's best response?
   a. "If you can't eat all the vegetables, make up for the difference by eating more fruit."
   b. "Be sure you take a daily multivitamin to provide the nutrients that may be missing from your diet."

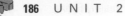 

    **c.** "Set a goal of eating larger quantities of the vegetable servings you currently eat and gradually increase the servings and variety as you become more skillful in adding vegetables to your diet."

    **d.** "No one can. The recommendations are only a guide. Just eat what you can."

**6.** The nurse knows her instructions about portion sizes have been effective when the client verbalizes that ½ cup cooked cereal looks like:
    **a.** A scoop of ice cream
    **b.** An adult handful
    **c.** A ping-pong ball
    **d.** A softball

**7.** Which of the following would contribute to "discretionary calories?"
    **a.** Whole milk
    **b.** Wheat bread
    **c.** Orange juice
    **d.** Sweet potatoes

**8.** A client demonstrates understanding of the "plate method" by devoting two-thirds or more of her dinner plate to:
    **a.** Vegetables
    **b.** Vegetables, whole grains, fruits, and beans
    **c.** Animal protein, vegetables, whole grains, and beans
    **d.** Animal protein

## KEY CONCEPTS

- A healthy diet provides optimal amounts of all essential nutrients to prevent deficiency symptoms and not excessive amounts that may cause nutrient toxicities or increase the risk of chronic diseases such as heart disease, cancer, stroke, and diabetes.

- Healthy People 2010 is a comprehensive blueprint for monitoring the nation's progress toward becoming healthier. The goal under nutrition is to promote health and reduce the risk of chronic diseases.

- DRIs are a set of reference values: the new RDAs, EAR, AIs, and UL. Individual nutrients do not have each of these reference values; a nutrient has either an EAR plus RDA or an AI. ULs are not established for all nutrients.

- The RDAs are amounts of essential nutrients considered adequate to meet the nutritional needs of 97% to 98% of healthy people in a gender or life stage group. The AIs are similar to the RDA, but it is not known what percentage of people are meeting nutritional needs by consuming the AI.

- UL is the highest intake of a nutrient over time that does not pose a risk. There is no benefit to consuming amounts between the RDA and UL of a nutrient.

- The DRIs are primarily for professional use because they deal with quantities of nutrients as opposed to amounts of food.

- The Dietary Guidelines for Americans are intended to help the public choose diets that are nutritionally adequate, promote health, and reduce the risk of chronic disease. They are revised every 5 years.

- The major messages conveyed by the Dietary Guidelines for Americans are to consume a variety of foods while staying within calorie needs; control calorie intake to manage body weight; be physically active every day; increase intake of fruits, vegetables, whole grains, and nonfat or low-fat milk and milk products; choose fats wisely; choose carbohydrates wisely; choose and prepare foods with little salt; if you drink alcohol, do so in moderation; and keep food safe to eat.

● MyPyramid is the newest generation of the graphic illustration of the Dietary Guidelines for Americans. To emphasize a personal approach to healthy eating and physical activity, MyPyramid is actually a series of pyramids providing 12 different calorie levels for individualization based on a person's age, gender, and level of activity.

● MyPyramid is designed to convey the concepts of daily physical activity, moderation, personalization, proportionality, variety, and gradual improvement.

● Consumers need to understand that it may be necessary to monitor their weight because MyPyramid calorie recommendations are population-based estimates, not individual requirements.

● Discretionary calorie allowances are small, and if not strictly adhered to, total calorie intake will exceed recommended levels.

● Portion control is vital to staying within calorie restraints. Consumers may benefit from learning to estimate portion sizes using common household items.

● Because a "healthy" diet not only limits excess calories but also provides adequate amounts of all essential nutrients, wise food choices are necessary, and variety within the Vegetable and Fruit groups is imperative.

● The pyramidal shape is not necessarily superior to other food guide graphics. Circles, a rainbow, a pagoda, and a plate are used as food graphics in other countries. Worldwide, food guides consistently recommend a high intake of whole grains, fruits, and vegetables.

● The American Heart Association, the American Cancer Society, and the American Institute for Cancer Research each recommend a plant-based diet to reduce the risk of chronic disease. The New American Plate, a nutrition campaign of the American Institute for Cancer Research, uses a plate to depict how a plant-based diet is achieved. It recommends two-thirds or more of the plate be devoted to plant foods and one-third or less feature animal protein.

## ANSWER KEY

1. **TRUE** The RDAs are intended for healthy people only.

2. **FALSE** The DRIs are most often used by dietitians to plan and evaluate menus and by researchers studying nutrition. Because they focus on nutrients, not foods, they are of limited value in teaching people how to choose healthy diets.

3. **FALSE** The Tolerable Upper Intake Level is the highest intake of a nutrient that does not produce any adverse effects. There is no advantage in consuming amounts greater than the RDA.

4. **TRUE** The Dietary Guidelines for Americans are intended to promote wellness and decrease the risk of chronic disease in healthy Americans 2 years of age and older.

5. **TRUE** MyPyramid, like its predecessor, is the graphic designed to illustrate the Dietary Guidelines for Americans.

6. **TRUE** MyPyramid is actually a group of 12 different pyramids so that dietary advice can be personalized for a person's gender, age, and activity patterns.

7. **FALSE** Unlike its predecessor, MyPyramid specifies how many cups or ounces a person should consume from each group instead of using the vague term "servings."

8. **TRUE** Too much variety can contribute to overeating, depending on how variety is achieved. Variety in fruit and vegetables has a positive impact on the nutritional adequacy of the diet without promoting excessive calorie intake. Conversely, variety in snacks, entrees, and high-carbohydrate foods may contribute to overeating. Isn't it generally harder to limit food intake at a buffet than a traditional restaurant?

9. **TRUE** MyPyramid recommends at least 30 minutes of physical activity on most days of the week. More than 30 minutes of activity may be needed to prevent weight gain or sustain weight loss.

10. **TRUE** Discretionary calories can be "extras," but extra may not translate to extra food if selections within the food plan are not ones that are lowest in fat and added sugars. Discretionary calories may be used to choose higher–calorie density foods within the existing plan instead of adding extra food.

## WEBSITES

American Cancer Society at **www.cancer.org**
American Heart Association at **www.americanheart.org**
American Institute for Cancer Research at **www.aicr.org**
Dietary Reference Intakes from the National Academy Press are found at **www.nap.edu**
Dietary Guidelines for Americans at **www.health.gov/dietaryguidelines**
Healthy People 2010 at **www.healthypeople.gov**
International Dietary Guidelines, under Topics A-Z available at **www.nal.usda.gov/fnic**
MyPyramid: Steps to a Healthier You at **www.mypyramid.gov**

## REFERENCES

American Cancer Society. (2006). *The complete guide—Nutrition and physical activity.* Available at www.cancer.org/docroot/PED/content/PED_3_2X_Diet_and_Activity_Factors_That_Affect_Risks.asp. Accessed on 7/9/07.

American Dietetic Association. (2007). Position of the American Dietetic Association: Total diet approach to communicating food and nutrition information. *Journal of the American Dietetic Association, 107*(7), 1224–1232.

American Heart Association. (2006). *Our 2006 diet and lifestyle recommendations.* Available at www.americanheart.org/presenter.jhtml?identifier=851. Accessed on 7/4/07.

Britten, P., Haven, J., & Davis, C. (2006). Consumer research for development of educational messages for the MyPyramid food guidance system. *Journal of Nutrition Education and Behavior, 38*(6 suppl), S108–S123.

Centers for Disease Control and Prevention, National Center for Health Statistics (last update 2007). *About Healthy People 2010.* Available at www.cdc.gov/nchs/about/otheract/hpdata2010/abouthp.htm. Accessed on 7/11/07.

Gao, X., Wilde, P. E., Lichtenstein, A. H., & Tucker, K. L. (2006). The 2005 USDA Food Guide Pyramid is associated with more adequate nutrient intakes within energy constraints than the 1992 pyramid. *The Journal of Nutrition, 136*, 1341–1346.

International Food Information Council. (2006). *Food & Health Survey: Consumer attitudes toward food, nutrition & health.* Available at www.ific.org/research/foodandhealthsurvey.cfm. Accessed on July 6, 2007.

Kennedy, E. (2006). Evidence for nutritional benefits in prolonging wellness. *The American Journal of Clinical Nutrition, 83*(suppl), 410S–414S.

Krebs-Smith, S., & Kris-Etherton, P. (2007). How does MyPyramid compare to other population-based recommendations for controlling chronic disease? *Journal of the American Dietetic Association, 107*(5), 830–837.

McCrory, A., Fuss, P., McCallum, J., Yao, M., Vinken, A. G., Hays, N. P., et al. (1999). Dietary variety within food groups: Association with energy intakes and body fatness in men and women. *The American Journal of Clinical Nutrition, 69*, 440–447.

Minino, A., Heron, M., & Smith, B. (2006). Deaths: Preliminary data for 2004. *National Vital Statistics Reports, 54*(19). Available at www.cdc.gov/nchs/products/pubs/pubd/hestats/prelimdeaths04/preliminarydeaths04.htm.

Otten, J., Hellwig, J., & Meyers, L. (Eds.). (2006). *Dietary reference intakes. The essential guide to nutrient requirements.* Washington, DC: National Academy Press.

United States Department of Agriculture, Center for Nutrition Policy and Promotion. (2005). *MyPyramid—Steps to a healthier you food guidance system.* Available at www.MyPyramid.gov. Accessed 7/20/07.

United States Department of Health and Human Services, United States Department of Agriculture. (2005). *Dietary guidelines for Americans* (7th ed.). Available at www.cnpp.usda.gov/ dietaryguidelines.htm. Accessed 7/30/07.

Wansink, B. (2006). *Mindless eating: Why we eat more than we think.* New York: Bantam Dell.

Wansink, B., & Ittersum, K. (2007). Portion size me: Downsizing our consumption norms. *Journal of the American Dietetic Association, 107*(7), 1103–1106.

World Cancer Research Fund, American Institute for Cancer Research. (2007). *Food, nutrition, physical activity, and the prevention of cancer: A global perspective.* Washington DC: AICR.

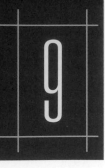

# 9 Consumer Issues

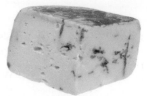

## UPON COMPLETION OF THIS CHAPTER, YOU WILL BE ABLE TO

- Analyze a nutrition or health claim for credibility.
- Evaluate a "Nutrition Facts" label to make better food choices.
- Compare how the regulation and marketing of dietary supplements differs from drugs.
- Advise clients of what questions to consider before using a supplement.
- Implement practices to help retain the nutritional value of food.
- Discuss functional foods.
- Interpret labeling on organic products.
- Teach clients about the four simple steps to keep food safe.
- Debate whether genetically modified food is safe.
- Explain the reason why some foods are irradiated.

**Functional Foods:** commonly (not legally) defined as foods that provide health benefits beyond basic nutrition.

The proliferation of cyberspace information—and misinformation—gives millions of Americans ready access to nutritional concepts. Advances in food technology have brought us **functional foods**, bioengineering, and **food irradiation** as well as new questions about food safety and optimal nutrition. The ever-evolving science of nutrition has progressed from three square meals a day and a well-rounded diet to MyPyramid. The baby

**Food Irradiation:** treatment of food with approved levels of ionizing radiation for a prescribed period of time and a controlled dose to destroy bacteria and parasites that would otherwise cause foodborne illness.

boomers' inspired quest for health and eternal youth has thrust nutrition into the spotlight not only as a means to prevent chronic health problems but also as a way to delay aging. This is an era that presents old and new challenges for health professionals.

This chapter explores how to identify and combat nutrition misinformation, with emphasis placed on how to read a food label. Dietary supplements are discussed. Consumer issues regarding food quality and safety are presented, namely organic foods, functional foods, foodborne illnesses, biotechnology, and irradiation.

# ▶ INFORMATION AND MISINFORMATION

### 🍎 QUICK BITE

Where Americans turn for nutrition information

| | |
|---|---|
| News media | 72% |
| Internet | 54% |
| Medical sources | 44% |
| Friends/family | 20% |
| Diet and health books | 13% |
| Researchers and scientists | 4% |

*Source:* International Food Information Council. (2006). 2005 *Consumer attitudes toward functional foods/foods for health. Executive summary.* Available at www.ific.org/research/upload/2005funcfoodsresearch.pdf. Accessed on 7/18/07.

Although almost all Americans believe that weight, diet, and physical activity impact health, surveys indicate that for many people, eating behaviors may be at odds with nutrition knowledge and beliefs (Table 9.1) (International Food Information Council, 2006). Consumers are often confused by nutrition messages and grow skeptical when what seems like fact today is considered fiction tomorrow. Sources of consumer confusion include the media, the Internet, and the food industry.

## The Media

The media, namely magazines, television, books, and newspapers, is a significant source of nutrition information as well as misinformation. "Breaking news" may be little more than spin or incomplete coverage of preliminary results from scientific studies, which are often

| TABLE 9.1 | "Diet Disconnects": What Americans Believe Versus What They Do | |
|---|---|---|
| | **What Americans Say...** | **What They Do...** |
| | 70% are trying to eat healthier to lose weight | 9% are reducing their calorie intake or eating less |
| | 69% believe food and nutrition play a "great role" in maintaining or improving overall health | 29% have made changes to their diet |
| | 72% are concerned about the amount and types of fats they eat | 19% are trying to consume less fat |
| | 90% named breakfast as the most important meal of the day | 49% claim to eat breakfast everyday |
| | 88% believe that certain foods and beverages can provide health benefits beyond basic nutrition and may reduce the risk of disease | 25% are adding healthier foods to their diet |

*Source:* International Food Information Council. (2007). *Calories count, but consumers don't: Food and health survey highlights six "diet disconnects".* Available at www.ific.org/newsroom/releases/2007foodandhealthsurvey.cfm. Accessed on 7/13/07.

International Food Information Council. (2006). *2005 Consumer attitudes toward functional foods/foods for health. Executive summary.* Available at www.ific.org/research/upload/2005funcfoodsresearch.pdf. Accessed on 7/18/07.

discounted later as more research is completed. Consumers may fail to make the distinction between correlation and causation and may draw inappropriate conclusions from study results. Articles that fail to identify how much or little of a food should be eaten, how often it should be eaten, or to whom the advice applies do not give consumers enough information to appropriately judge what the study means to them personally. Other types of media inaccuracy include generalizing a study to a broader population than was actually studied and overstating the size of the effect. Consumers may not even suspect that media reports may not be accurate, balanced, or complete.

## The Internet

The Internet is a vast and ever-growing source of nutrition and health information. According to the Pew Internet Project's 2006 study of online health searching, 113 million people have searched the Internet for information on at least one health topic, with 49% of the users seeking information on diet, nutrition, vitamins, or nutritional supplements (Fox, 2006). Although the information available on the Internet is vast, there are no regulatory safeguards in place to ensure that the information is accurate. Junk science coexists with legitimate data. It is the responsibility of each individual consumer to evaluate the reliability of information.

## The Food and Supplement Industry

Although ingredient listings and "Nutrition Facts" labels are reliable and accurate by law, advertising made to resemble newsworthy articles or featuring celebrity endorsements can blur the line between false advertising and freedom of speech. Sometimes ads fall short of the expectations of being truthful, substantiated, and not misleading. For example, an ad for a weight loss product may feature before and after photos with the claim of "I lost 20 pounds in 6 weeks using 'xyz.'" And although the fine print at the bottom of the ad may say "results will vary," a more honest disclaimer would be "Results not typical. Average weight loss is 4 pounds/month."

## Judging Reliability

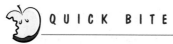 QUICK BITE

Red flags that a health or nutrient claim may
  be fraudulent
  Breakthrough
  Easy
  Enzymatic process
  Discovered in Europe
  New
  Mysterious
  Quick
  Secret
  Absolutely safe
  Miraculous cure
  Ancient formula
  All natural
  Exclusive formula
  Scientifically proven

To protect yourself and your clients from misinformation, be cautious and skeptical about what you hear and read about nutrition. Test the validity and reliability of nutrition "news" by asking who, what, when, where, and why.

*Who is promoting the message?* Anyone who stands to benefit economically by promoting a food, supplement, or diet is not likely to be an objective resource.

*What is the message?* Generally, if it sounds too good to be true, it usually is.

*When was the study conducted, the results published, the website updated?* Even seemingly legitimate information can become quickly outdated.

*Where was the study conducted?* Was the site a reputable research institution or an impressive-sounding but unknown facility?

Internet addresses ending in .edu (educational institutions), .org (organizations), or .gov (government agencies) are more credible than those ending in .com (commercial), whose main objective may be to sell a product.

*Why was the article written—to further the reader's awareness and knowledge or to sell or promote a product?* Question objectivity when the author or site has a financial interest.

## Combating Nutrition Misinformation

Determining if information is valid and reliable may be easier than persuading a client that he or she has been a victim of hype. Many people assume that anything that appears in print form (e.g., in a book, magazine, or newspaper) is accurate and not everyone recognizes the shortcomings of the World Wide Web. If clients' beliefs are unsupported but harmless, you may risk alienating them for no reason by waging a war to convince them they're misinformed. Determine how much of an emotional investment the client has in believing the misinformation. Be aware that casual or judgmental dismissal of misinformation can cause clients to become defensive and distrustful; clients may conclude that you are not as up-to-date as they are about nutrition, and they may reject you as a credible reference.

# ▶ FOOD LABELS

Food labels can help consumers make healthier food choices. Information provided on a label includes Nutrition Facts and an ingredient list; nutrient content claims, health claims, and structure/function claims may also be found.

## Nutrition Facts

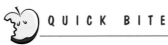

**QUICK BITE**

Measurement equivalents
  1 tsp = 5 mL
  1 tbsp = 15 mL
  1 cup = 240 mL
  1 fluid oz = 30 mL
  1 oz = 28 g

The "Nutrition Facts" label gives consumers "facts" they need to know to make informed decisions as they shop for food. Figure 9.1 lists facts about the "Nutrition Facts" label.

### Everything Hinges on Portion Size

All information that appears on the "Nutrition Facts" label is specific for the size portion listed. So if the actual portion size eaten differs from that listed, all the "facts" are incorrect. Because different varieties of a food differ in weight, there may be slight differences in the serving size among different manufacturers. For instance, the serving size of Barbara's Bakery Puffins cereal is ¾ cup, 30 g; Kellogg's Special K is 1 cup, 31 g; Kellogg's Rice Krispies is 1¼ cup, 33 g. Food label serving sizes may also differ from size equivalents used in MyPyramid.

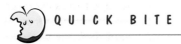

**QUICK BITE**

Serving size variations

|  | Nutrition Facts serving size | 1 oz equivalents in MyPyramid |
|---|---|---|
| Peanut butter | 2 tbsp | 1 tbsp |
| Cooked kidney beans | ½ cup | ¼ cup |
| Bread | 2 slices | 1 slice |

**Sample Label for
Macaroni and Cheese**

The Nutrition Facts information is based on one serving, but the size of a serving can vary among brands and varieties of some foods

Other voluntary information may be included, such as the amount of polyunsaturated fat and monounsaturated fat

# Nutrition Facts

Serving Size 1 cup (228g)
Servings Per Container  2

**Amount Per Serving**

**Calories** 250          Calories from Fat 110

|  | % Daily Value* |
|---|---|
| **Total Fat** 12g | **18%** |
| Saturated Fat 3g | **15%** |
| *Trans* Fat 3g | |
| **Cholesterol** 30mg | **10%** |
| **Sodium** 470mg | **20%** |
| **Potassium** 700mg | **20%** |
| **Total Carbohydrate** 31g | **10%** |
| Dietary Fiber 0g | **0%** |
| Sugars 5g | |
| **Protein** 5g | |
| Vitamin A | **4%** |
| Vitamin C | **2%** |
| Calcium | **20%** |
| Iron | **4%** |

Limit these nutrients

Includes both natural and added sugars

Get enough of these nutrients

Footnote

Quick guide to %DV
5% or less is low
20% or more is high

Trans fat does not have a DV; eat as little as possible because it increases the risk of heart disease

The %DV represents the contribution to a 2,000 calorie diet, not the percentage of calories in that food from each nutrient

If the food is enriched or fortified with nutrients or if a health claim is made, pertinent information must be listed

\* Percent Daily Values are based on a 2,000 calorie diet.
Your Daily Values may be higher or lower depending on
your calorie needs.

| | Calories: | 2,000 | 2,500 |
|---|---|---|---|
| Total Fat | Less than | 65g | 80g |
| Sat Fat | Less than | 20g | 25g |
| Cholesterol | Less than | 300mg | 300mg |
| Sodium | Less than | 2,400mg | 2,400mg |
| Total Carbohydrate | | 300g | 375g |
| Dietary Fiber | | 25g | 30g |

**F I G U R E  9 . 1**  "Nutrition facts" label. (*From:* Food and Drug Administration.)

## Percent Daily Value May Not Be Accurate for an Individual

**Percent Daily Value (%DV):** the percentage of how much of a particular nutrient or fiber a person should consume based on a 2000-calorie diet.

The **Percent Daily Value (%DV)** stated on the label may underestimate or overestimate the contribution to an individual's diet, depending on how many calories the individual actually needs. For nutrients whose amounts are based on a percent of total calories (e.g., carbohydrates, fiber, fat, saturated fat), the %DV is calculated on the basis of a 2000-calorie diet. For people who need less than 2000 calories daily, such as most women and elderly men, the %DV listed on the label actually *underestimates* the contribution a serving makes to the total needed daily. For young active men who need more than 2000 cal/day, the %DV *overestimates* actual contribution.

A wrinkle in the usefulness of the "Nutrition Facts" label is that the nutrient amounts used to calculate the %DV are not all based on current Dietary Reference Intakes (DRIs).

The %DV for vitamin A, vitamin D, calcium, iron, vitamin E, folate, and zinc are based on the 1968 Recommended Dietary Allowances. Similarly, the value used for sodium is 2400 mg even though the new Adequate Intake set for sodium intake in adults is 1500 mg.

## Ingredient List

Ingredients are listed in descending order *by weight*. The further down the list an item appears, the less of that ingredient is in the product. This information gives the consumer a relative idea of how much of each ingredient is in a product, but not the proportion.

## Nutrient Content Claims

**Daily Values (DVs):** are reference values established by the FDA for use on food labels. For some nutrients (e.g., sodium), they are amounts that should not be exceeded; for others (e.g., fiber), they are amounts to strive toward. For nutrient intakes that are based on the percentage of calories consumed, 2000 calories is the standard used.

Terms such as "low," "free," and "high" describe the level of a nutrient or substance in a food. The terms are legally defined and so they are reliable and valid. Nutrient claims may also compare the level of a nutrient to that of comparable food with terms such as "more," "reduced," or "light." Box 9.1 defines the terms used in nutrient claims.

## Health Claims

The U.S. Food and Drug Administration (FDA) has approved certain health claims about the relationship between specific nutrients or foods and the risk of a disease or health-related conditions that meet significant scientific agreement (SSA) (Box 9.2). Items that make one of these claims also meet other requirements: (1) they do not exceed specific levels for total fat, saturated fat, cholesterol, and sodium and (2) they contain at least 10% of the **Daily Value** (before supplementation) for any one or all of the following: protein, dietary fiber, vitamin A, vitamin C, calcium, and iron. Additional health claim criteria are specific for the claim made. For instance, the claim regarding calcium and osteoporosis is only allowed

---

**BOX 9.1** **DEFINITIONS OF TERMS USED IN NUTRIENT CLAIMS**

**Free** means the product contains virtually none of that nutrient. " Free" can refer to calories, sugar, sodium, salt, fat, saturated fat, and cholesterol.

**Low** means there is a small enough amount of a nutrient that the product can be used frequently without concern about exceeding dietary recommendations. Low sodium, low calorie, low fat, low saturated fat, and low cholesterol are all defined as to the amount allowed per serving. For instance, to be labeled low cholesterol, a product must have no more than 20 mg cholesterol/serving.

**Very low** refers to sodium only. The product cannot have more than 35 mg sodium/serving.

**Reduced or less** means the product has at least a 25% reduction in a nutrient compared to the regular product.

**Light or lite** means the product has ⅓ fewer calories than a comparable product or 50% of the fat found in a comparable product.

**Good source** means the product provides 10% to 19% of the Daily Value for a nutrient.

**High, rich in, or excellent source** means the product has at least 20% of the Daily Value for a nutrient.

**More** means the product has at least 10% more of a desirable nutrient than does a comparable product.

**Lean** refers to meat or poultry products with less than 10 g fat, less than 4 g saturated fat, and less than 95 mg cholesterol per standardized serving and per 100 g.

**Extra lean** refers to meat or poultry products with less than 5 g fat, less than 2 g saturated fat, and less than 95 mg cholesterol per standardized serving and per 100 g.

| BOX 9.2 | GRADE "A" HEALTH CLAIMS BASED ON SIGNIFICANT SCIENTIFIC AGREEMENT |

**Cancer Risk**
- Dietary fat
- Fruits and vegetables
- Fiber-containing grain products
- Whole grain foods and certain cancers

**Coronary Heart Disease Risk**
- Saturated fat and cholesterol
- Fruits, vegetables, and grain products that contain fiber, particularly soluble fiber
- Plant sterol/stanol esters
- Soluble fiber, such as that found in whole oats and psyllium seed husk
- Soy protein
- Whole grain foods

**Decreased Risk of Dental Caries**
- Sugar alcohols

**Hypertension Risk**
- Sodium
- Potassium (also decreased risk of stroke)

**Neural Tube Defect Risk**
- Folate

**Osteoporosis Risk**
- Calcium

on foods that have at least 20% DV for calcium. These claims are sometimes referred to as *unqualified* health claims because they do not require a qualifying statement about the strength of evidence supporting the claim.

The FDA allows certain qualified health claims when the relationship between food, a food component, and a supplement is not strong enough to meet SSA or published authoritative standards. Specific FDA-approved labeling language must be used for qualified health claims and companies must petition the FDA for prior written permission to make a qualified health claim. The weakest claim is as follows: "Very limited and preliminary scientific research suggests [health claim]. The FDA concludes that there is little scientific evidence supporting this claim." Examples of qualified health claims are listed in Box 9.3.

| BOX 9.3 | SELECTED QUALIFIED HEALTH CLAIMS |

**Cancer Risk**
- Green tea
- Selenium

**Cardiovascular Disease Risk**
- Nuts
- Monounsaturated fatty acids from olive oil

**Hypertension Risk (and Pregnancy-Induced Hypertension and Preeclampsia)**
- Calcium

## Structure/Function Claims

Structure/function claims offer the possibility that a food may improve or support body function, which is a fine distinction from the approved health claims that relate a food or nutrient to a disease. An example of disease claim needing approval is "suppresses appetite to treat obesity," whereas a function claim that does not need approval is "suppresses appetite to aid weight loss." These structure claims had previously been used primarily by supplement manufacturers with the disclaimer that "These statements have not been evaluated by the FDA. This product is not intended to diagnose, treat, cure or prevent any disease." Structure/function claims are now appearing on food labels and do not require a disclaimer. Unlike health claims that can only appear on foods that meet other nutritional criteria (e.g., they cannot be high in fat, cholesterol, sodium), structure/function claims can appear on "junk" foods. Structure/function claims do not require FDA approval, so there may be no evidence to support the claim. See Box 9.4 for structure/function claims that do not need prior approval.

## Future Directions

Some food manufacturers and retailers have begun adding symbols to food packages to show how nutritious they are. PepsiCo uses the "Smart Pot" symbol on baked Lay's potato chips and other products. The New England supermarket chain Hannaford Brothers uses a 0 to 3 star system to rate more than 25,000 items it sells. Some food companies in Britain have adopted a traffic light label system that shows by red, yellow, or green lights if a food is low, medium, or high in fat, sodium, and sugar. Although action may be years away, the FDA is considering amending labeling laws to include a front of the label symbol system to help shoppers identify healthy choices. Such a system would compliment the "Nutrition Facts" label, not replace it.

---

| BOX 9.4 | **STRUCTURE/FUNCTION CLAIMS THAT DO NOT NEED APPROVAL** |

Improves memory
Improves strength
Improves digestion
Boosts stamina
For common symptoms of PMS
For hot flashes
Helps you relax
Helps enhance muscle tone or size
Relieves stress
Helps promote urinary tract health
Maintains intestinal flora
For hair loss associated with aging
Prevents wrinkles
For relief of muscle pain after exercise
To treat or prevent nocturnal leg muscle cramps
Helps maintain normal cholesterol levels
Provides relief of occasional constipation
Supports the immune system

# ► DIETARY SUPPLEMENTS

**Herbs:** plants or parts of plants used to alleviate health problems or promote wellness.

The term dietary supplement is a group name for products that contain one or more dietary ingredients including vitamins, minerals, **herbs** or other botanicals, amino acids, and other substances. They are intended to *add to* (supplement) the diets of some people, not to replace a healthy diet. Supplements are taken by mouth as a capsule, tablet, lozenges, liquid, or "tea." Labeling laws require the front label to state that the product is a dietary supplement. Figure 9.2 depicts a supplement label.

The FDA estimates that there are more than 29,000 supplements on the market with more added daily. At least half of American adults take a dietary supplement, collectively spending about $23 billion/year (National Institutes of Health State-of-the Science Panel, 2007). Although the majority of supplements used are multivitamin/multimineral supplements, other products are also popular. The top ten selling herbal supplements in food, drug, and mass marketing retail channels in the United States are summarized in Table 9.2.

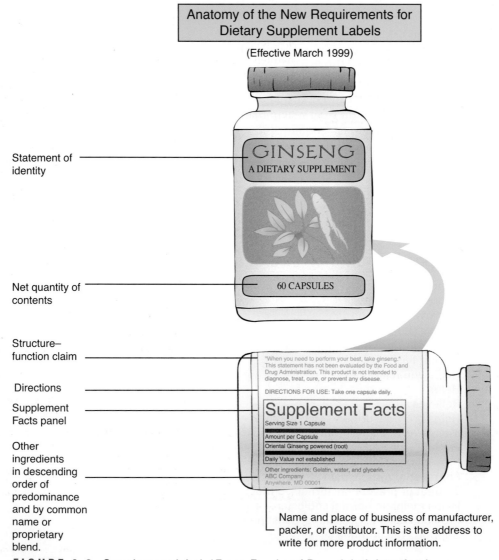

**Anatomy of the New Requirements for Dietary Supplement Labels**

(Effective March 1999)

Statement of identity

GINSENG
A DIETARY SUPPLEMENT

Net quantity of contents

60 CAPSULES

Structure–function claim

"When you need to perform your best, take ginseng." This statement has not been evaluated by the Food and Drug Administration. This product is not intended to diagnose, treat, cure, or prevent any disease.

Directions

DIRECTIONS FOR USE: Take one capsule daily.

Supplement Facts panel

## Supplement Facts
Serving Size 1 Capsule

Amount per Capsule

Oriental Ginseng powered (root)

Daily Value not established

Other ingredients in descending order of predominance and by common name or proprietary blend.

Other ingredients: Gelatin, water, and glycerin.
ABC Company
Anywhere, MD 00001

Name and place of business of manufacturer, packer, or distributor. This is the address to write for more product information.

**F I G U R E 9 . 2** Supplement label. (*From:* Food and Drug Administration.)

| TABLE 9.2 | | Top 10 Selling Herbal Supplements in the United States in the Food, Drug, and Mass Market Channels | | | |
|-----------|----------------|------|-----------------------------|--------------------------|-------------------------------|
| **Supplement** | **Forms Available** | **Uses** | **Potential Side Effects** | **People Who Should Not Use** | **Potential Herb–Drug Interactions** |
| Cranberry | Capsules, tablets | Prevention and treatment of urinary tract infections | Prolonged or high use of concentrated tablets may increase risk of kidney stones | People at high risk for kidney stones | No reported adverse interactions |
| Soy isoflavones | Capsules, powder, tablets | To lessen symptoms of menopause such as hot flashes, to lower serum cholesterol levels | The safety of concentrated sources of isolated isoflavones in pill form is not known | Women with a history of or at high risk for breast cancer. People with altered thyroid function | May reduce the absorption of thyroid medications when taken concurrently |
| Garlic | Capsules, liquid, powder, tablets | To lower cholesterol and/or triglyceride levels; may be useful in the treatment of bacterial and fungal infections, digestive ailments, and hypertension | Large quantities may cause heartburn, flatulence, and GI distress | People about to have surgery, due to increased bleeding | May increase bleeding time when taken with other blood thinning supplements or anticoagulants; may decrease effectiveness of cyclosporine, some calcium channel blockers, chemotherapeutic agents, antifungals, glucocorticoids, and others; may interfere with the effectiveness of oral contraceptives; avoid if used with NNRTI antiretroviral drugs |
| Saw palmetto | Capsules, liquid, tablets | To prevent or relieve symptoms of enlarged prostate | Mild GI upset (rare) | Should be avoided for 2 weeks prior to surgery; people with bleeding disorders | May increase bleeding time when taken with anticoagulants, aspirin, supplements of vitamin E or *Ginkgo*; may interfere with hormone and contraceptive drug therapies |
| Ginkgo biloba | Capsules, infusions, liquid, tablets | To improve memory, to treat peripheral vascular disease | Mild headache, GI upset, constipation, allergic skin reactions. Consumption of *ginko* seeds can be fatal | Should be avoided at least 36 hours prior to surgery; people with bleeding disorders or diabetes | Anticoagulants, aspirin, vitamin E or garlic supplements, trazodone, Prozac, antidiabetics, thiazide diuretics |

*(table continues on page 200)*

| TABLE 9.2 | Top 10 Selling Herbal Supplements in the United States in the Food, Drug, and Mass Market Channels (continued) | | | | |
|---|---|---|---|---|---|
| **Supplement** | **Forms Available** | **Uses** | **Potential Side Effects** | **People Who Should Not Use** | **Potential Herb–Drug Interactions** |
| Echinacea | Capsules, liquid, tablets; also sold in herbal teas and throat lozenges | To prevent or treat colds and the flu | Minor GI upset, increased urination, allergic reactions (especially in people allergic to grass pollens) | People with autoimmune diseases such as multiple sclerosis, lupus. Not recommended to be used >8 successive weeks | May decrease effectiveness of immune-suppressing drugs, such as cyclosporine, azathioprine, prednisone, and other corticosteroids |
| Milk thistle | Capsules, tablets, softgel, liquid, tincture | To treat alcoholic liver cirrhosis, to reduce the risk of cancers of the prostate and skin | Minimal occurrence of side effects that include GI upset and skin rash | None known | May increase clearance of glucuronidated drugs, such as select statin medications, acetaminophen, diazepam, digoxin, morphine |
| St. John's wort | Capsules, liquid, tea, tablets, powders | To treat depression, anxiety, seasonal affective disorder, sleep disorders | Dry mouth, dizziness, GI symptoms, increased sensitivity to sunlight, fatigue | People sensitive to sunlight or taking UV treatment. People with bipolar disorder; people scheduled for surgery; may increase dementia in people with Alzheimer's disease | Do not use with antidepressant medications; may decrease the effectiveness of oral contraceptives, theophylline, digoxin, and numerous other drugs for epilepsy, heart disease, immunosuppression, and psychosis |
| Ginseng | Capsules, gel caps, tablets, tea | To improve mental alertness or increase energy. As an aphrodisiac or stress reliever | Generally not associated with adverse side effects | People with untreated hypertension. Women with a history of breast cancer | May increase bleeding time when taken with other blood-thinning supplements or medications; when used with caffeine may stimulate hypertension; may interfere with corticosteroids, digoxin, diabetes medications, and estrogen therapy |
| Black cohosh | Capsules, liquid, tablets, teas | Relief of menopausal symptoms, PMS, dysmenorrhea | GI upset, headaches, dizziness, weight gain, cramping, feeling of heaviness in the legs | Women with a history of breast cancer or at risk of breast cancer (an animal study showed black cohosh promoted cancer metastasis) | May increase the risk of liver damage in people taking potentially hepatotoxic drugs or supplements |

*Source:* FDM market sales data for herbal supplements, 52 weeks ending January 1, 2006. Chicago, Il: Information Resources, Inc. Available at http://cms.herbalgram.org/herbalgram/issue82/article3400.html?issue=82

Fragakis, A., & Thomson, C. (2007). *The health professional's guide to popular dietary supplements* (3rd ed.). Chicago: The American Dietetic Association.

Whereas the functions and requirements of vitamins and minerals are fairly well understood, scientific research is lacking for many herbal products. Many people mistakenly believe "natural" is synonymous with "safe"; they assume that herbs must be harmless because they come from flowers, leaves, and seeds. In truth, herbs are not guaranteed to be safe or effective.

In June 2007, the FDA announced a final rule establishing current good manufacturing practice requirements (CGMPs) for dietary supplements. For the first time, identity, purity, quality, and composition of dietary supplements are required to be accurately reflected on the label. The final rule is a significant step in protecting consumers by ensuring supplements that

- Are free of contaminants or impurities such as natural toxins, bacteria, pesticides, glass, lead, or other substances.
- Contain the stated amount of a dietary ingredient.
- Are properly packaged.
- Are made from ingredients that were properly handled.

In addition, the final rule requires that manufacturers report all serious dietary supplement adverse events to the FDA. Still, there are major differences between how supplements and drugs are regulated and marketed.

## Supplement Regulation

In their medicinal sense, herbs are technically unapproved drugs; approximately 30% of drugs used today originated from plants (e.g., paclitavel, aspirin, digoxin). In the United States, dietary supplements are regulated by the FDA as *foods,* which mean they do not have to meet the same standards as drugs and over-the-counter medications. Supplements differ greatly from conventional drugs in how they are marketed and regulated.

## Safety and Effectiveness Are Not Proven

**New Dietary Ingredient:** supplement ingredient not marketed in the United States before October 15, 1994.

Before a drug can be marketed, the FDA must authorize its use based on the results of clinical studies performed to determine safety, effectiveness, possible interactions with other substances, and appropriate doses. In contrast, the regulations regarding dietary supplements are lax. Supplement ingredients sold in the United States before October 15, 1994 are assumed to be safe and so do not require FDA review for safety before they are marketed. Dietary supplement manufacturers that want to market a **new dietary ingredient** must submit information to the FDA that supports their conclusion that *reasonable* evidence exists that the product is safe for human consumption. Manufacturers do not have to *prove* to the FDA that dietary supplements are safe or effective; however, they are not supposed to market unsafe or ineffective products.

Once a product is marketed, the responsibility lies with the FDA to prove danger rather than with the manufacturer to prove safety. They do this through adverse event monitoring and research. When the FDA determines a supplement is unsafe, it issues a consumer advisory discouraging its use. Only one supplement, ephedra, has actually been banned by the FDA in an unprecedented move culminating a 7-year review of tens of thousands of public comments and peer reviewed scientific literature on the safety of ephedra. Despite the ban, consumers are still able to buy ephedra.

**Standardization:** a manufacturing process that ensures product consistency from batch to batch.

## Strength Is Not Standardized

Dietary supplements are not required to be standardized in the United States. In fact, there is no legal definition of **standardization** as it applies to supplements, so the concentration of active compounds in different batches of supposedly identical plant material can vary greatly. The difference in concentration may be related to several factors such as the variety of plant used and the part of the plant used (e.g., the stems or leaves).

## Dosages Are Not Standardized

Recommended dosages vary among manufacturers because there is no premarket testing to determine optimum dosage or maximum safe dosage. Other than the manufacturers' responsibility to ensure safety, there are no regulations that limit a "serving size" of any supplement.

## Claims on Packaging Do Not Require FDA Approval

Although dietary supplements cannot claim to be used for the diagnosis, treatment, cure, or prevention of disease, they can be labeled with statements explaining their purported effect on the structure or function of the human body (e.g., "alleviates fatigue") or their role in promoting well-being (e.g., "improves mood"). These statements do not require FDA approval but the label must include the following disclaimer: "This statement has not been evaluated by the FDA. This product is not intended to diagnose, treat, cure, or prevent any disease."

## Warnings Are Not Required

Unlike drugs, supplements are not required to carry warning labels about potential side effects, adverse effects, or supplement–drug interactions. Nor are there advisories about who should not use the product.

## Supplements Are Self-Prescribed

A major concern with self-medication is that consumers may misdiagnose their condition or forsake effective conventional medical care to treat themselves "naturally." Another problem with self-medicating is that patients may not inform their physicians about their use of herbs, so side effects and herb–drug interactions go undiagnosed and unreported.

## Advice for Supplement Users

Clients who choose to use supplements should ask critical questions beforehand, such as whether there is any scientific evidence to support the use of the product or if there are any potential adverse side effects associated with its use. Consumers should check with the FDA website for consumer advisories on supplements to avoid and discuss supplement use with the physician. To prevent and manage adverse side effects and supplement–drug interactions, only single supplement products should be used and the dose should be small. Supplements should be taken at different times from prescribed medications to help reduce the potential for supplement–drug interactions; supplements should be discontinued immediately if adverse side effects or supplement–drug interactions occur. Pregnant or lactating women and children under the age of 6 should not use herbs and other botanical supplements.

## ▶ FOOD QUALITY CONCERNS

The following section deals with issues of food quality, namely proper food handling, functional foods, and organic foods.

## Retaining the Nutrient Content of Food

Even when it is carefully planned, an eating plan may not provide optimal amounts of all nutrients if the food has been improperly stored or overly processed. Food generally begins to lose its nutrients the moment harvesting or processing begins; the more it is done to a food before it is eaten, the greater the loss of naturally present nutrients. Heat, light, air, soaking in water, mechanical injury, dry storage, and acidic or alkaline food processing ingredients can all hasten nutrient losses. Vitamins, minerals, and fibers are particularly vulnerable to the effects of food processing. Tips to retain the nutrient value of foods are featured in Box 9.5.

## Functional Foods

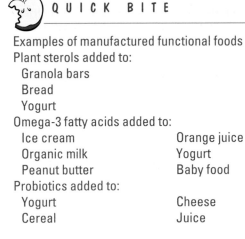

**QUICK BITE**

Examples of manufactured functional foods
Plant sterols added to:
    Granola bars
    Bread
    Yogurt
Omega-3 fatty acids added to:
    Ice cream            Orange juice
    Organic milk        Yogurt
    Peanut butter       Baby food
Probiotics added to:
    Yogurt               Cheese
    Cereal               Juice

Functional foods are one of the fastest growing segments of the food industry. The term generally applies to foods that provide health benefits beyond basic nutrition. Functional foods may be natural (Table 9.3) or manufactured.

Manufactured functional foods are a blend of food and pharmacy ("phoods") in which food has one or more functional ingredients added such as vitamins, minerals, phytochemicals, or herbs. New functional foods with unique combinations of ingredients are being introduced in the marketplace faster than science can provide information

---

| BOX 9.5 | TIPS FOR RETAINING THE NUTRIENT VALUE OF FOODS |
|---|---|

- Don't buy produce that is damaged or wilted or that has been improperly stored. Produce picked when fully ripe is higher in nutrients than produce picked when green.
- Refrigerate most fruits and vegetables immediately to slow enzyme activity and retain nutrients. Keep produce in the refrigerator crisper or in moisture-proof bags.
- Wash, don't soak, produce to avoid leaching nutrients.
- Avoid peeling and paring vegetables before cooking because a valuable layer of nutrients is stored directly beneath the skin. If necessary, scrape or pare as thin a layer as possible.
- Avoid cutting produce into small pieces: the more surface area exposed, the greater the nutrient loss.
- Prepare vegetables as close to serving time as possible to avoid excessive exposure to light and air . Don't thaw frozen vegetables before cooking.
- Eat some fruits and vegetables raw.
- Cook produce in as little water as possible to avoid leaching vitamins. Stir-fry, steam, microwave, or pressure-cook vegetables to retain nutrients. If water is used in cooking, save and use it as stock for soups, gravies, or sauces.
- Shorten cooking time as much as possible. Cook vegetables to the tender crunchy, rather than to the mushy, stage of doneness; cover the pan to retain heat; and preheat the pan or water before adding foods to speed heating time.
- Cook only as many vegetables as are needed at a time because reheating causes considerable loss of vitamins.

| TABLE 9.3 | Natural Functional Foods | | | |
|---|---|---|---|---|
| Food | Active Ingredient | Effective Level | Potential Health Benefits | Strength of Evidence* |
| Soy foods | Soy protein | 25 g/day | Lower total and LDL cholesterol | ***** |
| Oats | Soluble fiber (beta-glucan) | 3 g beta-glucan/day (1½ servings oats/day) | Lower total and LDL cholesterol | ***** |
| Fatty fish | Omega-3 fatty acids | 6 oz/week | Lower triglycerides, lower heart disease, cardiac deaths, and fatal and nonfatal heart attacks | **** |
| Purple grape juice or red wine | Resveratrol | 8–16 oz/day | Decrease platelet aggregation | *** |
| Cranberry juice | Proanthocyanidins | 300 mL/day | Reduces the risk of urinary tract infections | ** |
| Green tea | Catechins | 4–6 cups/day | Reduces the risk of certain cancers | ** |
| Tomatoes and tomato products | Lycopene | ½ cup/day or 10 servings/week | Reduce the risk of prostate cancer | ** |
| Yogurt and fermented dairy products | Probiotics | 1–2 billion colony-forming units/day | Promote gastrointestinal health | ** |
| Nuts | Monounsaturated fatty acids and vitamin E | 1–2 oz/day | Reduce the risk of cardiovascular disease | ** |
| Cruciferous vegetables (e.g., broccoli, cauliflower, cabbage) | Sulforaphane | >½ cup/day | Reduce the risk of certain types of cancer | * |
| Garlic | Sulfur compounds | Approximately 1 fresh clove/day | Lowers total and LDL cholesterol | * |
| Spinach, kale, collard greens | Lutein | 6 mg/day as lutein | Lower risk of age-related macular degeneration | * |

Very strong = *****
Strong to moderate = ****
Moderate to strong = ***
Moderate = **
Weak to moderate = *

*Source:* American Dietetic Association. (2004). Position of the American Dietetic Association: Functional foods. *Journal of the American Dietetic Association, 104*(5), 814–826.

on their safety. Like supplements, once functional foods are marketed, adverse effects are brought to light only if consumers alert the FDA to suspected problems.

As scientific evidence mounts in the role of specific nutrients or food substances in preventing chronic diseases such as heart disease, cancer, diabetes, hypertension, and osteoporosis, it is likely that more foods will be considered functional and the supply of manufactured functional foods will expand exponentially. It is the position of the American Dietetic Association that functional foods have a potentially beneficial effect on health when consumed as part of a varied diet on a regular basis (American Dietetic Association, 2004). Functional foods should be viewed as an option in the continuum of good nutrition, not as a "magic bullet" to cure all dietary ills.

# Organically Grown Foods

**Organic:** in a chemical sense, organic means carbon containing. Generally, organic refers to living organisms; as such, all foods are technically organic.

**Organically Grown or Organically Produced:** foods produced with little or no synthetic fertilizers or pesticides (e.g., plants) and no antibiotics or hormones (e.g., livestock).

**QUICK BITE**

The following items comprise 75% of total organic food sales in the United States:
Fresh fruit and vegetables
Bread and grains
Packaged and prepared foods
Dairy products

***Source:*** Economic Research Service, USDA. (2003). *Organic farming and marketing. Questions and answers. What is the size of the U.S. market for organic foods.* June 24, 2003. Available at www.ers.usda.gov/Briefing/ Organic/Questions/orgqa5.htm. Accessed on 7/20/07.

The demand for **organic** foods has soared over the last decade, with a sales growth rate of approximately 20% annually (EWG, 2007). Reasons Americans give for buying organic foods are: (1) to limit consumption of chemicals, (2) because they are "better" for them, and (3) because they are concerned about the environment.

Organic farming uses "natural" products to fertilize crops, such as manure, compost, and other organic wastes. Chemicals that occur naturally in the environment, such as sulfur, nicotine, and copper, may be used as pesticides. Insects that do not harm a particular crop may be used to control other insects known to cause crop damage. Crop rotation, tillage, and cover crops are used to manage soil. Food irradiation, sewage sludge, and bioengineered plants cannot be used.

Regulations are also in place for raising organically grown livestock. **Organically produced** feed must be used for a specified period of time toward the end of gestation; animals may be given vitamin and mineral supplements but the use of growth hormones and antibiotics is prohibited; and animals treated with medication cannot be sold as organic.

The United States Department of Agriculture (USDA) ensures that the production, processing, and certification of **organically grown** foods adhere to strict national standards and organic labeling meet criterion that define the four official organic categories (Fig. 9.3). Most consumers assume that produce sold at local farmers' markets is grown locally and organic but neither is necessarily true.

Organic food is usually more expensive because of higher production costs, greater losses, and smaller yields. However, the difference in price between organic and conventionally processed food varies considerably among items. For instance, a gallon of organic milk typically costs twice as much as a gallon of store brand or name brand milk. Other organic products, such as oranges and bread, tend to be priced closer to their conventional counterparts (Dunlop, 2007).

Are organically produced foods superior to their conventionally raised counterparts? The USDA maintains that organic foods are not safer than conventional foods. However, a study published in the journal *Food Additives and Contaminants* showed that organically grown produce consistently had only one-third as many pesticide residues as produce grown conventionally and that organic produce was far less likely to contain residues of more than

**FIGURE 9.3** Sample cereal boxes showing four labeling categories for organic labeling. From left: cereal with 100% organic ingredients; cereal with 95% to 100% organic ingredients; cereal made with at least 70% organic ingredients; and cereal with less than 70% organic ingredients. (***Source:*** USDA website.)

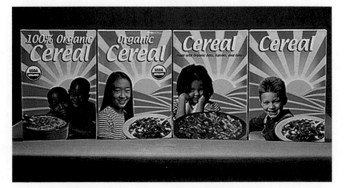

one residue (Baker, Benbrook, Groth, & Lutz Benbrook, 2002). Even data from the USDA and FDA show that conventionally grown produce routinely has higher pesticide levels than organically grown produce, but the amount is still well below the level the Environmental Protection Agency deems as unsafe. What is not known is whether chronic ingestion of pesticides at low levels over years or decades is a health risk (Shardt, 2007).

Based on results of nearly 43,000 tests for pesticide residue on produce collected by the USDA and FDA, the Environmental Working Group created a ranking of produce from worst (most pesticide residues) to best (least pesticide residues) (Environmental Working Group, 2006). Although they urge consumers to buy organic whenever possible, they contend that consumers can reduce their exposure to pesticides by 90% by avoiding the 12 most contaminated fruits and vegetables and substituting them with the 12 least contaminated (Table 9.4). Whether produce is grown organically or conventionally, experts agree that thoroughly rinsing all fruits and vegetables under running water and discarding the outer leaves, where appropriate, are vital to reduce exposure to natural dangers such as bacteria and man-made risks such as chemical residues.

While the USDA contends that organically produced food is not nutritionally better than its conventional counterpart, a 10-year study found that organically grown tomatoes have a higher content of certain phytochemicals than conventionally grown tomatoes, possibly because the fertility of the soil changed over time due to changes in farming practices (Mitchell et al., 2007). Time will tell if organically produced food has a significantly better nutritional profile than foods produced by conventional methods.

| TABLE 9.4 | **Produce with the Highest and Lowest Pesticide Residues** |
|---|---|
| **The Highest Pesticide Load** | **Ranking is based on** |
| Peaches<br>Apples<br>Sweet bell peppers<br>Celery<br>Nectarines<br>Strawberries<br>Cherries<br>Lettuce<br>Imported grapes<br>Pears<br>Spinach<br>Potatoes | • The percentage of samples with detectable pesticides<br>• The percentage of samples with 2 or more pesticides<br>• The average number of pesticides found on a sample<br>• The average concentration of all pesticides found<br>• The maximum number of pesticides found on a single sample<br>• The total number of pesticides found |
| **The Lowest Pesticide Load (in Ascending Order)** | |
| Onions<br>Avocado<br>Sweet corn (frozen)<br>Pineapples<br>Mango<br>Asparagus<br>Sweet peas (frozen)<br>Kiwi<br>Bananas<br>Cabbage<br>Broccoli<br>Papaya | |

*Source:* Environmental Working Group Food News. (2006). *Shoppers guide.* Available at www.foodnews.org/walletguide.php. Accessed on 7/13/07.

## ▶ FOOD SAFETY CONCERNS

Food safety concerns include preventing foodborne illnesses that can occur from improperly handled or stored food. Other current issues of food safety include biotechnology and irradiation.

### Foodborne Illness

**Foodborne Illness:** an illness transmitted to humans via food.

QUICK BITE

Foods implicated in foodborne illnesses in the United States, 1990–2004 (includes *E. coli* 0157:H7)

| Food | Number of people sickened |
| --- | --- |
| Greens, salad based | 7555 |
| Turkey | 5832 |
| Chicken | 3979 |
| Ground beef | 3425 |
| Shellfish | 3399 |
| Berries | 3330 |
| Tomatoes | 2852 |
| Lettuce | 2380 |
| Eggs | 2117 |
| Ham | 2107 |

*Source:* Liebman, B. (2006). Fear of fresh. How to avoid foodborne illness from fruits and vegetables. *Nutrition Action Heatlh Letter, 33* (10), 1, 3–6.

In the United States, as many as 76 million illnesses and 5000 deaths per year are attributed to consumption of contaminated food or water ( Centers for Disease Control, 2007). The microorganisms that cause **foodborne illness** are found widely in nature and are transmitted to people from within the food (e.g., meat and fish), on the food (e.g., eggshell or vegetables), from unsafe water, or from human or animal feces.

Bacteria are responsible for more than 90% of all foodborne illnesses. To spread, bacteria simply need food, moisture, a favorable temperature, and time to multiply. The remainder of cases are blamed on viruses, parasites, food toxins, and unknown causes.

Although foodborne illness can be caused by any food, foods containing animal proteins are the most frequent vehicles. Table 9.5 outlines common foodborne illnesses caused by bacteria. Table 9.6 features foodborne illnesses caused by viruses.

The most common symptoms of foodborne illness may be mistaken for the flu, diarrhea, nausea, vomiting, fever, abdominal pain, and headaches. Most cases are self-limiting and run their course within a few days. Symptoms that warrant medical attention include bloody diarrhea (possible *E. coli* 0157:H7 infection), a stiff neck with severe headache and fever (possible meningitis related to *Listeria*), excessive diarrhea or vomiting (possible life-threatening dehydration), and any symptoms that persist for more than 3 days. Infants, pregnant women, the elderly, and people with compromised immune systems (people with acquired immunodeficiency syndrome [AIDS] or cancer, organ transplant recipients, people taking corticosteroids) are particularly vulnerable to the effects of foodborne illness.

The major cause of foodborne illnesses is unsanitary food handling. To reduce the risk of contamination, proper personal hygiene and handwashing must be practiced by all food handlers. Steps must be taken to prevent cross-contamination between raw and cooked foods and through food handlers. Because heat kills most bacteria, thorough cooking of meat and fish is vital, as is pasteurization of all milk products. Adequate refrigeration inhibits the growth of bacteria. Figure 9.4 depicts the four simple steps to keep food safe, promoted by the Fight BAC! (as in bacteria) campaign of the Partnership for Food Safety Education. See the Partnership for Food Safety Education website for additional food safety tips.

TABLE 9.5

## Common Foodborne Illnesses in the United States Caused by Bacteria

| Bacteria (illness) | Common Food Vehicles | Onset | Symptoms | Other |
|---|---|---|---|---|
| *Bacillus cereus* (bacillus) | Meat products, soups, vegetables, puddings, sauces, milk and milk products | 8–16 hours | Abdominal pain, watery diarrhea, nausea | Symptoms last for 24 hours in most cases |
| *Campylobacter jejuni* (campylobacter enteritis) | Raw milk, undercooked poultry, raw beef, unchlorinated water | 1–7 days | Diarrhea, muscle pain, fever, nausea, abdominal pain | Leading cause of diarrhea in the United States: rarely life-threatening symptoms. Symptoms may last 7–10 days |
| *Clostridium botulinum* (botulism) | Underheated, low-acid home canned foods (corn, peppers, green beans, mushrooms, tuna), vacuum-packed meats, sausage, fish, honey (in infants only) | Usually 18–36 hours after ingesting toxin, but onset may range from 4 hours to 8 days | Nausea, vomiting, diarrhea, fatigue, headache, dry mouth, double vision, difficulty speaking and swallowing, muscle paralysis, difficulty breathing | Fatal in 3–10 days if not treated |
| *Clostridium perfringens* (perfringens food poisoning) | Meat, poultry, stuffing, gravy and cooked foods held or stored at inappropriate temperature | 8–22 hours | Intense abdominal cramps, diarrhea, headache, the chills | The "cafeteria germ," associated with steam table foods not kept hot enough. Illness usually over within 24-hours. One of most common foodborne illnesses in the United States |
| *Cryptosporidium parvum* (intestinal, tracheal, or pulmonary cryptosporidiosis) | Any food touched by an infected food handler | Approximately 2 days | Intestinal: severe watery diarrhea or no symptoms at all. Pulmonary/tracheal: cough, low grade fever; often accompanied by severe intestinal distress | Incidence is higher in day care centers that serve food. Outbreaks often related to contaminated water supplies. Microbe is resistant to chlorine |
| *Cyclospora cayetanesis* (cyclosporidiosis) | Food or water contaminated with infected stool | 1 week | Explosive, watery diarrhea with fatigue, nausea, vomiting, cramping, myalgia, significant weight loss | Some people infected with Cyclospora are symptom-free |
| *Escherichia coli* (*E. coli* 0157-H7; hemorrhagic colitis, hemolytic, uremic syndrome) | Undercooked beef, especially ground beef; raw milk; unpasteurized fruit juice and cider; alfalfa and radish sprouts; plant foods fertilized with raw manure or irrigated with contaminated water | 2–5 days | Severe abdominal cramps and diarrhea. Hemorrhagic colitis may lead to hemolytic-uremic syndrome (severe anemia and renal failure) | |

(table continues on page 209)

TABLE 9.5

**Common Foodborne Illnesses in the United States Caused by Bacteria** (continued)

| Bacteria (illness) | Common Food Vehicles | Onset | Symptoms | Other |
|---|---|---|---|---|
| *Listeria mono-cytogenes* (listeriosis) | Raw milk, deli-type salads, processed meats, soft cheese, undercooked poultry, ice cream, raw vegetables, raw and cooked poultry | 2 days to 3 weeks | Sudden fever, chills, headache, backache, occasional abdominal pain, and diarrhea<br>Septicemia and meningitis may lead to death<br>May cause spontaneous abortion or stillbirth during pregnancy | This bacterium thrives in cold temperatures and appears to be able to survive short-term pasteurization<br>Mortality from listeric meningitis may be as high as 70% |
| *Salmonella* species (salmonellosis) | Raw and undercooked eggs, poultry, meats, milk and dairy products, raw sprouts (alfalfa, bean), shrimp, sauces, and salad dressings | 6–48 hours | Nausea, vomiting, cramps, fever, diarrhea, headache<br>Arthritic symptoms may occur 3–4 weeks after onset of acute infection | Can be fatal<br>Incidence is increasing in the United States |
| *Shigella* species (shigellosis) | Salads (potato, tuna, shrimp, macaroni, chicken), raw vegetables, untreated water | 12–50 hours | Severe diarrhea that may be bloody, abdominal pain, fever, vomiting | Fecally contaminated water and unsanitary food handling are most common causes of contamination |
| *Staphylococcus aureus* (staphylococcal food poisoning) | Custard- or cream-filled baked goods, sandwich fillings; poultry and egg products; salad made of egg, tuna, chicken, potato, and macaroni | 1–6 hours | Severe nausea, vomiting, abdominal cramps, prostration | Of healthy people, 40–50% are carriers. Most frequently found in the nose, throat, on skin, and in infected boils, pimples, cuts, and burns<br>Frequently transmitted to foods by human carriers |
| *Vibrio vulnificus* (Vibrio infection) | Raw or undercooked shellfish, especially oysters. Organism is easily killed by cooking | Abrupt | Fever, chills, skin lesions, nausea, vomiting, diarrhea, hypotension, shock<br>May lead to septicemia | Infection can occur in coastal waters through open wounds<br>Infection rarely occurs in healthy people; those at risk include people with compromised immune systems, achlorhydria, and chronic liver disease<br>Mortality rate about 50% in immunocompromised people including those with liver disease |
| *Yersinia enterocolitica* (yersiniosis) | Pork and raw milk | 1–3 days | Enterocolitis with diarrhea and/or vomiting; fever, abdominal pain | May mimic acute appendicitis |

| TABLE 9.6 | Common Foodborne Illnesses in the United States Caused by Viruses | | | | |
|---|---|---|---|---|---|
| **Virus (Illness)** | **Common Food Vehicles** | **Onset** | **Symptoms** | **Other** |
| Hepatitis A virus (hepatitis) | Food contaminated by infected food handlers, water, shellfish, and salads are the most common vehicles | 10–50 days (average is 28–30 days) | Fever, malaise, nausea, vomiting, muscle pain, jaundice | Illness usually subsides after a few weeks; but may last for months |
| Norwalk virus (food poisoning; viral gastroenteritis) | Untreated water, shellfish, raw or undercooked clams, and oysters | 24–48 hours | Nausea, vomiting, diarrhea, abdominal pain, headache, low-grade fever | Severe illness is rare |

*Source:* International Food Information Council. (2007). *A consumer's guide to food safety risks.* Available at http://www.ific.org/publications/other/consumersguideom.cfm. Accessed on 7/18/07.

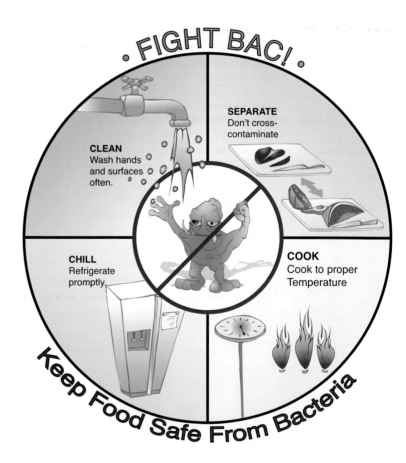

**FIGURE 9.4** Fight BAC! infographic. (*Source:* Partnership for Food Safety Education.)

## "Mad Cow Disease" (Bovine Spongiform Encephalopathy)

Mad cow disease is the common name for bovine spongiform encephalopathy (BSE), a slowly progressive, degenerative, fatal disease affecting the central nervous system of adult cattle. Although the exact cause is unknown, BSE is believed to be caused by prions, an infectious form of a type of protein. BSE was first reported in 1986 in the United Kingdom and is believed to have originated when scrapie-infected sheep meat and bone meal were fed to cattle (scrapie is the sheep version of BSE). Evidence suggests the disease proliferated when BSE-contaminated cattle protein was fed to calves. Unlike bacteria, prions are resistant to heat and so are not destroyed by cooking. Eating BSE-infected beef products is believed to cause a variant form of Creutzfeldt–Jakob disease (vCJD), which is the human version of BSE.

Although the FDA and other federal agencies have had regulatory measures in place since 1989 to prevent BSE from entering the United States' food supply, the first case of BSE in the United States was identified in December 2003. Fortunately, the animal's organs infected with prions never entered the food supply and the rest of the meat from that cow was successfully recalled from the marketplace. Since then, the USDA has enacted additional rules to enhance safeguards against BSE. Research is ongoing to better understand prion transmission and the diseases it causes.

# Food Biotechnology

**Food Biotechnology:** a process that involves taking a gene with a desirable trait from one plant and inserting it into another with the goal of changing one or more of its characteristics. Also called genetically engineered food.

**Food biotechnology** combines plant science with genetics to improve food. Genes associated with desirable characteristics are moved from one plant to another—a quicker and more precise version of old-fashioned "crossbreeding." The positive results are numerous and varied:

- Healthier crops and greater yields. Some plants are genetically modified to increase their resistance to plant viruses and other diseases; this means they can be raised using fewer pesticides to help reduce production costs and environmental residues.
- Greater resistance to severe weather, which reduces crop losses and increases year-round availability of fresh crops.
- Longer shelf life and increased freshness. Plants can be made to ripen more slowly, staying fresher longer—a big plus for transportation.
- Higher nutritional value. Plants can be genetically modified to contain more vitamins, minerals, or protein, or less fat.
- Better flavor. Genetic modification has produced sweeter melons and sweeter strawberries.
- Improved characteristics such as celery without strings.
- New food varieties through crossbreeding such as broccoflower (a blend of broccoli and cauliflower) and tangelos (a tangerine–grapefruit hybrid).
- Potential benefits to alleviate world hunger through stronger crops with enhanced nutritional value.

The United States is the leader in biotech farming: over 85% of the soybeans, 76% of the cotton, and 45% of the corn grown are genetically modified (Biotechnology Industry Organization, 2007). Ingredients made from these top crops, such as soybean oil, corn oil, and corn syrup, are estimated to be found in 60% to 70% of processed foods available in U.S. grocery stores, from cereals and frozen pizza to hot dogs and soft drinks (Biotechnology Industry Organization, 2007). In addition to permeating the food supply, biotechnology has created more than 200 new therapies and vaccines, beginning with FDA approval of recombinant human insulin in 1982 (Biotechnology Industry Organization, 2007).

## QUICK BITE

Main crops produced from biotechnology
Corn
Soybeans
Cotton
Potatoes
Rapeseed (grown for canola oil)

**Source:** American Dietetic Association. (2006). Position of the American Dietetic Association: Agricultural and food biotechnology. *Journal of the American Dietetic Association, 106,* 285–293.

The FDA asserts that genetically engineered foods do not pose a health or safety risk and, therefore, do not require mandatory labeling unless the food contains new allergens, has a modified nutritional profile, or represents a new plant (Chapman, 1997). Despite the relative consensus among the scientific community that it is safe (ADA, 2006), biotechnology has not been used long enough to know if long-term complications may develop. People who do not want to consume genetically engineered foods can avoid these products by using organically produced foods.

## Food Irradiation

To many consumers, the term irradiated food conjures up visions of radioactive fallout. In truth, irradiation used on approved foods does not produce radioactive food but does enhance food safety by reducing or eliminating pathogens, controlling insects, or killing parasites.

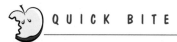 **Q U I C K   B I T E**

Foods allowed to be irradiated in the United States include
Wheat and wheat flour to control mold
White potatoes to inhibit sprouting
Pork to kill trichina parasites
Fresh produce to control insects
Many spices and dry vegetable seasonings for sterilization
Fresh meat and poultry to reduce bacterial pathogens
Fresh shell eggs

*Source:* USDA, Food Safety and Inspection Service. (2005). *Irradiation and food safety. Answers to frequently asked questions.* Available at www.fsis.usda.gov/Fact_Sheets/Irradiation_and-Food_Safey/index.asp. Accessed on 7/19/07.

Irradiation does not use heat and so is sometimes referred to as "cold pasteurization." Bacteria, mold, fungi, and insects are destroyed as the food is exposed to radiant energy, including gamma rays, electron beams, and x-rays. A small amount of new compounds are formed that are similar to the changes seen in food as it is cooked, pasteurized, frozen, or otherwise prepared. Except for a slight decrease in thiamin, the nutrient content is essentially unchanged. Because irradiation kills any living cells that may be contained in the food, such as in seeds or potatoes, shelf life may be prolonged. For instance, irradiated potatoes do not sprout during storage. However, irradiation does not hide spoilage or eliminate the need for safe food handling; irradiated food can still become contaminated through cross-contamination.

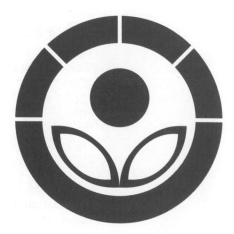

**FIGURE 9.5** Radura: international symbol for irradiation.

Irradiation is the most extensively studied food-processing technique available in the world and is used by 37 countries on more than 40 foods (USDA, FSIS, 2005). The FDA first approved the use of radiation in 1963 and is responsible for establishing the maximum radiation dose allowed on foods. Federal law requires irradiated food to be labeled with the international symbol, the radura (Fig. 9.5), and state "Treated with irradiation" or "Treated by irradiation." Research on irradiation as a part of an overall system of ensuring food safety is ongoing.

## ▶ HOW DO YOU RESPOND?

**Is "sugars" on the "Nutrition Facts" label just added sugar?** Sugars on the label refer to both added and natural sugars, which is why plain milk lists 12 g of sugar—all of it is naturally occurring lactose.

**Can you prevent foodborne illness by washing produce?** While washing produce—even varieties that you peel—is recommended, it cannot guarantee food safety. For instance, it is difficult to remove sticky bacteria from leafy greens like spinach. Even "triple" or thoroughly washed ready-to-eat bags of spinach, lettuce, and mixed greens may be contaminated with bacteria, because the cleaning process using chlorinated water kills only 90–95% of microbes when performed correctly. And with other produce, such as melon, mango, or apple, if bacteria have migrated to the inside of the fruit, such as traveling through the apple core to the interior, washing will not remove it. Safe food handling at home is important, but cannot guarantee safety.

**If the FDA has banned the sale of dietary supplements containing ephedra (also known as Ma Huang), why is it still available for sale over the Internet?** Although the national ban on the sale of ephedra remains in effect, a Federal District Court in Utah overturned the ban there in 2005, calling into question the FDA's authority to completely ban the product without conclusively demonstrating that it is dangerous at low levels. Because the burden of proof lies with the FDA to prove danger than with the supplement industry to prove safety, the FDA has the ethical dilemma of how to prove danger through human studies if it truly believes the product is dangerous. At this point it is unclear whether the national ban will be overturned. In the meantime, consumers need to understand that dangerous side effects (heart attack, stroke, and death) may occur, particularly at high doses. Unfortunately "high dose" is subjectively defined and the concentration of active ingredient varies considerably among products and from lot to lot. For instance, supplements containing ephedra alkaloids have been shown to have 5- to 75-mg ephedrine alkaloids, compared to 24-mg ephedrine hydrochloride in asthma medications (Fragakia & Thomson, 2007). To complicate matters, the absorption rate from extracts (found in supplements) is much quicker than formulations made from ground stem and aerial portions of the plant. Critical safety issues remain unanswered.

## ▶ CASE STUDY

Maria is 52 years old, has a normal BMI, and does not have any health problems. She prides herself on being "into" holistic treatments and goes to the doctor only when her attempts to treat herself fail. She occasionally takes one aspirin a day because she has heard that it can prevent heart attacks. She tries to eat a healthy diet and uses supplements to give her added protection against chronic diseases, especially heart disease, which runs in her family. Currently, she takes *Ginkgo biloba* to prevent memory loss, garlic to prevent heart disease, and fish oil supplements to keep her blood thin. She routinely drinks omega-3 fortified orange juice and organic milk. She attributes the bruises on her legs to being clumsy. She is thinking about adding vitamin E to her regimen because she heard it may also lower the risk of heart disease. To save money, she is thinking about discontinuing her use of garlic pills and fish oil supplements and instead eating more of each in her diet.

- What are the dangers of her present regimen? What may be responsible for the bruising she is experiencing?
- What would you tell Maria about the use of supplements in general? About the types and combination of supplements she is currently using? What specific changes would you suggest she make?
- What would you tell her about using omega-3 fortified milk and juice?
- Is it safer for her to eat more garlic and fish instead of taking them as supplements? Is it as "effective" as taking them as supplements? Could she "overdose" on garlic and fish oil from food?
- What questions would you ask about her diet to see if there are any improvements in her eating habits she could make to reduce the risk of heart disease?

## STUDY QUESTIONS

1. Which statement indicates that the client needs further instruction about reading nutrition labels?
   a. "The %DV is the contribution of a serving of a food to a 2000-calorie diet."
   b. "The %DV represents the percentage of calories in that food from each nutrient."
   c. "The amount of sugar on the label includes both natural and added sugars."
   d. "The serving size listed on the label can vary among brands and varieties of the same food."

2. The client asks if a tea that claims to "improve memory" really works. Which of the following would be the nurse's best response?
   a. "If the tea claims to improve memory, it has been tested and proven effective at improving memory."
   b. "Claims on food labels are not regulated by law and cannot be trusted."
   c. "Function claims like 'improve memory' can be used on labels without supporting proof that they are accurate."
   d. "That type of claim is illegal and should not appear on any food label."

3. Which statement about supplements is accurate?
   a. "All supplements must be tested for safety and effectiveness before they can be marketed."
   b. "Supplement dosages are standardized."
   c. "Proper handling of supplement ingredients is required by law."
   d. "Warnings about potential side effects or interactions must be stated on the packaging."

4. Which supplement should be used with caution by people taking anticoagulants?
   a. Echinacea
   b. St. John's wort
   c. Cranberry
   d. Garlic

5. A client asks how she can minimize her risk of foodborne illness. Which of the following should the nurse expect to include in the response as the best way to reduce the risk? Select all that apply.
   a. "Wash your hands before and after handling food."
   b. "Rely on organically grown foods as much as possible."
   c. "Cook foods thoroughly."
   d. "Avoid cross-contamination by using separate surfaces for meats and foods that will be eaten raw."

6. The best response to a client's question about whether organic food is worth the extra cost is:
   a. "Is there anything more important to spend money on than your health?"
   b. "There is no difference in pesticide levels and nutritional value of organically grown foods than conventional foods."
   c. "Buying organic foods is an individual decision; some may be more nutritious than their conventional counterparts and they do have lower pesticide levels, but current levels of pesticide residues on foods are not known to cause health problems."
   d. "It is worth it to buy organic produce but not organic milk and dairy products."

7. Which of the following practices helps preserve the nutritional value of produce?
   a. Refrigerating vegetables in the crisper.
   b. Adding baking soda to the water when steaming vegetables.
   c. Cutting vegetables into small pieces before boiling to hasten the cooking time.
   d. Thawing frozen vegetables prior to cooking.

8. A client asks how she can avoid buying foods that are genetically engineered. The nurse's best response is:
   a. "Foods labeled as 'organic' cannot be genetically engineered."
   b. "There is no way to avoid genetically engineered foods."
   c. "Buy foods that have the radura symbol on them; they cannot be genetically engineered."
   d. "Genetically engineered food must have that fact stated on the front label where consumers can clearly see it."

## KEY CONCEPTS

- The field of nutrition is rapidly changing and growing. New challenges in nutrition stem from advances in food technology, the explosion of information available on the World Wide Web, and the aging baby boom generation's quest for quality of life.

- To judge the validity and reliability of nutrition "news," ask who, what, when, where, and why. Beware of claims that sound too good to be true, quick fixes, and recommendations that are intended to help sell a product.

- Nutrition misinformation is everywhere and can be difficult to refute in a client who is convinced that what he or she knows is accurate.

- The "Nutrition Facts" label is intended to provide consumers with reliable and useful information to help avoid nutritional excesses such as fat, saturated fat, cholesterol, and sodium.

- The %DV listed on food labels for fat, saturated fat, carbohydrate, and dietary fiber is based on a 2000-calorie diet. The %DV for these nutrients underestimates the contribution in diets containing fewer than 2000 calories.

- Ingredients are listed in order of descending weight.

- Grade "A" health claims on food labels are based on SSA and include statements such as "calcium may help prevent osteoporosis" and "low sodium may help prevent high blood pressure." The evidence supporting claims graded as "B," "C," or "D" is less conclusive.

- Structure/function claims, such as "improves mood," "relieves stress," and "for hot flashes," can be used without FDA approval and do not have to carry a disclaimer.

- A dietary supplement is a product (other than tobacco) intended to supplement the diet and that contains one or more of the following: vitamins; minerals; herbs, or other botanicals; amino acids; or any combination of these ingredients.

- Dietary supplements are regulated by the FDA-like food; proof of their safety and effectiveness is not required before marketing. When a dietary supplement is deemed to be unsafe by the FDA, consumer advisories are issued and the manufacturer is requested, not ordered, to stop selling the product. As such, harmful supplements may remain on the market.

- People choosing to use supplements should first check with the FDA for consumer advisories and consult with their physicians. Many supplements can render certain drugs ineffective or potentiate the effectiveness of drugs.

- Pregnant and lactating women and children under the age of 6 should not use dietary supplements.

- To help retain their nutrient value, plants should be purchased fresh, stored properly, and cooked for a minimum amount of time in a minimum amount of water.

- Functional foods contain substances that appear to enhance health beyond their basic nutritional value. Incorporating more natural functional foods into the diet is prudent; the use of manufactured functional foods may pose risks.

- Organically grown foods are comparable to conventionally grown foods in taste and nutritional value. Because of production costs, higher losses, and lower yields, they are generally more expensive than other foods. They consistently have lower levels of pesticides but it is not known whether that offers any real health benefits.

- The majority of foodborne illnesses are caused by bacteria. Other causes include viruses, parasites, and molds.

- The foods most commonly contaminated with bacteria are animal proteins—meat, fish, poultry, eggs, milk, and foods containing these items. Improper food handling, such as inadequate cooking and poor personal hygiene, is the major cause of food-borne illness.

- Food biotechnology uses genetic modification to improve the characteristics of a food. Biotechnology has created plant foods that are more resistant to disease, stay fresher longer, have higher nutritional value, or are more resistant to severe weather. The FDA considers biotechnology safe.

- Irradiation is used to reduce or eliminate pathogens that can cause foodborne illness. The food remains uncooked and completely free of any radiation residues. Strict regulations and ongoing research protect consumers from potential risks regarding irradiation.

## ANSWER KEY

1. **TRUE** Most Americans believe food and nutrition are important for good health but have trouble changing their eating habits.

2. **TRUE** The serving sizes used on the "Nutrition Facts" label are based on amounts typically eaten. However, they may not represent what an *individual* consumes.

3. **TRUE** The %DVs for fat, saturated fat, carbohydrate, and fiber listed on the "Nutrition Facts" label are based on a 2000-calorie diet. The values are not accurate percentages for anyone who eats more or less than 2000 cal/day. The %DV for other nutrients, such as cholesterol and sodium, are based on Daily Reference Values that are constant for all people over the age of 4 regardless of total calorie intake.

4. **FALSE** Structure/function claims are not regulated by the FDA; their use does not require prior approval nor is a disclaimer necessary.

5. **FALSE** Supplement manufacturers do not have to prove safety or effectiveness before marketing a product, although they are not supposed to sell dangerous or ineffective products.

6. **FALSE** Warning labels about potential side effects or supplement–drug interactions are not required. Nor is a statement regarding who should *not* use the product such as pregnant and lactating women, children under 6 years of age, people with certain chronic illnesses, etc.

7. **FALSE** While some organically grown foods may have higher nutritional profiles than their conventionally grown counterparts, it is not known whether the difference is significant in terms of overall intake. Likewise, organically grown produce does have fewer pesticides than conventionally grown fruits and vegetables, but the health implications are not clear.

8. **TRUE** Bacteria are responsible for more than 90% of all foodborne illnesses.

9. **FALSE** Genetically modified foods are not labeled as such unless the food contains new allergens, modified nutritional profiles, or represents a new plant.

10. **FALSE** Irradiated food is completely free of radiation residues.

## WEBSITES

### *Reliable nutrition information*

American Cancer Society at **www.cancer.org**
American Diabetes Association at **www.diabetes.org**
American Dietetic Association at **www.eatright.org**
Cancer Net, National Cancer Institute, National Institutes of Health at **www.nci.nih.gov**
Case Western Reserve consumer health information at **www.netwellness.org**
Center for Science in the Public Interest at **www.cspinet.org**
Government site for nutrition at **www.nutrition.gov**
Health On the Net Foundation at **www.hon.ch**
International Food Information Council at **www.ific.org**
Mayo Clinic at **www.mayohealth.org**
National Council Against Health Fraud, Inc. at **www.ncahf.org**
National Heart, Lung, and Blood Institute, National Institutes of Health at **www.nhlbi.nih.gov**
Office of Disease Prevention and Health Promotion, U.S. Department of Health and Human Services at **www.odphp.osophs.dhhs.gov**
PubMed, National Library of Medicine at **www.ncbi.nlm.nih.gov/Pubmed/**
U.S. Department of Agriculture Food and Nutrition Information Center at **www.nal.usda.gov/fnic**
U.S. Department of Health and Human Services Healthfinder at **www.healthfinder.gov**
U.S. Food and Drug Administration Center for Safety and Applied Nutrition at **www.cfsan.fda.gov**
World Health Organization at **www.who.int**

### *Supplement information*

Food and Nutrition Information Center Dietary Supplements Resource list at **www.nal.usda.gov/fnic/pubs/bibs/gen/dietsupp.html**
Office of Dietary Supplements (ODS) of the National Institutes of Health at **http://dietarysupplements.info.nih.gov**
SupplementWatch, Inc. (free subscription) at **www.supplementwatch.com/**
The International Bibliographic Information on Dietary Supplements (IBIDS) NIH-Office of Dietary Supplements at **http://ods.od.nih.gov**
The NCCAM Clearinghouse provides information on complementary and alternative medication at **www.nccam.nih.gov**
U.S. Food and Drug Administration Center for Food Safety and Applied Nutrition at **www.cfsan.fda.gov.** Check out "Tips for the Savvy Supplement User: Making informed decisions and evaluating information."
U.S. Pharmacopeia at **www.usp.org**

*Food safety*

International Food Information Council at **www.ific.org**
Partnership for Food Safety Education at **www.fightbac.org**
U.S. Food and Drug Administration at **www.fda.gov**

# REFERENCES

American Dietetic Association. (2004). Position of the American Dietetic Association: Functional foods. *Journal of the American Dietetic Association, 104*(5), 814–826.

American Dietetic Association. (2006a). Position of the American Dietetic Association: Food and nutrition misinformation. *Journal of the American Dietetic Association, 106*(4), 601–607.

American Dietetic Association. (2006b). Position of the American Dietetic Association: Agricultural and food biotechnology. *Journal of the American Dietetic Association, 106*(2), 285–293.

Baker, B., Benbrook, C., Groth, E., & Lutz Benbrook, K. (2002). Pesticide residues in conventional, integrated pest management (IPM)-grown and organic foods: Insights from three US data sets. *Food Additives and Contaminants, 19*(5), 427–446.

Biotechnology Industry Organization. (2007). *Biotech industry facts.* Available at www.bio.org/speeches/pubs/er/statistics.asp. Accessed on 10/29/07.

Biotech Industry Organization. (2007). *Frequently asked questions on agricultural biotechnology.* Available at www.bio.org/foodag/faq.asp#8. Accessed on 10/29/07.

Centers for Disease Control. (2007). *Preliminary FoodNet Data on the incidence of infection with pathogens transmitted commonly through food—10 states, United States, 2006.* Available at www.cdc.gov/mmwr/preview/mmwrhtml/mm5614ahtm?s_cid=mm5614a4_e. Accessed on 10/24/07.

Chapman, N. (1997). Developing new foods through biotechnology. *Prepared Foods, 166*(2), 34.

Dunlop, M. (2007). *Shoppers are hungry for organic foods.* Published on www.ewg.org. Accessed on 7/20/07.

Economic Research Service, USDA. (2003). *Organic farming and marketing. Questions and answers. What is the size of the US market for organic foods.* June 24, 2003. Available at www.ers.usda.gov/Briefing/Organic/Questions/orgqa5.htm. Accessed on 7/20/07.

Environmental Working Group. (2006). *Shoppers guide to pesticides in produce.* Available at www.foodnews.org/walletguide.php. Accessed on 7/13/07.

Fox, S. (2006). *Online health search 2006. Pew Internet & American Life Project,* October 29, 2006. Available at www.pewinternet.org/pdfs/PIP_on-line_Health_2006.pdf. Accessed on 7/19/07.

Fragakia, A., & Thomson, C. (2007). *The health professional's guide to popular dietary supplements* (3rd ed.). Chicago: The American Dietetic Association.

International Food Information Council. (2006a). *2005 Consumer attitudes toward functional foods/food for health.* Available at www.ific.org/research/upload/2005funcfoodsresearch.pdf. Accessed on 7/18/07.

International Food Information Council. (2006b). *Food biotechnology.* Available at www.ific.org/food/biotechnology/index.cfm. Accessed on 7/18/07.

International Food Information Council. (2007). *A consumer's guide to food safety risks.* Available at www.ific.org/publications/other/consumerguideom.cfm. Accessed on 7/18/07.

International Food Information Council. (2007a). *A report on the global status of biotech crops.* Available at www.ific.org/foodinsight/2007/jf/biotechnbfi107.cfm?renderforprint=1. Accessed on 10/29/07.

International Food Information Council. (2007b). *Calories count, but consumers don't: Food & health survey highlights six "diet disconnects".* Available at www.ific.org/newsroom/raleases/2007foodandhealthsurveycfm?renderforprint=1. Accessed on 7/13/07.

Liebman, B. (2006). Fear of fresh. How to avoid foodborne illness from fruits and vegetables. *Nutrition Action Health Letter, 33*(10), 1, 3–6.

Mitchell, A., Hong, Y., Koh, E., Barrett, D. M., Bryant, D. E., Denison, R. F., et al. (2007). Ten-year comparison of the influence of organic and conventional crop management practices on the content of flavonoids in tomatoes. *Journal of Agricultural and Food Chemistry, 55*(15), 6154–6159.

National Institutes of Health State-of-the Science Panel. (2007). National Institutes of Health State-of-the-Science Conference Statement: Multivitamin/mineral supplements and chronic disease prevention. *American Journal of Nutrition, 85*(Suppl.), 257S–264S.

Schardt, D. (2007). Organic food. Worth the price? *Nutrition Action Health Letter, 34*(6), 1, 3–8.

USDA, FSIS. (2005). *Irradiation and food safety. Answers to frequently asked questions.* Available at www.fsis.usda.gov/Fact_Sheet?Irradiation_and_Food_Safety/index.asp. Accessed on 7/19/07.

# 10

# Cultural and Religious Influences on Food and Nutrition

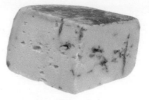

| TRUE | FALSE | |
|------|-------|---|
| ☐ | ☐ | **1** Culture defines what normal food behaviors are. |
| ☐ | ☐ | **2** Race and ethnicity are synonymous with culture. |
| ☐ | ☐ | **3** Core foods tend to be complex carbohydrates, such as cereal grains, starchy tubers, and starchy vegetables. |
| ☐ | ☐ | **4** Most Americans are willing to pay more for healthy restaurant food. |
| ☐ | ☐ | **5** The hot–cold theory of health and diet refers to the temperature of the food eaten. |
| ☐ | ☐ | **6** First-generation Americans tend to adhere more closely to their cultural food patterns than subsequent generations. |
| ☐ | ☐ | **7** For many ethnic groups who move to the United States, breakfast and lunch are more likely than dinner to be composed of new "American" foods. |
| ☐ | ☐ | **8** People who eat out or get take-out food many times a week tend to eat more calories, fat, and sodium than people who eat out less often. |
| ☐ | ☐ | **9** Dietary acculturation always produces unhealthy changes in eating. |
| ☐ | ☐ | **10** Like restaurant food, the portion sizes listed on convenience meals are much larger than they should be. |

### UPON COMPLETION OF THIS CHAPTER, YOU WILL BE ABLE TO

- Debate the value of using convenience foods to prepare home-cooked meals.
- Select the healthiest choices from a restaurant menu.
- Give examples of how culture influences food choices.
- Explain the general ways in which people's food choices change as they become acculturated to a new area.
- Contrast American cultural values with those of traditional cultures.
- Assess a person's dietary acculturation.
- Summarize dietary laws followed by major world religions.

The nutritional requirements among people of similar age and gender are essentially the same throughout the world, yet an infinite variety of food and food combinations can satisfy those requirements. How a person chooses to satisfy nutritional requirements is influenced by many variables, including culture, socioeconomic status, personal factors, and religion.

**Culture:** encompasses the total way of life of a particular population or community at a given time.

This chapter discusses what America eats and the impact of **culture** on food choices. Traditional food practices of major cultural subgroups in the United States are presented, as are religious food practices.

# ▶ AMERICAN CUISINE

**Foodway:** an all-encompassing term that refers to all aspects of food including what is edible, the role of certain foods in the diet, how food is prepared, the use of foods, the number and timing of daily meals, how food is eaten, and health beliefs related to food.

American cuisine is a rich and complex melting pot of foods and cooking methods that have been adapted and adopted from cuisines brought to the United States by immigrants. Early settlers from northern and southern Europe came with their own established **foodway** that changed in response to what was available in the New World. Native Americans made significant contributions to American cuisine by introducing items such as corn, squash, beans, cranberries, and maple syrup. Later, West African slaves brought okra, watermelon, black-eyed peas, and taro, and influenced the regional cuisine in the southeastern United States with fried, boiled, and roasted dishes made with pork and pork fat. Likewise, American southwest cuisine was shaped by flavors and ingredients brought across the border by Mexican Indians and Spanish settlers.

## QUICK BITE

| **Ethnic restaurant trends** | | **Examples of convenience items with a positive impact on nutrition** |
|---|---|---|
| • Curry | • Pasta with shrimp | Fresh fruits and vegetables from the salad bar |
| • Fajitas | • Quesadillas | Washed spinach |
| • Fish tacos | • Ravioli | Presliced mushrooms |
| • Lasagna | • Satay/skewers | Bagged salad mixes |
| • Noodle bowls | • Stir-fry | Frozen vegetables |
| | | Fresh sushi |

*Source:* Perlick, A. (2007). *R & I's 2007 menu census: Variety show. Restaurants & Institutions,* 11/1/07. Available at www.rimag.com/archives/2007/11/menu-census-main.asp. Accessed on 2/10/08.

Whole grain rolls from the bakery section
Prepared hummus
Fully cooked roasted chickens
Lean deli meats

In the early 1850s, the first wave of Chinese immigrants came to the United States to join the gold rush. They brought stir-fry, a novel cooking method, and new foods such as egg rolls, fried rice, and spare ribs. The first wave of Italian immigrants arrived around 1880 and, although they were unable to replicate their native foods, they utilized the available ingredients to create Americanized versions of lasagna, manicotti, veal parmigiana, and meatballs. Today, Italian food is mainstream American fare.

The influx of immigrants continued and cuisines from around the globe melded. Today, it is difficult to determine which foods are truly American and which are an adaptation from other cultures. Swiss steak, Russian dressing, and chili con carne are American inventions. And although ethnic restaurants and ethnic foods sections in grocery stores offer distinct fare, cross-cultural food creations such as Tex-Mex wontons and tofu lasagna reaffirm the ongoing melting pot nature of American cuisine.

Although a "typical American diet" is difficult to define, Box 10.1 offers a snapshot view of what and how America eats. Driven by expediency and ease, convenience foods and restaurant-sourced meals (either eat in or take-out) are a driving force in current food trends.

## Convenience Foods

According to Gallup reports, on a typical night in 2007, 89% of meal preparers made dinner at home (Sloan, 2008). Although 57% of those made dinner from scratch, 24% made their

## BOX 10.1  A SNAPSHOT VIEW OF WHAT AND HOW AMERICA EATS

Pizza, Chinese food, and hamburgers/other sandwiches are the top three take-out items.
Chicken/turkey and hamburgers are the most frequently served items for dinner.
Hamburgers are the item most frequently ordered at restaurants by men; French fries top the list for women.
Convenience stores are the most popular place for buying prepared foods.
33 meals per person were eaten in a car in 2006.
60% of office workers spend lunch breaks at their desks.
28% of consumers have used home meal delivery services; the trend is growing.
55% of snackers do so in the evening.
*Requires little effort* or *easy to make* is the top reason people give for deciding what to make for dinner.
57% of Americans make dinner from scratch (no mixes), 24% make "homemade meals" using a combination of home cooking and convenience products, and 8% use only frozen or heat-and-serve prepackaged foods.
Only 46% of Americans plan their meals in advance.

*Source:* Sloan, A. (2008). What, when, and where America eat. *Food Technology.* Available at www.ift.org. Accessed on 1/2/08.

**Convenience Food:** broadly defined as any product that saves time in food preparation, ranging from bagged fresh salad mixes to frozen packaged complete meals.

"home-cooked" meals with prepackaged foods that require some preparation, and 8% used only frozen or heat-and-serve prepackaged foods. When asked what factors were important in defining a **convenience food,** *helps me maintain a healthy diet* topped the list of responses at 48% of those polled (GfK Roper, 2007).

Convenience products range from convenient ingredients used to make home-cooked meals to complete, heat-and-serve meals. Generally, the more convenient the meal is, the greater the impact all around on time, budget, and nutritional value. When time is short, frozen complete or nearly complete meals or boxed "helper" type entrées earn their designation as "convenient." They generally cost more than "from scratch" items and lack that "homemade" taste but are less expensive than take-out and are easy and quick to prepare. And variety abounds, from typical American fare such as meatloaf and pot roast to vegetarian, Mexican, Chinese, Southwestern, and Italian cuisines. On the downside, these products tend to be high in sodium, relatively low in fiber, and provide little to no fruit, vegetables, and whole grains. The 1 to 2 cup portion sizes listed on the label may leave many people hungry. Yet, they are here to stay. With a little planning and effort, they can be part of a healthy diet. See Box 10.2 for tips on balancing convenience with nutrition.

### QUICK BITE

**Healthy restaurant trends**
- Fruit plates
- Grilled chicken breast
- Oatmeal/hot cereal
- Organic cold cereals
- Lentils
- Salads
- Smoothies
- Stir-fried vegetables
- Whole wheat pasta
- Yogurt/yogurt parfaits

*Source:* Perlick, A. (2007). *R & I's 2007 menu census: Variety show. Restaurants & Institutions,* 11/1/07. Available at www.rimag.com/archives/2007/11/menu-census-main.asp. Accessed on 2/10/08.

## Restaurant-Sourced Meals

In 2006, the average American reported to eat out approximately five times a week (*Science Daily,* 2007). Fast food restaurants are the most popular establishments for breakfast and

| BOX 10.2 | **TIPS FOR BALANCING CONVENIENCE WITH NUTRITION** |

*Read the label to comparison shop.* Calories, fat, saturated fat, and sodium can vary greatly among different brands of similar items. A rule-of-thumb guideline is to limit sodium to less than 800 mg and fat to no more than 10 to 13 g in a meal that provides 300 to 400 calories.

*Look for "healthy" on the label.* The government allows "healthy" on the label of meals or entrées that limit sodium to 140 mg/100 g of food. And "healthy" foods must also provide 3 g or less of total fat or 1 g of saturated fat per 100 g of food. They are a better choice than the products not labeled "healthy," yet may still lack adequate fiber.

*Add additional ingredients to "stretch" the meal.* For instance, adding a bag of frozen vegetables, a can of tomatoes, or a can of garbanzo or black beans provides nutrients and increases volume.

*Add healthy side dishes.* A convenience "meal" that provides 300 to 400 calories may leave many people hungry. Adding quick and easy side dishes, such as bagged salad mixes, raw vegetables, whole grain rolls, an instant cup of soup, or piece of fresh fruit, can greatly increase nutritional and satiety values.

*Adjust the seasoning when possible.* Some frozen meal solutions contain a separate seasoning packet; using half satisfies taste while cutting sodium.

lunch; for dinner, fast food restaurants and casual dining are most popular (*Science Daily,* 2007). Compared to 3 years ago, Americans say they are less willing to pay more for healthy dishes, less knowledgeable about healthy menu items, and more likely to consider healthy items bland-tasting; they go for value/combo meals because they are easy, convenient, and inexpensive (*Science Daily,* 2007).

### QUICK BITE

**From a prominent fast food restaurant**

| | Sodium* (mg) | Calories |
|---|---|---|
| Double cheeseburger | 780 | 380 |
| Crispy chicken sandwich | 810 | 340 |
| Fish fillet sandwich | 1020 | 450 |
| Small French fries | 340 | 330 |
| Large French fries | 550 | 540 |
| Bacon and cheese stuffed baked potato | 920 | 440 |

*Adult Adequate Intake (AI) for sodium is 1200–1500 mg.

Meals ordered out tend to be higher in calories, fat, and sodium than home-cooked meals, partly because portion sizes are bigger. Conversely, the fiber and calcium content of restaurant meals is usually lower. Because eating out has evolved from a special treat to an everyday occurrence, planning and menu savvy are needed to ensure that eating out is consistent with, not contradictory to, eating healthy. Tips for eating healthy while eating out appear in Box 10.3. "Best bet" choices from various ethnic restaurants are listed in Box 10.4.

| BOX 10.3 | TIPS FOR EATING HEALTHY WHILE EATING OUT |
|---|---|

**Plan Ahead**
- Choose the restaurant carefully so you know there are reasonable choices available.
- Call ahead to inquire about menu selections. This is an especially important strategy when the location is not a matter of choice but, rather, a requirement such as for business luncheons or conferences. It may be possible to make a special request ahead of time.

**Don't Arrive Starving**
People become much less discriminating in their food choices when they are hungry.

- Eating a small, high-fiber snack an hour or so before going out to dinner, such as whole wheat crackers with peanut butter or a piece of fresh fruit with milk, can take the edge off hunger without bankrupting healthy eating.

**Balance the Rest of the Day**
- When eating out *is* an occasion, such as for a birthday or anniversary celebration, make healthier choices the rest of the day to compensate for a planned indulgence.

**Practice Portion Control**
- Order the smallest size meat available.
- Create a doggie bag *before eating;* if you wait until the end of the meal, there may not be any left.
- Order regular size, not biggie size or super size.
- Order a la carte. Is a value meal a "better value" if it undermines your attempt to eat healthily?
- Order a half portion, when available.
- Order two (carefully chosen) appetizers in place of an entrée or order an appetizer and split an entrée with a companion.

**Know the Terminology**
"Fatty" words to watch out for include:

- buttered
- battered
- breaded
- deep fried
- au gratin
- creamy
- crispy

- alfredo
- bisque
- hollandaise
- parmigiana
- béarnaise
- en croute

- escalloped
- French fried
- pan fried
- rich
- sautéed
- with gravy, with mayonnaise, with cheese

Less fatty terms are: baked, braised, broiled, cooked in its own juice, grilled, lightly sautéed, poached, roasted, steamed.

**Beware of Hidden Fats, Such As**
- high-fat meats
- nuts
- cream and full-fat milk
- full-fat salad dressings and mayonnaise

**Make Special Requests**
- Order sauces and gravies "on the side" to control portions.
- Ask that lower fat items be substituted for high-fat items (e.g., a baked potato instead of French fries).
- Request an alternate cooking method (e.g., broiled instead of fried).

| BOX 10.4 | BEST BET CHOICES FROM FAST FOOD AND ETHNIC RESTAURANTS |

**Fast Foods**
English muffins or bagels with spreads on the side
Butter, margarine, or syrups on the side—not added to food
Baked potato—plain or with reduced fat or fat-free dressings or salsa
Pretzels or baked chips
Regular, small, or junior sizes
Ketchup, mustard, relish, BBQ sauce, and fresh vegetables as toppings
Grilled chicken sandwiches without "special sauce"
Veggie burger
Small roast beef on roll
Fruit 'n yogurt parfait
Lean, 6-inch subs on whole grain rolls
Side salads with reduced fat or fat-free dressings
Salads with grilled chicken
Low-fat or nonfat milk
Fresh fruit
Specialty coffees with skim milk

**Salad Bars**
Dark, leafy greens
Plain raw vegetables
Chickpeas, kidney beans, peas
Low-fat cottage cheese
Hard-cooked egg
Fresh fruit
Lean ham, turkey
Reduced fat or fat-free dressings

**Pizza**
Thin crust
Vegetables: onions, spinach, tomatoes, broccoli, mushrooms, peppers
Lean meats: Canadian bacon, ham, grilled chicken, shrimp, crab meat
Half-cheese pizza
Salad as a side dish

**Buffet**
Survey the buffet before beginning
Use a small plate
Pile food no thicker than a deck of cards
Practice the "plate method:" one-quarter meat, three-quarters plants

**Mexican**
Sauces: salsa, mole, picante, enchilada, pico de gallo
Guacamole and sour cream on the side
Black bean soup, gazpacho
Soft, nonfried tortillas as in bean burritos or enchiladas
Refried beans (without lard)
Arroz con pollo (chicken with rice)
Grilled meat, fish, or chicken
Steamed vegetables

*(box continues on page 226)*

Soft-shell chicken or veggie tacos
A la carte or half entrée
Fajitas: chicken, seafood, vegetable, beef
Flan (usually a small portion)

**Chinese**
Hot-and-sour soup, wonton soup
Chicken chow mein
Chicken or beef chop suey
Szechuan dishes
Shrimp with garlic sauce
Stir-fried and teriyaki dishes
Noodles: lo mein, chow fun, Singapore noodle
Steamed rice instead of fried
Steamed spring rolls
Tofu
Steamed dumplings and other dim sum instead of egg rolls
Fortune cookies
Use chopsticks
No MSG

**Italian**
Minestrone
Garden salad; vinegar and oil dressing
Breadsticks, bruschetta, Italian bread
Sauces: red clam, marinara, wine, cacciatore, fra diavlo, marsala
Shrimp, veal, chicken without breading
Choose vegetables for a side dish instead of pasta or potatoes
Limit "unlimited" bread or breadsticks
Italian ice or fruit

**Indian**
Raw vegetable salads, Mulligatawny soup (lentil soup)
Tandoori meats
Condiments: fruits and vegetable chutneys, raita (cucumber and yogurt sauce)
Lentil and chickpea curries
Chicken and vegetables
Chicken rice pilaf
Basmati rice
Naan (bread baked in tandoori oven)
Dal

**Japanese**
Boiled green soybeans, miso soup, bean soups
Sushi—cooked varieties include imitation crab, cooked shrimp, scrambled egg
Most combinations of grilled meats or seafood
Teriyaki chicken or seafood
Steamed rice, rice noodles
Green tea

| BOX 10.4 | **BEST BET CHOICES FROM FAST FOOD AND ETHNIC RESTAURANTS** (continued) |
| --- | --- |

**Greek**
Lentil soup
Greek salad, tabouli
Chicken, lamb, pork souvlaki salad or sandwich
Shish kebabs
Pita bread

Make a meal of appetizers: baba ghanoush (smoked eggplant), hummus (mashed chickpeas), dolma (stuffed grape leaves), tabouli (cracked wheat salad). Olive oil is often poured on the baba ghanoush, hummus, and other foods so ask for it on the side.

# ▶ THE IMPACT OF CULTURE

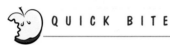

**QUICK BITE**

**Culture**
- Has an inherent value system that defines what is "normal"
- Is learned, not instinctive
- Is passed from generation to generation
- Has an unconscious influence on its members
- Resists change but is not static

Culture has a profound and unconscious effect on food choices. Yet, within all cultures, individuals or groups of individuals may behave differently from the socially standardized foodway because of age, gender, state of health, household structure, or socioeconomic status. Race, ethnicity, and geographic region are often inaccurately assumed to be synonymous with culture. This misconception leads to stereotypic grouping, such as assuming that all Jews adhere to orthodox food laws or that all Southerners eat sausage, biscuits, and gravy. **Subgroups** within a culture display a unique range of cultural characteristics that affect food intake and nutritional status. What is edible, the role of food, how food is prepared, the symbolic use of food, and when and how food is eaten are among the many things defined by culture.

**Subgroups:** a unique cultural group that coexists within a dominant culture.

## Culture Defines What Is Edible

**Edible:** foods that are part of an individual's diet.

**Inedible:** foods that are usually poisonous or taboo.

Culture determines what is **edible** and what is **inedible**. To be labeled a food, an item must be readily available, safe, and nutritious enough to support reproduction. However, cultures do not define as edible all sources of nutrients that meet those criteria. For instance in the United States, horse meat, insects, and dog meat are not considered food, even though they meet the food criteria. Culture overrides flavor in determining what is offensive or unacceptable. For example, you may like a food (e.g., rattlesnake) until you know what it is; this reflects disliking the *idea* of the food rather than the actual food itself. An unconscious food selection decision process appears in Figure 10.1.

## The Role of Certain Foods in the Diet

Every culture has a ranking for its foods that is influenced by cost and availability. Major food categories include core foods, secondary foods, and occasional foods.

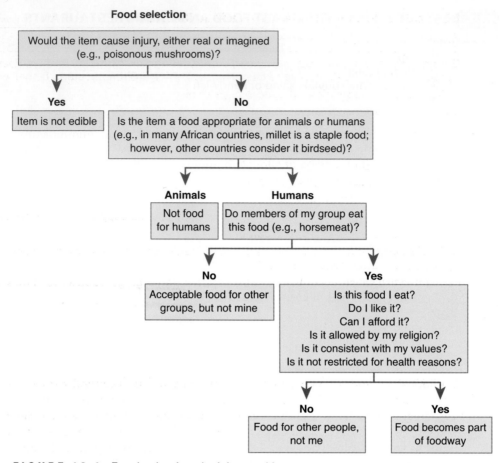

**Food selection**

Would the item cause injury, either real or imagined (e.g., poisonous mushrooms)?

**Yes** → Item is not edible

**No** → Is the item a food appropriate for animals or humans (e.g., in many African countries, millet is a staple food; however, other countries consider it birdseed)?

**Animals** → Not food for humans

**Humans** → Do members of my group eat this food (e.g., horsemeat)?

**No** → Acceptable food for other groups, but not mine

**Yes** → Is this food I eat?
Do I like it?
Can I afford it?
Is it allowed by my religion?
Is it consistent with my values?
Is it not restricted for health reasons?

**No** → Food for other people, not me

**Yes** → Food becomes part of foodway

**F I G U R E   1 0 . 1**   Food selection decision making.

## Core Foods

**Core Foods:** the important and consistently eaten foods that form the foundation of the diet; they are the dietary staples.

**Core foods** provide a significant source of calories and are regularly included in the diet, usually on a daily basis. Core foods are typically complex carbohydrates, such as cereal grains (rice, wheat, millet, corn) starchy tubers (potatoes, yams, taro, cassava), and starchy vegetables (plantain or green bananas).

## Secondary Foods

**Secondary Foods:** foods that are widespread in the diet but not eaten consistently.

Foods widely consumed, but not on a daily basis, are considered **secondary foods,** such as vegetables, legumes, nuts, fish, eggs, and meats. Secondary foods used by a culture vary with availability. For instance, the types of legumes used in Chinese culture include mung beans and soybeans, whereas those used in Latin American culture include black beans and pinto beans.

## Peripheral Foods

**Peripheral or Occasional Foods:** foods that are infrequently consumed.

**Peripheral foods,** eaten sporadically, are typically based on an individual's preferences, not cultural norms. They may be foods that are reserved for special occasions, not readily available, or not generally well tolerated, as is the case with milk among Asian Americans.

| TABLE 10.1 | Examples of Seasonings Used by Various Cultures |
|---|---|
| **Cultural Group** | **Distinguishing Flavors** |
| Asian Indian | Garam masala (curry blend of coriander, cumin, fenugreek, turmeric, black pepper, cayenne, cloves, cardamom, and chile peppers), mint, saffron, mustard, fennel, cinnamon |
| Brazilian (Bahia) | Chile peppers, dried shrimp, ginger root, palm oil |
| Chinese | Soy sauce, rice wine, ginger root |
| French | Butter, cream, wine, bouquet garni (tarragon, thyme, bay leaf) |
| German | Sour cream, vinegar, dill, mustard, black pepper |
| Greek | Lemon, onions, garlic, oregano, olive oil |
| Italian | Tomato, garlic, basil, oregano, olive oil |
| Japanese | Soy sauce, sugar, rice wine vinegar |
| Korean | Soy sauce, garlic ginger root, black pepper, scallions, chile peppers, sesame seeds, or oil |
| Mexican | Tomatoes, onions, chile peppers, cumin |
| Puerto Rican | Sofrito (seasoning sauce of tomatoes, onions, garlic, bell peppers, cilantro, capers, pimento, annatto seeds, and lard) |
| Thai | Fermented fish sauce, coconut milk, chile peppers, garlic, ginger root, lemon grass, tamarind |

*Source:* Kittler, P., & Sucher, K. (2008). *Food and culture* (5th ed.). Belmont, CA: Thomson/Wadsworth.

## How Food Is Prepared

Traditional methods of preparation vary between and within cultural groups. For instance, vegetables often are stir-fried in Asian cultures but boiled in Hispanic cultures. Traditional seasonings also vary among cultures and may be the distinguishing feature between one culture's foods and another's (Table 10.1). The choice of seasonings varies among geographic regions and between seasons, based on availability. With home-prepared meals, seasonings are adjusted to suit the family's preferences.

## Symbolic Use of Foods

Each culture has food customs and bestows symbolism on certain foods. Custom determines what foods are served as meals versus snacks and what foods are considered feminine versus masculine. Symbolically, food can be used to express love, to reward or punish, to display piety, to express moral sentiments, to demonstrate belongingness to a group, or to proclaim the separateness of a group. On a personal level, food may be used inappropriately to relieve anxiety, reduce stress, ease loneliness, or to substitute for sex. Culture also determines which foods are used in celebration and which provide comfort. People who move to other cultures may retain their own cultural comfort foods as a link with the past.

## When and How Food Is Eaten

All cultures eat at least once a day. Some may eat five or more meals each day. Dinner may start at 6 p.m. in Australia and 7 to 9 p.m. in Kenya. A Lebanese custom is to arrive anytime when invited for dinner, even as early as 9 or 10 a.m. Food may be eaten with chopsticks, a knife and fork, or fingers. In the United States, bad manners in eating may be associated with animal behavior, as in "He eats like a pig," "She chews like a cow," or "Don't wolf down your food."

## Cultural Values

Cultural values define desirable and undesirable personal and public behavior and social interaction. Understanding the client's cultural values and their impact on health and food choices facilitates cross-cultural nutrition care. Table 10.2 highlights the contrast between selected American cultural values and values of more traditional cultures.

## Health Beliefs

Each culture has a unique point of view on life, health, and illness, and the meaning of each in society (Kittler & Sucher, 2008). Almost all cultures define certain foods that promote wellness, cure disease, or impart medicinal properties. For instance, hot oregano tea seasoned with salt is used to treat an upset stomach in Vietnamese culture. Some cultures define foods that create equilibrium within the body and soul (Kittler & Sucher, 2008).

Culture also shapes body image. In the United States, "you can never be too thin" and thinness, particularly in women, is equated with beauty and status. Overweight and obesity may be viewed as a character flaw. Conversely, thinness has historically been a risk factor for poor health or associated with poverty. In many cultures today, including those of some Africans, Mexicans, American Indians, and Caribbean Islanders, being overweight is a sign of health,

| TABLE 10.2 | A Contrast of Cultural Values | |
| --- | --- | --- |
| **American Values** | **Traditional Values** | **Potential Considerations** |
| **Personal Control** Individuals believe they have personal control over their future | **Fate** Individuals may accept what happens to them as out of their control | Clients may not consider themselves active participants in their own healing but rather as recipients |
| **Individualism** Interests of the individual have preference over the interests of the group | **Group Welfare** The group is valued over the individual; decisions may be made by the group, not the individual | Involve family in planning Emphasize the good of the entire family rather than individual benefits |
| **Time Dominates** "Being on time" and "not wasting time" are virtues | **Human Interaction Dominates** Personal interaction is more important than time management | Expediency and efficiency may be counterproductive Pause while talking Avoid interruptions |
| **Informality** Informality is viewed as a sign of friendliness | **Formality** Informality may be equated with disrespect | Use a formal tone, especially with older people |
| **Directness** Honest, open communication is considered effective communication | **Indirectness** Straightforwardness may be rude or too personal | It may be appropriate to avoid eye contact Talking in the third person, such as "someone who wants to eat less sodium may choose fresh vegetables over canned" is valued over "you should . . ." Asking questions may be considered disrespectful |

beauty, and prosperity (Kittler & Sucher, 2008). To some people, "healthy eating" is synonymous with eating large quantities of food rather than making more nutritious food choices.

## Dietary Acculturation

**Dietary Acculturation:** the process that occurs as members of a minority group adopt the eating patterns and food choices of the host country.

**Acculturation:** the process that occurs as people who move to a different cultural area adopt the beliefs, values, attitudes, and behaviors of the dominant culture; not limited to immigrants but affects anyone (to varying degrees) who moves from one community to another.

**Dietary acculturation** occurs when eating patterns of people who move change to resemble those of the host country. In the United States, **acculturation** is linked to increased risk of chronic disease and obesity, which may be related to a decreased intake of fruits and vegetables and a higher intake of fat (Stimpson & Urrutia-Rojas, 2007). Americans born elsewhere are more likely to meet dietary guidelines for fat, fiber, vitamins, and minerals than those born in the United States (Stimpson & Urrutia-Rojas, 2007). Data from National Health Interview Survey found that years of U.S. residence was positively associated with risk of obesity (Kaplan, Newsom, & McFarland, 2004). Although acculturation can include positive changes, various studies show that it increases the prevalence of unhealthy eating practices (Archer, 2005).

Generally, food habits are one of the last behaviors people change through acculturation, possibly because eating is done in the privacy of the home, not in full view of the majority culture. Usually, first-generation Americans adhere more closely to cultural food patterns and have at least one native meal daily (Brown, 2005). They may cling to traditional foods to preserve their ethnic identity. Second-generation Americans do not have the direct native connection and may follow cultural patterns only on holidays and at family gatherings, or they may give up ethnic foods but retain traditional methods of preparation. Children tend to adopt new ways quickly as they learn from other children at school. Points to keep in mind regarding dietary acculturation appear in Box 10.5.

Interrelated changes in food choices that occur as part of acculturation are as follows:

- *New foods are added to the diet.* Status, economics, information, taste, and exposure are some of the reasons why new foods are added to the diet. Eating "American" food may symbolize status and make people feel more connected to their new culture. Frequently, new foods are added because they are relatively inexpensive and widely available.
- *Some traditional foods are replaced by new foods.* This often occurs because traditional foods may be difficult to find, are too expensive, or have lengthy preparation times. For many

---

| BOX 10.5 | **POINTS TO KEEP IN MIND REGARDING DIETARY ACCULTURATION** |
|---|---|

- Generally with acculturation, the intake of sweets and fats increases, neither of which has a positive effect on health.
- Because dietary acculturation is most likely to change food choices for breakfast and lunch rather than dinner, focus on promoting healthy "American" food choices for those meals.
- Portion control is a better option than advising someone to eliminate an important native food from their diet. Lower fat or lower sodium options, when available, may also be an acceptable option for the client. While giving up soy sauce may not be an option for a Chinese American, using a reduced sodium version may be doable.
- It is essential to determine how often a food is consumed in order to determine the potential impact of that food. For instance, lard is unimportant in the context of the total diet if it is used in cooking only on special occasions.
- Don't assume the client knows what American foods are considered healthy.
- Suggest fruits and vegetables that are similar in texture to those that are familiar but unavailable to the client.

ethnic groups who move to the United States, breakfast and lunch are most likely to be composed of convenient American foods, whereas traditional foods are retained for the major dinner meal, which has greater emotional significance.

- *Some traditional foods are rejected.* To become more like their peers, children and adolescents are more likely than older adults to reject traditional foods. Traditional foods may also be rejected because of an increased awareness of the role of nutrition in the development of chronic diseases. For instance, one reason why Indians who have resided in the United States for a relatively long period tend to eat significantly less ghee (clarified butter served with rice or spread on Indian breads) may be that they are trying to decrease their intake of saturated fat.

## Understanding Acculturation

It is important to understand acculturation so that interventions to promote healthy food choices can be tailored to be culturally and individually appropriate. Ideally, clients will retain healthy traditional food practices, adopt healthy new food behaviors, and avoid forming less healthy American dietary habits. While first-generation citizens usually need help choosing American replacements for their native foods, second-generation citizens may need help selecting healthy American foods. The art of asking the right questions, rather than making general assumptions, is key to understanding the client's level of acculturation (ElGindy, 2004).

- What native foods do you eat daily?
- What native foods do you no longer eat?
- What new foods do you eat? Remember that new immigrants may not know the name of American foods.
- What foods do you eat to keep you healthy?
- What foods do you avoid to prevent illness?
- Do you balance some foods with other foods?
- Are there foods you will not eat? Is it because of personal preference, cultural norms, or religious mandate?
- For hospitalized clients, are there any special customs or religious practices you want performed before or after a meal?

Suggestions for conducting effective cross-cultural nutrition counseling are listed in Box 10.6.

---

**BOX 10.6** **SUGGESTIONS FOR CONDUCTING EFFECTIVE CROSS-CULTURAL NUTRITION COUNSELING**

- Establish rapport; respect cultural differences
- Be knowledgeable of cultural food habits and health beliefs
- Be sensitive to verbal and nonverbal communication
- Determine the primary written and spoken language used in the client's home
- Use trained interpreters when necessary
- Determine whether the client prefers direct or indirect communication
- Pare down information to only what the client needs to know
- Emphasize the positive food practices of traditional health beliefs and food customs
- Provide written material only after determining reading ability
- Communicate consistent messages

# ▶ TRADITIONAL DIETS OF SELECTED CULTURAL SUBGROUPS IN THE UNITED STATES

The U.S. Census Bureau projects that by the year 2060, less than 50% of the U.S. population will be white (CDC-OMHD, 2007a). The nutritional implication of this shift in cultural predominance is that cultural sensitivity will become increasingly important to nursing care. Nutrition information that is technically correct but culturally inappropriate does not produce behavior change. Cultural awareness facilitates nutrition care consistent with the individual's needs, desires, and lifestyle.

Three major cultural subgroups in the United States are highlighted in the following sections. Their leading causes of death appear in Table 10.3. Although generalizations can be made about traditional eating practices and dietary changes related to acculturation, actual food choices vary greatly within a subgroup on the basis of national, regional, ethnic, and individual differences.

## African Americans

The majority of African Americans can trace their ancestors to West Africa, although some have immigrated from the Caribbean, Central America, and East African countries. Because most are many generations away from their original homeland, much of their native heritage has been assimilated, lost, or modified.

## Traditional Food Practices

"Soul food" describes traditional southern African-American foods and cooking techniques that evolved from West African, slave, and post-abolition cuisine. Many soul food customs and practices are shared by white Americans in the southern United States, particularly those of lower socioeconomic status or living in rural areas (Kulkarni, 2004).

| TABLE 10.3 | Leading Causes of Death of Selected Groups in the United States | | | |
|---|---|---|---|---|
| Cause of Death Rank | African Americans | Hispanic/Latino Americans | Asian Americans | White Americans |
| 1 | Heart disease | Heart disease | Cancer | Heart disease |
| 2 | Cancer | Cancer | Heart disease | Cancer |
| 3 | Stroke | Unintentional injuries | Stroke | Stroke |
| 4 | Diabetes | Stroke | Unintentional injuries | Chronic lower respiratory disease |
| 5 | Unintentional injuries | Diabetes | Diabetes | Unintentional injuries |
| 6 | Homicide | Chronic liver disease and cirrhosis | Influenza and pneumonia | Alzheimer's disease |
| 7 | Nephritis, nephrotic syndrome, and nephrosis | Homicide | Chronic lower respiratory disease | Diabetes |
| 8 | Chronic lower respiratory disease | Chronic lower respiratory disease | Suicide | Influenza and pneumonia |
| 9 | HIV/AIDS | Influenza and pneumonia | Nephritis, nephrotic syndrome, and nephrosis | Nephritis, nephrotic syndrome, and nephrosis |
| 10 | Septicemia | Certain conditions originating in the perinatal period | Alzheimer's disease | Suicide |

*Source:* CDC, Office of Minority Health and Health Disparities. Available at www.cdc.gov/omhd/populations/definitions.htm. Accessed on 1/30/08.

| TABLE 10.4 | Traditional Soul Foods and the Effects of Acculturation | |
|---|---|---|
| **Food Group** | **Foods Commonly Consumed** | **Effects of Acculturation** |
| Grains | Rice, grits, cornbread, biscuits, muffins, dry and cooked cereals, macaroni | Substitution of commercially made bread for homemade biscuits |
| Vegetables | Green leafy vegetables (collard, mustard, turnip, and dandelion greens), kale, spinach, and pokeweed are collectively known as "greens"<br>Corn, sweet and white potatoes | Vegetable intake remains low; is based on availability. Greens remain popular |
| Fruit | Apples, bananas, berries, peaches, and watermelon, eaten based on availability | Fruit intake remains low; is based on availability |
| Milk | Whole milk (commonly referred to as "sweet milk") and buttermilk | Greater consumption of milk, at least among blacks living in urban areas |
| Meat and Beans | A variety of beef, pork, poultry, and fish; oxtail, tripe, tongue<br>Dried beans (pinto, navy, lima, butter, kidney); fresh or dried peas (black-eyed, field, green, crowder, butter); beans with pork; succotash (corn with lima beans) | Packaged and luncheon meats are popular; intake of fatty meats, such as sausage and bacon, is high |
| Fats | Butter, lard, bacon, fatback, salt pork, meat drippings, vegetable shortening | |
| Beverages | Coffee, fruit drinks, fruit wine, soft drinks, tea | |

*Source:* Kittler, P., & Sucher, K. (2008). *Food and culture* (5th ed.). Belmont, CA: Thomson/Wadsworth.

Traditional soul foods tend to be high in fat, cholesterol, and sodium and low in protective nutrients such as potassium (fruits and vegetables), fiber (whole grains and vegetables), and calcium (milk, cheese, and yogurt). Corn and corn products (grits and cornmeal) are the primary grain. Meats are often breaded and fried. A variety of beef and pork cuts are consumed, as is poultry, oxtail, trip, and tongue. Table 10.4 highlights traditional soul foods and the impact of acculturation on food choices.

Although soul food has become a symbol of African-American identity and African heritage, today African Americans' food habits usually reflect their current socioeconomic status, geographic location, and work schedule more than their African or southern heritage (Kittler & Sucher, 2008). Soul food may be reserved for special occasions and holidays.

## Health Beliefs

The health beliefs and practices of some African Americans are a blend of traditional African concepts as well as those encountered through early contact with both Native Americans and whites (Kittler & Sucher, 2008). Some African Americans believe that ill health is due to bad luck or fate; home remedies and natural therapies may be frequently used.

## Nutrition-Related Health Problems

African Americans score just slightly below the national population average on the Healthy Eating Index (HEI), a tool developed by the USDA Center for Nutrition Policy and Promotion that measures dietary factors such as the intake of total fat, saturated fat, cholesterol, and sodium as well as dietary variety. However, a greater proportion of African Americans are considered to have "poor" diets when compared to the general population. In general African Americans have

- Diets low in fruits, vegetables, whole grains, and dairy products and high intakes of sodium (Fig. 10.2). Fat intake is also high, related to a high meat intake, the popularity of frying, and high intake of fast foods.

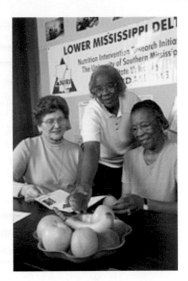

**FIGURE 10.2**  In general, African Americans should increase their intake of fruits, vegetables, whole grains, and dairy products and reduce their sodium intakes (USDA).

- A high prevalence of obesity. The National Center for Health Statistics (NCHS) data for 2001–2004 indicate, the prevalence of obesity (BMI ≥ 30) among adult black American men is 31.2%; among black women the prevalence is 51.6% (NCHS, 2006). For overweight, defined as BMI ≥25, the prevalence is 67% for black males and 79.6% for black females. The high incidence may be related to a permissive attitude regarding obesity and a sedentary lifestyle, which is not associated with income, education, occupation, marital status, poverty, or other indicators of social class (Kittler & Sucher, 2008).
- A disproportionately high prevalence of hypertension. 37.8% of adult black males and 40.3% of adult black females have hypertension compared to 26.7% of the total adult population (NCHS, 2006). African Americans are also more likely to develop complications related to hypertension, such as heart disease, stroke, and end-stage renal disease.
- A rate of type 2 diabetes that is 1.6 times higher than that of the total U.S. population (Kulkarni, 2004).
- Higher rates of iron deficiency anemia than whites at every age, regardless of gender or income level (Kittler & Sucher, 2008).
- Disproportionately high morbidity and mortality for mothers and infants. African-American women are two times more likely than white women to deliver a low birth weight infant, and their infant death rate is two times higher (NCHS, 2006). Dietary factors, particularly low folate intake, may be partially to blame.

## Mexican Americans

The Office of Minority Health and Health Disparities (OMHD) describe Hispanics or Latinos as people of Cuban, Mexican, Puerto Rican, South or Central American, or other Spanish culture or origin regardless of race (CDC, OMHD, 2007b). They are a diverse group differing in native language, customs, history, and foodways and have become the largest ethnic minority in the United States. By 2040, they are expected to comprise approximately 22% of the U.S. population (CDC, OMHD, 2007b). According to the 2000 U.S. census, 66% of Latinos are of Mexican origin.

## Traditional Food Practices

The traditional Mexican diet, influenced by Spanish and Native American cultures, is generally a low-fat, high-fiber diet, rich in complex carbohydrates and vegetable proteins, with an emphasis on corn, corn products, beans, and rice. Tortillas are a staple and may be consumed at every meal. Pork, goat, and poultry are the most used animal proteins; they are usually served ground or chopped as part of a mixed dish. Vegetables are also rarely served separately; they are incorporated into soups, rice, pasta, and tortilla-based dishes. Milk is not widely used, and lactose intolerance is common. Table 10.5 highlights traditional Mexican food practices and the impact of acculturation.

## Health Beliefs

Traditional health beliefs are a blend of European folk medicine introduced from Spain and Native American rituals. Health is viewed as a gift from God, and illness is caused by outside forces unless it is punishment from God for sin (Kittler & Sucher, 2008). Illness is inevitable and to be endured. Certain foods may be considered "cold" or "hot" for healing purposes.

| TABLE 10.5 | Traditional Mexican Foods and the Effects of Acculturation | |
|---|---|---|
| **Food Group** | **Foods Commonly Consumed** | **Effects of Acculturation** |
| Grains | Corn, rice | Rice eaten as part of a mixed dish with vegetables decreases; intake of plain rice increases<br>Flour tortillas are used more often than corn tortillas<br>Intake of white bread and sweetened cereals increases |
| Vegetables | Avocados, cactus, calabaza cricolla (green pumpkin), chili peppers, corn, jicama, lettuce, onions, peas, plantains, potatoes, squash, tomatillos, tomatoes, yams, yuca | Intake of most vegetables decreases |
| Fruit | Bananas, carambala, cherimoya, coconut, passion fruit, guava, lemons, limes, mangoes, melon, oranges, papaya, pineapple, strawberries | Intake of bananas, apples, oranges, orange juice, and cantaloupe remains relatively constant |
| Milk | Goat and cow's milk (whole is preferred), evaporated milk, café con leche, hot chocolate, cheese | Milk intake increases related to its use with a new food, such as ready-to-eat breakfast cereal; whole milk is replaced with low-fat or non fat milk |
| Meat and Beans | Beef, goat, pork, chicken, turkey, shrimp, eggs<br>Legumes: black beans, chickpeas, kidney beans, pinto beans | Red meat intake increases<br>Legume intake falls<br>Intake of traditional meat and vegetable preparations declines drastically |
| Fats | Butter, lard, Mexican cream | Butter, margarine, and salad dressing intake increases related to introduction of cooked vegetables and salads |
| Beverages | Fruit-based beverage | Severe decline in fruit-based beverage consumption; increased use of highly sweetened drinks (e.g., Kool Aid, soft drinks) and caffeinated beverages<br>Alcohol intake increases |

*Source:* Kittler, P., & Sucher, K. (2008). *Food and Culture* (5th ed.). Belmont, CA: Thomson/Wadsworth.

Prayer is appropriate for all illnesses and lighting of candles on behalf of a sick person is common (Kittler & Sucher, 2008).

## Nutrition-Related Health Problems

Mexican Americans have the highest HEI scores of all ethnic groups, especially in terms of dietary variety and a high intake of fruit. Acculturation generally *decreases* the quality of the diet: fat and cholesterol intake increases related to an increased intake of high-fat snacks, animal protein, and fried foods. The intake of fiber decreases due to a decrease in the intake of legumes, fruits, and vegetables (Murtaugh, Herrick, Sweeney et al., 2007). In general Mexican Americans have

- A high prevalence of overweight and obesity. Based on statistics for 2001 to 2004, the prevalence of obesity is 30.5% among Mexican males and 40.3% among Mexican females, with obesity defined as BMI ≥ 30. For overweight (BMI ≥ 25), the prevalence is 75.8% among Mexican males and 73.2% among Mexican females (NCHS, 2006). Leisure time physical inactivity and low socioeconomic status may contribute to high rates of overweight (Kittler & Sucher, 2008). Compared to whites, the concept of ideal weight may be higher for Mexican Americans.
- A high prevalence of type 2 diabetes, which is not explained by the incidence of obesity, age, or education (Haffner, Hazuda, Mitchell et al., 1991). The prevalence among Mexicans is 14.9%; among whites it is 8.9% (NCHS, 2006).
- Cavities and gingivitis are common. Nearly one-third of all Mexican immigrants never receive any dental care (Kittler & Sucher, 2008).
- High alcohol use. Compared to Mexican Americans who were born in Mexico, the first generation of Mexican Americans born in the U.S. have a 47% higher intake of alcohol (Monroe, Hankin, Pike et al., 2003).

## Chinese Americans

The term "Asian Americans" encompasses a diverse population originating from at least 25 countries, including China, Japan, Hong Kong, South Korea, India, Thailand, Vietnam, Cambodia, Indonesia, Malaysia, the Philippines, and other Pacific Rim areas. Two dietary commonalities exist between these diverse cultures: (1) emphasis on rice and vegetables with relatively little meat and (2) cooking techniques that include meticulous attention to preparing ingredients before cooking. Chinese food practices and health and nutrition status are described below.

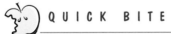 QUICK BITE

**While native Chinese food is healthy, Chinese restaurant food is not necessarily so**

|  | Calories | Sodium (mg) |
|---|---|---|
| 1 egg roll | 200 | 400 |
| 1 pork dumpling | 500 | 900 |
| Dinner sized: |  |  |
| Eggplant in garlic sauce | 1000 | 2000 |
| Kung Pao chicken | 1400 | 2600 |
| Orange (crispy) beef | 1500 | 3100 |
| Combination (house) fried rice | 1500 | 2700 |

*Source:* Hurley, J., & Liebman, B. (2007). Chinese restaurant food. *Nutrition Action Health Letter, 34*(3), 13–15.

| TABLE 10.6 | Traditional Chinese Foods and the Effects of Acculturation | |
|---|---|---|
| **Food Group** | **Foods Commonly Consumed** | **Effects of Acculturation** |
| Grains | Rice, wheat, buckwheat, corn, millet, sorghum | Rice remains a staple but the intake of wheat bread and cereals increases |
| Vegetables | Amaranth, asparagus, bamboo shoots, bean sprouts, bitter melon, cassava, cauliflower, celery, bok choy, Napa cabbage, chile peppers, Chinese broccoli, Chinese long beans, eggplant, flat beans, garlic, lily root, dried and fresh mushrooms, okra, onions, seaweed, spinach, taro | Raw vegetable and salad intake increases Traditional vegetables are replaced by more commonly available ones |
| Fruit | Apples, bananas, coconut, dates, figs, kumquats, lime, litchi, mango, oranges, passion fruit, pineapple, pomegranates, tangerines, watermelon | Intake of temperate fruits increases (e.g., apples, grapes, pears, peaches) |
| Milk | Cow's milk, buffalo milk | Milk, ice cream, and cheese intake increases |
| Meat and Beans | Almost all sources of protein are eaten | Intake of meat and ethnic dishes increases |
| Fats | Butter, lard, corn oil, peanut oil, sesame oil, soybean oil, suet | Fat intake increases as fast food intake increases |
| Beverages | Tea (southern China), soup (northern China), wine, beer | |

*Source:* Kittler, P., & Sucher, K. (2008). *Food and culture* (5th ed.). Belmont, CA: Thomson/Wadsworth.

## Traditional Food Practices

Traditional Chinese foods and the effect of acculturation are highlighted in Table 10.6. The foundation of the traditional diet are grains—predominately rice in southern China and wheat, in the form of noodles, dumplings, pancakes, and steamed bread, in northern China. A variety of vegetables are used extensively; other foods commonly consumed include sea vegetables, nuts, seeds, beans, soy foods, vegetable and nut oils, herbs and spices, tea, wine, and beer. A variety of animal proteins are consumed; the use of fish and seafood depends on availability. Most Chinese food is cooked; the exception is fresh fruit, which is eaten infrequently. Few dairy products are consumed because lactose intolerance is common. Calcium is provided by tofu, small fish (bones are eaten), and soups made with bones that have been partially dissolved by vinegar in making stock. Sodium intake is generally assumed to be high because of traditional food preservation methods (salting and drying) and condiments (e.g., soy sauce).

## Health Beliefs

Asian cultures believe that health and illness are related to the balance between yin and yang forces in the body. Yin represents female, cold, and darkness; yang represents male, hot, and light. Digested foods turn into air that is either yin or yang. Diseases caused by yin forces are treated with yang foods, and diseases caused by yang forces are treated with yin foods. Pregnancy is considered a yang or "hot" condition, so women following traditional practices during pregnancy eat yin foods such as most fruits and vegetables, seaweed, cold drinks, juices, and rice water. Yang foods include chicken, meat, pig's feet, meat broth, nuts, fried food, coffee, and spices. The hot–cold theory of foods and illness also exists in Puerto Rico and Mexico, but the food designations are not universal within or across cultures.

## Nutrition-Related Health Problems

The traditional Chinese diet is low in fat and dairy products and high in complex carbohydrates and sodium (Kittler & Sucher, 2008). With Americanization, the diet becomes higher in fat, protein, sugar, and cholesterol and lower in complex carbohydrates. In general

- Asian-American women have the highest life expectancy of all ethnic groups in the United States (USDHHS, Office of Minority Health, 2008). Life expectancy varies among Asian subgroups: Filipino women (81.5 years), Japanese women (84.5 years), and Chinese women (86.1 years).
- The prevalence of overweight and obesity are low among Chinese Americans, but goes up in U.S. born subjects compared to those who are foreign born (Kittler & Sucher, 2008).
- When adjusted for BMI, Asians are 60% to 74% more likely than whites to develop diabetes (McNeely & Boyko, 2004).
- The leading cause of death among Asian Americans is cancer. Compared to whites, Asian men and women have higher incidence and mortality rates for stomach and liver cancer; Asian women are less likely to have breast cancer but are more likely to have cervical cancer (USDHHS, Office of Minority Health, 2008).

# ▶ FOOD AND RELIGION

**Kosher:** a word commonly used to identify Jewish dietary laws that define "clean" foods, "unclean" foods, how food animals must be slaughtered, how foods must be prepared, and when foods may be consumed (e.g., the timing between eating milk products and meat products).

Religion tends to have a greater impact on food habits than nationality or culture does (e.g., Orthodox Jews follow **kosher** dietary laws regardless of their national origin). However, religious food practices vary significantly even among denominations of the same faith. National variations also exist. How closely an individual follows dietary laws is based on his or her degree of orthodoxy. An overview of religious food practices follows. Table 10.7 outlines major features of various religious dietary laws.

| TABLE 10.7 | **Summary of Dietary Laws of Selected Religions** | | | |
|---|---|---|---|---|
| | **Orthodox Judaism** | **Islam** | **Hinduism** | **Buddhism** |
| Meat | Cannot be eaten with dairy products | | Beef is prohibited | Avoided by the most devout |
| Pork and pork products | Prohibited | Prohibited | Avoided by the most devout | Avoided by the most devout |
| Lacto-ovo vegetarianism | | | Encouraged | Practiced by many |
| Seafood | Only fish with fins and scales are allowed | | Restricted | Avoided by the most devout |
| Alcohol | | Prohibited | Avoided by the most devout | |
| Coffee/tea | | Strongly discouraged | | |
| Ritual slaughter of animals | Yes | Yes | | |
| Moderation | | Practiced | | Practiced |
| Partial or total fasting | Practiced | Practiced | Practiced | Practiced |

*Sources:* ElGindy, G. *Cultural competence. Understanding Buddhist patient's dietary needs.* Available at MinorityNurse.com. Accessed on 2/6/08.
ElGindy, G. *Cultural competence. Hindu dietary practices: Feeding the body, mind and soul.* Available at MinorityNurse.com. Accessed on 2/6/08.
ElGindy, G. *Cultural competence. Meeting Jewish and Muslim patients' dietary needs.* Available at MinorityNurse.com. Accessed on 2/6/08.

## Christianity

The three primary branches of Christianity are Roman Catholicism, Eastern Orthodox Christianity, and Protestantism. Dietary practices vary from none to explicit.

- Roman Catholics do not eat meat on Ash Wednesday or on Fridays of Lent. Food and beverages are avoided for 1 hour before communion is taken. Devout Catholics observe several fast days during the year.
- Eastern Orthodox Christians observe numerous feast and fast days throughout the year.

The only denominations in the Protestant faith with dietary laws are the Mormons (Church of Jesus Christ of Latter-Day Saints) and Seventh-Day Adventists.

- Mormons do not use coffee, tea, alcohol, or tobacco. Followers are encouraged to limit meats and consume mostly grains. Some Mormons fast one day a month.
- Most Seventh-Day Adventists are lacto-ovo vegetarians; those who do eat meat avoid pork. Overeating is avoided, and coffee, tea, and alcohol are prohibited. An interval of 5 to 6 hours between meals is recommended with no snacking between meals. Water is consumed before and after meals. Strong seasonings, such as pepper and mustard, are avoided.

## Judaism

In the United States there are three main Jewish denominations: Orthodox, Conservative, and Reform. Hasidic Jews are a sect within the Orthodox. These groups differ in their interpretation of the precepts of Judaism. Orthodox Jews believe that the laws are the direct commandments of God, so they adhere strictly to dietary laws. Reform Jews follow the moral law but may selectively follow other laws; for instance, they may not follow any religious dietary laws. Conservative Jews fall between the other two groups in their beliefs and adherence to the laws. They may follow the Jewish dietary laws at home but take a more liberal attitude on social occasions. Because Jews have diverse backgrounds and nationalities, their food practices vary widely.

Because dietary laws are rigid, Orthodox Jews rarely eat outside the home except at homes or restaurants with kosher kitchens. Milk and dairy products are used widely but cannot be consumed at the same meal with meat or poultry. Dairy products are not allowed within 1 to 6 hours after eating meat or poultry, depending on the individual's ethnic tradition. Meat and poultry cannot be eaten for 30 minutes after dairy products have been consumed. Margarine labeled **pareve**, nondairy creamers, and oils may be used with meats. Fruits, vegetables, plain grains, pastas, plain legumes, and eggs are considered kosher and can be eaten with either dairy or meat products.

**Pareve:** dairy-free.

Food preparation is prohibited on the Sabbath. Religious holidays are celebrated with certain foods. For example, only unleavened bread is eaten during Passover, and a 24-hour fast is observed on Yom Kippur.

## Islam

**Halal:** Islamic dietary laws.

**Haram:** foods that are prohibited.

Muslims eat as a matter of faith and for good health. Basic guidance concerning food laws is revealed in the Quran (the divine book) from Allah (the Creator) to Muhammad (the Prophet). For Muslims, health and food are considered acts of worship for which Allah must be thanked (ElGindy, 2005a). There are 11 generally accepted rules pertaining to **halal** (permitted) and **haram** (prohibited) foods. Islam also stresses certain hygienic practices, such as washing hands before and after eating and frequent teeth cleaning.

## Hinduism

A love of nature and desire to live a simple natural life are the basis of Hinduism (ElGindy, 2005b). A number of health beliefs and dietary practices stem from the idea of living in harmony with nature and having mercy and respect for all God's creations. Generally, Hindus avoid all foods that are believed to inhibit physical and spiritual development. Eating meat is not explicitly prohibited, but many Hindus are vegetarian because they adhere to the concept of **ahimsa**.

**Ahimsa:** nonviolence as applicable to foods.

Another influential concept is that of purity. Some foods, such as dairy products (e.g., milk, yogurt, ghee [clarified butter]) are considered to enhance spiritual purity. When prepared together, pure foods can improve the purity of unpure foods. Some foods, such as beef or alcohol, are innately polluted and can never be made pure.

Jainism, a branch of Hinduism, also promotes the nonviolent doctrine of ahimsa. Devout Jains are complete vegetarians and may avoid blood-colored foods (e.g., tomatoes) and root vegetables (because harvesting them may cause the death of insects).

## Buddhism

In the Buddhist faith, life revolves around nature with its two opposing energy systems of yin and yang (ElGindy, 2005c). Examples of these opposing energy systems are heat/cold, light/darkness, good/evil, and sickness/health. Illnesses may result from an imbalance of yin and yang. Most Buddhists subscribe to the concept of ahimsa, so many are lacto-ovo vegetarians. Some eat fish; some avoid only beef. Buddhist dietary practices vary widely depending on the sect and country. Buddhist monks avoid eating solid food after the noon hour.

### ▶ HOW DO YOU RESPOND?

**Is all fast food bad?** No, not all fast foods are "bad." "Bad" is a relative term that depends on how often and how much. But even when "healthy" selections are made, such as a grilled chicken sandwich or a plain baked potato, fast food meals tend to be low in fiber, fruit, vegetables, and milk/dairy products. While an occasional fast food meal will not jeopardize someone's nutritional status, a steady diet of it can be detrimental for what it provides (too much fat, calories, and sodium) and for what it lacks.

### ▶ CASE STUDY

Elizabet moved to the Midwest at the age of 26 from her native country, Iceland, where she ate seafood almost every evening for dinner. She ate fruit and vegetables daily, but the variety was limited. In her new home, she complains that good seafood is hard to find—that it is not as fresh as it is at home, it tastes different, and it is more expensive. She also misses the dark brown and black breads she is accustomed to; she is willing to try American breads, but is unsure what variety is "good." American fast food is well known to her but she does not want to rely on that to satisfy her need for familiar foods. She wants to eat foods that are healthy, tasty, and affordable.

• What questions would you ask Elizabet before coming up with suggestions about foods she could try?
• What would you say to her about her frustration with the seafood available locally? What suggestions would you make to her?
• What would you tell her about healthy breads? What fruits would you recommend as healthy, tasty, and affordable? What vegetables?

1. Which of the following items would be the healthiest choice from a Mexican restaurant?
   a. Cheese quesadillas
   b. Arroz con pollo
   c. Taco salad
   d. Guacamole with taco chips

2. A descriptive word that indicates a low-fat cooking technique is:
   a. Au gratin
   b. Breaded
   c. Roasted
   d. Battered

3. A first-generation Chinese American has been advised to consume less sodium. What native food would the nurse ask about to get an idea of how much sodium he consumes?
   a. Soybeans
   b. Soy sauce
   c. Wonton
   d. Bok choy

4. A negative impact of acculturation on Mexican-American food choices is often a decrease in fiber intake related to a decrease in the intake of (select all that apply):
   a. Legumes
   b. Whole grain cereals
   c. Whole wheat bread
   d. Vegetables
   e. Fruit

5. What are the nutritional characteristics of a traditional soul food diet? Select all that apply.
   a. High in fat
   b. High in sodium
   c. High in fiber
   d. High in cholesterol
   e. Low in calcium

6. Which of the following is a healthy traditional food practice of Chinese Americans that should be encouraged?
   a. None; an American diet is healthier
   b. High intake of milk and dairy products
   c. Frequent use of fresh fruit
   d. Extensive use of vegetables in mixed dishes

7. When developing a teaching plan for an overweight woman from Mexico, which approach would be best?
   a. Tell the client she will feel better if she loses some of the extra weight she is carrying around
   b. Encourage more "nutritious" food choices
   c. Advise the client that "healthy eating" will help her shed inches
   d. Provide a low-calorie diet and encourage her to eat low-calorie American foods, such as artificially sweetened soda and low-fat ice cream

8. Muslims are prohibited from consuming:
   a. Alcohol
   b. Eggs
   c. Beef
   d. Shellfish

KEY CONCEPTS

● American cuisine has evolved from a melting pot of food, flavors, and cooking techniques contributed by immigrants over the course of U.S. history. It continues to undergo change.

● Convenience foods range from pre-prepared ingredients to use to make a home-cooked meal (e.g., fresh cut vegetables and bagged salad) to complete, heat-and-serve meals. Convenience "meals" tend to be high in sodium and low in fiber, fruit, vegetables, and whole grains. Portion sizes are smaller than most people normally consume.

● The average American eats out approximately five times a week. Fast food restaurants are the most popular type of restaurant for breakfast and lunch; fast food restaurants and casual dining are favored for dinner. Fast food "value" meals are high in calories, fat, and sodium, in part because the portion sizes are large.

● Suggestions to help control portion sizes while eating out include ordering two appetizers as a meal, splitting an entrée with a companion, ordering a "child" sized meal, or creating a doggie bag before beginning to eat.

● Culture defines what is edible; how food is handled, prepared, and consumed; what foods are appropriate for particular groups within the culture; the meaning of food and eating; attitudes toward body size; and the relationship between food and health. Yet, food habits vary considerably among individuals and families within a cultural group based on personal factors, socioeconomic factors, and religious factors.

● Core foods are an indispensable part of the diet and consist of grains or starchy vegetables. Secondary foods are nutrient rich and add variety and ethnic identity to meals. Occasional or peripheral foods are used infrequently.

● Cultural values identify behavior that is desirable and define how people should interact within society. American values are often very different from values of other cultures. Understanding a client's cultural values facilitates communication.

● Culture defines body image and desirable weight. In the United States, thinness is valued, particularly for women. In some other cultures, thinness is equated with poverty; heavier weight is considered desirable and a sign of prosperity.

● Dietary acculturation occurs as people who move to a new area change their food habits to some degree. New foods are added to their diet or substituted for traditional foods, and some traditional foods are rejected. Availability and cost influence food choices.

● Acculturation can have a negative or positive effect on nutrition and health. Generally, as immigrants adopt the "typical American diet," their intake of fat, sugar, and calories goes up, and their intake of fiber, fruits, vegetables, and vegetable protein goes down. New Americans should be encouraged to retain the healthy eating practices of their native diet.

● Generalizations can be made about traditional eating practices of subcultures within the United States. However, an individual's food choices deviate from these based on personal preferences, socioeconomic status, and degree of acculturation.

● Traditional soul food is high in fat, cholesterol, and sodium and low in fiber, fruit, vegetables, and calcium. Socioeconomic factors, geographic area, and work schedules have a greater impact on the intake of African Americans than does the traditional soul food diet.

● African Americans have a higher prevalence of overweight/obesity, hypertension, type 2 diabetes, and iron deficiency anemia than whites. Morbidity and mortality for mothers and infants is also higher. The leading cause of death for African Americans and whites is heart disease.

● Mexican Americans have a higher prevalence of overweight/obesity, type 2 diabetes, and cavities/gingivitis than whites. Alcohol use is higher in Mexican Americans born in the United States than those born in Mexico. The leading cause of death is heart disease.

● Asian women have the longest life expectancy of all ethnic groups in the United States. The prevalence of overweight/obesity among Asian Americans is lower than in whites. Cancer is the leading cause of death.

● Religion tends to have a greater impact on food habits than nationality or culture. People are more likely to eat ethnic food from a different culture than they are to eat food that is prohibited by the mandates of their religion.

## ANSWER KEY

1. **TRUE** Each culture has its own socially standardized food behaviors that dictate what is edible, the role of certain foods in the diet, how food is prepared, the use of foods, the number and timing of daily meals, how food is eaten, and health beliefs related to food.

2. **FALSE** Race, ethnicity, and geographic region are often inaccurately assumed to be synonymous with culture. This misconception leads to stereotyping.

3. **TRUE** Core foods tend to be complex carbohydrates, such as cereal grains, starchy tubers, and starchy vegetables. These core foods are the indispensable foundation of the diet and provide significant calories.

4. **FALSE** Americans want healthier restaurant choices but are generally not willing to pay more for them. The allure of "value" wins out over health.

5. **FALSE** The hot–cold theory of health and diet refers to Asian cultures' belief that health and illness are related to the balance between yin and yang forces in the body. Yin represents female, cold, and darkness; yang represents male, hot, and light.

6. **TRUE** Usually, first-generation Americans adhere more closely to cultural food patterns to preserve their ethnic identity, compared with subsequent generations.

7. **TRUE** For many ethnic groups who move to the United States, breakfast and lunch are most likely to be composed of convenient American foods while traditional foods are retained for the major dinner meal, which has greater emotional significance.

8. **TRUE** People who eat at restaurants or buy take-out food tend to eat more calories, fat, and sodium than people who eat home-prepared meals.

9. **FALSE** Dietary acculturation can lead to positive or negative changes in food choices. For instance, Mexican Americans dramatically reduce their intake of lard and Mexican cream through the process of acculturation, which is a positive change. However, substituting sweetened drinks (e.g., Kool Aid and soft drinks) for the traditional beverage made from fruit has a negative impact on nutritional intake.

10. **FALSE** Although restaurant portions tend to be much larger than the standard serving size, the same is not true for convenience foods. The portion sizes listed on the label of convenience meals tend to be much smaller than what Americans typically consume in a meal.

## WEBSITES

*Cultural/Ethnic Food Guide Pyramids*

The Department of Anthropology and Geography at Georgia State University for materials developed by the Nutrition Education for New Americans project at **www.multiculturalhealth.org**
Oldways Preservation & Exchange Trust at **www.oldwayspt.org**

*Ethnic Medicine Information Including Nutrition Information*

Harborview Medical Center, University of Washington at **www.ethnomed.org**
USDA Food and Nutrition Information Center available at **www.nal.usda.gov/fnic**

*Website for information on fast food and eating out*

Center for Science in the Public Interest at **www.cspinet.org**

*Nutrition facts of 10 popular fast food restaurant chains*

**www.fatcalories.com**

# REFERENCES

Archer, S. (2005). Acculturation and dietary intake. *Journal of the American Dietetic Association, 105,* 411–412.

Brown, D. (2005). Dietary challenges of new Americans. *Journal of the American Dietetic Association, 105,* 1704–1706.

CDC, Office of Minority Health and Health Disparities. (2007a). *White populations.* Available at www.cdc.gov/omhd/Populations/White.htm. Accessed on 1/30/08.

CDC, Office of Minority Health and Health Disparities. (2007b). *Hispanic or Latino populations.* Available at www.cdc.gov/omhd/Populations/HL/HL.htm. Accessed on 1/30/08.

ElGindy, G. (2004). *Cultural competence Q & A: Dietary needs.* Available at www.minoritynurse.com/features/health/10-20-04h.html. Accessed on 2/6/08.

ElGindy, G. (2005a). *Cultural competence Q & A: Meeting Jewish and Muslim patients' dietary needs.* Available at www.minoritynurse.com/features/health/03-01-05f.html. Accessed on 2/6/08.

ElGindy, G. (2005b). *Cultural competence Q & A: Hindu dietary practices: feeding the body, mind and soul.* Available at www.minoritynurse.com/features/health/10-25-05b.html. Accessed on 2/6/08.

ElGindy, G. (2005c). *Cultural competence Q & A: Understanding Buddhist patients' dietary needs.* Available at www.minoritynurse.com/features/health/05-03-05a.html. Accessed on 2/6/08.

GfK Roper. (2007). *Gfk Roper Consulting's Roper Reports, New York.* Available at www.gfkamerican.com. Accessed on 2/4/08.

Haffner, S. M., Hazuda, H. P., Mitchell, B., et al. (1991). Increased incidence of Type II diabetes mellitus in Mexican Americans. *Diabetes Care, 14,* 102–108.

Hurley, J., & Liebman, B. (2007). Chinese restaurant food: Wok carefully. *Nutrition Action Health Letter, 34*(3), 13–15.

Kaplan, M., Newsom, J., & McFarland, B. (2004). The association between length of residence and obesity among Hispanic immigrants. *American Journal of Preventive Medicine, 27,* 323–326.

Kittler, R., & Sucher, K. (2008). *Food and culture.* (5th ed.). Belmont, CA: Thomson Wadsworth.

Kulkarni, K. (2004). Food, culture, and diabetes in the United States. *Clinical Diabetes, 22,* 190–192.

McNeely, M., & Boyko, E. (2004). Type 2 diabetes prevalence in Asian Americans. *Diabetes Care, 27,* 66–69.

Monroe, K. R., Hankin, J. H., Pike, M. C., et al. (2003). Correlation of dietary intake and colorectal cancer incidence among Mexican-American migrants: The Multiethnic Cohort Study. *Nutrition and Cancer, 45,* 133–147.

Murtaugh, M. A., Herrick, J. S., Sweeney, C., et al. (2007). Diet composition and risk of over-weight and obesity in women living in the southwestern United States. *Journal of the American Dietetic Association, 107,* 1311–1321.

National Center for Health Statistics, United States. (2006). *Health, United States, 2006. DHHS publication # 2006-1232.* Available at www.cdc.gov/nchs/data/hus/hus06.pdf#073. Accessed on 2/12/08.

Perlick, A. (2007). *R & I's 2007 menu census: variety show. Restaurants & Institutions,* Nov 1, 2007. Available at www.rimag.com/archives/2007/11/menu-census-main.asp. Accessed on 2/10/08.

Science Daily. (2007). *Price and taste trump nutrition when Americans eat out.* Available at www.sciencedaily.com/releases/2007/10/071022120256.htm. Accessed on 2/10/08.

Sloan, A. (2008). What, when, and where America eats. *Food Technology.* Available at www.ift.org. Accessed on 1/2/08.

Stimpson, J., & Urrutia-Rojas, X. (2007). Acculturation in the United States is associated with lower serum carotenoid levels: Third National Health and Nutrition Examination Survey. *Journal of the American Dietetic Association, 107,* 1218–1223.

United States Department of Health and Human Services, The Office of Minority Health. (2008). *Asian Americans profile.* Available at www.ombrc.gov/templates/broswe.aspx?lvl=2&lvlID=32. Accessed on 2/11/08.

# 11

# Healthy Eating for Healthy Babies

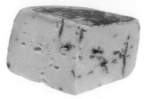

| TRUE | FALSE | |
|---|---|---|
| ☐ | ☐ | **1** Adequate weight gain during pregnancy ensures delivery of a normal-weight baby. |
| ☐ | ☐ | **2** Obese women should not gain weight during pregnancy. |
| ☐ | ☐ | **3** An important source of folic acid is ready-to-eat breakfast cereals. |
| ☐ | ☐ | **4** Weight gain in excess of the recommended ranges is likely to lead to an increase in maternal fat stores and so increase the risk of postpartum weight retention. |
| ☐ | ☐ | **5** To get enough calcium during pregnancy, women need to double their usual intake of milk. |
| ☐ | ☐ | **6** Pregnant and lactating women are advised to eliminate fish and seafood from their diets to avoid mercury contamination. |
| ☐ | ☐ | **7** Calorie needs do not increase during pregnancy until the second trimester. |
| ☐ | ☐ | **8** Lactation increases calorie requirements more than pregnancy does. |
| ☐ | ☐ | **9** An inadequate maternal intake of nutrients decreases the quantity of breast milk produced, not the quality. |
| ☐ | ☐ | **10** Thirst is a good indicator for the need for fluid in most lactating women. |

### *UPON COMPLETION OF THIS CHAPTER, YOU WILL BE ABLE TO*

- Evaluate a woman's pattern and amount of weight gain during pregnancy based on her prepregnancy BMI.
- Assess a woman's intake of folic acid for adequacy in the preconception period and during pregnancy.
- Assess whether a woman may benefit from a multivitamin and mineral supplement during pregnancy.
- Plan a day's intake for a pregnant woman based on her MyPyramid food intake pattern.
- Give examples of nutrition interventions used for nausea, constipation, and heartburn during pregnancy.
- Compare nutrition guidelines for healthy eating during pregnancy with the guidelines for lactation.
- Identify risk factors for poor nutritional status during pregnancy.
- List benefits of breastfeeding for mother and infant.

Although an optimal diet before and during pregnancy cannot *guarantee* a successful outcome of pregnancy, it can improve the chance of a healthy newborn baby, a healthy mom, and a healthy future for both. A woman who is well nourished and within her healthy weight range prior to conception provides an environment conducive to normal fetal growth and development during the critical first trimester of pregnancy. Recent studies suggest that nutritional deficiencies during this period increase the risk of certain chronic diseases later in the infant's life (Fowles, 2006). During pregnancy, the fetus cannot meet its genetic potential for development if the supply of energy and nutrients is inadequate. For the mother, adequate but not excessive weight gain reduces the risk of complications during pregnancy and delivery and lowers the risk of postpartum weight retention (Ricciotti, 2008). An optimal diet provides enough, but not too many, calories and nutrients to optimize maternal and fetal health.

This chapter discusses dietary guidelines for women before, during, and after pregnancy. Weight gain recommendations, common problems of pregnancy, and nutrition interventions for maternal health conditions are presented.

# ► PREPREGNANCY NUTRITION

The basic principles of healthy eating that apply to healthy people are also appropriate before, during, and after pregnancy: eat plenty of fruits and vegetables of various kinds and colors; whole-grain bread and cereals; lean meats; low-fat or fat-free milk and dairy products; and healthy fats in moderation. The amount of food recommended from each MyPyramid food group is individualized according to a woman's age and activity level.

**Neural Tube Defect:** a serious central nervous system birth defect, such as anencephaly (absence of a brain) and spina bifida (incomplete closure of the spinal cord and its bony encasement).

The Institute of Medicine (IOM), Centers for Disease Control and Prevention (CDC), Dietary Guidelines for Americans, and March of Dimes (MOD) are among the many experts who recommend synthetic folic acid be consumed prior to pregnancy to prevent **neural tube defects** (CDC, 2006; IOM, 1998; MOD, 2006a; USDHHS, USDA, 2005). Among other preconception care recommendations of the CDC that are proven to improve pregnancy outcomes is that obesity should be controlled (Box 11.1). Both these recommendations are presented below. Key recommendations within the 2005 Dietary Guidelines for Americans are listed in Box 11.2. Alcohol use is addressed under the section on "Nutrition during Pregnancy."

## Folic Acid Supplementation

**Folic Acid:** synthetic form of folate found in multivitamins, fortified breakfast cereals, and enriched grain products.

### QUICK BITE

**Good sources of folic acid and folate**

*Folic acid:*
100% fortified ready-to-eat breakfast cereals
White bread, rolls, pasta, and crackers (In the United States and Canada, enriched flour is required to be fortified with folic acid.)
*Naturally occurring folate:*
Leafy green vegetables, such as spinach
Citrus fruits
Dried peas and beans, such as lentils, soybeans, pinto beans

It is well established that daily supplements of **folic acid** taken prior to pregnancy decrease the risk of neural tube defects by as much as two-thirds (CDC, 2006). Adequate folic acid may also decrease the risk of preterm delivery, low birth weight, and poor fetal growth (Mayo Clinic, 2007). Because neural tube defects originate in the first month of pregnancy before a woman may even know she is pregnant, all women of childbearing age who are capable of becoming pregnant are urged to consume 400 micrograms of synthetic folic

| BOX 11.1 | CDC RECOMMENDATIONS: PRECONCEPTION INTERVENTIONS WITH PROVEN HEALTH EFFECTS |

- Folic acid supplementation
- Vaccinations: rubella, hepatitis B
- Screening and treatment of: HIV/AIDS, sexually transmitted diseases
- Medication management: oral anticoagulant, antiepileptic drugs, Accutane
- Disease management: diabetes, hypothyroidism, maternal PKU
- Lifestyle management: smoking cessation, eliminating alcohol use, obesity control

*Source:* Centers for Disease Control and Prevention (CDC). (2006). *Preconception and health care.* CDC website: www.cdc.gov/ncbddd/preconception/default.htm. Accessed 3/14/08.

| BOX 11.2 | 2005 DIETARY GUIDELINES FOR AMERICANS AND KEY RECOMMENDATIONS |

**All adults, including women who may become pregnant, are pregnant, or are breastfeeding, are urged to**

- Eat a variety of nutrient-dense food and beverages among the basic food groups.
- Limit the intake of saturated fat, trans fats, cholesterol, added sugars, salt, and alcohol.
- Meet recommended intakes for nutrients within calorie needs.
- Follow a balanced plan, such as an individualized MyPyramid food plan.

**Additional Key Recommendations**
*Women of childbearing age who may become pregnant:*
- Consume adequate synthetic folic acid daily (from fortified foods or supplements) in addition to food forms of folate from a varied diet.
- Eat foods high in heme-iron and/or consume iron-rich plant foods or iron-fortified foods with an enhancer of iron absorption, such as vitamin C–rich foods.
- Alcoholic beverages should not be consumed.

*Pregnant women:*
- Ensure appropriate weight gain as specified by a health care provider.
- In the absence of medical or obstetric complications, incorporate 30 minutes or more of moderate-intensity physical activity on most, if not all, days of the week. Avoid activities with a high risk of falling or abdominal trauma.
- Alcoholic beverages should not be consumed.
- Do not consume unpasteurized milk or any products made from unpasteurized milk, raw or partially cooked eggs or foods containing raw eggs, raw or undercooked meat and poultry, raw or undercooked fish or shellfish, unpasteurized juices, and raw sprouts. Eat only certain deli meats and frankfurters that have been reheated to steaming hot.

*Breastfeeding women:*
- Moderate weight reduction is safe and does not compromise weight gain of the nursing infant.
- Be aware that neither acute nor regular exercise adversely affects the mother's ability to successfully breastfeed.
- Alcoholic beverages should not be consumed.

*Source:* USDHHS, USDA. (2005). *Dietary Guidelines for Americans.* Available at www.health.gov/dietaryguidelines/dga2005/document/default.htm. Accessed 3/20/08.

**Folate:** natural form of the B vitamin involved in the synthesis of DNA; only one-half is available to the body as synthetic folic acid.

acid every day in addition to consuming natural **folate** in a varied diet. Synthetic folic acid in supplements and fortified foods is recommended because it is better absorbed and has greater availability than natural folate in foods. The CDC recommends daily supplementation for at least 3 months prior to conception.

## Obesity Control

**"Ideal" Weight (Healthy Weight):** BMI of 18.5 to 24.9

The CDC recommends that overweight women try to get within 15 pounds of their ideal weight prior to conception. Attaining healthy weight before conception reduces the risk of neural tube defects, preterm delivery, diabetes, cesarean section, and hypertensive disease related to obesity (CDC, 2006). Because prepregnancy body mass index (BMI) is the strongest predictor of excess gestational weight gain and future obesity, weight management is recommended before or between pregnancies (Krummel, 2007). Once a woman becomes pregnant, weight reduction should never be undertaken.

## ▶ NUTRITION AND LIFESTYLE DURING PREGNANCY

Pregnant women are urged to continue eating a healthy diet and to increase their intake of synthetic folic acid to 600 micrograms/day (USDHHS, USDA, 2005). Folic acid has a vital role in DNA synthesis and thus is essential for the synthesis of new cells and transmission of inherited characteristics. Key recommendations for pregnant women are listed in Box 11.2.

## Amount of Weight Gain

Current weight gain recommendations for pregnancy are based on prepregnancy BMI (Table 11.1). Recommended weight gain is 25 to 35 pounds in women of normal weight, 28 to 40 pounds for underweight women, 15 to 25 pounds for overweight women, and 11 to 20 pounds for women who are obese at the time of conception (IOM, in press). Women pregnant with twins need to gain somewhat more weight than that recommended for single births but not double the amounts.

Despite the increased prevalence of overweight and obesity over the last 20 years since the last weight gain guidelines issued by the IOM, the new guidelines show only modest change: obese women were advised to limit weight gain to 11–20 pounds. Among the

**TABLE 11.1**   **Recommended Weight Gain Ranges Based on Maternal Prepregnancy BMI**

| Prepregnancy BMI | Category | Gestational Weight Gain (lb) | |
|---|---|---|---|
| | | Single Fetus | Twins |
| <18.5 | Underweight | 28–40 | *37–54 |
| 18.5–24.9 | Normal weight | 25–35 | 31–50 |
| 25–29.9 | Overweight | 15–25 | 25–42 |
| ≥30 | Obese | 11–20 | |

*No guideline due to insufficient data

**Source:** Institute of Medicine (IOM). (in press). Weight Gain during Pregnancy: Examining the Guidelines. Available at www.nap.edu/catalog/1258.htm. Washington, DC: National Academies Press.

guideline's key findings are that 1) women should enter pregnancy with a normal BMI to reduce the risks of adverse pregnancy outcomes associated with excess prepregnancy weight and 2) although record numbers of American women have BMI values >35, there is insufficient data available to issue specific weight gain recommendations for this population. The report emphasizes the need for increased nutrition and exercise counseling to help women attain a normal BMI.

All too often—in an estimated 30% to 40% of pregnancies—women gain more or less weight than recommended, increasing risks to both mother and infant (Ricciotti, 2008). Overweight women are more likely to gain more than the recommended amount, increasing the risk of gestational diabetes, cesarean deliveries, complications during delivery, and postpartum weight retention (Ricciotti, 2008); risks to the infant include hypoglycemia, large for gestational age, a low Apgar score, seizures, and childhood obesity (ADA, 2008). In one of the few randomized controlled trials designed to prevent excessive weight gain during pregnancy, interventions decreased the prevalence of excess weight gain in normal-weight women but actually *increased* the prevalence of excess weight in women who were overweight at the time of conception (Polley et al., 2002). Unfortunately, there are no evidence-based dietary recommendations to control excessive maternal weight gain (Ricciotti, 2008).

In contrast, underweight women are more likely to gain less than the recommended amount, which increases the risk of a **low birth weight (LBW)** infant. LBW infants have a high incidence of postnatal complications and mortality and are at increased risk for coronary heart disease, type 2 diabetes, and hyperlipidemia later in life (Hanson et al., 2004).

**Low Birth Weight (LBW):** a baby weighing less than 2500 g or 5.5 pounds.

## Weight Gain Pattern

Assuming a 1.1–4.4 pound weight gain in the first trimester of pregnancy, normal-weight women are urged to gain 3–4 pounds per month thereafter. Weight gain recommendations after the first trimester for other women are as follows: 1 pound/week for underweight women, 0.6 pound/week for overweight women, and 0.5 pounds/week for obese women (IOM, 2009). Although slightly higher or lower rates of weight gain can be considered normal, obvious or persistent deviations warrant further investigation.

## Calorie Requirements

According to Dietary Reference Intakes (DRIs), pregnant women do not need any additional calories until the second trimester. Even then, the increase is surprisingly small: an extra 340 cal/day is recommended during the second trimester and an additional 452 cal/day in the third (IOM, 2005). Most pregnant women need a total of 2200 to 2900 cal/day (ADA, 2008). Throughout pregnancy, adequacy of calorie intake is measured by adequacy of weight gain.

Figure 11.1 illustrates a sample MyPyramid for Moms food plan for a woman who normally requires 2000 cal/day and whose due date is in November. A 2000-calorie meal plan

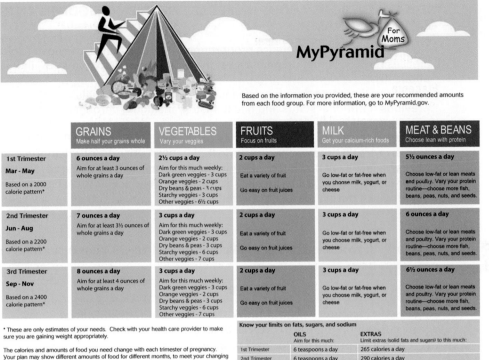

**FIGURE 11.1** MyPyramid for Moms food plan. (USDA, Center for Nutrition Policy and Promotion (2005). MyPyramid—Steps to Healthier You Food Guidance System. Available at www.MyPyramid.gov.)

is shown for the first trimester, a 2200-calorie pattern for the second trimester, and a 2400-calorie pattern for the third trimester. Notice that from the beginning to end of pregnancy, the additional food needed is very small: 2 ounces of grains, ½ cup of vegetables, and 1 ounce of meat/beans. The discretionary calorie allowance shows a modest increase of 95 cal/day. For someone needing 2400 calories at baseline, the three food patterns would be 2400, 2600, and 2800 calories for the first, second, and third trimesters, respectively.

## Vitamin and Mineral Supplements

Generalizations about nutrient requirements during pregnancy are listed in Box 11.3.

Although most nutrients are needed in greater amounts during pregnancy (Table 11.2), most women who are at low nutritional risk can meet their nutrient needs throughout pregnancy from food alone (ADA, 2008). Folic acid is one possible exception: as previously noted, fortified foods or supplements containing 600 micrograms of folic acid are recommended during pregnancy. The other notable exception is iron. The need for other supplements is based on individual circumstances.

## Iron

The DRI for iron increases by 50% during pregnancy to support the increase in maternal blood volume and to provide iron for fetal liver storage, which sustains the infant for the first 4 to 6 months of life. Even with careful selections, women are not likely to consume adequate

| BOX 11.3 | GENERALIZATIONS ABOUT INCREASED NUTRIENT REQUIREMENTS DURING PREGNANCY |
|---|---|

- Nutrient needs do not increase proportionately. For instance, the need for iron increases by 50% during pregnancy, yet the requirement for vitamin $B_{12}$ increases by only about 10%.
- Actual requirements during pregnancy vary among individuals and are influenced by previous nutritional status and health history including chronic illnesses, multiple pregnancies, and closely spaced pregnancies.
- The requirement for one nutrient may be altered by the intake of another. For instance, women who do not meet their calorie requirements need higher amounts of protein.
- Nutrient needs are not constant throughout the course of pregnancy. Nutrient needs generally change little during the first trimester (folic acid is an exception) and are at their highest during the last trimester.

| TABLE 11.2 | Selected Nutritional Needs for Women (Aged 19–30 Years) During Pregnancy and Lactation |
|---|---|

| Nutrient | Nonpregnant Women | Pregnancy | Lactation |
|---|---|---|---|
| Calories* | Individualized | 1st tri: +0<br>2nd tri: +340<br>3rd tri: +450 | 1st 6 month: +330<br>2nd 6 month: +400 |
| Protein (g) | 46 | 71 | 71 |
| Vit A (micrograms) | 700 | 770 | 1300 |
| Vit C (mg) | 75 | 85 | 120 |
| Vit D (micrograms) | 5.0* | 5.0* | 5.0* |
| Vit E (mg) | 15 | 15 | 19 |
| Vit K (micrograms)* | 90* | 90* | 90* |
| Thiamin (mg) | 1.1 | 1.4 | 1.4 |
| Riboflavin (mg) | 1.1 | 1.4 | 1.6 |
| Niacin (mg) | 14 | 18 | 17 |
| Vit $B_6$ (mg) | 1.3 | 1.9 | 2.0 |
| Folate (micrograms) | 400 | 600 | 500 |
| Vit $B_{12}$ (micrograms) | 2.4 | 2.6 | 2.8 |
| Calcium (mg) | 1000* | 1000* | 1000* |
| Iron (mg) | 18 | 27 | 9 |
| Magnesium (mg) | 310 | 350 | 310 |
| Selenium (micrograms) | 55 | 60 | 70 |
| Zinc (mg) | 8 | 11 | 12 |

Recommended Dietary Allowances are in **bold;** Adequate Intakes (AIs) in ordinary type followed by an asterisk (*).
tri, trimester; Vit, Vitamin.

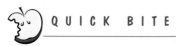

**QUICK BITE**

**Good sources of iron***
Heme iron
  Lean red meat, poultry, fish
Nonheme iron
  100% iron-fortified ready-to-eat cereals
  Dried peas and beans, such as soybeans, lentils, lima beans

Baked potato with skin
Dried fruit

*Heme iron is well absorbed and not influenced by the presence of other dietary factors. Nonheme iron absorption is enhanced when eaten at the same time as foods high in vitamin C, such as citrus fruits or juices, tomato products, red peppers, cantaloupe, or strawberries.

amounts of iron during pregnancy from food alone. Infants born to women who have iron deficiency anemia have an increased risk of LBW and possibly preterm delivery and perinatal mortality (ADA, 2008). It is recommended that pregnant women take an iron supplement of 27 mg of iron daily; women who are anemic may need 60 mg of iron daily until the anemia is resolved (ADA, 2008).

Some women experience **pica**, a craving for nonfood items such as laundry starch, clay, or ice. Pica can be a strongly rooted social tradition and is more prevalent among African Americans and rural residents. Iron deficiency was thought to be a risk factor for pica, but it may be a consequence. Eating clay or soil may displace the intake of iron-rich foods from the diet and may interfere with iron absorption.

**Pica:** a psychobehavioral disorder characterized by the ingestion of nonfood substances such as dirt, clay, starch, and ice.

## Other Supplements

A multivitamin and mineral supplement is recommended for pregnant women who (ADA, 2008)

- Have iron deficiency anemia
- Consume a poor-quality diet
- Do not consume enough foods from animal sources
- Smoke or abuse alcohol or drugs
- Are carrying two or more fetuses
- Have HIV, especially if access to antiretroviral treatment is limited

### QUICK BITE

**Vegan sources of B$_{12}$: reliable and unreliable**

B$_{12}$-fortified foods are reliable sources:
   Yeast extracts
   Vegetable stock
   Veggie burgers
   Textured vegetable protein
   Soymilk
   Vegetable and sunflower margarines
   Ready-to-eat breakfast cereals
Unreliable sources:
   Tempeh
   Sea vegetables
   Algae

**Source:** Ricciotti, H. (2008). Nutrition and lifestyle for a healthy pregnancy. *American Journal of Lifestyle Medicine, 2,* 151–158.

Specific supplements that may be needed based on individual circumstances are as follows:

- Complete vegans who are pregnant or breastfeeding should take supplements of vitamin B$_{12}$ if a reliable dietary source is not consumed. All other nutrient needs can be met through a well-planned lacto-ovo vegetarian or vegan diet.
- Women who do not consume adequate vitamin D or have insufficient sunlight exposure should consume supplemental vitamin D to reduce the risk of low serum calcium in the infant and abnormal neonatal bone metabolism (ADA, 2008). Amounts greater than the Recommended Dietary Allowances (RDA) do not appear to provide added benefits.

**Fetal Alcohol Syndrome (FAS):** a condition characterized by varying degrees of physical and mental growth failure and birth defects caused by maternal intake of alcohol.

**Teratogen:** anything that causes abnormal fetal development and birth defects.

## Alcohol

Alcohol use during pregnancy can cause physical and neurodevelopmental problems, such as mental retardation, learning disabilities, and **fetal alcohol syndrome**. Alcohol does its damage by dehydrating fetal cells, leaving them dead or functionless, or by causing secondary nutrient deficiencies. Because alcohol is a potent **teratogen** and a "safe" level of consumption is not known, women are advised to completely avoid alcohol before and during pregnancy.

## Avoiding Foodborne Illness

Foodborne risks are more dangerous for pregnant women than for most other adults. During pregnancy, listeriosis, caused by the bacterium *Listeria monocytogenes,* may cause only mild, flu-like illness in the mother but may lead to miscarriage, stillbirth, premature delivery, or neonatal infection (Ricciotti, 2008). Pregnant women are 20 times more likely to get listeriosis than other healthy adults, and approximately one-third of all listeriosis cases occur during pregnancy. To reduce the risk of listeriosis, pregnant women should *not* consume the following foods:

• Unpasteurized milk or products made with it
• Raw or undercooked meat, poultry, eggs, fish, or shellfish
• Refrigerated pâtés or meat spreads
• Certain soft cheeses such as feta, Brie, bleu, and Camembert
• Leftover foods and ready-to-eat foods, including hot dogs and deli meats, unless heated until steaming hot

An infection caused by the parasite *Toxoplasma gondii* may be asymptomatic in healthy people or may bring about flu-like symptoms. During pregnancy, the consequences are more serious: if transmitted from mother to fetus in the first trimester, toxoplasmosis can cause mental retardation, blindness, and epilepsy. Eating raw meat is the cause of approximately half of toxoplasmosis infections (Ricciotti, 2008). Pregnant women should be instructed on how to prevent transmission of the parasite, including:

• Cook meat thoroughly
• Peel or wash fresh fruits and vegetables before eating
• Avoid cross contamination in the kitchen by cleaning surfaces and utensils exposed to raw food
• Avoid changing cat litter (cats pass an environmentally resistant form of the organism in their feces)

## Caffeine

A high caffeine intake is associated with spontaneous miscarriage and LBW, but not with birth defects (ADA, 2008). The ADA recommends pregnant women limit their intake of caffeine to 300 mg/day or less.

## Nonnutritive Sweeteners

The use of nonnutritive sweeteners during pregnancy has been studied extensively. Acesulfame potassium (Sunette, Sweet One), aspartame (NutraSweet, Spoonful, Equal), saccharin (Sweet'N Low), sucralose (Splenda), and neotame are all deemed to be safe during pregnancy when consumed at levels within the U.S. Food and Drug Administration (FDA) Acceptable Daily Intake (ADI) guidelines (ADA, 2008). The exception is that women with PKU should not use aspartame because it is made from phenylalanine.

## Herbal Supplements

Because little is known about the safety and efficacy of herbal supplements during pregnancy, it is generally recommended that they not be used during pregnancy and lactation. Herbal

QUICK BITE

Caffeine content of selected beverages and foods

| | *Average Caffeine Content (mg)* |
|---|---|
| 8 oz coffee, generic brewed | 133 (range 102–200) |
| 16 oz coffee, generic brewed | 266 |
| 16 oz Starbucks brewed coffee (Grande) | 320 |
| 8 oz coffee, generic instant | 93 (range 27–173) |
| 8 oz coffee, generic decaffeinated | 5 (range 3–12) |
| 8 oz brewed tea | 53 (range 40–120) |
| 16 oz Snapple, lemon (and diet version) | 42 |
| 12 oz Pepsi | 38 |
| 12 oz Coca-Cola Classic | 35 |
| 7-Up, Sprite | 0 |
| 8.3 oz Red Bull | 80 |
| 8 oz Ben & Jerry's coffee-flavored ice cream | 68 |
| 1 stick Jolt caffeinated gum | 33 |
| 1.55 oz Hershey's chocolate bar | 9 |
| 1 Hershey kiss | 1 |
| 8 oz hot cocoa | 9 (range 3–13) |

**Source:** Center for Science in the Public Interest. *Caffeine content of food & drugs.* Available at www.cspinet.org/new/cafchart.htm. Accessed on 3/28/08.

products are technically unapproved drugs; most drugs cross the placental barrier to some degree, exposing the fetus to potentially teratogenic effects. Unlike approved drugs, little animal or human testing has been done to determine if herbs can cause birth defects or potentially harm mothers and infants.

## Fish

The FDA has issued advisories regarding fish and shellfish consumption during pregnancy due to the risk of methylmercury contamination. Mercury occurs naturally in the environment, including waterways. Bacteria in the water convert mercury to methylmercury, which is absorbed by fish low on the food chain and becomes concentrated in larger, longer-living predatory fish at the top of the food chain. Nearly all fish contain trace amounts of mercury; it accumulates in humans primarily by eating fish.

Mercury can be toxic, particularly to developing brains in fetuses and young children. Mercury poisoning in a fetus can result in learning delays in walking or talking to more severe problems such as cerebral palsy, seizures, and mental retardation. To reduce the risk of methylmercury poisoning, it is recommended that pregnant women, lactating women, and women who may become pregnant:

- Do not eat shark, swordfish, king mackerel, and tilefish
- Limit total intake of seafood to 12 oz/week
- Limit albacore ("white") tuna to 6 oz/week
- Check with the local health department or Environmental Protection Agency to determine which fish from local waters are safe to eat

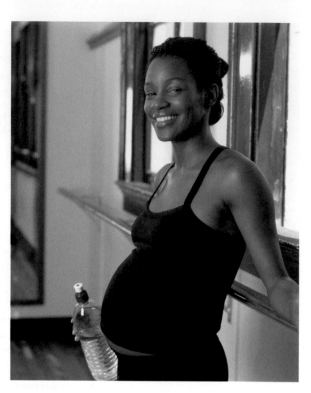

**FIGURE 11.2** Pregnant women are urged to get at least 30 minutes of moderate, safe exercise daily throughout their pregnancies.

## Physical Activity

Healthy pregnant women who do not have medical or obstetric complications are urged to follow the advice for all healthy adults: get at least 30 minutes of moderate exercise on most days of the week. Safe exercise should be encouraged, with attention paid to fall risk and avoiding supine positions during the second and third trimesters (Fig. 11.2). Exercise may play a role in preventing and managing gestational diabetes and fetal macrosomia (ACOG Committee Opinion, 2002).

## Maternal Health

Common complaints associated with pregnancy, such as nausea, heartburn, and constipation, may be prevented or alleviated by nutrition interventions (Table 11.3). More serious health conditions in the mother, whether preexisting or gestational, can greatly impact the course of pregnancy and infant health. Diabetes mellitus, gestational hypertension, and maternal PKU are discussed in the following sections.

### Diabetes Mellitus

Preexisting diabetes increases the risk of congenital malformations (ADA, 2008). Gestational diabetes, which appears in the latter half (after 24 weeks) of pregnancy, increases the risk of macrosomia and can make delivery difficult, increasing the risk of infant shoulder dislocation and cesarean delivery. Although symptoms of gestational diabetes disappear after delivery, women who have had gestational diabetes, especially those who continue to have impaired glucose tolerance in the postpartum period, are at high risk for type 2 diabetes later in life. In the long term, children born to mothers with diabetes are at increased risk for hypertension and high BMI in childhood.

Diabetes mellitus requires nutrition management regardless of whether it was present before conception or developed during gestation as a result of the metabolic changes of

| TABLE 11.3 | Common Complaints Associated with Pregnancy | | |
|---|---|---|---|
| | **Complaint** | **Possible Causes** | **Nutrition Interventions** |
| | Nausea and vomiting (common during the first trimester) | Hypoglycemia, decreased gastric motility, relaxation of the cardiac sphincter, anxiety | Eat easily digested carbohydrate foods (e.g., dry crackers, melba toast, dry cereal, hard candy) before getting out of bed in the morning<br>Eat frequent, small snacks of dry carbohydrates (e.g., crackers, hard candy) to prevent drop in glucose<br>Eat small frequent meals<br>Avoid liquids with meals<br>Limit high-fat foods because they delay gastric emptying<br>Eliminate individual intolerances and foods with a strong odor |
| | Constipation | Relaxation of gastrointestinal muscle tone and motility related to increased progesterone levels<br>Increasing pressure on the GI tract by the fetus<br>Decrease in physical activity<br>Inadequate fiber and fluid intake<br>Use of iron supplements | Increase fiber intake, especially intake of whole-grain breads and cereals. Look for breads that provide at least 2 g fiber/slice and cereals with at least 5 g fiber/serving<br>Drink at least eight 8-oz glasses of liquid daily<br>Try hot water with lemon or prune juice upon waking to help stimulate peristalsis<br>Participate in regular exercise |
| | Heartburn | Decrease in GI motility<br><br>Relaxation of the cardiac sphincter<br>Pressure of the uterus on the stomach | Eat small, frequent meals and eliminate liquids immediately before and after meals to avoid gastric distention<br>Avoid coffee, high-fat foods, and spices<br>Eliminate individual intolerances<br>Avoid lying down or bending over after eating |

pregnancy. Women with preexisting diabetes should achieve glycemic control prior to conception. All women should be screened for gestational diabetes between 24 and 28 weeks of pregnancy. Nutrition recommendations for managing diabetes during pregnancy appear in Box 11.4.

## BOX 11.4    NUTRITIONAL MANAGEMENT OF DIABETES DURING PREGNANCY

- The goals of diet are to achieve weight gain within the recommended range, keep blood glucose levels within the goal range, and to avoid ketosis.
- Total calories required are determined on an individual basis on the basis of an individual's goals.
- Carbohydrates are controlled, but a minimum of 175 g are needed daily.
- Clinical measures such as blood glucose levels and ketones determine how carbohydrates are distributed during the day.
- Glucose control may be improved by allowing less carbohydrates at breakfast and more at other meals.
- Exercise is encouraged if there are no medical or obstetrical complications.

*Source:* American Dietetic Association (ADA). (2008). Position of the American Dietetic Association: Nutrition and lifestyle for healthy pregnancy outcome. *The Journal of the American Dental Association, 108,* 553–561.

## Gestational Hypertension

**Gestational Hypertension:** blood pressure of greater than or equal to 140 or greater than or equal to 90 that develops in the second half of pregnancy and ends with childbirth.

**Gestational hypertension** disease develops in 5% to 8% of pregnancies (MOD, 2006b). It is defined as a systolic blood pressure of greater than or equal to 140 or a diastolic reading of greater than or equal to 90 with onset after 20 weeks gestation. Often gestational hypertension does not occur until 30 weeks or later.

Approximately one-fourth of the gestational hypertension cases progress to **preeclampsia**, a potentially serious disorder characterized by proteinuria. Although most cases are mild and asymptomatic, edema of the hands and face, weight gain greater than or equal to 5 pounds/week, visual disturbances, severe headaches, dizziness, and pain in the upper right abdominal quadrant may occur. Preeclampsia increases maternal and infant morbidity and mortality (ADA, 2008). In rare cases, preeclampsia progresses to **eclampsia**, characterized by grand mal seizures and sometimes coma.

**Preeclampsia:** a toxemia of pregnancy characterized by hypertension accompanied by proteinuria, edema, or both.

**Eclampsia:** a toxemia of pregnancy that develops with the occurrence of one or more convulsions resulting from preeclampsia.

Risk factors for eclampsia include a history of chronic hypertension or preeclampsia in a prior pregnancy, primaparity, multiple pregnancy, maternal age of less than 20 or greater than 35 years, African-American race, and maternal obesity (ADA, 2008).

There is no way to prevent gestational hypertension or preeclampsia. In most cases, delivery "cures" preeclampsia. In high-risk women with low-calcium intakes, high amounts of calcium appear to reduce the risk of preeclampsia (ADA, 2008). Fish oils are being investigated for their potential blood pressure–lowering effects; currently there is no evidence to support the use of omega-3 fatty acid supplements for the prevention of preeclampsia.

## Maternal PKU

**Phenylketonuria (PKU):** an inborn error of phenylalanine (an essential amino acid) metabolism that results in retardation and physical handicaps in newborns if they are not treated with a low-phenylalanine diet beginning shortly after birth.

**Microcephaly:** abnormally small head.

Women who have **phenylketonuria (PKU)** and who consume a normal diet before and during pregnancy have very high blood levels of phenylalanine, which are devastating to the developing fetus. As many as 90% of babies born to mothers with PKU who do not control their phenylalanine intake have mental retardation, and many also have **microcephaly**, heart defects, and LBW. Most of these infants do not inherit PKU and cannot benefit from a low-phenylalanine diet after birth.

To prevent mental retardation and other problems associated with maternal PKU, a rigid low-phenylalanine diet is necessary at least 3 months before conception and throughout the duration of the pregnancy to strictly control blood phenylalanine levels and eliminate risks to the developing fetus. General diet guidelines are listed in Box 11.5.

---

| BOX 11.5 | DIET GUIDELINES FOR PREGNANT WOMEN WITH PKU |
|---|---|

Pregnant women with PKU should be advised that:

- Complete understanding and strict adherence to the diet are vital.
- Protein foods such as meat, fish, poultry, eggs, dairy products, and nuts are high in phenylalanine and must be eliminated.
- Diet drinks and foods sweetened with aspartame (NutraSweet) are strictly forbidden.
- The special PKU formula is expensive and often offensive to adult palates, but it must be consumed in adequate amounts to support fetal growth and to prevent maternal tissue breakdown that would have results similar to those caused by cheating on the diet.
- An adequate calorie intake is necessary for normal protein metabolism.
- Close monitoring of blood phenylalanine levels is essential.

| BOX 11.6 | **FACTORS ASSOCIATED WITH HIGH-RISK PREGNANCIES** |

**Age**
Teens (especially 15 years or younger) and women 35 years or older

**Anthropometric Data**
Prepregnancy BMI <18.5 or >25
Inadequate or excessive weight gain during pregnancy

**Dietary Data**
Nutrient deficiencies or excesses
Disordered eating
Use of a therapeutic diet
Use of alcohol, tobacco, or drugs

**Medical-Psychosocial Data**
Chronic preexisting medical problems such as diabetes, heart disease, pulmonary disease, renal disease, maternal PKU
Development of gestational disorders, such as gestational diabetes and gestational hypertension
Poor obstetric history (LBW, stillbirth, abortion, fetal anomalies), high parity, multipara
Repetitive pregnancies at short intervals (younger than 18 months)
Low socioeconomic status, lack of family support, low level of education, problems with food availability

## Nutrition Care: Assessment and Counseling

The first prenatal visit should identify clients who present with a high-risk pregnancy (Box 11.6). A high-risk pregnancy is likely to produce an LBW infant; LBW infants are more likely to experience complications during delivery and have a higher risk of physical and mental defects. Monitoring continues throughout pregnancy to identify high-risk criteria that may develop during gestation, such as excessive or inadequate weight gain or the development of gestational diabetes.

Many women are motivated during pregnancy to adopt healthy lifestyle changes, which have the potential to make a long-lasting impact on the health of mother and infant. All women should receive prenatal nutrition advice that includes guidelines for healthy eating and diet strategies for preventing or treating common problems as appropriate (Table 11.3). Health care providers are urged to incorporate obesity assessment and counseling into clinical practice before, during, and after pregnancy to help avoid postpartum weight retention (ACOG, 2005).

## ▶ NUTRITION FOR LACTATION

The World Health Organization (WHO) recommends that infants be exclusively breastfed for the first 6 months of life with the introduction of complementary foods thereafter as breastfeeding continues for the first 2 years of life (WHO, 2003). In the United States, both the American Academy of Pediatrics (AAP) and the ADA recommend infants be exclusively

| BOX 11.7 | BENEFITS OF BREASTFEEDING |
|---|---|

**For the Mother**
- Promotes optimal maternal–infant bonding
- Simulates uterine contractions to help control postpartum bleeding and regain prepregnant uterus size
- Provides breast milk, which is readily available and requires no mixing or dilution
- Is less expensive than purchasing bottles, nipples, sterilizing equipment, and formula
- Decreases risk of breast and ovarian cancer
- Delays resumption of menstruation, though not reliable for birth control
- Conserves iron stores by prolonging amenorrhea
- Improves bone density and reduces risk for hip fracture
- Improves glucose profile in gestational diabetes

**For the Infant**
- Increases bonding with mother
- Optimal "natural" nutrition that contains no artificial colorings, flavorings, preservatives, or additives
- Enhances immune system
- Protects against infectious and noninfectious diseases
- Protects against allergies and intolerances
- Decreases the risk of diarrhea and respiratory infections
- Promotes better tooth and jaw development than bottle-feeding because the infant has to suck harder
- Lowers risk of childhood obesity
- Increases cognitive function
- Reduces the risk of heart disease

*Source:* American Dietetic Association (ADA). (2005). Position of the American Dietetic Association: Promoting and supporting breastfeeding. *Journal of American Diet Association, 105*, 810–818.

breastfed for the first 6 months of life and that breastfeeding continue with complementary foods until 1 year of age (AAP, 2005; ADA, 2005). The benefits of breastfeeding for both mother and infant are well recognized (ADA, 2005) (Box 11.7).

## Promoting Breastfeeding

Although almost all women have the potential to successfully breastfeed, lactation may fail for a variety of reasons (Box 11.8). As a learned behavior, not a physiologic response, the ability to successfully breastfeed and the duration of lactation can be positively impacted by counseling. Preparation for breastfeeding should begin prenatally with counseling, guidance, and support for both the woman and her partner and continue throughout the gestational period. Hospital practices that promote breastfeeding appear in Box 11.9. Contraindications to breastfeeding are listed in Box 11.10.

Although almost 70% of newborns are breastfed, only 36% of all infants are still breastfed at 6 months of age (MOD, 2005). Breastfeeding for at least 12 weeks is highly beneficial to both the infant and mother (Krummel, 2007) and is associated with lower maternal BMI later in life (Rooney et al., 2005). However, even a short period of breastfeeding is better than not breastfeeding at all. Women should be encouraged to breastfeed for as long as they are able and not be made to feel guilty if they fall short of the recommendations.

| BOX 11.8 | FACTORS THAT IMPAIR LACTATION |

**Impaired Letdown, Related to**
Embarrassment or stress
Fatigue
Negative attitude, lack of desire, lack of family support
Excessive intake of caffeine or alcohol
Smoking
Drugs

**Failure to Establish Lactation, Related to**
Delayed or infrequent feedings
Weak infant sucking because of anesthesia during labor and delivery
Nipple discomfort or engorgement
Lack of support especially from baby's father

**Decreased Demand, Related to**
Supplemental bottles of formula or water
Introduction of solid food
Infant's lack of interest

| BOX 11.9 | HOSPITAL PRACTICES THAT PROMOTE BREASTFEEDING |

- Offer the infant the breast within 1 hour of birth and at frequent intervals thereafter. Hospital procedures should allow for immediate maternal–infant contact after delivery and for true demand feedings preferably through rooming-in.
- Inform all pregnant women about the benefits and management of breastfeeding.
- Show mothers how to breastfeed and maintain lactation even if they are separated from their infants.
- Give newborn infants no food or drink other than breast milk unless medically indicated.
- Give no artificial teats or pacifiers (e.g., dummies, soothers) to breastfeeding infants.
- Foster the establishment of breastfeeding support groups and refer mothers to them upon discharge from the hospital or clinic.

*Source:* American Dietetic Association (ADA). (2005). Position of the American Dietetic Association: Promoting and supporting breastfeeding. *Journal of American Diet Association, 105*, 810–818.

| BOX 11.10 | CONTRAINDICATIONS TO BREASTFEEDING |

- Galactosemia in the infant
- Illegal drug use in the mother
- Active tuberculosis
- HIV/AIDS (In some countries, the risk of infant mortality from not breastfeeding may outweigh the risk of acquiring HIV through breast milk.)
- Use of certain drugs, such as radioactive isotopes, antimetabolites, cancer chemotherapy agents, lithium, ergotamine

*Source:* American Dietetic Association (ADA). (2005). Position of the American Dietetic Association: Promoting and supporting breastfeeding. *Journal of American Diet Association, 105*, 810–818.

# Maternal Diet

Nutritional needs during lactation are based on the nutritional content of breast milk and the energy "cost" of producing milk. Compared with pregnancy, the need for some nutrients increases, whereas the need for other nutrients falls (Table 11.2). The healthy diet consumed during pregnancy should continue during lactation. Key recommendations during breast-feeding are listed in Box 11.2.

## Calories

Women use approximately 500 calories above their normal total daily calorie needs to produce breast milk. Approximately 100 to 150 of these calories come from fat stored during pregnancy, and the remaining ones come from extra calories consumed. An extra 330 cal/day are recommended for the first 6 months of lactation and an extra 400 calories for the second 6 months for women who exclusively breastfeed; partial breastfeeding uses fewer calories. In theory, mobilizing fat calories for the production of breast milk can contribute to a calorie deficit and weight loss over time. In reality, breastfeeding is not always associated with return to preconception weight, and some women actually gain weight during lactation (Lovelady et al., 2006).

For the sample woman used for the MyPyramid plan in Figure 11.1, the food plan recommended while she exclusively breastfeeds is 2200 calories for the first 6 months and 2400 calories for the second 6 months, representing a 200- and then 400-calorie increase above her nonpregnant calorie needs for the first and second 6 months of lactation, respectively. These calorie levels would allow her to mobilize fat accumulated during pregnancy to provide the additional calories needed to produce enough breast milk.

Adequacy of calorie intake is determined by changes in a woman's weight. Women who lose too much weight need to increase their calorie intake. Conversely, women who are not losing weight while lactating can reduce their calorie intake. A study by Lovelady et al. showed that overweight lactating women can successfully lose 1 pound/week without impeding the growth of their infants—the outcome of a decrease in milk production (Lovelady et al., 2000). Most women need at least 1800 cal/day to obtain adequate amounts of nutrients needed during pregnancy. Women who failed to gain enough weight during pregnancy or who have inadequate fat reserves have higher calorie requirements.

## Fluid

Another nutritional consideration during lactation is fluid intake. It is suggested that breastfeeding mothers drink a glass of fluid every time the baby nurses and with all meals. Thirst is a good indicator of need except among women who live in a dry climate or who exercise in hot weather. Fluids consumed in excess of thirst quenching do not increase milk volume.

## Vitamins and Minerals

For many vitamins and minerals, requirements during lactation are higher than during pregnancy. In general, an inadequate maternal diet decreases the *quantity* of milk produced, not the *quality*. The exceptions are thiamin, riboflavin, vitamin $B_6$, vitamin $B_{12}$, vitamin A, and iodine: low maternal intake or stores of these nutrients reduces their amount in breast milk and may compromise infant nutrition (Allen, 2005). Maternal supplements can correct inadequacies; their use may be prudent for the majority of lactating women in developing and industrialized nations (Allen, 2005). However supplements are made to "add to" a healthy diet, not replace it.

## Attaining Healthy BMI

The highest incidence of obesity in women is during the childbearing years (Krummel, 2007). In a study by Rooney et al., excess weight gain during pregnancy, insufficient weight loss at 6 months postpartum, and high prepregnancy BMI were predictive of BMI 15 years later, as well as for risk of diabetes, heart disease, and hypertension (Rooney et al., 2005). Women who had lost most of their pregnancy weight by 6 months postpartum, had breast-fed, and/or had participated in regular aerobic exercise tended to gain the least weight over the 15-year follow-up period. Many women do not realize that weight gained during their reproductive years affects their health in midlife (Krummel, 2006).

For many women, the last visit to the obstetrician is at 6 weeks postpartum in the absence of complications. At that time, over two-thirds of women have not achieved their prepregnancy weight (Krummel, 2007). Some women gain additional weight during the postpartum period. Increased food intake, greater access to food during the day, less exercise, an increase in television viewing, and less social support may all contribute to postpartum weight gain (Johnson et al., 2006).

Suggestions for managing postpartum weight are as follows (Krummel, 2007):

- Assess readiness to change. Many women say they want to lose weight but are not ready to make behavioral changes, such as avoid high-fat foods, eat more fiber, and exercise at least three times per week.
- Assess lactation status, dietary intake, and activity levels. Although 44% of nonpregnant women of childbearing age were trying to lose weight, only 21% were consuming fewer calories and engaging in at least 150 minutes of physical activity per week (Cogswell et al., 1999).
- Assess for stress or depressive symptoms, which complicate weight management.

## NURSING PROCESS: *Normal Pregnancy*

Jana is a 33-year-old professional who is 20 weeks pregnant with her first baby. Her prepregnancy BMI was 19.2. She has gained 7 pounds and complains of constipation. She plans on returning to work 6 weeks after delivery and wants to limit her weight gain so that she can fit into her clothes by the time she returns to work. She has asked you what she should eat that will be good for the baby but not cause her to get fat.

| Assessment |
| --- |

| Medical-Psychosocial History | • Medical history such as diabetes, hypertension, lactose intolerance, PKU, or other chronic disease |
| --- | --- |
| | • Use of medications and over-the-counter drugs |
| | • Adequacy of sunlight exposure |
| | • Symptoms of constipation including frequency, interventions attempted, and results |
| | • Other complaints related to pregnancy, such as heartburn |
| | • Usual frequency and intensity of physical activity |
| | • Attitude about pregnancy and weight gain; knowledge about normal amount and pattern of weight gain during pregnancy |

*(nursing process continues on page 264)*

## NURSING PROCESS: *Normal Pregnancy* (continued)

|  |  |
|---|---|
|  | • Attitude/plan regarding breastfeeding |
|  | • Level of family/social support |
| Anthropometric Assessment | Height, prepregnancy weight, pattern of 7-pound weight gain during pregnancy |
| Biochemical and Physical Assessment | • Hemoglobin to screen for iron deficiency anemia. (Many laboratory values change during pregnancy related to normal changes in maternal physiology and so cannot be validly compared with nonpregnancy standards.) |
|  | • Glucose, other laboratory values as available |
|  | • Blood pressure |
| Dietary Assessment | • How does the client describe her appetite? |
|  | • Does the client follow a balanced and varied diet that includes all food groups from MyPyramid in reasonable amounts? |
|  | • Does the client eat at regular intervals? |
|  | • How has the client modified her intake since becoming pregnant? |
|  | • Does the client eat nonfoods or have unusual eating habits? |
|  | • Does the client take a vitamin and/or mineral supplement? |
|  | • Does the client use alcohol, tobacco, caffeine, or herbal supplements? |
|  | • Is the client knowledgeable about nutrient needs during pregnancy? |
|  | • What cultural, religious, and ethnic influences affect the client's food choices? |

### Diagnosis

|  |  |
|---|---|
| Possible Nursing Diagnoses | • Constipation related to pregnancy |
|  | • Health-seeking behaviors, as evidenced by lack of knowledge of appropriate diet for pregnancy and a desire to learn |
|  | • Imbalanced nutrition: less than body requirements related to voluntary food restriction to limit weight gain |

### Planning

|  |  |
|---|---|
| Client Outcomes | The client will: |
|  | • Avoid constipation |
|  | • Identify measures that prevent constipation |
|  | • Explain the importance of nutrition for her health and for fetal growth and development |
|  | • Consume an adequate, varied, and balanced diet based on MyPyramid |
|  | • Explain the amount and pattern of recommended weight gain |
|  | • Gain approximately 1 pound of weight per week |

*(nursing process continues on page 265)*

## NURSING PROCESS: Normal Pregnancy (continued)

| Nursing Interventions | |
|---|---|
| Nutrition Therapy | • Increase fiber intake gradually to prevent constipation<br>• Provide an eating plan that includes all food groups and emphasizes ample fruits and vegetables; whole grains; lean protein; fat-free dairy; and healthy fats with total amounts/day based on her calorie needs<br>• Encourage adequate fluid intake due to increased fiber intake |
| Client Teaching | Instruct the client on:<br>• The role of nutrition and weight gain in the outcome of pregnancy<br>• The role of fiber and fluids in preventing and alleviating constipation<br>Eating plan essentials, including<br>• Choosing a variety of foods within each major food group<br>• Selecting the appropriate number of servings from each major food group<br>• Consuming sources of fiber such as bran and whole-grain breads and cereals, dried peas and beans, fresh fruits, and vegetables<br>Behavioral matters including<br>• Abandoning the idea of limiting weight gain to fit into clothes after pregnancy<br>• Eating small, frequent meals<br>• The importance of maintaining physical activity<br>Where to find more information (see websites at the end of this chapter) |

| Evaluation | |
|---|---|
| Evaluate and Monitor | • Monitor for complaints of constipation<br>• Monitor amount and pattern of weight gain<br>• Suggest changes in the food plan as needed<br>• Provide periodic feedback and support |

## ▶ How Do You Respond?

**Why don't pregnant women need to increase their calcium intake during pregnancy?** The DRI for women aged 19 to 50 years—whether pregnant or not—is 1000 mg. The reason why the DRI for calcium does not increase during pregnancy is that the body compensates for the increased need by more than doubling the rate of calcium absorption. If calcium intake was adequate before pregnancy, the amount consumed does not need to increase.

**Is it true that pregnant and breastfeeding women should avoid certain foods to prevent allergies from developing in their children?** According to a clinical report published by the AAP, there is insufficient evidence to a significant protective effect of maternal dietary restriction during pregnancy or lactation (Greer et al., 2008). There is no convincing evidence that women who avoid eating peanuts or other foods during pregnancy or lactation lower their child's risk of allergies.

▶ CASE STUDY

Sarah is 28 years old and 7 months pregnant with her third child. Her other children are aged 2½ and 1½ years. She had uncomplicated pregnancies and deliveries. Sarah is 5 ft. 6 in. tall; she weighed 142 pounds at the beginning of this pregnancy, which made her prepregnancy BMI 23. She has gained 24 pounds so far. Prior to her first pregnancy, her BMI was 20 (124 pounds). She is unhappy about her weight gain, but the stress of having two young children and being a stay-at-home mom made losing weight impossible.

She went online for her MyPyramid plan, which recommends she consume 2400 cal/day. She doesn't think she eats that much because she seems to have constant heartburn. She takes a prenatal supplement so feels pretty confident that even if her intake is not perfect, she is getting all the nutrients she needs through her supplement. A typical day's intake for her:

| | |
|---|---|
| **Breakfast:** | Cornflakes with whole milk (because the children drink whole milk)<br>Orange juice |
| **Snack:** | Bran muffin and whole milk |
| **Lunch:** | Either a peanut butter and jelly sandwich or tuna fish sandwich with mayonnaise<br>Snack crackers<br>Whole milk<br>Pudding or cookies |
| **Snack:** | Ice cream |
| **Dinner:** | Macaroni and cheese<br>Green beans<br>Roll and butter<br>Whole milk<br>Cake or ice cream for dessert |
| **Evening:** | Chips and salsa |

- Does she have any risk factors for a high-risk pregnancy?
- Evaluate her prepregnancy weight and weight gain thus far. How much total weight should she gain?
- Based on the 2400-calorie meal pattern in Figure 11.1, what does Sarah need to eat more of? What is she eating in more than the recommended amounts? How would you suggest she modify her intake to minimize heartburn?
- What would you tell her about weight gain during pregnancy? What strategies would you suggest to her after her baby is born that would help her regain her healthy weight?
- Is her attitude about supplements appropriate? What would you tell her about supplements?

▶ Devise a 1-day menu for her that would provide all the food she needs in the recommended amounts and alleviate her heartburn.

## STUDY QUESTIONS

1. A woman trying to become pregnant was told by her physician to take a daily supplement containing 400 micrograms of folic acid. She asks why a supplement is better than eating folic acid through food. Which statement is the nurses' best response?
   a. "There are few natural sources of folate in food."
   b. "Synthetic folic acid in supplements and fortified foods is better absorbed, more available, and a more reliable source than the folate found naturally in food."
   c. "Folate in food is equally as good as folic acid in supplements. It is just easier to take it in pill form and then you don't have to worry about how much you're getting in food."
   d. "If you are sure that you eat at least five servings of fruits and vegetables everyday, you don't really need to take a supplement of folic acid."

2. A woman who was at her healthy weight when she got pregnant is distraught by her 5-pound weight gain between 20 and 24 weeks of gestation. Prior to this office visit, her weight gain was right on target. What is the nurse's best response?

a. "Gaining slightly more or less than the recommended monthly gain is not a cause for concern when it happens one time. It is only when a pattern of abnormal weight gain occurs that it is viewed as a potential problem."

b. "Although it is slightly less than the recommended amount, it is not a cause for concern. Just be sure to follow your meal plan next month so you get enough calories and nutrients."

c. "I recommend you write down everything you eat for a few days so we can identify where the problem lies."

d. "A 6½-pound weight gain in one month at this point in your pregnancy may be a sign that you are at risk of preeclampsia. You should cut back on the 'extras' in your diet to limit your weight gain for next month."

3. Which of the following conditions are associated with a high-risk pregnancy? Select all that apply.
   a. Prepregnancy BMI of 20
   b. Prepregnancy BMI >25
   c. Maternal age of 30
   d. Pregnancies spaced <18 months apart
   e. Lack of family support
   f. Excessive weight gain

4. At her first prenatal visit, an overweight woman asks how much weight she should gain during the course of her pregnancy. What is the nurse's best response?
   a. "You should not gain any weight during your pregnancy. You have adequate calorie reserves to meet all the energy demands of pregnancy without gaining additional weight."
   b. "You should try to gain less than 15 pounds."
   c. "Aim for a 15- to 25-pound weight gain."
   d. "The recommended weight gain for your weight is 25 to 35 pounds."

5. Which of the following statements indicates that the pregnant woman understands the recommendations about caffeine intake during pregnancy?
   a. "I have to give up drinking coffee and cola."
   b. "I will limit my intake of coffee to about 2 cups a day and avoid other sources of caffeine."
   c. "As long as I don't drink coffee, I can eat other sources of caffeine because they don't contain enough to cause any problems."
   d. "Caffeine is harmless during pregnancy, so I am allowed to consume as much as I want."

6. What nutrient is not likely to be consumed in adequate amounts during pregnancy so a supplement is recommended?
   a. Iron
   b. Calcium
   c. Vitamin $B_{12}$
   d. Vitamin C

7. A woman at 5 weeks gestation is complaining of nausea throughout the day. What should the nurse recommend?
   a. Small frequent meals of easily digested carbohydrates
   b. Small frequent meals that are high in protein
   c. A liquid diet until the nausea subsides
   d. A low fiber intake

8. Which of the following statements is true?
   a. "Women who breastfeed almost always achieve their prepregnancy weight at 6 weeks postpartum."

b. "Weight loss during lactation is not recommended because it lowers the quantity and quality of breast milk produced."

c. "Breastfeeding women do not have to increase their intake by the full amount of calories it 'costs' to produce milk because they can mobilize fat stored during pregnancy for some of the extra energy required."

d. "Women do not need to increase their calorie intake at all for the first 6 months of breastfeeding because they can use calories stored in fat to produce milk."

## KEY CONCEPTS

- Although proper nutrition before and during pregnancy cannot guarantee a successful pregnancy outcome, it does profoundly affect fetal development and birth.

- A healthy diet based on MyPyramid food patterns is recommended before, during, and after pregnancy, with few modifications.

- Two nutrition-related preconception interventions with proven health benefits are folic acid supplementation and obesity control.

- All women of childbearing age who are capable of becoming pregnant are urged to consume 400 micrograms of synthetic folic acid daily—through fortified foods or supplements—to reduce the risk of neural tube defects. The most critical period for the development of neural tube defects is the first month after conception when a woman may not even know she is pregnant.

- Weight gain recommendations during pregnancy are based on a woman's BMI: 25 to 35 pounds for women of normal weight, 28 to 40 pounds for underweight women, 15 to 25 pounds for overweight women, and 11 to 20 pounds for obese women.

- The recommended pattern of weight gain for normal-weight women is 1.1 to 4.4 pounds in the first trimester and approximately 1 pound/week for the rest of pregnancy. This pattern is adjusted up or down for women who are not within their healthy weight range at the time of conception.

- Calorie requirements do not increase during the first trimester. In the second trimester, calorie needs increase by 340 cal/day and in the third trimester by 452 cal/day.

- A woman who eats a varied diet with adequate calories should be able to meet her increased need for vitamins and minerals through food alone except for iron. Iron supplements are recommended. Folic acid requirements increase to 600 micrograms during pregnancy; supplements and/or fortified foods can provide this amount. Multivitamin and minerals are recommended for specific situations, such as during iron deficiency, for women carrying two or more fetuses, and when intake is poor.

- Women are urged to avoid alcohol before and during pregnancy because a safe level is not known.

- The consequences of foodborne illness can be devastating for a developing fetus. Pregnant women are urged to take precautions to avoid foodborne illness.

- Pregnant women are advised to limit their caffeine intake to 300 mg/day or less—the equivalent of approximately 2 cups of coffee. Caffeine is associated with LBW, but not with birth defects.

- Nonnutritive sweeteners are safe to use during pregnancy with the amounts specified by the FDA.

- Herbal supplements should not be used during pregnancy because their safety has not been tested during pregnancy or lactation.

- Women are advised to limit their intake of predatory fish and to heed local advisories for fish consumption to limit their exposure to methylmercury. Mercury poisoning in a fetus can result in developmental delays, cerebral palsy, seizures, and mental retardation.

● Pregnant woman should engage in moderate physical activity for at least 30 min/day on most days of the week. Safe activities include those that do not have a risk of fall or require lying down in the supine position after the second trimester of pregnancy.

● Diabetes, gestational hypertension, and maternal PKU are maternal health conditions that can greatly impact fetal development and the course of pregnancy. Women with these conditions must be closely monitored.

● A screening preformed at the first prenatal visit can identify women at potential nutritional risk during pregnancy and provides baseline data for ongoing monitoring. Adequacy of weight gain is related to adequacy of calorie intake.

● Nutrition counseling should be initiated early in prenatal care and continue throughout the pregnancy. It should stress the importance of appropriate weight gain, ways to improve overall intake, and the benefits of breastfeeding.

● Breastfeeding is recommended for the first 12 months of life. In addition to being uniquely suited to infant growth and development, it imparts other significant benefits to both infant and mother.

● Almost all women are capable of breastfeeding.

● The healthy diet recommended during pregnancy should be continued during lactation. Although more calories are needed during lactation than pregnancy, women can eat less than the total calories needed and mobilize calories stored as fat to help regain prepregnancy weight.

● Thirst is a reliable indicator of fluid need for most women during lactation.

● Generally when maternal intake of nutrients is inadequate, the quantity, not the quality, of breast milk is diminished.

● In the postpartum period, attaining a health BMI is important for avoiding obesity and its health risks later in life.

## ANSWER KEY

1. **FALSE** The amount of weight a woman gains during pregnancy is an important indicator of fetal growth. However, adequate weight gain during pregnancy cannot by itself ensure the delivery of a normal-birth-weight infant.

2. **FALSE** Obese women should gain 11 to 20 pounds during pregnancy. It is not known how much weight severely obese women should gain during pregnancy.

3. **TRUE** Fortified cereals are a significant source of folic acid. In fact, the recommended amount of folic acid could easily be exceeded with fortified cereal.

4. **TRUE** Excessive weight gain is likely to result in an increase in maternal fat stores, increasing the likelihood that prepregnancy weight will not be restored after delivery.

5. **FALSE** The RDA for calcium does not increase during pregnancy because calcium absorption greatly increases. Calcium needs can be met with the equivalent of 3 cups of milk daily.

6. **FALSE** Pregnant and lactating women as well as women who may become pregnant are advised to eliminate only shark, swordfish, king mackerel, and tilefish from their diets; white albacore tuna should be limited to 6 oz/week, and other fish and shellfish can be consumed in amounts up to 12 oz/week as long as any one particular type of fish is not eaten more than once a week. Local advisories about fish caught in local waters should also be heeded.

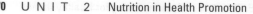 

7. **TRUE** Calorie requirements do not increase until the second trimester and even then the increase is small: an additional 340 calories for the second trimester and an additional 452 calories in the third trimester.

8. **TRUE** Lactation increases calorie recommendations by 500 for the first 6 months of breastfeeding and by 400 for the second 6 months. Women may eat fewer calories than this and still produce enough milk by mobilizing calories stored as fat.

9. **TRUE** An inadequate maternal intake of nutrients decreases the quantity of breast milk produced, not the quality.

10. **TRUE** Thirst is a good indicator of the need for fluids except among women who live in a dry climate or exercise in hot weather.

## WEBSITES

*Information on nutrition as it relates to pregnancy and lactation is available at*

March of Dimes at **www.marchofdimes.com**
Government nutrition information center at **www.nutrition.gov**
American Dietetic Association at **www.eatright.org**
LaLèche League International at **www.lalecheleague.org**
MyPyramid for Pregnancy and Breastfeeding at **www.mypyramid.gov**
American College of Obstetricians and Gynecologists at **www.acog.org**
American Academy of Pediatrics at **www.aap.org**
Supplemental Nutrition Program for Women, Infants, and Children (WIC) at
  **www.fns.usda.gov/fns**
FDA food information website for more on risks of mercury in fish and shellfish at
  **www.cfsan.fda.gov/seafood1.html**

## REFERENCES

Allen, L. (2005). Multiple micronutrients in pregnancy and lactation: An overview. *The American Journal of Clinical Nutrition, 81*(Suppl.), 1206S–1212S.

American Academy of Pediatrics (AAP). (2005). Breastfeeding and the use of human milk: Policy statement. *Pediatrics, 115*, 496–506.

American College of Obstetricians and Gynecologists. ACOG Committee Opinion. Number 267. (2002). Exercise during pregnancy and the postpartum period. *Obstetrics and Gynecology, 99*, 171–173.

American College of Obstetricians and Gynecologists. ACOG Committee Opinion. Number 315. (2005). Obesity in pregnancy. *Obstetrics and Gynecology, 106*, 671–675.

American Dietetic Association (ADA). (2005). Position of the American Dietetic Association: Promoting and supporting breastfeeding. *Journal of the American Dietetic Association, 105*, 810–818.

American Dietetic Association (ADA). (2008). Position of the American Dietetic Association: Nutrition and lifestyle for a healthy pregnancy outcome. *Journal of the American Dietetic Association, 108*, 553–560.

Centers for Disease Control and Prevention (CDC). (2006). *Preconception health and care.* Available at www.cdc.gov/ncbddd/preconception/default.htm. Accessed on 3/14/08.

Cogswell, M., Scanlon, K., Fein, S., et al. (1999). Medically advised, mother's personal target, and actual weight gain during pregnancy. *Obstetrics and Gynecology, 94*, 616–622.

Fowles, E. R. (2006). What's a pregnant woman to eat? A review of current USDA Dietary Guidelines and MyPyramid. *Journal of Perinatal Education, 15*, 28–33.

Greer, F. R., Sicherer, S. H., & Burks, A. W., and the Committee on Nutrition and Section on Allergy and Immunology. (2008). Effects of early nutritional interventions on the development of atopic disease in infants and children: The role of maternal dietary restriction, breastfeeding, timing of introduction of complementary foods, and hydrolyzed formulas. *Pediatrics, 121*, 183–191.

Hanson, M., Gluckman, P., Bier, D., et al. (2004). Report on the 2nd World Congress on Fetal Origins of Adult Disease. *Pediatric Research, 55*, 894–897.

Institute of Medicine (IOM). (in press). *Weight gain during pregnancy: Examining the guidelines.* Washington, DC: National Academies Press.

Institute of Medicine (IOM). (1998). *Dietary reference intakes for thiamin, riboflavin, niacin, vitamin B6, folate, vitamin B12, pantothenic acid, biotin, and choline.* Washington, DC: National Academies Press.

Institute of Medicine (IOM). (2005). *Dietary reference intakes for energy, carbohydrates, fiber, fat, fatty acids, cholesterol, protein, and amino acids (macronutrients).* Washington, DC: National Academies Press.

Johnson, D. B., Gerstein, D. E., Evans, A. E., et al. (2006). Preventing obesity: A life cycle perspective. *Journal of the American Dietetic Association, 106,* 97–102.

Krummel, D. (2007). Postpartum weight control: A vicious cycle. *Journal of the American Dietetic Association, 107,* 37–40.

Lovelady, C. A., Garner, K. E., Moreno, K. L., et al. (2000). The effect of weight loss in overweight, lactating women on the growth of their infants. *The New England Journal of Medicine, 342,* 449–453.

Lovelady, C. A., Stephenson, K. G., Kuppler, K. M., et al. (2006). The effects of dieting on food and nutrient intake of lactating women. *Journal of the American Dietetic Association, 106,* 908–912.

March of Dimes (MOD). (2005). *Quick reference and fact sheets: Breastfeeding.* Available at www.marchofdimes.com/printableArticles/14332_9148.asp. Accessed on 3/24/08.

March of Dimes (MOD). (2006a). *Preconception risk reduction: Folic acid.* Available at www.marchofdimes.com/printableArticles/19695_1151.asp. Accessed on 3/17/08.

March of Dimes (MOD). (2006b). *Quick reference: Fact sheets. High blood pressure during pregnancy.* Available at www.marchofdimes.com/printableArticles/14332_1222.asp. Accessed on 3/21/08.

Mayo Clinic. (2007). *Pregnancy nutrition: Essential nutrients when you're eating for two.* Available at www.mayclinic.com/health/pregnancynutrition/PR0110. Accessed on 3/17/08.

Polley, B. A., Wing, R. R., & Sims, C. J. (2002). Randomized controlled trial to prevent excessive weight gain in pregnant women. *International Journal of Obesity, 26,* 1494–1502.

Ricciotti, H. (2008). Nutrition and lifestyle for a healthy pregnancy. *American Journal of Lifestyle Medicine, 2,* 151–158.

Rooney, B., Schauberger, C., & Mathiason, M. (2005). Impact of perinatal weight change on long-term obesity and obesity-related illnesses. *Obstetrics and Gynecology, 106,* 1349–1356.

USDHHS, USDA. (2005). *Dietary Guidelines for Americans.* Available at www.health.gov/dietaryguidelines. Accessed on 3/26/08.

World Health Organization (WHO). (2003). *Global strategy for infant and young child feeding.* Geneva, Switzerland: World Health Organization.

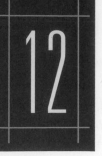

# Nutrition for Infants, Children, and Adolescents

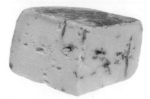

| TRUE | FALSE | |
|:---:|:---:|---|
| ☐ | ☐ | **1** Infants have higher requirements per kilogram of body weight for calories and most nutrients than adults do. |
| ☐ | ☐ | **2** If breastfeeding is discontinued before the infant's first birthday, it should be replaced with iron-fortified infant formula. |
| ☐ | ☐ | **3** Protein is the nutrient of most concern when solids are introduced into the diet. |
| ☐ | ☐ | **4** A potential problem with early introduction of solid foods is overfeeding. |
| ☐ | ☐ | **5** The risk of nutrient deficiencies among American toddlers is low. |
| ☐ | ☐ | **6** The *Dietary Guidelines for Americans* do not apply to children, only adolescents and adults. |
| ☐ | ☐ | **7** Iron deficiency in young children may be related to drinking too much milk. |
| ☐ | ☐ | **8** To decrease the risk of overweight, parents need to be in charge of how much food their children eat. |
| ☐ | ☐ | **9** Overweight youth are at risk for the same complications from overweight that afflict adults, namely type 2 diabetes, high blood pressure, and metabolic syndrome. |
| ☐ | ☐ | **10** Adolescents consume more soft drinks than milk. |

## *UPON COMPLETION OF THIS CHAPTER, YOU WILL BE ABLE TO*

- Compare breast feeding to formula feeding.
- Explain how adequacy of intake is assessed for the pediatric population.
- Give examples of feeding skills seen throughout the first year of life.
- Estimate a child's calorie requirements according to MyPyramid recommendations based on age and activity level.
- Describe common eating practices of children that may place them at nutritional risk.
- Summarize nutritional concerns that arise during childhood and adolescence.
- Evaluate a youth's diet according to MyPyramid food intake recommendations.

An intake of adequate calories and nutrients in children and adolescents promotes optimal physical, social, and cognitive growth and development (ADA, 2006). Children and adolescents who do not consume enough calories and nutrients are at increased risk of impaired health, such as iron deficiency anemia and growth retardation in childhood and an increased risk of certain chronic diseases in adulthood, such as cardiovascular disease, osteoporosis, and certain types of cancer (ADA, 2006).

Actual nutrient requirements vary according to health status, activity pattern, and growth rate. The greater the rate of growth, the more intense the nutritional needs. Although the focus of childhood nutrition has traditionally been on getting enough calories and nutrients, problems related to overconsumption are much more prevalent among today's American children. Nutritional guidance for children has expanded beyond "getting enough" to include recommendations for healthy eating to reduce the risk of chronic disease related to nutritional excesses.

# ▶ INFANCY (BIRTH TO 1 YEAR)

Excluding fetal growth, growth in the first year of life is more rapid than at any other time in the life cycle. Birth weight doubles by 4 to 6 months of age and triples by the first birthday. Length increases by approximately 10 in. during the first year. Adequate calories and nutrients are needed to support the unprecedented rate of growth.

Recommendations for the amount of calories, macronutrients, vitamins, and minerals infants should consume are based on the average intakes of healthy full-term newborns who are exclusively breast-fed by well nourished mothers. (IOM, 2002) Although the total amount of calories and nutrients are generally far less than what adults need, the infant's needs are much higher per kilogram of body weight. Proportionately, infants use large amounts of energy and nutrients to fuel their body processes and growth.

## Breast Milk

Breast milk is specifically designed to support optimal growth and development in the newborn and its composition makes it uniquely superior for infant feeding (Box 12.1)

---

| BOX 12.1 | COMPOSITION OF BREAST MILK |
| --- | --- |

- The protein content is adequate to support growth and development without contributing to an excessive renal solute load.
- The majority of the protein is easy-to-digest whey.
- Breast milk contains small amounts of amino acids that may be harmful in large amounts (e.g., phenylalanine) and high levels of amino acids that infants cannot synthesize well (e.g., taurine).
- The fat in breast milk is easily digested because of fat-digesting enzymes contained in the milk.
- The content of linoleic acid (an essential fatty acid) is high.
- The high level of cholesterol is believed to help infants develop enzyme systems capable of handling cholesterol later in life.
- Breast milk contains amylase (a starch-digesting enzyme), which may promote starch digestion in early infancy when pancreatic amylase is low or absent.
- Breast milk contains enough minerals to support adequate growth and development, but not excessive amounts that would burden immature kidneys with a high renal solute load.
- The minerals are mostly protein-bound and balanced to enhance bioavailability. For instance, the rate of iron absorption from breast milk is approximately 50% compared with about 4% for iron-fortified formulas. Zinc absorption is better from breast milk than from either cow's milk or formula.
- All vitamins needed for growth and health are supplied in breast milk, but the vitamin content of breast milk varies with the mother's diet.
- The renal solute load of breast milk is approximately one-half that of commercial formulas. The low renal solute load is suited to the immature kidneys' inability to concentrate urine.
- Although they are more abundant in colostrum, antibodies and antiinfective factors are present in mature breast milk. Bifidus factor promotes the growth of normal GI flora (e.g., *Lactobacillus bifidus*) that protect the infant against harmful GI bacteria.

(APA, 2005). Exclusive breast-feeding for the first 6 months of life followed by optimal complementary feeding are critical public health measures aimed at reducing and preventing morbidity and mortality in young children (Krebs & Hambidge, 2007). Adequacy of intake is determined by monitoring weight for height on growth charts. Research in developed and developing countries shows that breast-feeding decreases the incidence and/or severity of infectious diseases. Some studies suggest that older children and adults who were breast-fed have a lower risk of type 1 and type 2 diabetes, lymphoma, leukemia, Hodgkin disease, overweight, obesity, hypercholesterolemia, and asthma compared with individuals who were not breast-fed (APA, 2005). The maternal benefits of breast-feeding are presented in Chapter 11.

Because of the unquestionable benefits to both mother and infant, the American Academy of Pediatrics (AAP) recommends exclusive breast-feeding for the first 6 months of life, which, with few exceptions, is considered adequate to meet the needs of healthy, full-term infants (Box 12.2). Even after solid foods are introduced, breast-feeding should continue for at least the first 12 months of age. What the breast-feeding mother needs to know appears in Box 12.3.

| BOX 12.2 | AMERICAN ACADEMY OF PEDIATRICS RECOMMENDATIONS FOR SUPPLEMENTS FOR BREAST-FED, HEALTHY FULL-TERM INFANTS |

- IM vitamin K after the first feeding and within the first 6 hours of life.
- 200 IU of oral vitamin D drops daily beginning in the first 2 months of life and continuing daily until daily intake of vitamin D–fortified formula or milk is approximately 2 cups.
- Fluoride should not be given during the first 6 months of life; thereafter the decision to provide supplemental fluoride should be based on the fluoride content of the drinking water and other sources, including toothpaste.

*Source:* American Academy of Pediatrics. (2005). Policy statement. Breastfeeding and the use of human milk. *Pediatrics, 115,* 496–506.

| BOX 12.3 | WHAT THE BREAST-FEEDING MOTHER NEEDS TO KNOW |

- The infant should be allowed to nurse for 5 minutes on each side on the first day to achieve letdown and milk ejection. By the end of the first week, the infant should be nursing up to 15 minutes per side.
- In the first few weeks of breast-feeding, the infant may nurse 8 to 12 times every 24 hours. Mothers should offer the breast whenever the infant shows early signs of hunger, such as increased alertness, physical activity, mouthing, or rooting. After breast-feeding is well established, eight feedings every 24 hours may be appropriate.
- The first breast offered should be alternated with every feeding so both breasts receive equal stimulation and draining.
- Even though the infant will be able to virtually empty the breast within 5 to 10 minutes once the milk supply is established, the infant needs to nurse beyond that point to satisfy the need to suck and to receive emotional and physical comfort.
- The supply of milk is equal to the demand—the more the infant sucks, the more milk is produced. Infants aged 6 weeks or 12 weeks who suck more are probably experiencing a growth spurt and so need more milk.
- Water and juice are unnecessary for breast-fed infants in the first 6 months of life, even in hot climates.
- Early substitution of formula or introduction of solid foods may decrease the chance of maintaining lactation.
- Infants weaned before 12 months of age should be given iron-fortified formula, not cow's milk.
- Both feeding the infant more frequently and manually expressing milk will help to increase the milk supply.
- Breast milk can be pumped, placed in a sanitary bottle, and immediately refrigerated or frozen for later use. Milk should be used within 24 hours if refrigerated or within 3 months if stored in the freezer compartment of the refrigerator.

# Infant Formula

Infant formulas may be used in place of breast-feeding, as an occasional supplement to breast-feeding, or when exclusively breast-fed infants are weaned before 12 months of age. When compared to exclusively breast-fed infants, there are few, if any, differences in the rate of growth, blood components, or body composition in formula-fed infants up to 4 to 6 months of age (Treuth and Griffin, 2006). Thereafter, formula-fed infants grow slightly faster, confirming that formula adequately supports infant growth and development.

Routine formulas are prepared from cow's milk made to resemble human milk. Almost all formula used in the United States is iron-fortified, a practice that has greatly reduced the risk of iron deficiency in older infants (Krebs & Hambidge, 2007). The Infant Formula Act regulates the levels of nutrients in formulas, specifying both minimum and maximum amounts of each essential nutrient. Because the minimum recommended amount of each nutrient is more than the amount provided in breast milk, nutrient supplements are unnecessary.

Approximately 25% of the formulas used in the United States are made from soy, which offers an advantage only to infants intolerant of the protein lactose in cow's milk. A variety of formulas are available for infants with special needs, for instance, infants with inborn errors of metabolism such as phenylketonuria (PKU) or maple syrup urine disease. These specialized formulas are intentionally lacking or deficient in one or more nutrients, so they do not supply adequate nutrition for normal infants. They must be supplemented with small amounts of regular formula. Low birth weight (LBW) formulas intended for premature infants are higher in whey protein, vitamins, and minerals (except iron) and have less lactose than routine formulas.

The amount of formula provided per feeding and the frequency of feeding depend on the infant's age and individual needs. General parameters are provided in Table 12.1. Overfeeding is one of the biggest hazards of formula-feeding. Caregivers should recognize that infants cry for reasons other than hunger and should not be fed every time they cry, nor should an infant be forced to finish her or his bottle. To avoid nursing bottle caries, infants and children should not be put to bed with a bottle of formula, milk, juice, or other sweetened liquid (Fig. 12.1). Teaching points for formula-feeding are summarized in Box 12.4.

**QUICK BITE**

Examples of routine formulas
  Similac
  Enfamil
  SMA

**QUICK BITE**

Examples of soy-based formulas
  Prosobee
  Isomil

# Complementary Foods: Introducing Solids

Physiologically, complementary foods become a necessary source of nutrients at around 6 months of age because neonatal nutrient reserves become depleted and the concentrations of some nutrients in breast milk, such as zinc, decline over time (Krebs & Hambidge,

| TABLE 12.1 | General Parameters for Formula Feeding | |
| --- | --- | --- |
| Age | No. of Feedings in 24 hours | Amount per Feeding (oz) |
| 1 month | 6–8 | 2–4 |
| 2 months | 5–6 | 5–6 |
| 3–5 months | 4–5 | 6–7 |

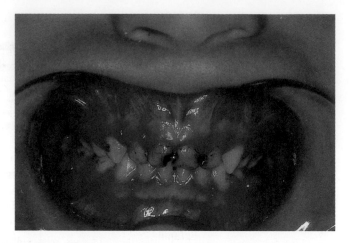

**FIGURE 12.1** Nursing bottle caries. Notice the extensive decay in the upper teeth. (© K. L. Boyd, DDS/Custom Medical Stock Photo.)

| BOX 12.4 | TEACHING POINTS FOR FORMULA FEEDING |
| --- | --- |

One of the greatest hazards of formula feeding is overfeeding. Never force the infant to finish a bottle or to take more than he or she wants. Signs that an infant is finished include biting the nipple, puckering the face, and turning away from the bottle. Discourage the misconception that "a fat baby = a healthy baby = good parents."

Each feeding should last 20 to 30 minutes.

Formula may be given at room temperature, slightly warmed, or directly from the refrigerator; however, always give formula at approximately the same temperature.

Spitting up of a small amount of formula during or after a feeding is normal. Feed the infant more slowly and burp more frequently to help alleviate spitting up.

Hold the infant closely and securely. Position the infant so that the head is higher than the rest of the body.

Avoid jiggling the bottle and making extra movements that could distract the infant from feeding.

Check the flow of formula by holding the bottle upside down. A steady drip from the nipple should be observed. If the flow is too rapid because of too large a nipple opening, the infant may overfeed and develop indigestion. If the flow rate is too slow because of too small a nipple opening, the infant may tire and fall asleep without taking enough formula. Discard any nipples with holes that are too large, and enlarge holes that are too small with a sterilized needle.

Reassure caregivers that there is no danger of "spoiling" an infant by feeding him when he or she cries for a feeding.

Burp the infant halfway through the feeding, at the end of the feeding, and more often if necessary to help get rid of air swallowed during feeding. Burping can be accomplished by gently rubbing or patting the infant's back as he or she is held on the shoulder, lies on his or her stomach over the caregiver's lap, or sits in an upright position.

After the teeth erupt, the baby should be given only plain water for a bedtime bottle-feeding. Never prop the bottle or put the infant to bed with a bottle.

2007). Developmentally, most infants exhibit readiness to spoon-feed around 4 to 6 months of age as reflexes disappear, head control develops, and the infant is able to sit. Over time, control of the head, neck, jaw, and tongue; hand-eye coordination; and the ability to sit, grasp, chew, drink, and self-feed evolve. The eruption of teeth indicates readiness to progress from strained to mashed to chopped fine to regular consistency foods. Guidelines for introducing solids on the basis of developmental readiness appear in Table 12.2.

For both breast- and formula-fed infants, iron-fortified infant cereal is generally the first solid food introduced. To increase the likelihood of acceptance, parents are urged to give a small amount of formula or breast milk to take the edge off hunger before beginning the cereal. Iron-fortified infant cereals are recommended until the infant is 12 to 18 months old because the iron in these cereals is absorbed more readily than that in other cereals.

| TABLE 12.2 | Sequence of Infant Development and Feeding Skills in Normal, Healthy Full-Term Infants* | | |
|---|---|---|---|
| | **Developmental Skills** | | |
| **Baby's Approx. Age** | **Mouth Patterns** | **Hand and Body Skills** | **Feeding Skills or Abilities** |
| Birth through 5 months | • Suck/swallow reflex<br>• Tongue thrust reflex<br>• Rooting reflex<br>• Gag reflex | • Poor control of head, neck, trunk<br>• Brings hands to mouth around 3 months | • Swallows liquids but pushes most solid objects from the mouth |
| 4 months through 6 months | • Draws in upper or lower lip as spoon is removed from mouth<br>• Up-and-down munching movement<br>• Can transfer food from front to back of tongue to swallow<br>• Tongue thrust and rooting reflexes begin to disappear<br>• Gag reflex diminishes<br>• Opens mouth when sees spoon approaching | • Sits with support<br>• Good head control<br>• Uses whole hand to grasp objects (palmer grasp) | • Takes in a spoonful of pureed or strained food and swallows it without choking<br>• Drinks small amounts from cup when held by another person, with spilling |
| 5 months through 9 months | • Begins to control the position of food in the mouth<br>• Up-and-down munching movement<br>• Positions food between jaws for chewing | • Begins to sit alone unsupported<br>• Follows food with eyes<br>• Begins to use thumb and index finger to pick up objects (pincer grasp) | • Begins to eat mashed foods<br>• Eats from a spoon easily<br>• Drinks from a cup with some spilling<br>• Begins to feed self with hands |
| 8 months through 11 months | • Moves food from side-to-side in mouth<br>• Begins to curve lips around rim of cup<br>• Begins to chew in rotary pattern (diagonal movement of the jaw as food is moved to the side or center of the mouth) | • Sits alone easily<br>• Transfers objects from hand to mouth | • Begins to eat ground or finely chopped food and small pieces of soft food<br>• Begins to experiment with spoon but prefers to feed self with hands<br>• Drinks from a cup with less spilling |
| 10 months through 12 months | • Rotary chewing (diagonal movement of the jaw as food is moved to the side or center of the mouth) | • Begins to put spoon in mouth<br>• Begins to hold cup<br>• Good eye-hand-mouth coordination | • Eats chopped food and small pieces of soft, cooked table food<br>• Begins self-spoon feeding with help |

*Developmental stages may vary with individual babies.

***Source:*** USDA Food Nutrition Service. Feeding Infants. A Guide for Use in Child Nutrition Programs. Available at www.fns.usda.gov/tn/Resources/feedinginfants-ch2.pdf. Accessed on 04/04/08.

Traditionally, the order of foods introduced after iron-fortified cereals was vegetables, fruits, meats, and then eggs. The order is no longer considered important, and some experts recommend offering meat as one of the first complementary foods because of its iron and zinc content (Heird & Cooper, 2006). The WHO and Pan American Health Organization (PAHO) recommend that "meat, poultry, fish or eggs should be eaten daily or as often as possible" (PAHO/WHO, 2003). The Institute of Medicine has proposed that meat be provided as part of the WIC food package for breast-fed infants at 6 months of age (IOM, 2006). Although easily chewed red meats such as baby food meat and home-pureed cooked meats are recommended, relatively few infants under 9 months are fed plain meats of any kind. Commercial baby food dinners are more commonly consumed. Chicken and turkey, which provide less heme iron than red meats, are the most popular meats. Other commonly consumed meats are hot dogs, sausages, and cold cuts, all of which are higher in fat and sodium and lower in iron and zinc than plain meats.

New foods should be introduced in plain and simple form one at a time for a period of 5 to 7 days to identify allergic reactions, such as rashes, fussiness, vomiting, diarrhea, or constipation. If there is a positive family history for food allergies, milk, eggs, wheat, and citrus fruits should be introduced cautiously. Peanuts and peanut butter should be avoided because of the potential for severe reaction.

Infants differ in the amount of food they want or need at each feeding. The amount of solid food taken at a feeding may vary from 1 to 2 teaspoons initially to ¼ to ½ cup as the infant gets older. To avoid overfeeding, infants and children should be allowed to self-regulate the amount of food consumed. Only healthy foods should be introduced; it may take 15 to 20 exposures before a new food is accepted (Johnson, 2000). Parents should be cautioned against introducing empty calorie foods simply to provide calories (American Heart Association (AHA), 2006). Tips for creating a positive eating environment are listed in Box 12.5.

Fruit juices were once considered essential complementary foods. Current recommendations are to delay introducing 100% fruit juice until after 6 months of age and to limit intake to 4 to 6 oz/day for children aged 1 to 6 (AHA, 2006). Excessive amounts of juice may displace the intake of nutrient-rich food and milk in the diet and contribute to an excessive calorie intake.

---

| BOX 12.5 | TIPS TO CREATE A POSITIVE EATING ENVIRONMENT |
|---|---|

- Keep in mind that it is not important if a child refuses to eat a particular food (e.g., spinach), so long as the child has a reasonable intake from each major food group.
- Offer a variety of foods, not just the ones you like. Repeated exposures may be needed before a child accepts a new food.
- Fat and cholesterol should not be limited in the diets of very young children, who need fat and cholesterol for their developing brains and nervous systems.
- Never force a child to eat; if a healthy child is hungry, he or she will eat.
- Do not use food to reward, punish, bribe, or convey love.
- Let toddlers explore and enjoy food, even if it means eating with their fingers.
- Space meals further apart and limit snacking so the child will be hungry at mealtimes.
- Keep mealtime relaxed, pleasant, and unhurried, allowing 20 to 30 minutes per meal.
- Eat with the child.
- Children may refuse to eat because they are (1) too excited or distracted, (2) seeking attention, (3) expressing independence, (4) too tired, or (5) simply not hungry. When any of these instances occur, remove the child's plate without comment. If the child wants a snack later, make it nutritious.

# ► NUTRITION FOR TODDLERS

The period between ages 1 and 2 is a time of transition between infancy and childhood. The dramatic decrease in growth rate is reflected in a disinterest in food, a "physiologic anorexia" due to lower calorie needs per kilogram of body weight. At age 1, the child should be drinking from a cup and eating many of the same foods as the rest of the family, although in smaller portions. Beginning around 15 months of age, food jags may develop as a normal expression of autonomy as the child develops a sense of independence. By the end of the second year, children can completely self-feed and can seek food independently.

At age 1, whole milk becomes a major source of nutrients. Milk intake should not exceed 2 to 3½ cups per day because at this level it may displace the intake of iron-rich foods from the diet and promote **milk anemia**. The AAP recommends that low-fat or nonfat milk not be started until after the age of 2. Although a Recommended Dietary Allowance (RDA) for fat has not been established, the Acceptable Macronutrient Distribution Range (AMDR) for total fat for 1 to 3 year olds is 30% to 40% of total calories, higher than the 25% to 35% recommended for youth aged 4 to 18 (IOM, 2005).

**Milk anemia:** an iron deficiency anemia related to excessive milk intake, which displaces the intake of iron-rich foods from the diet.

There is very little research on the best ways to achieve optimal nutritional intakes during this transition period, and no nutritional guidelines exist (AHA, 2006). Data from the Feeding Infants and Toddlers Study (FITS) show that American infants and toddlers consume a nutritionally adequate diet with little risk of nutrient deficiencies (Devaney, et al., 2004). However, the FITS also showed that sizable percentages of toddlers consumed high-calorie, high-fat, and salty snacks and carbonated beverages and sweetened fruit drinks. Among children aged 19 to 24 months, French fries are the most frequently consumed vegetable, and on a given day, one-third of children ate no fruit, 60% ate baked desserts, 20% ate candy, and 44% consumed sweetened beverages (Fox, et al., 2004).

### QUICK BITE

Foods that may cause choking in small children

| | |
|---|---|
| Hot dogs | Tough meat |
| Candy | Watermelon with seeds |
| Nuts | Celery |
| Grapes | Popcorn |
| Raw carrots | Peanut butter |

Until the age of 4, young children are at risk of choking. To decrease the risk of choking, foods that are difficult to chew and swallow should be avoided; meals and snacks should be supervised; foods should be prepared in forms that are easy to chew and swallow (e.g., cut grapes into small pieces and spread peanut butter thinly); and infants should not be allowed to eat or drink from a cup while lying down, playing, or strapped in a car seat.

# ► NUTRITION FOR CHILDREN

Childhood represents a more latent period of growth compared to infancy and adolescence. Before puberty, children annually grow 2 to 3 in. in height and gain about 5 pounds on average. Although there are individual differences, usually a larger child eats more than a smaller one, an active child eats more than a quiet one, and a happy, content child eats more than an anxious one. School-age children maintain a relatively constant intake in relation to their age group; children who are considered big eaters in second grade are also big eaters in sixth grade.

## Calories and Nutrients

Total calorie needs steadily increase during childhood, although calorie needs per kilogram of body weight progressively fall. The challenge in childhood is to meet nutrient requirements

| TABLE 12.3 | MyPyramid Food and Calorie Intake Levels Recommended for 2 to 18-Year-Olds | | | | | | | | |
|---|---|---|---|---|---|---|---|---|---|
| **Daily amount of calories and food recommended by age and gender for moderately active individuals*** | | | | | | | | | |
| **Age** | | | | | | | | | |
| Males | 2 | | 3–5 | 6–8 | 9–10 | 11 | 12–13 | 14 | 15 | 16–18 |
| Females | 2 | 3 | 4–6 | 7–9 | 10–11 | 12–18 | | | | |
| **Calorie level** | 1000 | 1200 | 1400 | 1600 | 1800 | 2000 | 2200 | 2400 | 2600 | 2800 |
| **Daily amount of food** | | | | | | | | | | |
| Fruits (cups) | 1 | 1 | 1.5 | 1.5 | 1.5 | 2 | 2 | 2 | 2 | 2.5 |
| Vegetables (cups) | 1 | 1.5 | 1.5 | 2 | 2.5 | 2.5 | 3 | 3 | 3.5 | 3.5 |
| Grains (oz-eq) | 3 | 4 | 5 | 5 | 6 | 6 | 7 | 8 | 9 | 10 |
| Meat and Beans (oz-eq) | 2 | 3 | 4 | 5 | 5 | 5.5 | 6 | 6.5 | 6.5 | 7 |
| Milk (cups) | 2 | 2 | 2 | 3 | 3 | 3 | 3 | 3 | 3 | 3 |
| Oils (tsp) | 3 | 4 | 4 | 5 | 5 | 6 | 6 | 7 | 8 | 8 |
| Discretionary calorie allowance | 165 | 171 | 171 | 132 | 195 | 267 | 290 | 362 | 410 | 426 |

*Calorie needs generally increase by 200/day at each age for active individuals and decrease by 200/day for people who are sedentary.

*Source:* www.MyPyramid.gov

without exceeding calorie needs (AHA, 2006). MyPyramid food and calorie level guidelines for ages 2 to 18 are shown in Table 12.3.

The *Dietary Guidelines for Americans* are intended for healthy people over the age of 2; thus, the content of childhood diets should be similar to that of adults. The basic messages are to choose whole grains for at least half the total grain intake; eat plenty of colorful fruit and vegetables; drink 2 to 3 cups of low-fat or nonfat milk per day; choose lean proteins; and limit fats and added sugars. These recommendations are illustrated in Figure 12.2, a MyPyramid for Kids graphic featuring an 1800-calorie diet.

The DRI for children are divided into two age groups: 1- to 3-year-olds and 4- to 8-year-olds. Thereafter, age groups are further divided by gender: for males and females the age groups through adolescence are 9 to 13 and 14 to 18. Generally, nutrient needs increase with each age grouping, and most nutrient requirements reach their adult levels at the 14 to 18 age group. Table 12.4 lists fiber and nutrients most likely to be deficient in the diets of American youth. Notice that except for fiber and potassium, the mean intake of the other nutrients listed is above the DRI for ages 1 to 3 and 4 to 8.

## Eating Practices

As children get older, they consume more foods from nonhome sources and have more outside influences on their food choices. School, friends' houses, child-care centers, and social events present opportunities for children to make their own choices beyond parental supervision. Children who are home alone after school prepare their own snacks and, possibly, meals. The "ideal" of children eating breakfast, dinner, and a snack at home, with a nutritious brown-bag or healthy cafeteria lunch at school is not representative of what most children are eating (AHA, 2006). Today, many children do not eat breakfast and get at least one-third of their calories from snacks, and many obtain a significant portion of their calories from sweetened beverages (AHA, 2006).

## Promoting Healthy Habits

Parents are the primary gatekeepers and role models for their young children's food intake and habits. Parents should decide what foods the child is offered, when the child eats, and where eating takes place; the child should decide whether he or she wants to eat and how

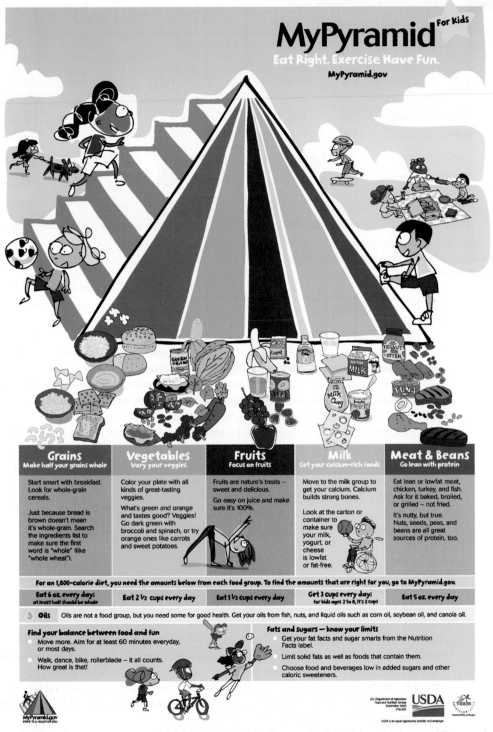

**FIGURE 12.2** MyPyramid for Kids. (USDA, Center for Nutrition Policy and Promotion (2005). MyPyramid—Steps to Healthier You Food Guidance System. Available at www .MyPyramid.gov

| TABLE 12.4 | DRIs* for Fiber and Nutrients Most Likely to be Deficient in the Diets of American Youth.** |||||||||||
|---|---|---|---|---|---|---|---|---|---|---|---|
| | Fiber (g) || Vit A (mg RAE) || Calcium (mg) || Iron (mg) || Potassium (mg) ||
| Age | DRI | Mean Intake | DRI | Mean Intake | DRI | Mean Intake | DRI | Mean Intake | DRI | Mean Intake |
| **Children** | | | | | | | | | | |
| 1–3 years | 19 | 9.5 | **300** | 532 | 500 | 972 | 7 | 11.0 | 3000 | 2086 |
| 4–8 years | 25 | 11.6 | **400** | 573 | 800 | 960 | **10** | 13.7 | 3800 | 2136 |
| **Males** | | | | | | | | | | |
| 9–13 years | 31 | 14.2 | **600** | 670 | 1300 | 1139 | 8 | 17.0 | 4500 | 2472 |
| 14–18 years | 38 | 15.3 | **900** | 638 | 1300 | 1142 | **11** | 19.1 | 4700 | 2774 |
| **Females** | | | | | | | | | | |
| 9–13 years | 26 | 12.3 | **600** | 536 | 1300 | 865 | 8 | 13.7 | 4500 | 2125 |
| 14–18 years | 26 | 11.7 | **700** | 513 | 1300 | 804 | **15** | 13.1 | 4700 | 2020 |

*values in bold represent RDA's; all others are Adequate Intakes (AI)

**shaded areas depict nutrients with mean intakes below the DRI

*Source:* Dietary Reference Intakes. Reports may be accessed via www.nap.edu.

Moshfegh, A., Goldman, J., Cleveland, L. (2005). What We Eat in America, NHANES 2002–2002: Usual nutrient intakes from food compared to dietary reference intakes. US Department of Agriculture, Agricultural Research Service. Available at http://www.ars.usda.gov/SP2UserFiles/Place/12355000/pdf/usualintaketables2001-02.pdf. Accessed on 4/14/08.

much to eat (AHA, 2006). A rule of thumb guideline to determine age-appropriate serving sizes is to provide 1 tablespoon of food per year of age (e.g., the serving size for a 3-year-old is 3 tablespoons). By age 4 to 6, recommended serving sizes are similar to those for adults.

Children who eat more meals with their families have healthier diets (Gable, Chang, & Krull, 2007). Family meals promote social interaction and allow children to learn food-related behaviors. Parents should provide and consume healthy meals and snacks and avoid or limit empty calorie foods (Fig. 12.3). Snacks, especially sweetened beverages, should be limited during sedentary activities. Forbidding the intake of certain foods and pressuring children to eat are counterproductive in that they may lead to overeating, dislikes, and an interest in eating forbidden foods (Fisher & Birch, 1999).

### QUICK BITE

Healthy snack ideas
- Unsweetened cereal with or without milk
- Meat or cheese on whole grain bread or crackers
- Graham crackers, fig bars
- Whole grain cookies or muffins made with oatmeal, dried fruit, or iron-fortified cereal
- Quick breads such as banana, date, pumpkin
- Raw vegetables, vegetable juices
- Fresh, dried, or canned fruits without sugar
- Pure fruit juice as a drink or frozen on a stick
- Low-fat yogurt with or without fresh fruit added
- Air-popped popcorn (not before age 4), pretzels
- Peanut butter on bread, crackers, celery, apple slices
- Milk shakes made with fruit and low fat ice cream or frozen yogurt
- Low-fat ice cream, frozen yogurt, low fat ice cream, sherbet, sorbet, fruit ice
- Animal crackers, ginger snaps
- Skim or 1% milk (after age 2)
- Low-fat cheese, low-fat cottage cheese
- Rice cakes or popcorn cakes

The *Dietary Guidelines for Americans* recommends children and adolescents engage in at least 60 minutes of physical activity on most, preferably all, days of the week (USDHHS, 2005).

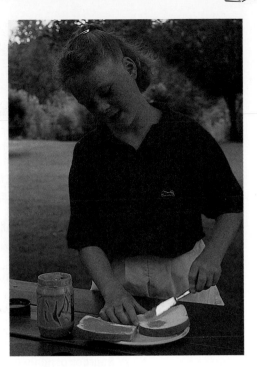

**FIGURE 12.3**  Good nutritional habits, such as eating healthy snacks, develop early in life. (© Bob Kramer.)

Physical activity should not be limited to organized sports, but should include a more active lifestyle such as walking the dog, flying a kite, joining the marching band, and riding a bike. Because there is a positive association between television/video use and BMI, the AAP recommends these types of sedentary activities be limited to no more than 1 to 2 hr/day (AHA, 2006).

# ▶ NUTRITION FOR ADOLESCENCE (12 TO 18 YEARS)

The slow growth of childhood abruptly and dramatically increases with pubescence until the rate is as rapid as that of early infancy. Adolescence is a period of physical, emotional, social, and sexual maturation. Approximately 15% to 20% of adult height and 50% of adult weight are gained during adolescence. Fat distribution shifts and sexual maturation occurs. Subsequently, calorie and nutrient needs increase, as does appetite, but exactly when those increases occur depends on the timing and duration of the growth spurt. Because there are wide variations in the timing of the growth spurt among individuals, chronological age is a poor indicator of physiological maturity and nutritional needs.

Gender differences are obvious. For instance, girls generally experience increases in growth between 10 to 11 years of age and peak at 12 years. Because peak weight occurs before peak height, many girls and parents become concerned about what appears to be excess weight. In contrast, boys usually begin the growth spurt at about 12 years of age and peak at 14 years. Stature growth ceases at a median age of 21.2 years (Treuth and Griffin, 2006). Nutritional needs increase later for boys than for girls.

## Calories and Nutrients

Table 12.3 lists MyPyramid recommended calorie intakes for adolescents, which are based on DRI estimated energy expenditure calculations that account for age, gender, weight, height, physical activity level, and energy deposition. Generally, nutrient requirements are higher during adolescence than at any other time in the life cycle, with the exception of

**QUICK BITE**

Sources of calcium
  Milk
  Yogurt
  Hard cheeses, such as cheddar
  Calcium-fortified orange juice
  Calcium-fortified breakfast cereals
  Canned fish with bones, such as salmon
  "Greens," such as Bok choy, collard
    greens, turnip greens, kale
  Broccoli
  Chinese/Napa cabbage
  Okra
  Tofu, soymilk
  Tortillas made from lime processed corn

**QUICK BITE**

Sources of nonheme iron
  Iron-fortified, ready-to-eat cereals
  Whole-wheat, enriched, or fortified bread
  Noodles, rice, or barley
  Canned plums
  Cooked dried apricots
  Raisins
  Bean dip
  Peanut butter

pregnancy and lactation. Notice that the calories suggested for moderately active females aged 12 to 18 is 2000, whereas for males the need ranges from 2200 to 2800 calories. Females require fewer calories than males because they have proportionally more fat tissue and lesser muscle mass due to the effects of estrogen. Girls also experience less bone growth than boys.

As indicated in Table 12.4, the requirements for calcium and iron (for males only) are higher during adolescence than at any other time in the life cycle. Approximately half of adult bone mass is accrued during adolescence; optimizing calcium intake during adolescence increases bone mineralization and may decrease the risk of fracture and osteoporosis later in life (Treuth and Griffin, 2006). In reality, mean calcium intake is less than the DRI for both males and females from age 9 onward (see Table 12.4).

Adolescents have increased needs for iron related to an expanding blood volume, the rise in hemoglobin concentration, and the growth of muscle mass. In boys, peak iron requirement occurs at 14 to 18 years of age as muscle mass expands. The requirement for iron in adolescent girls increases from 8 to 15 mg/day at the age of 14 to account for menstrual losses. For girls who are not menstruating at 14, the requirement for iron is 10.5 mg/day, not 15 mg/day. Girls tend to develop an iron deficiency slowly after puberty, particularly if menstrual losses are compounded by poor eating habits or chronic fad dieting. Heme iron, found in meats, is better absorbed than nonheme iron. Nonheme iron absorption increases when a source of vitamin C, such as orange juice or tomatoes, is consumed at the same time.

## Eating Practices

In early adolescence, peer pressure overtakes parental influence on food choices. As the adolescent becomes increasingly independent, more self-selected meals and snacks are purchased and eaten outside the home. A natural increase in appetite combined with fast food marketing practices geared for adolescents and a decrease in physical activity increase the risk of overeating (AHA, 2006). Generally, adolescents overconsume sweetened beverages, French fries, pizza, and fast food entrées, causing excessive intakes of fat, saturated fat, trans fats, and added sugars. (AHA, 2006). Conversely, they lack adequate fruits, vegetables, dairy foods, and whole grains. Nutrients most likely to be deficient in the diets of American adolescents are fiber, vitamin A, calcium, iron, and potassium (ADA, 2004a, 2004b) (Table 12.4). This represents a worsening of nutritional adequacy from the age of 8 and younger when only fiber and potassium are consumed, on average, in amounts less than recommended.

# ► NUTRITION CONCERNS DURING CHILDHOOD AND ADOLESCENCE

Indicators of nutrition risk for children and adolescents appear in Box 12.6. Nutrition concerns discussed next include breakfast skipping, sweetened beverage consumption, overweight, and adolescent pregnancy. Eating disorders are discussed in Chapter 14.

## Breakfast Skipping

Among children aged 6 to 13, an estimated 8% to 15% skip breakfast (Affenito, 2007). Adolescent females are more likely to skip breakfast than males of similar age, and African-American adolescents (24%) are more likely to skip breakfast than white adolescents (13%) (Nicklas, O'Neil, & Myers, 2004). Breakfast is missed more than any other meal (Utter et al., 2007).

Children who regularly skip breakfast have lower intakes of vitamins and minerals than those who routinely eat breakfast, and those nutrients are not made up for at other meals.

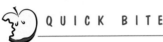

**QUICK BITE**

Nontraditional breakfast ideas
  Pizza
  Peanut butter sandwich
  Soup with crackers
  Yogurt parfait
  Smoothies
  Baked potato with cottage cheese
  Dinner leftovers

In the Bogalusa Heart Study, 10-year-old breakfast skippers failed to meet two-thirds the reference standards for vitamin A, vitamin B6, vitamin D, riboflavin, folate, calcium, iron, magnesium, phosphorus, riboflavin, and zinc (Nicklas, O'Neil, & Berenson, 1998). Eating breakfast is linked to better academic performance (Kleinman et al., 2002) and cognition among children (Pollitt & Mathews, 1998). Children who skip breakfast are significantly less likely to meet recommendations for fruit and vegetable intake and more likely to frequently eat unhealthy snacks (Utter et al., 2007). Although breakfast eaters tend to consume more calories than breakfast skippers, they are less likely to be overweight, according to most but not all studies (Affenito, 2007). Although a high-fiber, nutrient-fortified ready-to-eat cereal with skim milk and fruit may be an optimal choice for breakfast, nontraditional breakfasts may be more appealing to people who "don't like breakfast." Overall, breakfast skipping tends to increase with age and seems to be associated with other lifestyle factors that may be detrimental to health, such as dieting and infrequent exercise (Rampersaud et al., 2005).

## Increased Consumption of Soft Drinks

In the last 50 years, the ratio of milk to soft drink consumption has changed dramatically. In 1945, Americans drank four times more milk than soft drinks; in 1997 they drank

| BOX 12.6 | INDICATORS OF NUTRITION RISK IN CHILDREN AND ADOLESCENTS |
| --- | --- |

- Meal skipping three or more times per week
- Frequent breakfast skipping
- Eating fast food more than three times per week
- Eating from only one food group
- Poor appetite
- Frequently eating without family supervision

***Source:*** Melanson, K. (2008). Lifestyle approaches to promoting healthy eating for children. *American Journal of Lifestyle Medicine, 2,* 26–36.

| TABLE 12.5 | Prevalence of Overweight in Youth* | | |
|---|---|---|---|
| **Age** | | **1988–1994** | **2003–2004** |
| 2–5 | | 7.2% | 13.9% |
| 6–11 | | 11.3% | 18.8% |
| 12–19 | | 10.5% | 17.4% |

*Overweight is defined as greater than 95th percentile for weight in the CDC growth charts for children.

*Source:* CDC, National Center for Health Statistics (2006). Prevalence of overweight among children and adolescents: United States, 2003–2004. Available at www.cdc.gov/nchs/products/pubs/pubd/hestats/overweight/overwght_child_03.htm Accessed on 4/18/08.

almost two-and-a-half times more soft drinks than milk (ADA, 2004a). Soft drinks and sweetened beverages provide calories without nutrients and high soft drink consumption is linked to low intakes of vitamins A and C, some B vitamins, calcium, and phosphorus because they displace the intake of nutrient dense items such as milk, fruits, and vegetables (Johnson, 2000).

## Overweight and Obesity

In recent decades, the prevalence of obesity among youth has risen dramatically in the United States (Table 12.5). Children who are overweight may develop complications of excess weight seen in adults, such as glucose intolerance, type 2 diabetes, hypertension, hyperlipidemia, and metabolic syndrome (ADA, 2006). Overweight and obesity in childhood or adolescence increases the risk of several diseases in adulthood, such as cancer, insulin resistance, stroke, cardiovascular disease, and renal failure (LaFontaine, 2008). Among obese girls, the risk of premature death as an adult increases threefold (van Dam et al., 2006). Eighty percent of overweight and obese adolescents become obese adults (Dietz, 2004).

Overweight and obesity can have negative social and psychological consequences. A study that followed almost 11,000 American adolescents found that obese girls were half as likely to attend college, more likely to consider committing suicide and use alcohol and marijuana, and had a more negative self-image than normal weight girls (Crosnoe, 2007). Teasing and psychological abuse by peers and adults can lead to social isolation, depression, and low self-esteem. Overweight children may actually consume fewer calories than their thin counterparts; because they are social outcasts though, a perpetuating cycle of weight gain, inactivity, and further weight gain makes weight control difficult.

Although multifactorial in origin, the fundamental cause of overweight and obesity is an imbalance between caloric intake and caloric expenditure. Over the last 25 years, the average calorie intake of American children has increased, and portion sizes have grown. On the other side of the energy equation, physical inactivity is seen as a major contributor to weight gain in children.

### Healthy Lifestyles and Obesity Prevention

Prevention of obesity is critical because data on long-term successful treatment is limited (AAP, 2003). Parental support for a more healthful lifestyle is vital to initiating and sustaining changes in eating and exercise behaviors. Parents often recognize that they need to set an example for their children, but lack the time to do so. Still other parents who are overweight may feel they cannot set a good example because

**QUICK BITE**

Body Mass Index
BMI = weight (kg) ÷ height (m)$^2$

they do not practice what they preach. Other barriers to parents taking action are (1) a belief that children will outgrow their excess weight, (2) a lack of knowledge about how to help children control their weight, and (3) a fear they will cause eating disorders in their children. Even among adolescents, parents still have a major impact on food intake.

The AAP recommends that BMI be calculated and plotted once a year for all youth aged 2 and older as part of routine pediatric health visits (AAP, 2003). Gender specific BMI-for-age percentiles are used to screen for childhood overweight because BMI varies by age and gender (Figs. 12.4 and 12.5). All children and adolescents who are not in the healthy weight range should undergo further assessment and evaluation to identify contributing factors and help determine intervention strategies (AHA, 2006).

A key recommendation in the 2005 *Dietary Guidelines for Americans* is that the rate of weight gain be reduced in overweight children, while allowing for growth and development (USDHHS, 2005). The AAP advocates moderation rather than overconsumption and healthy choices over restrictive eating (AAP, 2003). The American Dietetic Association takes the position that pediatric overweight requires a combination of family- and school-based programs that include promoting physical activity, parent training/modeling, behavioral counseling, and nutrition education (ADA, 2006). While the importance of implementing obesity interventions for adolescents is clear, the most effective strategies for doing so are unknown (Shepherd et al., 2006). Providing nutrition and calorie related information, especially to adolescent girls, has the potential to inadvertently lead to weight preoccupation and unhealthful calorie counting.

## Adolescent Pregnancy

Adolescent pregnancy is associated with physiologic, socioeconomic, and behavioral factors that increase health risks to both infant and mother. Infants born to adolescent mothers are at higher risk of LBW and premature birth and are more likely to die within the first year of life than infants whose mothers are in their twenties or thirties (MOD, 2007). Pregnant adolescents are at higher risk for anemia, high blood pressure, and excessive postpartum weight retention (Nielsen, et al., 2006).

Compared with adult women, pregnant adolescents

- Are more likely to be physically, emotionally, financially, and socially immature. Low socioeconomic status may be a major reason for the high incidence of LBW infants and other complications of adolescent pregnancy.
- May not have adequate nutrient stores because they need large amounts of nutrients for their own growth and development. Although female adolescent growth is usually complete by the age of 15, physical maturity is not reached until 4 years after menarche, which usually occurs by age 17.
- May give low priority to healthy eating. A high sugar intake and low intake of iron, folate, zinc, and calcium may increase risks for poor pregnancy outcome (Neilsen, 2006). Dieting, erratic eating patterns, reliance on fast foods, and meal skipping (especially breakfast) are common adolescent practices.
- Younger adolescents often need to gain more weight for their BMI than older women to improve birth outcomes (IOM, 2009)
- Are more concerned with body image and confused about weight gain recommendations. Many do not understand why they should gain more than 7 pounds, the weight of the average baby at birth.

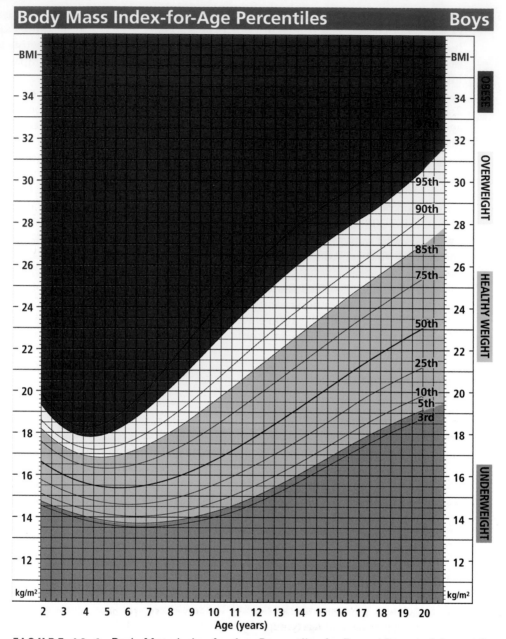

**FIGURE 12.4** Body Mass Index-for-Age Percentiles for Boys. (*Source:* Adapted from the Centers for Disease Control and Prevention (CDC) Growth Chart, New York State Department of Health.)

- Are more likely to smoke during pregnancy. Smoking doubles a woman's risk of delivering an LBW baby and increases the risk of complications, premature delivery, and stillbirth (USDHHS, 2004).
- Seek prenatal care later and have fewer total visits during pregnancy.

Appropriate weight gain and adequate nutrition are among the most important controllable factors that contribute to a healthful outcome of pregnancy for both mother and infant (Neilsen et al., 2006). Good nutrition has the potential to decrease the incidence of

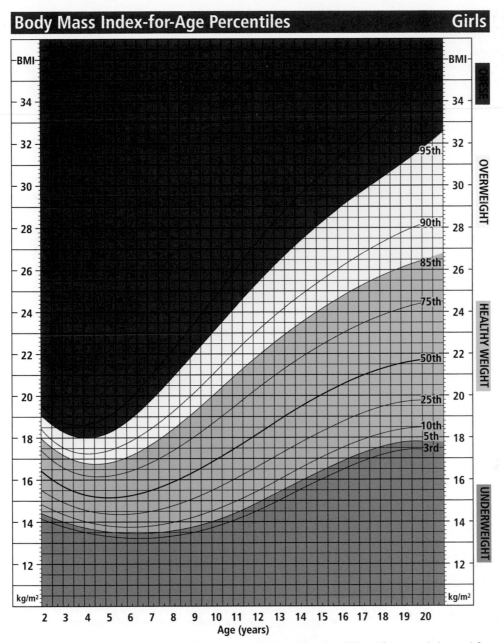

**Body Mass Index-for-Age Percentiles**                                    **Girls**

OBESE

OVERWEIGHT

HEALTHY WEIGHT

UNDERWEIGHT

95th

90th

85th

75th

50th

25th

10th
5th
3rd

Age (years)

**FIGURE 12.5**  Body Mass Index-for-Age Percentiles for Girls. (*Source:* Adapted from the Centers for Disease Control and Prevention (CDC) Growth Chart, New York State Department of Health.)

LBW infants and to improve the health of infants born to adolescents. Teenagers within the healthy BMI range should gain 25–35 pounds, more if they are very young (IOM, 2009). The MyPyramid recommendations in Table 11.3 can also be used by pregnant teens. MyPyramid is useful both in assessing dietary strengths and weaknesses and in providing a framework for implementing dietary changes in a way the teenager can understand. Because teens living with one or more adults may have little control over what food is available to them, parents and significant others should also be encouraged to attend counseling sessions.

## NURSING PROCESS: Well Child

Amanda is a 24-month-old girl who is regularly brought to the Well Baby Clinic for her check-ups and immunizations. At this visit you discover that her height and weight are in the 25th percentile for her age; records indicate that previously she had consistently ranked in the 75th percentile for weight and 50th percentile for height. The change has occurred over the last 6 months. Her mother complains that Amanda is "fussy" and has lost interest in eating.

| Assessment |
| --- |

**Medical–Psychosocial History**

- Medical history including prenatal, perinatal, and birth history; specifically assess for gastrointestinal (GI) problems such as slow gastric emptying, constipation, diarrhea, and allergies
- Use of medications that can cause side effects such as delayed gastric emptying, diarrhea, constipation, or decreased appetite
- Level of development for age
- Elimination and reflux patterns, if applicable
- Caregiver's ability to understand; attitude toward health and nutrition and readiness to learn
- Psychosocial and economic issues such as the living situation, who does the shopping and cooking, adequacy of food budget, need for food assistance, and level of family and social support
- Use of vitamins, minerals, and nutritional supplements: what, how much, and why they are given

**Anthropometric Assessment**

Obtain height and weight to calculate BMI; determine BMI-for-age percentile

Head circumference-for-age

Pattern of weight gain and growth

**Biochemical and Physical Assessment**

Laboratory values including hemoglobin, and hematocrit, and the significance of any other values that are abnormal

**Dietary Assessment**

- Food records, if available
- Interview the primary caregiver to assess:
  - What does Amanda usually eat in a 24-hour period, including types and amounts of food, frequency and pattern of eating, and texture of foods eaten?
  - How does her intake compare to a 1000-calorie (the calorie level appropriate for 2-year-olds) MyPyramid intake pattern?
  - What food groups is she consuming less than recommended amounts of?
  - Are self-feeding skills appropriate for Amanda's age?
  - Is the mealtime environment positive?
  - What is the caregiver's attitude about Amanda's current weight, recent weight loss, and eating behaviors?
  - Are the caregiver's expectations about how much Amanda should eat reasonable and appropriate? What is the problem according to the caregiver?
  - Are there cultural, religious, and ethnic influences on the family's eating habits?

*(nursing process continues on page 291)*

## NURSING PROCESS: *Well Child* (continued)

| Diagnosis | |
|---|---|
| Possible Nursing Diagnosis | Imbalanced nutrition, less than body requirements related to inadequate intake as evidenced by change of 2 percentile channels in growth charts. |

| Planning | |
|---|---|
| Client Outcomes | The client will<br>• Experience appropriate growth in height and weight<br>• Consume, on average, an intake consistent with MyPyramid recommendations for a 1000-calorie diet by eating a variety of foods within each food group<br>• Achieve or progress toward age-appropriate feeding skills |

| Nursing Interventions | |
|---|---|
| Nutrition Therapy | Promote MyPyramid food plan of 1000 calories, which is appropriate for her age |
| Client Teaching | Instruct the caregiver<br>• On the role of nutrition in maintaining health and promoting adequate growth and development, including the importance of adequate calories and protein<br>• On eating plan essentials, including the importance of<br>  • Choosing a varied diet to help ensure an average, adequate intake<br>  • Providing foods of appropriate texture for age<br>  • Providing three meals plus three or more planned snacks to maximize intake<br>  • Providing liquids after meals, instead of with meals, to avoid displacing food intake<br>  • Limiting low-nutrient-density foods (e.g., fruit drinks, carbonated beverages, sweetened cereals) because they displace the intake of more nutritious foods<br>  • The need to modify the diet, as appropriate, to improve elimination patterns<br>Address behavioral matters, such as<br>• Providing a positive mealtime environment (e.g., limiting distractions, having the child well-rested before mealtime)<br>• Not using food to punish, reward, or bribe the child<br>• Promoting eating behaviors and skills appropriate for the age<br>• Keeping accurate food records<br>• Modifying foods to increase their nutrient density, such as by fortifying milk with skim milk powder; using milk in place of water in recipes; melting cheese on potatoes, rice, or noodles; and so on |

| Evaluation | |
|---|---|
| Evaluate and Monitor | Monitor growth in height and weight<br>Evaluate food records to assess adequacy of intake according to a 1000-calorie MyPyramid plan<br>Progress toward age-appropriate feeding skills |

▶ **How Do You Respond?**

**Does early introduction of solid foods help infants sleep through the night?** A frequently given reason for introducing solids before 4 months of age is the unsupported belief that it will help infants to sleep through the night. A major objection to the early introduction of solids is that it may interfere with establishing sound eating habits and may contribute to overfeeding because infants less than 4 months old are unable to communicate satiety by turning away and leaning back.

**What foods are most likely to cause allergies?** Ninety percent of food allergy reactions are caused by these eight foods: milk, eggs, soy, peanuts, nuts (cashews, almonds), wheat, fish, and shellfish. Most people who have a food allergy are allergic to only one food.

**Does chocolate cause or aggravate acne?** There is no scientific evidence to correlate any dietary factors with the appearance or severity of acne. Although vitamin A is important for normal skin integrity, vitamin A supplements are not effective in treating acne and are toxic in large amounts. A compound related to vitamin A (13-*cis*-retinoic acid or Accutane) has been approved for treatment of severe cystic acne, but is available only through prescription and must be used with caution.

**Can diet be blamed for attention-deficit and hyperactivity disorder (ADHD)?** In the 1970s, the late Dr. Ben Feingold proposed that food additives and salicylates may be responsible for about 25% of cases of hyperactivity with learning disability among school-age children. Most controlled studies do not support the hypothesis that avoiding artificial colors and flavors; the preservatives beta-hydroxytheophylline [BHT] and butylated hydroxyanisole [BHA]; and salicylate-containing fruits, vegetables, and spices (the Feingold diet) helps to control hyperactivity (Marcason, 2005). Likewise, claims that sugar causes hyperactivity are not supported (ADA, 2004b). However, it is possible that a very small subset of children with ADHD have food sensitivities.

▶ **Case Study**

Andrew is 16 years old and sedentary. He is 5 ft. 8 in., weighs 218 pounds, and has a BMI of 33. He has been overweight for most of his life, as is most of his extended paternal family. His mother has tried "everything" over the years to get him to lose weight, from putting him on her own weight loss diet to hiding foods he shouldn't have, such as soft drinks and chips, to limit his access. He has a part-time job in a fast food restaurant, and is able to leave the school property at lunchtime to have lunch where he works. He is not good at sports but loves to play video games and watch movies. He hates that he's so big but feels hopeless about changing. His normal day's intake is as follows:

| | |
|---|---|
| **Breakfast:** | 2 doughnuts and a large glass of apple juice |
| **Lunch:** | a double cheeseburger, large fries, and a large shake |
| **Snacks:** | frozen mini pizzas, a large soft drink, and a handful of cookies |
| **Dinner:** | the same as lunch on nights he works. If he's home, he eats whatever is available, often pizza or sandwiches and chips, ice cream, and a soft drink |
| **Snacks:** | chips and salsa, and a soft drink |

• Using the BMI-for-age percentile for boys, what is Andrew's weight status? Is it an appropriate approach to limit Andrew's calories to outgrow his current weight status?

• How many calories should Andrew consume daily? Based on the MyPyramid intake levels, which food groups is he consuming the appropriate amounts of? Which groups is he overeating? Which groups is he not eating enough of? What are the sources of discretionary calories in his diet?

- What specific goals would you encourage Andrew to set regarding his intake, activity, and weight?
- What would you suggest his mother to do to support better eating habits and a healthier weight?

STUDY QUESTIONS

1. Which statement indicates the mother understands the nurse's instructions about breast-feeding?
   a. "Breast-feeding should only last 5 minutes on each breast."
   b. "Sometimes babies cry just because they are thirsty, so a bottle of water should be offered before breast-feeding begins to see if the infant is just thirsty."
   c. "The longer the baby sucks, the less milk I will have for the next feeding."
   d. "The first breast offered should be alternated with each feeding."

2. A mother asks why toddlers shouldn't drink all the milk they want. Which of the following is the nurse's best response?
   a. "Consuming more than the recommended amount of milk can displace the intake of iron-rich foods from the diet and increase the toddler's risk of iron deficiency anemia."
   b. "Consuming more than the recommended amount of milk increases the risk of milk allergy."
   c. "Too much milk can lead to overhydration."
   d. "Consuming more than the recommended amount of milk will provide too much protein."

3. The nurse knows her instructions about introducing solids into the infant's diet have been effective when the mother states:
   a. "Babies should be introduced to solid foods at 1 to 3 months of age."
   b. "New foods should be given for 5 to 7 days so that allergic responses can be easily identified."
   c. "Infants are more likely to accept infant cereal for the first time if it is mixed with breast milk or formula and given from a bottle."
   d. "The appropriate initial serving size for solids is 1 to 2 tablespoons."

4. Which of the following would be the best snack for a 2-year-old?
   a. Popcorn.
   b. Banana slices.
   c. Fresh cherries.
   d. Raw celery.

5. Which groups are adolescents most likely to eat in inadequate amounts? Select all that apply.
   a. Whole grains.
   b. Vegetables.
   c. Fruits
   d. Meat.

6. The client asks if her 10-year-old daughter needs a weight loss diet. Which of the following would be the nurse's best response?
   a. "Rather than a diet at this age, you should just forbid her to eat sweets and empty calories."
   b. "Because prevention of overweight is more effective than treatment, you should start to limit her calorie intake by only serving low-fat and artificially sweetened foods."
   c. "Ten-year-old girls are about to enter the growth spurt of puberty, and it is natural for her to gain weight before she grows taller. Diets are not recommended for children, although healthy eating and moderation are always appropriate."
   d. "She needs extra calories for the upcoming growth spurt so you should be encouraging her to eat more than she normally does."

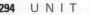 

**7.** Calorie and nutrient requirements during adolescence:
a. Are higher than during adulthood because of growth and developmental changes.
b. Peak early and then fall until adulthood is reached.
c. Are lower than during childhood.
d. Cannot be generalized because individual variations exist.

**8.** Nutrients most likely to be deficient in an adolescent's diet are
a. Vitamin D and folate.
b. Protein and vitamin C.
c. Zinc and vitamin E.
d. Iron and calcium.

## KEY CONCEPTS

- An optimal diet supports normal growth and development.

- Because of varying rates of growth and activity, nutritional requirements are less precise for children and adolescents than they are for adults.

- Exclusive breast-feeding is recommended for the first 6 months of life. Breast-feeding should continue up to the age of 1.

- Iron-fortified infant formula is an acceptable alternative or supplement to breast-feeding. The biggest hazard of formula-feeding is overfeeding.

- Adequacy of growth (height and weight) is the best indicator of whether or not an infant's intake is nutritionally adequate.

- Complementary foods should not be introduced before the infant is developmentally ready, usually around 4 to 6 months of age. Iron-fortified infant cereal is usually the first food introduced. New foods should be introduced one at a time for a period of 5 to 7 days so that any allergic reaction can be easily identified.

- Nutritional guidelines on how to achieve optimal nutritional intakes for toddlers do not exist. Infants and toddlers are at low risk of nutrient deficiencies, yet their diets may already be beginning to be high in added sugars and fats and low in fruits and vegetables.

- Parents are the primary gatekeepers of their children's nutritional intake. They should make healthy foods available and not introduce foods into their children's diet that have no other value than calories.

- The food groups most likely to be consumed in inadequate amounts by children and adolescents are fruits, vegetables, whole grains, and dairy products, resulting in inadequate intakes of calcium, iron, potassium, vitamin A, and fiber intakes.

- The *Dietary Guidelines* are intended for all healthy Americans over the age of 2. MyPyramid for Kids, crafted from the 2005 *Dietary Guidelines for Americans*, incorporates the principles of variety, moderation, proportionality, and activity.

- Compared to breakfast eaters, youth who skip breakfast eat less vitamins and minerals, have lower academic performance, frequently eat unhealthy snacks, and are more likely to be overweight.

- Soft drink consumption has increased over the last several decades as milk intake has decreased. Soft drinks are empty calories that may contribute to a positive calorie balance. They are associated with lower intakes of milk, vegetables, and fruit, and thus lower intakes of certain vitamins and minerals.

- The prevalence of overweight is increasing among youth. Children suffer greater social and psychological effects of obesity than adults. Disorders common in adults who are overweight, such as glucose intolerance, type 2 diabetes, hypertension, hyperlipidemia, and metabolic syndrome, may also develop in children who are overweight. Childhood overweight may increase the risk for cancer, insulin resistance, stroke, cardiovascular disease, and renal failure in adulthood.

- Adolescents may have unhealthy eating habits that increase their risk of poor pregnancy outcome, such as a high intake of sugar and inadequate intakes of iron, folate, zinc, and calcium.

## ANSWER KEY

1. **TRUE** The amount of calories and protein needed per unit of body weight is greater for infants than for adults because growth in the first year of life is more rapid than at any other time in the life cycle (excluding the fetal period).

2. **TRUE** If breastfeeding is discontinued before the infant's first birthday, it should be replaced with iron-fortified infant formula. Cow's milk is not recommended before the age of 1 year.

3. **FALSE** Iron is the nutrient of most concern when solids are introduced into the diet.

4. **TRUE** Overfeeding is a potential problem with early introduction of solid foods because young infants are unable to communicate satiety, the feeling of fullness.

5. **TRUE** The risk of nutrient deficiencies among American toddlers is negligible. However, the risks of overfeeding and eating empty calories are real.

6. **FALSE** The *Dietary Guidelines for Americans* are intended for all Americans over the age of 2 years.

7. **TRUE** Milk can displace the intake of iron-rich foods, increasing the risk of iron deficiency.

8. **FALSE** Parents should decide what their children eat; children should decide how much. Children who are not allowed to self-regulate the amount of food they consume may overeat.

9. **TRUE** An overweight child is more likely to develop complications of adult overweight, such as diabetes, hypertension, and metabolic syndrome.

10. **TRUE** Adolescents consume approximately two-and-a-half times more soft drinks than milk.

## WEBSITES

American Academy of Pediatrics at **www.aap.org**
Children's Nutrition Research Center at Baylor College of Medicine at **www.bcm.tcm.edu/cnrc**
Food and Nutrition Information Center for information on child care nutrition, WIC, and healthy school meals at **www.nal.usda.gov/fnic**
Kids Food CyberClub at **www.kidsfood.org**
KidsHealth at **www.kidshealth.org**
Nutrition Explorations at **www.nutritionexplorations.org**

## REFERENCES

Affenito, S. (2007). Breakfast: A missed opportunity. *Journal of the American Dietetic Association, 107,* 565–569.

American Academy of Pediatrics. (2003). Policy statement. Prevention of pediatric overweight and obesity. *Pediatrics, 112,* 424–430.

American Academy of Pediatrics. (2005). Policy Statement. Breastfeeding and the use of human milk. *Pediatrics, 115,* 496–506.

American Dietetic Association. (2004a). Position of the American Dietetic Association: Dietary guidance for healthy children ages 2–11 years. *Journal of the American Dietetic Association, 104,* 660–677.

American Dietetic Association. (2004b). Position of the American Dietetic Association. Use of nutritive and nonnutritive sweeteners. *Journal of the American Dietetic Association, 104,* 255–275.

American Dietetic Association. (2006). Position of the American Dietetic Association: Individual-, family-, school-, and community-based interventions for pediatric overweight. *Journal of the American Dietetic Association, 106,* 925–945.

American Heart Association (AHA). (2006). Dietary recommendations for children and adolescents: A guide for practitioners. *Pediatrics, 117,* 544–559.

Crosnoe, R. (2007). Gender, obesity, and education. *Sociology of Education, 80,* 241–260.

Devaney, B., Ziegle, P., Pac, S., et al. (2004). Nutrient intakes of infants and toddlers. *Journal of the American Dietetic Association, 104* (Suppl. 1), S14–S21.

Dietz, W. (2004). Oveweight in childhood and adolescence. *The New England Journal of Medicine, 350,* 855–857.

Fisher, J. & Birch, L. (1999). Restricting access to palatable foods affects children's behavioral response, food selection, and intake. *The American Journal of Clincal Nutrition, 69,* 1264–1272.

Fox, M., Pac, S., Devaney, B., et al. (2004). Feeding infants and toddlers study: What foods are infants and toddlers eating? *Journal of the American Dietetic Association, 104*(Suppl. 1), S22–S30.

Gable, S., Chang, Y., & Krull, J. L. (2007). Television watching and frequency of family meals are predictive of overweight onset and persistence in a national sample of school-aged children. *Journal of the American Dietetic Association, 107,* 53–61.

Heird, W., and Cooper, A. (2006). *Infancy and Childhood.* In: Shils, M., Shike, M., Ross, A. C., et al. (eds.) Modern Nutrition in Health and Disease. (10th ed.). Philadelphia: Lippincott, Williams & Wilkins.

Institute of Medicine. (2005). *Dietary Reference Intakes for energy, carbohydrate, fiber, fat, fatty acids, cholesterol, protein, and amino acids.* Washington, DC: National Academies Press.

Institute of Medicine. (2006). *WIC food packages: Time for a change.* Washington, DC: National Academies Press.

Johnson, R. (2000). Changing eating and physical activity patterns of US children. *The Proceedings of the Nutrition Society, 59,* 295–301.

Kleinman, R. E., Hall, S., Green, H., et al. (2002). Diet, breakfast, and academic performance in children. *Annals of Nutrition & Metabolism, 46*(Suppl. 1), 24–30.

Krebs, N., & Hambidge, M. (2007). Complementary feeding: Clinically relevant factors affecting timing and composition. *The American Journal of Clinical Nutrition, 85*(Suppl.), 639S–645S.

LaFontaine, T. (2008). The epidemic of obesity and overweight among youth: Trends, consequences, and interventions. *American Journal of Lifestyle Medicine, 2,* 30–36.

Marcason, W. (2005). Can dietary intervention play a part in the treatment of attention deficit and hyperactivity disorder? *Journal of the American Dietetic Association, 105,* 1161–1162.

March of Dimes. (2007). *Professionals & researchers. Quick reference: Fact sheets: Teenage pregnancy.* Available at www.marchofdimes.com/printableArticles/14332_1159.asp. Accessed on 4/21/08.

Nicklas, T., O'Neil, C., & Berenson, G. (1998). Nutrient contribution of breakfast, secular trends, and the role of ready-to-eat cereals: A review of data from the Bogalusa Heart Study. *American Journal of Clinical Nutrition, 67*(Suppl.), 757–763S.

Nicklas, T., O'Neil, C., & Myers, L. (2004). The importance of breakfast consumption to nutrition of children, adolescents, and young adults. *Nutrition Today, 1,* 30–39.

Nielsen, J. N., Gittelsohn, J., Anliker, J., et al. (2006). Interventions to improve diet and weight gain among pregnant adolescents and recommendations for future research. *Journal of the American Dietetic Association, 106,* 1825–1840.

PAHO/WHO. (2003). *Guiding principles for complementary feeding of the breastfed child.* Washington, DC: PAHO, WHO.

Pollitt, E. and Mathews, R. (1998). Breakfast and cognition: An integrative summary. *The American Journal of Clinical Nutrition, 67*(Suppl.), 804S–813S.

Rampersaud, G. C., Pereira, M. A., Girard, B. L., et al. (2005). Breakfast habits, nutritional status, body weight, and academic performance in children and adolescents. *Journal of the American Dietetic Association, 105,* 743–760.

Shepherd, L. M., Neumark-Sztainer, D., Beyer, K. M., et al. (2006). Should we discuss weight and calories in adolescent obesity prevention and weight-management programs? Perspectives of adolescent girls. *Journal of the American Dietetic Association, 106,* 1454–1458.

Shils, M. E., Shike, M., Ross, A. C., et al. (2006). *Modern Nutrition in Health and Disease* (10th ed.). Philadelphia: Lippincott Williams & Wilkins.

Treuth, M. & Griffin, I. (2006). "Adolescence." in Shils et al.

Utter, J., Scragg, R., Mhurchu, C. N., et al. (2007). At-home breakfast consumption among New Zealand children: Associations with body mass index and related nutrition behaviors. *Journal of the American Dietetic Association, 107,* 570–576.

USDHHS. (2004). *The health consequences of smoking: A report of the Surgeon General.* Atlanta: CDC, Office on Smoking and Health at www.cdc.gov/tobacco/data_statistics/sgr/sgr_2004/highlights/3.htm. Accessed 7/21/08.

USDHHS, USDA. (2005). *Dietary guidelines for Americans.* Available at www.health.gov/dietaryguidelines.

van Dam, R. M., Willet, W. C., Manson, J. E., et al. (2006). The relationship between overweight in adolescents and premature death in women. *Annals of Internal Medicine, 145,* 91–97.

# 13 Nutrition for Older Adults

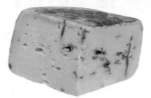

### UPON COMPLETION OF THIS CHAPTER, YOU WILL BE ABLE TO

- Give examples of physiological changes that occur with aging that have an impact on nutrition.
- Compare calorie and nutrient needs of older adults to those of younger adults.
- Compare MyPyramid with the Modified MyPyramid for Older Adults.
- Explain why older adults may need supplements of calcium, vitamin D, and vitamin $B_{12}$.
- Screen an older person for risk of nutrition problems.
- Debate the benefits of using a liberal diet in long-term care facilities.
- Propose strategies for enhancing food intake in long-term care residents.

With the exception of Chapters 11 and 12, which cover infants, children, and adolescents, this book implicitly addresses nutrition as it pertains to adults—nutrient and calorie basics in Section 1; food intake guidelines and consumer and cultural nutrition issues in Section 2; and the role of nutrition in the prevention and treatment of illness and disease in Section 3. Yet adulthood represents a wide age range, from young adults at 18 to the "oldest old." Adults over 50, and especially those over 70, have different nutritional needs than do younger adults. This chapter focuses on how aging impacts nutrition for older adults.

# ▶ AGING AND OLDER ADULTS

Aging is a gradual, inevitable, complex process of progressive physiologic, cellular, cultural, and psychosocial changes that begin at conception and end at death. As cells age, they undergo degenerative changes in structure and function that eventually lead to impairment of organs, tissues, and body functioning. Box 13.1 outlines the changes in physiology, income, health, and psychosocial well-being associated with aging that have nutritional implications. Exactly how and why aging occurs is unknown, although most theories are based on genetic or environmental causes.

## Aging Demographics

Older adults, especially those older than 75 years of age, represent the fastest-growing segment of the American population (Federal Interagency Forum on Aging-Related Statistics, 2008). In 2006, an estimated 37 million people, just over 12% of the population,

---

**BOX 13.1**     **CHANGES THAT MAY OCCUR WITH AGING**

**Body Composition and Energy Expenditure Changes**
- Decrease in lean body mass.
- Increase in fat tissue.
- Decrease in basal metabolic rate.
- Decrease in physical activity.

**Oral and GI Changes**
- Difficulty in chewing related to loss of teeth and periodontal disease.
- Constipation is more common and may be related to decreased peristalsis from loss of abdominal muscle tone; inadequate fluid and fiber intake; secondary reaction to drug therapy; or a decrease in physical activity.
- Digestive disorders may occur from a decreased secretion of HCl in the stomach and digestive enzymes; decreased GI motility; and decreased organ function.
- Prevalence of atrophic gastritis increases.
- Nutrient absorption may decrease because of decreased mucosal mass and decreased blood flow to and from the mucosal villi.

**Metabolic Changes**
- Altered glucose tolerance; the underlying reason may be a decrease in insulin secretion or a decrease in tissue sensitivity to insulin.
- Synthesis of vitamin D in the skin decreases with age.

**CNS Changes**
- Tremors, slowed reaction time, short-term memory deficits, personality changes, and depression may occur secondary to a decrease in the number of brain cells or the decrease in blood flow to the brain.

**Renal Changes**
- Ability to concentrate urine decreases.

**Sensory Losses**
- Hearing loss, loss of visual acuity, decreased sense of smell, decreased number of taste buds, and decreased sensation of thirst.

**Change in income related to retirement**

**Reliance on medications**

**Social isolation related to death of spouse, living alone, impaired mobility**

**Poor self-esteem related to change in body image, lack of productivity, feelings of aimlessness**

were 65 and over. By the year 2030, it is estimated that 71.5 million Americans, nearly 20% of the population, will be over 65. The number of Americans aged 80 and older is expected to increase from 9.3 million in 2000 to 19.5 million in 2030.

Life expectancies at both 65 and 85 have increased. People who live to age 65 can expect to live an average of 18.7 more years; among people who live to age 85, women will survive another 7.2 years on average and men will survive another 6.1 years (Federal Interagency Forum on Aging-Related Statistics, 2008). Adopting a healthy lifestyle early in life and maintaining it throughout life may help the elderly be independent and relatively healthy into their later years (Kennedy, 2006).

Despite the misconceptions and stereotypes that people have of older adults, they are a heterogeneous group that varies in age, marital status, social background, financial status, living arrangements, and health status. In the United States, approximately 80% of adults older than 65 years of age have one chronic health problem, such as arthritis, hypertension, heart disease, and diabetes (Fig. 13.1) (Federal Interagency Forum on Aging-Related Statistics, 2008). Yet during 2004–2006, 74% of people 65 and older considered their health to be good or better (Federal Interagency Forum on Aging-Related Statistics, 2008), possibly because people define wellness and illness differently as they age and may accept

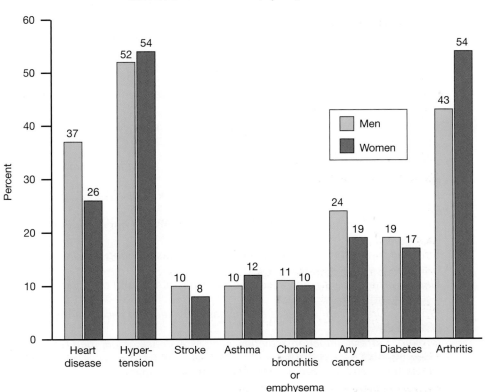

Percentage of people age 65 and over who reported having selected chronic conditions, by sex, 2005–2006

Note: Data are based on a 2-year average from 2005–2006.
Reference population: These data refer to the civilian noninstitutionalized population.
Source: Centers for Disease Control and Prevention, National Center for Health Statistics, National Health Interview Survey.

**FIGURE 13.1**  Chronic health conditions. (**Source:** Interagency Forum on Aging-Related Statistics. Older Americans 2008: Key Indicators of Well-Being. Washington, DC: U.S. Government Printing Office. March 2008.)

changes in health as a normal aspect of aging. Certainly differences exist between the "well" and the "frail" elderly, the latter group consisting of those with defined needs for support for activities of daily living. In 2004, only 3.5% of people 65 and older lived in nursing homes (Federal Interagency Forum on Aging-Related Statistics, 2008).

## Healthy Aging

Genetic and environmental "life advantages"—such as genetic potential for longevity, intelligence, motivation, curiosity, good socialization, religious affiliation, marriage and family, physical activity, avoidance of substance abuse, availability of health care, adequate sleep, sufficient rest and relaxation, and good eating habits—have positive effects on both length and quality of life. The CDC's tips for a healthy life for adults begins with the recommendation to "eat healthy" (Box 13.2).

Preventing disease is the key to healthy aging, and nutrition and exercise play a role in beginning life healthy, staying healthy, and maintaining a low risk of chronic disease throughout life (Dwyer, 2006). Good nutrition can enhance wellness, improve nutritional status, help avoid illness, and prevent or delay diseases and disability (Wellman, 2007). Exercise decreases the risk of diabetes, hypertension, cardiovascular diseases, osteoporosis, and sarcopenia (Kennedy, 2006). Although the earlier in life a healthy diet and lifestyle are adopted the better, evidence shows that even initiating healthy changes in one's 60s and 70s provides definite benefits in many categories of chronic disease (Rivlin, 2007).

## Nutritional Needs of Older Adults

Knowledge of the nutritional needs of older adults is growing. However, health status, physiologic functioning, physical activity, and nutritional status vary more among older adults (especially people older than 70 years of age) than among individuals in any other age group,

---

**BOX 13.2**  **TIPS FOR A HEALTHY LIFE FOR ADULT MEN AND WOMEN**

- Eat healthy
  *Eat at least five servings of fruits and vegetables a day and consume less saturated fat.*
- Maintain healthy weight
  *Eat better and exercise regularly to reduce the risk of disease.*
- Get moving
  *Get at least 30 minutes of moderate activity on most, if not all, days of the week.*
- Be smoke-free
  *Smoking triples the risk of dying from heart disease among middle aged people.*
- Get routine exams and screenings
  *Finding problems early increases the chance of successful treatment.*
- Get appropriate vaccinations
  *Protect yourself from illnesses and diseases by keeping vaccinations up to date.*
- Manage stress
  *Engage in stress reduction activities, such as exercise, yoga, meditation, or massage.*
- Know yourself and your risks
  *High risk may come from genetics, lifestyle, or occupation.*
- Protect yourself
  *Wear sunscreen, use seatbelts, and wash your hands.*
- Be good to yourself
  *Get enough sleep and balance work with play.*

*Source:* CDC. Tips for a healthy life. Available at www.cdc.gov/women/tips.htm and www.cdc.gov/men/tips.htm. Accessed on 5/13/08.

so nutrient recommendations may not be appropriate for all elderly individuals at all times. In general, calorie needs decrease, yet vitamin and mineral requirements stay the same or increase. Two Dietary Reference Intake (DRI) groupings exist for mature adults, one for people aged 51 to 70 and the other for adults over the age of 70. Calories and selected nutrients are discussed below.

## Calories

Calorie needs decrease with age due to a decrease in metabolic rate and a decrease in calorie expenditure (IOM, 2005). Changes in body composition, namely a decrease in muscle and bone mass and an increase in percentage of body fat, account for the decrease in metabolic rate of approximately 2% per decade beginning around the age of 30 (Elmadfa & Meyer, 2008). Physical activity also progressively declines from age 20 through age 80. Taken together, these changes lead to an estimated 5% decrease in total calorie needs each decade. However, neither the changes in body composition nor the decrease in physical activity is inevitable (Rivlin, 2007). These undesirable consequences of aging can be improved or reversed with an appropriate calorie intake, nutrient-dense food choices, and regular physical activity.

Table 13.1 shows MyPyramid calorie levels from young adulthood through age 76 and older. Among adults, daily calorie recommendations for men are lowest from age 66 on and are 600 cal/day less than peak calorie requirements for younger men aged 19 to 25. Calorie requirements for women are generally lowest from age 51 onward, 400 cal/day less than the peak requirements for women at ages 19 to 25.

## Protein

The Recommended Dietary Allowance (RDA) for protein remains constant at 0.8 g/kg for both men and women from the age of 19 on. According to data from the National Health

**TABLE 13.1    MyPyramid Food Intake Pattern Calorie Levels**

MyPyramid assigns Individuals to a calorie level based on their sex, age, and activity level.

| Males | | | | Females | | | |
|---|---|---|---|---|---|---|---|
| Activity Level | Sedentary* | Mod. Active* | Active* | Activity Level | Sedentary* | Mod. Active* | Active* |
| Age | | | | Age | | | |
| 19–20 | 2600 | 2800 | 3000 | 19–20 | 2000 | 2200 | 2400 |
| 21–25 | 2400 | 2800 | 3000 | 21–25 | 2000 | 2200 | 2400 |
| 26–30 | 2400 | 2600 | 3000 | 26–30 | 1800 | 2000 | 2400 |
| 31–35 | 2400 | 2600 | 3000 | 31–35 | 1800 | 2000 | 2200 |
| 36–40 | 2400 | 2600 | 2800 | 36–40 | 1800 | 2000 | 2200 |
| 41–45 | 2200 | 2600 | 2800 | 41–45 | 1800 | 2000 | 2200 |
| 46–50 | 2200 | 2400 | 2800 | 46–50 | 1800 | 2000 | 2200 |
| 51–55 | 2200 | 2400 | 2800 | 51–55 | 1600 | 1800 | 2200 |
| 56–60 | 2200 | 2400 | 2600 | 56–60 | 1600 | 1800 | 2200 |
| 61–65 | 2000 | 2400 | 2600 | 61–65 | 1600 | 1800 | 2000 |
| 66–70 | 2000 | 2200 | 2600 | 66–70 | 1600 | 1800 | 2000 |
| 71–75 | 2000 | 2200 | 2600 | 71–75 | 1600 | 1800 | 2000 |
| 76 and up | 2000 | 2200 | 2400 | 76 and up | 1600 | 1800 | 2000 |

*Calorie levels are based on the Estimated Energy Requirements (EER) and activity levels from the Institute of Medicine Dietary Reference Intakes Macronutrients Report, 2002.

SEDENTARY = less than 30 minutes a day of moderate physical activity in addition to daily activities.

MOD. ACTIVE = at least 30 minutes up to 60 minutes a day of moderate physical activity in addition to daily activities.

ACTIVE = 60 or more minutes a day of moderate physical activity in addition to daily activities.

and Nutrition Examination Survey (NHANES) 2001–2002, protein intake exceeds the RDA for both men and women among all age groups, although a steady decline in intake occurs with aging (Moshfegh et al., 2005). The mean protein intake in the age group of 71 and older is 1.04 g/kg for men and 0.95 g/kg for women. However, it is estimated that 7.2% to 8.6% of older adult women consume protein below their estimated average requirement (Fulgoni, 2008). Factors that may contribute to a low protein intake include the cost of high-protein foods, the decreased ability to chew meats, lower overall intake of food, and changes in digestion and gastric emptying (Paddon-Jones, D., Short, K., Campbell, W., et al., 2008). Groups at risk for inadequate protein intake include the oldest elderly, those with health problems, and those in nursing homes (Bales & Ritchie, 2006).

## Water

The adequate intake (AI) for water is constant from 19 years of age through more than 70 years old, with 3.7 L/day of total water recommended for men and 2.7 L/day for women (IOM, 2006). Both of these figures represent total water intake from beverages, drinking water, and water in solid foods. Like younger adults, the elderly are able to maintain fluid balance over a wide range of intakes. However, an altered sensation of thirst and an age-related decrease in the ability to concentrate urine may increase the risk of dehydration and hyponatremia, especially in hot weather or when water intake is impaired.

## Fiber

For all age groups, the AI for fiber is based on median intake levels observed to protect against coronary heart disease (CHD) (IOM, 2005). From the age of one on and for both genders, the AI for fiber is set at 14 g/1000 cal of intake. Based on median calorie intakes obtained from food surveys, the AI for fiber is 38 g/day for men through age 50 and 30 g/day thereafter. A similar decrease occurs in women, whose AI is 25 g/day from 19 to 50 and 21 g/day thereafter. Mean intake for men over 50 is 16 to 18 g, and for women it is approximately 14 to 15 g. Increasing fiber intake may help prevent constipation and decrease the risk of diabetes (Bales & Ritchie, 2006).

## Vitamins and Minerals

Most recommended levels of intake for vitamins and minerals do not change with aging. Significant exceptions to this generalization are calcium, vitamin D, and iron recommendations for women (Table 13.2). The DRI for sodium decreases with aging because the AI is extrapolated from younger adults based on median calorie intakes from food surveys.

### TABLE 13.2 — Important Nutrients Whose DRIS Change with Aging*

| Nutrient | Age 31–50 | Age 51–70 | Age >70 | Rationale for Change |
|---|---|---|---|---|
| Calcium (mg/day) | 1000 | 1200 | 1200 | The efficiency of calcium absorption decreases with age |
| Vitamin D (micrograms/day) | 5 | 10 | 15 | The ability to synthesize vitamin D on the skin from sunlight decreases with age |
| **Iron (mg/day) Females only** | **18** | **8** | **8** | Cessation of menstruation |

**Bold** items are Recommended Dietary Allowances (RDA), whereas Adequate Intakes (AI) appear in ordinary type.

*Values are for both males and females unless otherwise indicated.

*Source:* Institute of Medicine, Dietary Reference Intakes at www.nap.edu

Although the total amount of vitamin B₁₂ recommended does not change with aging, people over 50 are advised to consume most of their requirement from fortified food or supplements because 10% to 30% of older adults may not be able to absorb natural vitamin B₁₂ from food (IOM, 2000).

## Modified MyPyramid for Older Adults

**QUICK BITE**

Sources of vitamin D are
  Vitamin D-fortified milk or soy milk
  Fatty fish such as salmon, mackerel, and
    sardines
  Some fortified ready-to-eat cereals
  Sunshine

Modified MyPyramid for Older Adults, produced by Tufts University, is designed to help older adults choose a healthy diet (Fig. 13.2). It differs from MyPyramid in the following ways:

- Physical activity forms the base of the pyramid as a horizontal row. Activities enjoyed by older adults, such as walking, gardening, and group water activities, are featured. By increasing calorie expenditure, exercise can minimize the changes in body composition that occur with aging (Rivlin, 2007).
- Eight glasses of water appear in a horizontal row immediately above physical activity to highlight the importance of adequate fluid.
- Nutrient-dense food choices are used to illustrate each food group. As calorie needs decrease, there is less room for "extras," the discretionary calories from foods high in added fat or sugar.
- A flag appears at the top to alert older adults to their unique nutrient needs, namely the increased need for calcium and vitamin D and the recommendation that synthetic B₁₂ be consumed from supplements and/or fortified foods.
- The Modified MyPyramid for Older Adults is available in print form so that older adults who do not use a computer can still have easy access to nutrition guidance.

In addition to the graphic, the Modified MyPyramid for Adults comes with additional tips for healthy eating—limit foods with added sugar; choose healthy fats to limit the intake of saturated and trans fats; limit sodium by eating less salt and buying reduced sodium soups and frozen entrées; and choose high-fiber grains.

## Nutrient and Food Intake of Older Adults

In general, as calorie needs decrease with aging so does the quantity of food eaten and the amount of calories consumed (ADA, 2005a). Comparisons between 25-year-olds and 70-year-olds show that mean calorie intake falls by 1000 to 1200 cal/day in men and 600 to 800 cal/day in women (ADA, 2005a). Consuming less food translates to a lower intake of micronutrients (ADA, 2005a). According to data from **NHANES** 2001–2002, the nutrients with mean intakes less than the DRI among both the 51- to 70-year-old group and the 70+ age group are vitamin E, magnesium, fiber, calcium, and potassium (Box 13.3) (Moshfegh et al., 2005). (Vitamin D intake is not assessed through NHANES.)

**NHANES:** National Health and Nutrition Examination Survey; a survey conducted by the National Center for Health Statistics designed to assess the health and nutritional status of adults and children in the United States via personal interviews and physical exams.

**QUICK BITE**

Fruits and vegetables that are easily consumed by people who have difficulty chewing
  Ripe bananas          Canned fruit
  Baked winter squash   Soft melon
  Mashed potatoes       Citrus sections
  Stewed tomatoes       Cooked carrots
  Baked apples

Like younger adults, older Americans consume less fruit and vegetables than recommended and starchy vegetables account for about 80% of total vegetable intake on any given day (USDA, CNPP, 2007). According to the Healthy Eating Index (HEI) 2005, a tool designed to measure compliance of diets

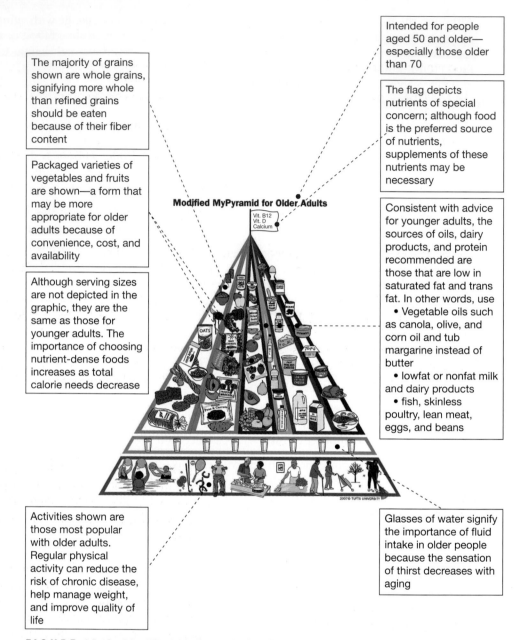

The majority of grains shown are whole grains, signifying more whole than refined grains should be eaten because of their fiber content

Packaged varieties of vegetables and fruits are shown—a form that may be more appropriate for older adults because of convenience, cost, and availability

Although serving sizes are not depicted in the graphic, they are the same as those for younger adults. The importance of choosing nutrient-dense foods increases as total calorie needs decrease

Intended for people aged 50 and older—especially those older than 70

The flag depicts nutrients of special concern; although food is the preferred source of nutrients, supplements of these nutrients may be necessary

Consistent with advice for younger adults, the sources of oils, dairy products, and protein recommended are those that are low in saturated fat and trans fat. In other words, use
• Vegetable oils such as canola, olive, and corn oil and tub margarine instead of butter
• lowfat or nonfat milk and dairy products
• fish, skinless poultry, lean meat, eggs, and beans

**Modified MyPyramid for Older Adults**

Vit. B12
Vit. D
Calcium

Activities shown are those most popular with older adults. Regular physical activity can reduce the risk of chronic disease, help manage weight, and improve quality of life

Glasses of water signify the importance of fluid intake in older people because the sensation of thirst decreases with aging

**FIGURE 13.2** Modified MyPyramid for Older Adults. (Journal of Nutrition. Online by Lichtenstein, A. © 2008 by American Society for Nutrition. Reproduced with permission.)

with the key diet-quality recommendations of the 2005 *Dietary Guidelines for Americans,* older adults need to improve their intakes of whole grains; dark green and orange vegetables; dried peas and beans; and fat-free and low-fat milk and milk products (Federal Interagency Forum on Aging-Related Statistics, 2008). Notice in Box 13.3 that for the nutrients most likely to be consumed in inadequate amounts by older adults, whole grains, vegetables (especially green leafy vegetables), dried peas and beans, and milk are listed as sources for three or more of these nutrients. Additional conclusions based on the HEI are that older adults need to eat more of all types of vegetables and fruits; should replace some solid fats with oils, including those in fish, nuts, and seeds; and should consume less sodium, saturated fat, and food

| BOX 13.3 | SOURCES OF NUTRIENTS THAT MAY BE LACKING IN THE DIETS OF OLDER ADULTS |
|---|---|

Vitamin E: vegetable oils, margarine, salad dressing made with vegetable oil, nuts, seeds, **whole grains, green leafy vegetables,** fortified cereals

Magnesium: **green leafy vegetables,** nuts, **dried peas and beans, whole grains,** seafood, chocolate, **milk**

Fiber: **whole grains; dried peas and beans;** fruit and **vegetables,** especially the skin and seeds

Calcium: **milk,** yogurt, cheese, fortified orange juice, **green leafy vegetables, dried peas and beans**

Potassium: Fruit and **vegetables; dried peas and beans, whole grains, milk,** meats

(**Bold** type used to illustrate the commonality of sources among these nutrients)

and beverages with added sugar, solid fats, and alcohol (Federal Interagency Forum on Aging-Related Statistics, 2008). Interestingly, the Healthy Eating Index is 64 out of 100 for adults aged 55 to 65 and improves to 68 for adults 65 and older.

While snacking may contribute to an excess calorie intake and obesity in other age groups, snacking in older adults may help ensure an adequate intake. In a study of adults aged 65 and older, those who snacked had significantly higher intakes of calories, protein, carbohydrate, and fat than non-snackers; snacking contributed almost 25% of their total calorie intake and 14% of their protein intake (Zizza et al., 2007). For older adults at risk of inadequate intake, encouraging snacking between meals may be more effective than urging them to eat more at each meal.

## Vitamin and Mineral Supplements

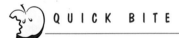

### QUICK BITE

**Demographics of older supplement users**

Among older women, supplement users tend to be:

- White
- From the western region of the country
- Nonsmokers
- Convinced that following a diet consistent with the *Dietary Guideline* recommendations is important

Among older men, supplement users tend to be:

- In the 71+ age group rather than the 51–70 year old group
- Living in metropolitan areas
- Better educated
- Convinced that following a diet consistent with the *Dietary Guideline* recommendations is important

*Source:* Sebastian, R., Cleveland, L., Goldman, J., et al. (2007). Older adults who use vitamin/mineral supplements differ from nonuser in nutrient intake adequacy and dietary attitudes. *Journal of the American Dietetic Association, 107,* 1322–1332.

In theory, older adults should be able to obtain adequate amounts of all essential nutrients through well-chosen foods. In practice, a large percentage of older adults do not obtain recommended amounts of many nutrients from food alone (Sebastian et al., 2007). A study by Sebastian et al. (2007), found that 50% of older adults had inadequate intakes of vitamin E and magnesium from food alone and that regular supplement use lowered the percentage of older adults with inadequate intakes by at least 75% for most nutrients. Folate intake was also noted to be inadequate in 50% of this population but that figure is believed to be overestimated because figures were based on folate absorption, which is lower than the absorption of synthetic folic acid found in fortified foods.

Supplements tend to have a positive impact on nutritional adequacy for adults 51 and older. While food is the preferred vehicle for providing nutrients, supplements can be valuable in helping older adults achieve nutritional adequacy (Sebastian et al.,

2007). Routine supplements of iron and vitamin A (in the form of retinol) should be avoided to prevent exceeding the upper limit. Interestingly, supplement users generally tend to eat more nutrient-dense diets than non-supplement users.

## Nutrition Screening for Older Adults

Older adults at greatest risk of consuming an inadequate diet are those who are less educated, live alone, and have low incomes. Frequently, food choices of older adults are based on considerations other than food preferences such as income; the client's physical ability to shop, prepare, chew, and swallow food; and the occurrence of food intolerances related to chronic disease or side effects of medications. Inadequate calorie intake can precipitate unintentional weight loss; weight loss in older adults is associated with functional limitations, nursing home admissions, and mortality (Zizza et al., 2007).

Identifying nutritional problems in older adults can be a challenge. Traditional assessment findings may be unreliable or invalid in older adults due to changes related to aging. Accurate weights are difficult to obtain in clients who are bedridden, and curvature of the spine interferes with accurate measurement of height. Likewise, age-related changes in physiology and function may mimic signs of a nutritional deficiency. For instance, loss of visual acuity in dim light occurs with aging and may not indicate a deficiency of vitamin A. Historical data are difficult to obtain from clients who have hearing loss or cognitive impairments. Box 13.4 lists screening criteria that may indicate nutritional risk.

---

**BOX 13.4    SCREENING CRITERIA FOR MALNUTRITION IN OLDER ADULTS**

**Disease**
*Do you have an illness that makes you change the kind and/or amount of food you eat?*

**Eating poorly**
*Do you eat fewer than two meals a day? Do you eat few fruits, vegetables, or milk products? Do you have three or more drinks of beer, liquor, or wine almost every day?*

**Tooth loss/mouth pain**
*Do you have tooth or mouth problems that make it hard for you to eat?*

**Economic hardship**
*Do you sometimes not have enough money to spend on the food you need?*

**Reduced social contact**
*Do you eat alone most of the time?*

**Multiple medications**
*Do you take three or more different prescribed or over-the-counter dugs a day?*

**Involuntary weight loss/gain**
*Have you gained or lost 10 pounds in the last 6 months without trying?*

**Needs assistance in self-care**
*Are you sometimes not physically able to shop, cook, and/or feed yourself?*

**Above age 80**
*Are you older than 80?*

*Source:* The Nutrition Screening Initiative, project of The American Academy of Family Physicians, The American Dietetic Association, the National Council on the Aging, Inc. The Nutrition Screening Initiative is funded in part by a grant from Ross Laboratories, a division of Abbott Laboratories.

# ► NUTRITION-RELATED CONCERNS IN OLDER ADULTS

Nutrition therapy for older adults should be client-centered and based on the individual's physiologic, pathologic, and psychosocial conditions. Overall goals of nutrition therapy for older adults are to maintain or restore maximal independent functioning and health and to maintain the client's sense of dignity and quality of life by imposing as few dietary restrictions as possible. Any necessary dietary changes should be incorporated into the client's existing food pattern because attempting to impose a completely new approach to eating could be counterproductive.

## Cataracts and Macular Degeneration

**Cataracts:** a clouding of the lenses of the eyes that impairs vision and can lead to blindness.

**Macular degeneration:** loss of central vision and eventually blindness that is related to the deterioration of the macular area of the eye.

The prevalence of **cataracts** and age-related **macular degeneration** (AMD) are increasing as the population of older Americans increases (Seddon, 2007). By age 80, more than half of all Americans either have a cataract or have had cataract surgery (National Eye Institute, 2006). AMD is the major cause of legal blindness in North America, Australia, and Western European countries (Tomany et al., 2004). Cataracts and macular degeneration were commonly assumed to be inevitable consequences of aging.

QUICK BITE

Sources of lutein and zeaxanthin (carotene pigments in plants):

- Kale
- Spinach
- Collard greens
- Mustard greens
- Turnip greens
- Broccoli
- Brussels sprouts

Over the last 25 years, researchers have been studying whether diet or supplements can slow or prevent the progression of cataracts and AMD. The hypothesis was that oxidative stress from pollution, smoking, sunlight, or normal metabolism generates free radicals that damage the eye when they are oxidized and that antioxidant nutrients, such as vitamin C, vitamin E, and beta-carotene, may offer protection. Trials are still ongoing but it appears that a multivitamin–multimineral supplement containing vitamin C, vitamin E, beta-carotene, and zinc is effective for AMD but not cataracts (Seddon, 2007). Observational studies show that a diet rich in antioxidants, especially lutein and zeaxanthin, and omega-3 fatty acids benefits AMD and possibly cataracts (Seddon, 2007). A long-term prospective study by Chiu et al. showed that people who eat diets high in refined carbohydrates (high glycemic index) are at greater risk of AMD progression than people who eat less refined carbohydrates (Chiu et al., 2007). They hypothesize that a high glycemic index diet creates a chronically high level of oxidative stress as high levels of glucose enter the cells after eating. In contrast, low glycemic index diets appear to decrease oxidative stress. At the very least, a diet rich in fruits, vegetables, and whole grains is healthy and may help prevent age-related vision loss.

## Functional Limitations

**Instrumental activities of daily living (IADL) limitations:** difficulty performing (or unable to perform for a health reason) one or more of the following tasks: using the telephone, light housework, heavy housework, meal preparation, shopping, or managing money.

**Activities of daily living (ADL) limitations:** difficulty performing (or unable to perform for a health reason) one or more of the following tasks: bathing, dressing, eating, getting in/out of chairs, walking, or using the toilet.

Aging causes a progressive decline in physical function that is related to a decrease in muscle mass and strength (Villareal et al., 2005). Between 1992 and 2005, the age-adjusted proportion of people aged 65 and older with a functional limitation (previously called disability) actually decreased from 49% to 42% (Federal Interagency Forum on Aging-Related Statistics, 2008). Twelve percent of this population had difficulty performing one or more **instrumental activities of daily living (IADL)** without any **activities of daily living (ADL)** limitation and 18% had difficulty with one to two ADLs. Major causes of functional limitations among older adults include arthritis, osteoporosis, and sarcopenia.

## Arthritis

Osteoarthritis (OA), the most common form of arthritis, can lead to joint degeneration, chronic pain, muscle atrophy, impaired mobility, and poor balance. Arthritis is a leading cause of functional limitation among older adults (ADA, 2005a). Among adults aged 70 and older who have arthritis, 50% need help with ADLs compared to only 23% of people in the same age group who do not have arthritis (ADA, 2005a). Older adults with arthritis rely on Meals On Wheels, among other services, more than older adults who do not have arthritis (ADA, 2005a).

OA is associated with aging and normal "wear and tear" on joints; the knee is the most commonly affected joint. Excess body weight is the greatest known modifiable risk factor (Haq et al., 2003); chronic overweight or obesity translates to chronic mechanical stress on the weight-bearing joints. Other risk factors for OA include genetics, age, ethnicity, gender, occupation, exercise, trauma, and bone density (Haq et al., 2003). Symptoms of OA usually appear after the age of 40 and by 65 years or more of age, the prevalence of OA is 68% in women and 58% in men (Villareal et al., 2005).

The objective of treatment is to control pain, improve function, and reduce physical limitations. Weight loss and appropriate exercise seem to have a positive effect on the prevention and treatment of OA (Greenstone, 2007). Data from the Arthritis, Diet, and Activity Promotion Trial (ADAPT) study of overweight and obese older adults with knee OA showed that the combination of a weight loss diet and exercise improved both subjective and objectives measures of physical function and quality of life, and the benefits were greater than when either diet or exercise were used alone (Messier et al., 2004). Losing weight reduces strain on the weight bearing joints; exercise improves strength, mobility, and joint stability and may also reduce pain and improve function (Roddy et al., 2005).

## Osteoporosis

**Peak bone mass:** the most bone mass a person will ever have.

Throughout life, bone tissue is constantly being destroyed and rebuilt, a process known as remodeling. In the first few decades of life, net gain exceeds net loss as bone mass is accrued. Between 30 and 35 years of age, **peak bone mass** is attained. Thereafter, more bone is lost than is gained. During the first 5 years or so after onset of menopause, women experience rapid bone loss related to estrogen deficiency. After that, bone loss continues at a slower rate.

Osteoporosis is a disease characterized by a decrease in total bone mass and deterioration of bone tissue which leads to increased bone fragility and risk of fracture. It affects almost 44 million American men and women aged 50 and older (ADA, 2005a). Estimated direct care costs of osteoporotic fractures are $12 to $18 billion annually (ADA, 2005a).

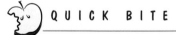 **Q U I C K   B I T E**

**Sources of phytoestrogens**

More than 20 compounds in more than 300 plants, including herbs, grains, and fruits, are classified as phytoestrogens:

| | |
|---|---|
| Soy beans and | Flaxseed oil |
| soy products | Cereal bran |
| Chickpeas | Alfalfa |
| Other legumes | Clover |

***Source:*** NIH, Osteoporosis and Related Bone Diseases-National Resource Center. Phytoestrogens and Bone Health. 2005. Available at http://www.niams.nih.gov/Health_Info/Bone/Osteoporosis/Menopause/bone_phyto.pdf. Accessed on 5/19/08.

Although osteoporosis manifests itself in older adults, the process actually begins much earlier in life. The peak period for calcium retention—and, therefore, the period during which measures to prevent osteoporosis can have their greatest impact—is between 4 and 20 years of age. The greater the peak bone mass, the less damaging the inevitable loss of bone mass.

However, results of studies show that interventions implemented late in life can effectively slow or halt bone loss. A study by Dawson-Hughes showed that in noninstitutionalized men and women 65 and older, consuming a supplement of 500 mg of

**Phytoestrogens:** naturally occurring plant compounds from plants that are functionally and structurally similar to human estrogen. Phytoestrogens tend to have weaker effects than most estrogens, are not stored in the body, and can be easily broken down and eliminated (NIH, 2005).

elemental calcium with 700 IU of vitamin D for a 3-year period reduced the rate of bone loss in the hip, spine, and total body and thus reduced or even halted the incidence of a first non-vertebral fracture (Dawson-Hughes et al., 1997). The Surgeon General's report on bone health and osteoporosis recommends Americans consume adequate amounts of calcium and vitamin D, maintain healthy body weight, and be physically active (USDHHS, 2004). People who cannot or will not consume the equivalent of three cups of milk daily should obtain the remaining calcium they need from calcium supplements. Calcium from supplements is absorbed best in doses of 500 mg or less, so if multiple doses are required, they should be spread out over the day. Other nutrients that are important for bone health include vitamin A, vitamin K, magnesium, vitamin C, and **phytoestrogens** (ADA, 2005a)—nutrients that can be obtained through a healthy diet that contains at least five servings of fruits and vegetables daily (Nieves, 2005).

## Sarcopenia

**Sarcopenia:** the loss of muscle mass with aging.

**Sarcopenia** is the loss of muscle mass and strength; advanced sarcopenia is characterized by physical frailty, increased likelihood of falls, and impaired ability to perform ADLs (Paddon-Jones, D., Short, K., Campbell, W., et al., 2008). Chronic muscle loss is estimated to affect 30% of people over the age of 60 and may affect more than 50% of those over 80. The loss of muscle mass is a process that begins in both men and women in their 40s and 50s (Schardt, 2007).

Sarcopenia is related to a sedentary lifestyle and less than optimal diet. Muscle protein synthesis decreases with age, probably because of a decreased response to the anabolic effects of insulin (Paddon-Jones, D., Short, K., Campbell, W., et al., 2008). Currently, strength training using progressive resistance is the best intervention shown to slow down or reverse sarcopenia (Fig. 13.3) (ADA, 2005a). An adequate protein intake is also essential and may be one of the few options available for older adults who are unable to exercise because of functional limitations or chronic disease. At least one study shows that older adults who consume the RDA for

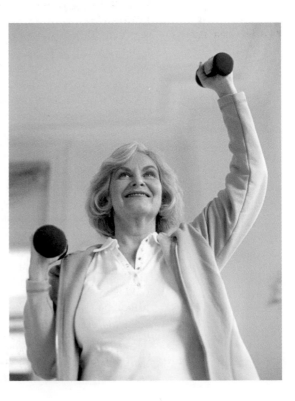

**FIGURE 13.3** An older woman exercising with dumbbells. Resistance training, such as weight lifting, is important for maintaining and building muscle mass.

protein will continue to lose muscle, despite strength training, and that to gain muscle mass, protein intake should be as much as 50% more than the current RDA (Chernoff, 2006).

## Alzheimer Disease

Alzheimer disease (AD) is the most common form of dementia in the United States, affecting an estimated 4.5 million Americans (NIA, 2007). Although not a normal consequence of aging, the risk of AD increases with age. Approximately half of all people over the age of 85 have AD (NIA, 2007).

The cause of AD is unknown, and there is no cure. AD appears to result from a complex series of events in the brain that occur over time. Disruptions in nerve cell communication, metabolism, and repair eventually cause many nerve cells to stop functioning, lose connections with other nerve cells, and die. Genetic and nongenetic factors (e.g., inflammation of the brain, stroke) have been identified in the etiology of AD. Like CHD, AD is at least partially a vascular problem, but plaques that form with AD are filled with beta-amyloid, an indissoluble protein, not fat and cholesterol. Researchers speculate that many of the risk factors for CHD may also increase the risk of AD: elevated homocysteine levels, hypercholesterolemia, high blood pressure, diabetes, and overweight.

The development of AD may also be related to oxidative stress. Some population and laboratory studies show that antioxidants from food or supplements offer some protective benefit while others do not (NIA, 2007). Clinical trials are underway to determine if vitamin E and C or vitamin E and/or selenium can help prevent dementia.

Another promising area of research is with omega-3 fatty acids, the predominate type of fat in fish oils. The Zutphen Elderly Study showed that people who eat fish had less cognitive decline than people who do not eat fish (vanGelder et al., 2007). It may be that omega-3 fatty acids provide protection against AD through their **anti-thrombosis** and anti-inflammatory activity, because inflammation is part of the AD syndrome (Connor & Connor, 2007). The omega-3 fatty acid docosahexaenoic acid (DHA) is the most prominent fat in the brain but it is diminished in the brain cell membranes of people with AD; consuming DHA through food or supplements may protect against AD by replacing missing DHA (Liebman, 2007). Although studies show an association between omega-3 fatty acids and AD, clinical trials are needed to establish evidence. Eating two servings of fatty fish per week is recommended for the prevention of heart disease; time will tell if it also protects against AD.

**Antithrombosis:** against the formation of a thrombosis or blood clot.

AD can have a devastating impact on an individual's nutritional status. Early in the disease, impairments in memory and judgment may make shopping, storing, and cooking food difficult. The client may forget to eat or may forget that he or she has already eaten and consequently eat again. Changes in the sense of smell may develop, a preference for sweet and salty foods may occur, and unusual food choices are not uncommon. Agitation increases energy expenditure and weight loss is common. Choking may occur if the client forgets to chew food sufficiently before swallowing or hoards food in the mouth. Eating of nonfood items may occur, and eventually self-feeding ability is lost. Clients in the latter stage of AD no longer know what to do when food is placed in the mouth. When this occurs, a decision regarding the use of other means of nutritional support (i.e., nasogastric or percutaneous endoscopic gastrostomy tube feedings) must be made.

## Obesity

Obesity is a major public health problem that is increasing in prevalence among all age groups (Table 13.3). It increases the risk of hypertension, diabetes, cardiovascular disease, certain cancers, and osteoarthritis—disorders that become more prevalent with aging.

| TABLE 13.3 | Increasing Prevalence of Obesity in American Adults | |
|---|---|---|
| | **Percentage of Adults with BMI ≥30** | |
| **Age Group (Years)** | **2000** | **2005** |
| 18–29 | 13.5 | 17.7 |
| 30–39 | 20.0 | 24.4 |
| 40–49 | 22.9 | 26.5 |
| 50–59 | 25.6 | 29.5 |
| 60–69 | 22.0 | 28.1 |
| ≥70 | 15.5 | 18.3 |

*Source:* CDC. (2006). State-Specific Prevalence of Obesity Among Adults-United States, 2005. *MMWR Weekly,* September 15, 2006. Available at www.cdc.gov/mmwr/preview/mmrhtml/mm5536a1.htm. Accessed on 5/21/08.

Obesity impairs quality of life because of its negative effect on mobility and self-perceived vitality. It also exacerbates age-related decline in physical function (Villareal et al., 2005). Conversely, weight loss can improve obesity-related medical complications, quality of life, and physical function.

The appropriateness of treating obesity in older adults is controversial because obesity may pose less of a health risk for older adults than younger adults, and a high BMI may help older adults to withstand the metabolic demands of illness. Complicating the issue is that loss of weight is not synonymous with, nor does it have the same benefit as, loss of fat; weight loss can be harmful to older adults if it results in muscle and bone loss. Also, promoting weight loss in obese older adults presents unique challenges. Many older people may not feel a need to make changes at this point in life. Active participation in physical activity may be difficult because of medical problems, financial limitations, or impaired hearing or vision. Diminished sense of taste, living alone, depression, and limited food budget may impede changes in intake.

Unlike weight loss therapy for younger adults that is intended to prevent or treat the medical complications of obesity, the goal of weight loss therapy for older adults should be to improve physical function and quality of life. A lifestyle approach that includes diet, physical activity, and behavior modification may be just as effective in older adults as it is in younger adults (Banks et al., 2005). In fact, data from the Diabetes Prevention Program show that older adults were more compliant with lifestyle therapy and achieved more weight loss than did younger adults (Wing, R., Hamman, R., Bray, G., et al., 2004). A modest reduction in calories by 500–750 cal/day, an adequate protein intake, and a multivitamin and mineral supplement that ensures nutrient needs are met is recommended along with exercise to improve physical function (Villareal et al., 2005).

## Social Isolation

Eating alone is a risk factor for poor nutritional status among older adults; therefore, efforts should be made to eat with friends and relatives whenever possible. Other potential options are the federally funded nutrition programs—congregate meals and Meals on Wheels. These programs are designed to provide low-cost, nutritious, hot meals; education about food and nutrition; opportunities for socialization and recreation; and information on other health and social assistance programs. The congregate meal program provides a hot, balanced, mid-day meal and the opportunity to socialize in senior citizen centers and other public or private facilities. Those who choose to pay may do so; otherwise, the meal is free. Meals on Wheels is a home-delivered meal program for elderly persons who are unable to get to congregate meal centers because they live in an isolated area or have a chronic illness or physical limitations. Usually a hot meal is served at midday and a bagged lunch is included to be used as the evening meal. Modified diets, such as diabetic diets and low-sodium diets, are provided as needed.

# ▶ LONG-TERM CARE

Long-term care residents tend to be frail elderly with multiple diseases and conditions, including psychosocial, functional, and medical problems. An estimated 23% to 85% of long-term care residents suffer from malnutrition or dehydration; poor nutritional status may be the cause or effect of physical decline (ADA, 2005b). Malnutrition has a negative impact on both the quality and length of life and is an indicator of risk for increased mortality (ADA, 2005b). While the screening criteria listed in Box 13.4 were designed for older adults living independently, many also apply to long-term care residents, such as the presence of illness or chronic disease; an inadequate food intake; dental problems; the use of multiple medications; and significant, unintentional weight loss. Additional risks among long-term care residents include:

- Loss of appetite. "Anorexia of aging" is a term used to describe the natural decrease in food intake that occurs even in healthy older adults in response to a decrease in physical activity and metabolic rate. Illness, medications, unfamiliar foods, and changes in the senses of taste and smell can contribute to anorexia, unintentional weight loss, and malnutrition in long-term care residents.
- Pressure ulcers may be a symptom of inadequate food and fluid intake. They produce a fourfold increase in the risk of death (ADA, 2005b).
- Dysphagia affects 30% to 50% of residents in long-term care (ADA, 2005). It contributes to inadequate food intake and decreased eating enjoyment.
- The loss of independence, depression, altered food choices, and cognitive impairments can negatively impact food intake.

## The Downhill Spiral

Loss of appetite is a major cause of undernutrition in long-term care (ADA, 2005b). An inadequate intake of food means the supply of calories, protein, vitamins, and minerals is reduced, which can lead to weight loss and depletion of essential nutrients. Undernutrition increases the risk of illness and infection. If an infection develops, metabolic rate increases, which increases the need for calories and protein. Undernutrition is exacerbated, and a downward spiral ensues.

To prevent malnutrition, ongoing monitoring of residents' intakes is vital so that prompt action can be taken. The **Minimum Data Set (MDS)** requires food intake be assessed so that residents at risk from inadequate intake (e.g., eating <75% of food at most meals) can be identified. Usually nursing assistants assess food items on a meal tray as a whole and assign a value to the amount eaten, such as 0%, 25%, 50%, or 100%. In practice, this system is fraught with many shortcomings such as:

- Food intake records may be neglected because of time constraints or personnel shortages.
- Lack of skill in accurately judging percentage of food consumed. Without adequate training, the reliability of a judgment cannot be guaranteed.
- A practical approach to convert individual item estimates into meaningful estimates of overall meal intake has yet to be determined. For instance, 50% may mean the resident ate

**Minimum data set (MDS):** a component of a federally mandated process of comprehensive assessment of the functional capabilities of all residents living in Medicare- and Medicaid-certified long-term care facilities for the purpose of identifying health problems.

half of everything served *or* ate all of half the items served (e.g., all the fruit punch, diced peaches, and green beans) and none of the other half (e.g., chicken rice casserole, milk, and whole grain muffin). In terms of estimating calories and nutrients consumed, there are significant differences between these two scenarios.

Although the system is far from perfect, it has the potential to yield accurate estimations of individual food and fluid intake when staff is adequately trained and the importance of monitoring intake is understood by the whole health care team.

## Preventing Malnutrition

Preventing malnutrition is a quality of life issue. Efforts should be made to optimize food and fluid intake at each meal and snack. Mealtime should be made as enjoyable an experience as possible. Encourage independence in eating, and supervise dining areas so that proper feeding techniques are used when residents are assisted or fed by certified nursing assistants. Food preferences should be honored whenever possible. Family involvement increases residents' intake. Additional strategies to promote food intake appear in Box 13.5.

Commercial supplements are often given between meals to increase the calorie and protein contents of a resident's diet. Although they may be temporarily useful, these supplements are generally not well accepted or tolerated on a long-term basis. Taste fatigue and lack of hunger for the meal that follows often occur. Use of supplements as a substitute for food deprives residents of the enjoyment of eating foods of their choice. The potential benefits must be weighed against the potential negative consequences. Another option is to increase the nutrient density of foods served with commercial modules or added ingredients: the nutritional value increases while the volume of food served remains the same.

## The Use of Diets

The use of restrictive diets as part of medical care in long-term care facilities is controversial. Although carbohydrate- or calorie-controlled diets may be theoretically beneficial for older adults with diabetes or obesity, the goals of preventing malnutrition and maintaining quality of life are of greater priority for most long-term care residents. Restrictive diets have the potential to negatively affect quality of life by eliminating personal choice in meals, dampening appetite, and promoting unintentional weight loss, thereby compromising functional status.

| BOX 13.5 | STRATEGIES TO PROMOTE INTAKE IN LONG-TERM CARE RESIDENTS |
|---|---|

Provide neat and comfortable dining environment.
Use simple verbal prompts to eat.
Provide small frequent meals rather than three large meals.
Provide specialized utensils such as a scoop plate, nosey cup, etc.
Place food on placemat directly in front of resident.
Avoid staff interruptions during feeding of residents.
Minimize noise and distractions in the dining room.
Use tactile prompt such as hand-over-hand.
Offer finger foods.
Encourage family involvement. Honor individual preferences.

---

**BOX 13.6** **SAMPLE LIBERAL DIET FOR OLDER ADULTS**

---

**Breakfast**
Orange juice
Oatmeal
One soft-cooked egg
One slice buttered whole wheat toast
Low-fat milk
Coffee/tea

**Dinner**
Roast pork
Oven roasted potatoes
Baked acorn squash
Fresh fruit salad
Ice cream
Coffee/tea

**Lunch**
Turkey sandwich made with two slices
   whole wheat bread, tomato, romaine,
   and low-fat salad dressing
Vegetable soup
Sliced strawberries over angel food cake
One cup low-fat milk
Coffee/tea

**Snack**
One cup low-fat yogurt

---

Restrictive diets should be used only when a significant improvement in health can be expected, such as in cases of ascites or constipation.

## A Liberal Diet Approach

To meet the needs of individual residents, a holistic approach is advocated that includes the individual's personal goals, overall prognosis, risk/benefit ratio, and quality of life. A liberalized approach has been shown to promote a better intake, lower the incidence of unintentional weight loss, and improve quality of life in long-term care residents (ADA, 2005b). A liberal diet is basically a healthy diet of nutrient-dense foods that contains neither excessive nor restrictive amounts of fat, cholesterol, sugar, and sodium (Box 13.6). The risks of a restrictive diet (e.g., decreased intake and weight loss) must be weighed against the potential benefits, especially when potential benefits may be lacking in older adults. Consider the following:

* Low-sodium diets used in the treatment of hypertension are often poorly tolerated by older adults and may lead to loss of appetite, hyponatremia, or confusion (ADA, 2005b). There is some controversy regarding whether the benefits of antihypertensive therapy apply to older adults (Gambassi et al., 1998).
* According to the American Diabetes Association, imposing dietary restrictions on long-term care residents with diabetes is unwarranted (ADA, 2007). It recommends that residents receive a regular diet that is consistent in the amount and timing of carbohydrates. The use of "no concentrated sweets" or "no sugar added" diets is not supported by evidence. Caution is urged in the use of weight loss diets because undernutrition is common.
* Epidemiological studies indicate that the importance of hypercholesterolemia as a risk factor for CHD decreases after age 44 and virtually disappears after the age of 65 (ADA, 2005b). Thus, the validity of a low-cholesterol diet in treating long-term care residents is questionable. Malnutrition is a greater threat to the majority of older adults than is hypercholesterolemia. Prudent measures for long-term residents with cardiac disease include using 1% or lower fat milk; substituting trans fat–free margarines for regular margarine and butter; and providing lean cuts of meat in place of fatty meats.

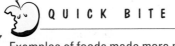

**QUICK BITE**

Examples of foods made more nutrient/calorie dense

Mashed potatoes made with a glucose module

Milk fortified with nonfat dry milk powder

Oatmeal made with added butter, nonfat dry milk, and sugar

Coffee with a commercial supplement similar to cream that adds calories and protein

Scrambled eggs with added cheese

Fruit juice with a glucose module added

A liberal diet can be modified to meet the requirements of residents with increased needs, such as those who have pressure ulcers. A liberal diet with extra meat and/or milk will provide increased amounts of calories, protein, and fluid. Foods may be made more nutrient dense with the addition of skim milk powder, cream in place of milk, or through modular products. Supplemental vitamin C and zinc may be ordered to promote healing. As with any nutritional intervention, frequent and accurate monitoring of the resident's intake, weight, and hydration status is vital to prevent or treat nutrition-related problems.

## NURSING PROCESS: *Older Adult*

Harold Hausman is a regular participant of the monthly congregational nursing program sponsored at his church. He is a sedentary 82-year-old widower who lives alone. You have noticed that he has lost weight over the last several months. He has asked you to answer a few questions he has about the low-sodium, low-cholesterol diet his doctor recommended.

| Assessment | |
|---|---|
| Medical–Psychosocial History | • Medical history including hyperlipidemia, hypertension, cardiovascular disease, or gastrointestinal complaints |
| | • Ability to understand, attitude toward health and nutrition, and readiness to learn |
| | • Attitude about his present weight and recent weight loss |
| | • Usual activity patterns |
| | • Use of prescribed and over-the-counter drugs |
| | • Functional limitations such as impaired ability to shop, cook, and eat |
| | • Psychosocial and economic issues such as who does the shopping and cooking, adequacy of food budget, need for food assistance, and level of family and social support |
| Anthropometric Assessment | • Height, current and usual weight |
| | • % weight change |
| | • Determine BMI |
| Biochemical and Physical Assessment | • Cholesterol level, if available |
| | • Blood pressure |
| | • Dentition and ability to swallow |

*(nursing process continues on page 316)*

## NURSING PROCESS: Older Adult (continued)

Dietary Assessment

- Why did your doctor give you this low-sodium, low-cholesterol diet?
- How many daily meals and snacks do you usually eat?
- What is a normal day's intake for you?
- What changes have you made in implementing this diet? For instance, did you stop using the saltshaker at the table or are you reading labels for sodium content? Did you change the type of butter/margarine you use? The type of salad dressing?
- Do you prepare food with added fat or do you bake, broil, steam, or boil your food?
- How does your intake compare to a 2000 cal/day meal plan recommended by MyPyramid for people your age?
- Do any cultural, religious, or ethnic considerations influence your eating habits?
- Do you use vitamins, minerals, or nutritional supplements? If so, which ones, how much, and why are they taken?
- Do you use alcohol, tobacco, and caffeine?
- How is your appetite?

### Diagnosis

Possible Nursing Diagnosis

- Imbalanced Nutrition: less than body requirements related to an inadequate intake as evidenced by weight loss.
- Readiness for enhanced knowledge.
- Knowledge deficit of low-cholesterol, low-sodium diet

### Planning

Client Outcomes

The client will:

- Attain/maintain a "healthy" weight
- Consume, on average, a varied and balanced diet that meets the recommended number of servings from the 2000 calorie MyPyramid meal plan
- Implement healthy low-sodium, low-cholesterol changes to his usual intake without compromising nutritional or caloric adequacy

### Nursing Interventions

Nutrition Therapy

Encourage a varied and balanced diet that meets the recommended number of servings from each of the major MyPyramid food groups for a 2000 calorie diet

Client Teaching

Instruct the client on:

- The role of nutrition in maintaining health and quality of life, including
  - A balanced diet based on the major food groups helps maximize the quality of life

*(nursing process continues on page 317)*

## NURSING PROCESS: Older Adult *(continued)*

- Avoiding excess salt is prudent for all people; recommendations on sodium intake should be made on an individual basis according to the client's cardiac and renal status, appetite, and use of medications
- Although it is wise to avoid high-fat, nutrient-poor foods such as most cakes, cookies, pastries, pies, chips, full fat dairy products, and fried foods, observing too severe a fat restriction compromises calorie intake and may result in undesirable weight loss

- Eating plan essentials, including the importance of
  - Choosing a varied diet to help ensure an average adequate intake; limiting food choices or skipping a food group increases the risk of both nutrient deficiencies and excesses
  - Eating enough food to avoid unfavorable weight loss
  - Eating enough high-fiber foods such as whole grain breads and cereals, dried peas and beans, and fresh fruits and vegetables
  - Drinking adequate fluid
  - Behavioral matters, including
  - The importance of discussing the rationale for the low-sodium, low-cholesterol diet with his physician, particularly because he has had an unfavorable weight loss
  - How to read labels to identify low-sodium foods
- Physical activity goals that may help improve appetite and intake

| Evaluation |
|---|

| Evaluate and Monitor | • Monitor weight and blood pressure<br>• Provide periodic feedback and reinforcement on food intake and questions about diet |
|---|---|

## ▶ How Do You Respond?

**Do glucosamine and chondroitin work for arthritis pain?** The Glucosamine/Chondroitin Arthritis Intervention Trial (GAIT), a multicenter, large-scale study funded by the National Institutes of Health, was launched to determine whether these two supplements are safe and effective treatments for knee pain from osteoarthritis (Clegg et al., 2006). The results showed decreased pain in:

- 70% of participants given 200 mg of Celebrex daily
- 60% taking a placebo
- 64% taking 1500 mg glucosamine daily
- 65% taking 1200 mg of chondroitin sulfate daily
- 67% of those taking glucosamine and chondroitin combined

Researchers concluded that glucosamine alone and chondroitin alone do not relieve knee pain from osteoarthritis and that together, the supplements do not help people with mild arthritis pain. But in a small subgroup of people with moderate to severe arthritis pain, glucosamine and chondroitin together helped decrease pain, although the results may have been due to chance because the sample size was small. If the supplements taken together seem to help, there is no reason to stop using them because they are harmless and relatively inexpensive.

**What makes weight change "significant"?** Significant weight change is defined as 5% or more in 30 days or 10% or more in 180 days. Most often, significant unintentional *weight* *gain* reflects fluid accumulation, not weight per se, and although it may indicate a serious health threat, eating too many calories is not to blame. Conversely, significant unintentional *weight loss* is much more common, and even if nutrition is not the cause, it is part of the solution. Because weight loss is one of the most important and sensitive indicators of malnutrition, it is vital to accurately weigh residents at least on a monthly basis.

## ▶ CASE STUDY

Annie is an 80-year-old widow who lives alone. She has a long history of hypertension and diabetes and suffers from the complications of CHD and neuropathy. She has diabetic retinopathy, which has left her legally blind. She has never been compliant with a diabetic diet but takes insulin as directed. She is 5 ft. 5 in. and weighs 170 pounds, down from her usual weight of 184 pounds 5 months ago.

Annie reluctantly agreed to receive Meals on Wheels so she does not have to prepare lunch and dinner except on weekends. Her daughter buys groceries for Annie every week, and her grocery list generally consists of milk, oatmeal, two cans of soup, two bananas, a bag of chocolate candy, a layer cake, two doughnuts, and mixed nuts. Her weekend meals consist of whatever she has available to eat.

- What is Annie's BMI? How would you assess her weight status?
- Is her recent weight loss significant? Is it better for her to lose weight, maintain her present weight, or try to regain what she has lost?
- What would you recommend Annie eat for breakfast? For snacks? For weekend meals? Would you discourage her from eating sweets?
- What arguments would you make for her to eat better?

## STUDY QUESTIONS

1. A 68-year-old man who has steadily gained excess weight over the years complains that it is too late for him to make any changes in diet or exercise that would effectively improve his health, particularly the arthritis he has in his knees. Which of the following would be the nurse's best response?
   a. "You're right. You should have made changes long ago. You cannot benefit from a change in diet and exercise now."
   b. "It is too hard for older people to change their habits. You should just continue what you've been doing and know that it's a quality of life issue to enjoy your food."
   c. "It may not help to change your diet and exercise but it certainly wouldn't hurt. Why don't you give it a try and see what happens?
   d. "It is not too late to make changes, and losing weight through diet and exercising are more effective at relieving arthritis pain than either strategy is alone. And older people often are better at making lifestyle changes than are younger adults."

2. The nurse knows her instructions about vitamin $B_{12}$ are effective when the client verbalizes he will:
   a. Consume more meat.
   b. Consume more fruits and vegetables.
   c. Eat vitamin $B_{12}$–fortified cereal.
   d. Drink vitamin $B_{12}$–enriched milk.

3. A client complains that she is not eating any more than she did when she was 30 years old and yet she keeps gaining weight. Which of the following would be the nurse's best response?
   a. "As people get older they lose muscle mass, which lowers their calorie requirements, and physical activity often decreases too. You can increase the number of calories you burn by building muscle with resistance exercises and increasing your activity."

b. "You may not think you are eating more calories but you probably are because the only way to gain weight is to eat more calories than you burn."

c. "Weight gain is an inevitable consequence of getting older related to changes in your body composition. Do not worry about it because older people are healthier when they are heavier."

d. "You need fewer calories now than when you were 30. The only way to lose weight is to eat less than you are currently eating."

**4.** A mineral likely to be consumed in inadequate amounts by older adults is:

a. Iron
b. Magnesium
c. Zinc
d. Sodium

**5.** The best dietary advice for the possible prevention of Alzheimer disease is to:

a. Consume a high-fiber diet.
b. Eat a heart healthy diet including two servings of fish per week.
c. Take antioxidant supplements every day.
d. Avoid foods with a high glycemic index.

**6.** Risk factors for malnutrition in older adults include (select all that apply):

a. Age over 80.
b. Decreased social contact.
c. Tooth pain.
d. Use of more than three prescriptions or over-the-counter medications per day.
e. Involuntary weight change.
f. BMI >25.

**7.** Older adults doing resistance exercises to rebuild lost muscle may also need to increase their intake of what nutrient to achieve their objective?

a. Calories
b. Carbohydrate
c. Protein
d. Iron

**8.** Which of the following would be most appropriate to promote the intake of a resident in long-term care? Select all that apply.

a. Use simple verbal prompts to eat.
b. Provide three meals a day; avoid snacks.
c. Minimize noise and distractions in the dining room.
d. Offer finger foods.
e. Honor individual preferences; solicit input from resident and family.

## KEY CONCEPTS

● Aging begins at birth and ends in death. Exactly how and why aging occurs is not known.

● Good eating habits developed early in life promote health in old age.

● As a group, older adults are at risk for nutritional problems because of changes in physiology (including changes in body composition, gastrointestinal tract, metabolism, central nervous system, renal system, and the senses), changes in income, changes in health, and psychosocial changes.

● Older adults represent a heterogeneous population that varies in health, activity and nutritional status. Generalizations about nutritional requirements are less accurate for this age group than for others.

● Generally, calorie needs decrease but the need for nutrients stays the same or increases with aging. Requirements increase for calcium and vitamin D. Older adults need to obtain their RDA for vitamin $B_{12}$ from the synthetic form found in supplements or fortified foods. The DRI for sodium decreases due to the decrease in calorie requirement. The RDA for iron in women decreases when menses stops.

● Modified MyPyramid for Older Adults has physical activity across the bottom of the pyramid to emphasize the important of exercise. Eight glasses of water form the next horizontal row. The remaining pyramid is composed of vertical bands like MyPyramid, but features the types of foods most likely to be consumed by older adults, such as the addition of frozen fruits and vegetables. On the top of the pyramid is a flag with calcium, vitamin D, and vitamin $B_{12}$ on it; it represents the nutrients most likely to be needed through supplements.

● Generally, older adults do not consume enough vitamin E, magnesium, fiber, calcium, potassium, and probably vitamin D. They should be encouraged to eat more whole grains; dark green and orange fruits and vegetables; dried peas and beans; and milk and milk products.

● Older adults should be screened for malnutrition, by asking questions such as "do you have enough money to buy the food you need?" and "do you sometimes eat fewer than 2 meals a day?"

● Cataracts and macular degeneration were once thought to be inevitable consequences of aging but studies are testing whether diet can help prevent both disorders. Omega-3 fatty acids, vitamin C, vitamin E, beta-carotene, and zinc may help prevent macular degeneration as may a diet low in foods with a high glycemic index. A diet rich in antioxidants, especially lutein and zeaxanthin, and omega-3 fatty acids may also benefit cataracts.

● Weight loss is the most effective dietary strategy against osteoarthritis. The benefits of weight loss and exercise combined are greater than when either method is used alone. Benefits include improvements in physical function and quality of life.

● Even interventions begun late in life can slow or halt bone loss characteristic of osteoporosis. The equivalent of 3 glasses of milk is needed to meet calcium requirement in older adults. Calcium supplements may be necessary to achieve the recommended amount. Other nutrients important for bone health include vitamin D, vitamin A, vitamin K, magnesium, vitamin C, and phytoestrogens.

● Sarcopenia is the loss of muscle mass and strength that occurs with aging. It is not inevitable and can be reversed with resistance training and adequate protein intake. To build muscle in older adults, more protein than the RDA may be required.

● Many known risk factors for Alzheimer disease are similar to those for CHD. Although the role of diet has not clearly been established, a heart healthy diet that includes 2 servings of fish per week may help prevent AD.

● The treatment of obesity in older adults is controversial. Weight loss can be counterproductive if it comes from a loss of muscle and bone, not fat. For many older adults, malnutrition presents more of a risk than overweight.

● Social isolation has a negative impact on appetite and intake and may contribute to unintentional weight loss. Older adults should be encouraged to eat with family and friends whenever possible. Meals on Wheels and congregate dining are 2 federal programs designed to assist older adults with obtaining an adequate diet.

● Long-term care residents are at high risk for malnutrition. Preventive efforts should focus on maintaining an adequate calorie and protein intake. Honor special requests, encourage food from home, and provide assistance with eating as needed.

● Goals of diet intervention for older adults are to maintain or restore maximal independent functioning and to maintain quality of life. Restrictive diets may not be appropriate for older adults and may actually promote malnutrition except when a significant improvement in health can be expected.

● A liberal diet approach may help prevent malnutrition and improve quality of life.

● Pressure ulcers increase the need for calories, protein, and other nutrients. Increasing nutrient density without increasing the volume of food served may be the most effective method of delivering additional nutrients. Between-meal supplements may also be needed to maximize intake.

## ANSWER KEY

1. **TRUE** Seventy-four percent of adults aged 65 and older rated their health as good or better during the period 2004–2006. Self-assessment of health status is important because poor ratings correlate with higher risks of mortality (Federal Interagency Forum on Aging-Related Statistics, 2008).

2. **TRUE** In general, calorie needs in older adults decrease due to a decrease in lean body mass and physical activity, while the need for other nutrients stays the same or increases.

3. **FALSE** The AI for water does not change for men or women from the age of 19 onward. Older adults have a blunted sense of thirst, yet if they are healthy, normal drinking and eating habits are considered adequate to guide fluid intake.

4. **TRUE** Older adults do not need more vitamin $B_{12}$ than younger adults, but their ability to absorb the natural form of $B_{12}$ from food may be impaired. Adults over the age of 50 are urged to consume the RDA for vitamin $B_{12}$ from fortified foods or supplements to ensure adequacy.

5. **FALSE** Most older adults consume adequate amounts of iron. In fact, they are cautioned against consuming supplements that contain iron so as not to exceed the upper limit for iron.

6. **FALSE** Snacking in older adults tends to have a positive impact on their overall calorie and nutrient intake. It should be encouraged for older adults at risk of inadequate intake.

7. **TRUE** Weight loss in older adults is associated with functional limitations, nursing home admissions, and mortality.

8. **FALSE** While it is true that peak calcium retention—the period when calcium intake has the greatest impact on bone density—occurs between the ages of 4 and 20, the efficiency of absorption decreases with age, so the AI for calcium for older adults is higher than that of younger adults.

9. **FALSE** The prevalence of malnutrition or dehydration among residents of long-term care facilities is from 23% to 85%.

10. **TRUE** A major cause of undernutrition among long-term care residents is loss of appetite. Monitoring of intake is essential to identify problems early, before a downhill spiral develops.

## WEBSITES

Alzheimer's Association at **www.alz.org**
American Association of Retired Persons at **www.aarp.org**
American Geriatrics Society at **www.americangeriatrics.org**
Arthritis Foundation at **www.arthritis.org**
National Institute of Aging Information Office at **www.nih.gov/nia**

## REFERENCES

American Diabetes Association (ADA). (2007). Nutrition recommendations and interventions for diabetes. A position statement of the American Diabetes Association. *Diabetes Care*, *30*(Suppl. 1), S48–S65.

American Dietetic Association (ADA). (2005a). Position of the American Dietetic Association: Nutrition, aging, and the continuum of care. *Journal of the American Dietetic Association, 105,* 616–633.

American Dietetic Association (ADA) (2005b). Position of the American Dietetic Association: Liberalization of the diet prescription improves quality of life for older adults in long-term care. *Journal of the American Dietetic Association, 105,* 1955–1965.

Arthritis Foundation. (2007). Osteoarthritis. Available at www.arthritis.org/disease-center.php? disease_id=32. Accessed on 5/19/08. Banks, M., Klein, S., Sinacore, D., et al. (2005). Effects of weight loss and exercise on frailty in obese elderly subjects. *Journal of the American Geriatrics Society, 53,* S16 (abstract).

Bales, C., & Ritchie, C. (2006). *The Elderly.* In: Shils, M., Shike, M., Ross, A., et al. (eds). Modern Nutrition in Health and Disease. (10th ed.). Philadelphia: Lippincott Williams and Wilkins.

Chernoff, R. (2006). Geriatric Nutrition: The Health Professional's Handbook. Sudbury, MA: Jones and Bartlett.

Chiu, C. J., Milton, R. C., Klein, R., et al. (2007). Dietary carbohydrate and the progression of age-related macular degeneration: A prospective study from the Age-Related Eye Disease Study. *The American Journal of Clinical Nutrition, 86,* 1210–1218.

Clegg, D. O., Reda, D. J., Harris, C. L., et al. (2006). Glucosamine, chondroitin sulfate, and the two in combination for painful knee osteoarthritis. *The New England Journal of Medicine, 354,* 795–808.

Connor, W., & Connor, S. (2007). The importance of fish and docosahexaenoic acid in Alzheimer disease. *The American Journal of Clinical Nutrition, 85,* 929–930.

Dawson-Hughes, B., Harris, S., Krall, E., et al. (1997). Effect of calcium and vitamin D supplementation on bone density in men and women 65 years of age or older. *The New England Journal of Medicine, 337,* 670–676.

Dwyer, J. (2006). Starting down the right path: Nutrition connections with chronic diseases of later life. *American Journal of Clinical Nutrition, 83*(Suppl.), 415S–420S.

Elmadfa, I., & Meyer, A. (2008). Body composition, changing physiological functions and nutrient requirements of the elderly. *Annals of Nutrition & Metabolism, 52*(Suppl. 1), 2–5.

Federal Interagency Forum on Aging-Related Statistics. Older Americans 2008: Key Indicators of Well-Being. Federal Interagency Form on Aging-Related Statistics. Washington, CD: US Government Printing Office. March 2008.

Fulgoni, V. (2008). Current protein intake in America: Analysis of the National Health and Nutrition Examination Survey, 2003–2004. *American Journal of Clinical Nutrition, 87,* S1554–1557.

Gambassi, G., Lapane, K., Sgadari, A., et al. (1998). Prevalence, clinical correlates, and treatment of hypertension in elderly nursing home residents. *Archives of Internal Medicine, 158,* 2377–2383.

Greenstone, C. (2007). Osteoarthritis: A lifestyle medicine assessment of risks, prevention, and treatment. *American Journal of Lifestyle Medicine, 1*(4), 256–259.

Haq, I., Murphy, E., & Dacre, J. (2003). Osteoarthritis. *Postgraduate Medical Journal, 79,* 377–383.

Institute of Medicine (IOM). (2000). *Dietary reference intakes for thiamin, riboflavin, niacin, vitamin B$_6$, folate, vitamin B$_{12}$, pantothenic acid, biotin, and choline.* Washington, DC: The National Academies Press.

Institute of Medicine (IOM). (2005). *Dietary reference intakes for energy, carbohydrates, fiber, fat, fatty acids, cholesterol, protein, and amino acids (macronutrients).* Washington, DC: The National Academies Press.

Institute of Medicine (IOM). (2006). *Dietary reference intakes. The essential guide to nutrient requirements.* Washington, DC: The National Academies Press.

Kennedy, E. (2006). Evidence for nutritional benefits in prolonging wellness. *The American Journal of Clinical Nutrition, 83*(Suppl.), 410S–414S.

Liebman, B. (2007). Staying sharp. How to avoid brain drain as you age. *Nutrition Action Health Letter, 34*(5), 1, 3–7.

Messier, S. P., Loeser, R. F., Miller, G. D., et al. (2004). Exercise and dietary weight loss in overweight and obese older adults with knee osteoarthritis: The Arthritis, Diet, and Activity Promotion Trial. *Arthritis Rhuem, 50,* 1501–1510.

Moshfegh, A., Goldman, J., & Cleveland, L. (2005). What We Eat in America, NHANES 2001–2002: Usual Nutrient Intakes from Food Compared to Dietary Reference Intakes. US Department of Agriculture, Agricultural Research Service.

National Eye Institute, US National Institutes of Health. (2006). Cataract. Available at http://www.nei.nih.gov/health/cataract/cataract_facts.asp. Accessed on 5/23/08.

National Institute on Aging, National Institutes of Health (NIA). (2007). Alzheimers. Available at http://www.nia.nih.gov. Accessed on 5/23/08.

Nieves, J. (2005). Osteoporosis: the role of micronutrients. *The American Journal of Clinical Nutrition, 81*(Suppl.), 1232S–1239S.

Paddon-Jones, D., Short, K., Campbell, W., et al. (2008). Role of dietary protein in the sarcopenia of aging. *American Journal of Clinical Nutrition, 87*(suppl), 1562C–1566S.

Rivlin, R. (2007). Keeping the young-elderly healthy: is it too late to improve our health through nutrition? *The American Journal of Clinical Nutrition, 86*(Suppl.), 1572S–1576S.

Roddy, E., Zhang, W., Doherty, M., et al. (2005). Evidence-based recommendations for the role of exercise in the management of osteoarthritis of the hip or knee—the MOVE consensus. *Rheumatology, 44,* 67–73.

Sebastian, R. S., Cleveland, L. E., Goldman, J. D., et al. (2007). Older adults who use vitamin/mineral supplements differ from nonusers in nutrient intake adequacy and dietary attitudes. *Journal of the American Dietetic Association, 107,* 1322–1332.

Seddon, J. (2007). Multivitamin–multimineral supplements and eye disease: Age-related macular degeneration and cataract. *The American Journal of Clinical Nutrition, 85*(Suppl.), 304S–307S.

Schardt, D. (2007). Saving muscle: How to stay strong and healthy as you age. *Nutrition Action Healthletter, 34*(3), 1, 3–6. Shils, M., Shike, M., & Ross, A. (2006). *Modern nutrition in health and disease* (10th ed.). Philadelphia: Lippincott Williams & Wilkins.

Tomany, S. C., Wang, J. J., Leeuwen, R., et al. (2004). Risk factors for incident age-related macular degeneration: Pooled findings from 3 continents. *Ophthalmology, 111,* 1280–1287.

USDA, Center for Nutrition Policy and Promotion (CNPP). (2007). Fruit and Vegetable Consumption by Older Americans. Nutrition Insight 34. Available at http://www.cnpp.usda.gov. Accessed on 5/1/08.

USDHHS. Bone Health and Osteoporosis: A report of the Surgeon General. (2004). Rockville, MD: USDHHS, Office of the Surgeon General.

vanGelder, B., Tijhuis, M., & Kalmijn, S. (2007). Fish consumption, n-3 fatty acids, and subsequent 5-y cognitive decline in elderly men: The Zutphen Elderly Study. *The American Journal of Clinical Nutrition, 85,* 1142–1147.

Villareal, D. T., Apovian, C. M., Kushner, R. F., et al. (2005). Obesity in older adults: Technical review and position statement of the American Society for Nutrition and NAASO, The Obesity Society. *The American Journal of Clinical Nutrition, 82,* 923–934.

Wellman, N. (2007). Prevention, prevention, prevention: Nutrition for successful aging. *Journal of the American Dietetic Association, 107,* 741–743.

Wing, R., Hamman, R., Bray, G., et al. (2004) Achieving weight and activity goals among diabetes prevention program lifestyle participants. *Obesity Research, 12,* 1426–1434.

Zizza, C, Tayie, F., & Lino, M. (2007). Benefits of snacking in older Americans. *Journal of the American Dietetic Association, 107,* 800–806.

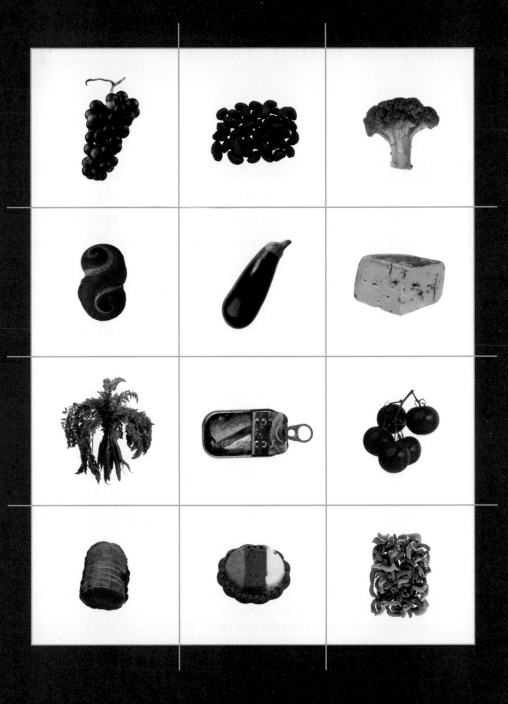

# UNIT THREE

## Nutrition in Clinical Practice

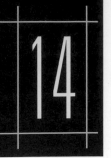

# 14

# Obesity and Eating Disorders

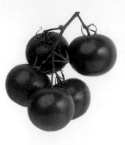

| TRUE | FALSE | |
|------|-------|---|
| ☐ | ☐ | **1** Eating in the evening causes weight gain. |
| ☐ | ☐ | **2** Skipping meals is an effective strategy for cutting calories. |
| ☐ | ☐ | **3** It is easier to lose weight than to maintain a lower weight after weight loss. |
| ☐ | ☐ | **4** Milk promotes weight loss. |
| ☐ | ☐ | **5** Obesity-related health problems improve only after BMI is lowered to normal. |
| ☐ | ☐ | **6** If a person will try only one strategy, lowering calories is more effective at promoting short-term weight loss than increasing activity is. |
| ☐ | ☐ | **7** Even if weight loss does not occur, increasing activity helps to lower blood pressure and improves glucose tolerance. |
| ☐ | ☐ | **8** People who eat fewer than 1200 calories may need a multivitamin and mineral supplement. |
| ☐ | ☐ | **9** For weight loss, it is better to cut carbohydrates than to cut fat grams. |
| ☐ | ☐ | **10** Bulimia poses fewer nutritional problems than anorexia does. |

---

### *UPON COMPLETION OF THIS CHAPTER, YOU WILL BE ABLE TO*

- Give examples of complications of obesity.
- Propose obesity treatment recommendations on the basis of an individual's BMI and the presence of comorbidities.
- Suggest an appropriate calorie intake to promote weight loss based on gender.
- Discuss optimal macronutrient distribution for weight loss.
- Create a sample weight loss meal plan based on MyPyramid intake patterns.
- Compare strategies to promote weight loss with those that are effective in maintaining weight loss.
- Contrast nutrition therapy for anorexia nervosa with that of bulimia nervosa.

---

ssues of weight are a pervasive concern in American culture. The prevalence of obesity is commonly described as being of epidemic proportions: over the past 40 years, the prevalence of obesity (BMI ≥30) in American adults aged 20 and older has almost tripled from 13% to 31.4% (USDHHS, NIH, NIDDK, WIN, 2007). The prevalence of obesity has climbed in both men and women, in all age groups, and in all racial, ethnic, and

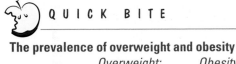

**The prevalence of overweight and obesity**

|  | Overweight:<br>BMI >25 | Obesity:<br>BMI ≥30 |
|---|---|---|
| All adults (%) | 66 | 31.4 |
| Women (%) | 61.6 | 33.2 |
| Men (%) | 70.5 | 29.5 |

*Source:* USDHHS, NIH, NIDDK, WIN. (2007). *Statistics related to overweight and obesity.* Available at http://www.win.niddk.nih.gov/statistics/index.htm. Accessed on 1/27/08.

socioeconomic groups (Cope & Allison, 2006). Obesity is one of the most common causes of preventable death.

A far less common weight issue is disordered eating manifested as anorexia nervosa (AN) or bulimia nervosa (BN). Historically, the study of obesity and eating disorders has been separate: the former has been rooted in medicine, and the latter has been the focus of psychiatry and psychology. Yet there are commonalities between them such as questions of appetite regulation, concerns with body image, and similar etiologic risk factors.

This chapter focuses on obesity—its causes, complications, and treatment approaches. The section on diet modification discusses how many calories are recommended for low-calorie diets, whether low fat or low carbohydrate is the best approach to cutting calories, and what clients need to know to implement a healthy low-calorie diet. Successful strategies for weight maintenance after weight loss are presented. Eating disorders and their nutrition therapy are described.

# ▶ OBESITY

**Overweight:** a BMI greater than or equal to 25.

**Obesity:** a BMI greater than or equal to 30.

**Overweight** is defined as having a BMI ≥25. It is related to an excessive body weight, not necessarily excessive body fat. Muscle, bone, fat, and water all contribute to body weight. **Obesity** is defined as having a BMI ≥30, which is generally assumed to be related to an excessive amount of body fat.

## Causes of Obesity

Obesity occurs when people eat more calories than they expend over time. Although we know *how* obesity occurs, *why* it occurs is not fully understood. In some people the body seemingly compensates for variations in calorie intake by adjusting the rate at which it burns calories during inactivity. The "set point" theory of weight control has long proposed that when weight falls below what the body has determined to be "ideal," metabolic rate is adjusted downward to reduce energy expenditure and conserve fat stores. Conversely, when calorie intake increases, some people are able to burn hundreds of extra calories in the activities of daily living to help control weight. This phenomenon suggests that the reason some people gain weight from overeating and others do not is related to whether this compensatory increase in nonexercise energy expenditure occurs. It is likely that a combination of genetic and environmental factors is involved.

### Genetics

More than 300 genes have been linked to obesity (Chagnon et al., 2003), and although estimates vary, approximately 30% to 40% of the variance in BMI is attributed to genetics and 60% to 70% to environment (Pi-Sunyer, 2002). Genetics does not cause obesity but are involved in how likely a person is to gain or lose weight in response to changes in calorie intake by influencing basal metabolic rate, where body fat is distributed, and response to overeating (O'Neil & Nicklas, 2007). Supporting the case for a genetic basis to weight management is the tendency of adopted children to have similar weights to their biological parents, not their adoptive parents.

## Environment

Yet the dramatic rise in obesity in the U.S. population over the last three decades has occurred without changes in the gene pool, suggesting the root cause is lifestyle and environment, not biology (Pi-Sunyer & Kris-Etherton, 2005). Environmental influences include an abundance of low cost, palatable, high–calorie density foods that are readily available in prepackaged forms and in fast food restaurants; increasing consumption of soft drinks and snacks; a great proportion of food expenditures spent on food away from home; the growing portion size of restaurant meals; low levels of physical activity; increases in television watching; and the widespread use of electronic devices in the home, such as computers and video games, that promote a sedentary lifestyle.

## Gene–Environment Interaction

Clearly there is a gene–environment interaction. In people with a genetic predisposition to obesity, the severity of the disease is largely determined by lifestyle and environmental conditions (Loos & Rankinen, 2005). Conversely, genetics accounts for the individual differences in weight loss that occur in response to calorie restriction (Loos & Rankinen, 2005).

## Complications of Obesity

Obesity significantly increases mortality and morbidity. The most common complications of obesity are insulin resistance, type 2 diabetes, hypertension, dyslipidemia, cardiovascular disease, stroke, gallstones and cholecystitis, sleep apnea, respiratory dysfunction, and increased incidence of certain cancers (NHLBI, 1998). Obesity increases the risk of complications during and after surgery and the risk of complications during pregnancy, labor, and delivery. Higher weights are associated with higher mortality from all causes. Obesity is considered to be a major contributor to preventable deaths in the United States.

Obesity presents psychological and social disadvantages. In a society that emphasizes thinness, obesity leads to feelings of low self-esteem, negative self-image, and hopelessness. Negative social consequences include stereotyping, prejudice, stigmatization, social isolation, and discrimination in social, educational, and employment settings.

## Goals of Treatment

Ideally, treatment would "cure" overweight and obesity; that is, weight would fall to the healthy BMI category and would be maintained there permanently. This would be gradually accomplished with a 1- to 2-pound loss every week for the first 6 months of weight-loss therapy, for a total of 10% weight loss. After 6 months, when the rate of weight loss usually decreases, then plateaus, the focus would shift to maintaining that weight loss. After 6 months of weight maintenance, weight loss efforts would be repeated. The cycle would continue until healthy weight is achieved.

In reality, this ideal is seldom achieved. The goal of losing large amounts of weight is unrealistic and overwhelming and from a health perspective does not appear necessary to achieve health benefits. A modest weight loss of 5% to 10% of initial body weight is associated with significant improvements in blood pressure, cholesterol and plasma lipid levels, and blood glucose levels (Moyers, 2005). Intervention studies show that 5% to 10% weight loss is effective in preventing or delaying the onset of type 2 diabetes and hypertension in high-risk people, even if "healthy" weight is not achieved (Knowler et al., 2002; Stevens et al., 2001). Compared with dramatic weight loss, modest weight loss (1) is more attainable, (2) is easier to maintain over the long term, and (3) sets the stage for subsequent weight loss.

Setting a modest weight loss goal and keeping that weight off are far more realistic than striving for thinness. Yet for some people, even modest weight loss may be unattainable. A more appropriate weight management goal for clients unable to lose weight is to prevent additional weight gain. Although this may sound like a passive approach, it requires active intervention, not simply maintaining the status quo.

## Evaluating Motivation to Lose Weight

Objectively identifying who may benefit from weight loss is not the only criterion to be considered before beginning treatment; assessing the client's level of motivation is crucial because weight loss is not likely to occur in people who are not motivated or committed to lifestyle change. Even worse, imposing treatment on an unmotivated or unwilling client may preclude subsequent attempts at weight loss when the client may be more likely to succeed. It is essential to assess the client's level of motivation before beginning weight loss therapy. Factors to consider appear in Box 14.1.

## Treatment Approaches

A lifestyle approach that includes diet modification, exercise, and behavior modification is the basis of treatment for all people whose BMI is ≥30. The lifestyle approach is also recommended for people with a BMI of 25 to 29.9 who have two or more comorbidities

---

| BOX 14.1 | ASSESSING MOTIVATION TO LOSE WEIGHT |
| --- | --- |

What are the client's reasons and motivation for weight loss?

• Is the client ready to make a lifelong commitment to lifestyle change?
• Is the client's goal realistic or based on an "ideal" weight that may never be achieved?

Does the client have a previous history of successful and unsuccessful attempts at weight loss?

• What does the client see as reasons why previous attempts failed or succeeded?

Does the client have a social support system that may help the client to achieve his or her goals?
Does the client have an understanding of the causes of obesity and its impact on disease risk?

• Is the client concerned about disease risks?

What is the client's attitude toward physical activity?

• What is the client's current level of physical activity (frequency, intensity, duration)?
• Is the client motivated to increase activity?
• Is the client willing to commit time to exercise consistently?
• In what activities is the client physically capable of participating?

Is the client able to commit the time necessary to interact with health professionals for weight loss therapy?
Is the client able and willing to pay for weight loss therapy that is not covered by health insurance?
What or who does the client anticipate will hinder his or her ability to succeed?

| TABLE 14.1 | A Guide to Treatment for Overweight and Obese People | | | |
|---|---|---|---|---|
| **BMI Category and Classification** | **Diet, Physical Activity, and Behavior Modification** | **Pharmacotherapy** | **Surgery** | |
| 25–26.9 Lower range of overweight | With comorbidities | | | |
| 27–29.9 Upper range of overweight | With comorbidities | With comorbidities | | |
| 30–34.5 Obesity class 1 | Yes | Yes | | |
| 35–39.9 Obesity class 2 | Yes | Yes | With comorbidities | |
| ≥40 Obesity class 3 | Yes | Yes | | |

Prevention of weight gain is indicated in all patients with a BMI ≥25; for people with BMI of 25–29.9, weight loss is not necessarily recommended unless comorbidities are present.

*Source:* National Heart, Lung, and Blood Institute, North American Association for the Study of Obesity. (2000). *The practical guide: Identification, evaluation, and treatment of overweight and obesity in adults.*

(USDHHS et al., 2000). Pharmacotherapy and surgery may be used in conjunction with lifestyle interventions, based on the individual's BMI and the presence of comorbidities (Table 14.1).

## Diet Modification

Diet modification is the cornerstone of most weight loss programs (O'Neil & Nicklas, 2007). Factors to consider when modifying the diet include total calories, macro- and micronutrient composition, and nutrition education.

**Fewer Calories.** A low-calorie diet is the foundation of the dietary component to weight management. The appropriate calorie level may be determined by subtracting 500 to 1000 calories from the client's estimated total energy needs, which is the sum of calories used for basal metabolic rate and physical activity (see Chapter 7). A more general approach is to choose a specific calorie level based on gender. The NIH recommends low-calorie diets of 1000 to 1200 cal/day for overweight women and 1200 to 1600 cal/day for overweight men and heavier (>165 pounds) or more active women (USDHHS et al., 2000). These intake goals are intended to produce a 1- to 2-pound weight loss per week.

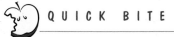 QUICK BITE

**One pound of body fat equals approximately 3500 calories**

To lose 1 lb/week, 3500 fewer cal/week should be consumed

3500 calories ÷ 7 days/week = 500 calorie deficit/day

To lose 2 lb/week, 7000 fewer cal/week should be consumed

7000 calories ÷ 7 days/week = 1000 calorie deficit/day

If 1500 calories can promote a 1- to 2-pound loss per week, will a bigger cut in calories speed the weight loss process? Clients often think that the more drastically they cut calories, the quicker they'll lose weight. In reality, cutting calories too much may result in higher proportions of lean tissue loss, leading to a compensatory decrease in basal energy expenditure and a reduction in exercise tolerance (Melanson, 2007). This makes weight loss and eventual weight maintenance more difficult. Highly restrictive diets also increase the risk of hunger, which makes compliance a challenge. For these reasons, fasting and very low–calorie diets (600 to 800 cal/day) are not recommended.

**Macronutrient Composition.** Weight loss diets are typically classified as (1) low fat/high carbohydrate, (2) high fat/low carbohydrate, or (3) moderate fat/high carbohydrate (Table 14.2). The optimal type of weight loss diet is the subject of debate (Fabricatore, 2007). Research shows that initial weight loss is greater on a low-carbohydrate diet than a low-fat diet, but the difference disappears over time (Hill & Wyatt, 2005). Low-carbohydrate diets severely limit fruit, vegetables, and whole grains, and may be deficient in micronutrients and fiber. The long-term effects of a low-carbohydrate diet are unknown. In addition, researchers speculate that it is the high protein, and not the low or modest carbohydrate, content that promotes short-term weight loss; protein increases **satiety**, leaving people feeling fuller and better able to adhere to a low calorie intake, which causes weight loss (Schoeller & Buchholz, 2005). Any type of hypocaloric diet can produce weight loss, whether the calorie reduction is achieved by limiting carbohydrates, limiting fat, or a more moderate approach (Hill & Wyatt, 2005). When total calories are the same, the macronutrient distributions of the diet do not affect the amount of weight lost. What matters with weight loss is *the amount of calories consumed, not the source of those calories*. Sample menus for each type of diet appear in Table 14.3.

**Satiety:** the feeling of fullness.

| TABLE 14.2 | A Comparison of Low-Fat, Low-Carbohydrate, and Moderate-Fat/High-Carbohydrate Diets | | | | | |
|---|---|---|---|---|---|---|
| Type | Examples | Total Calories | Calories from CHO (Average %) | Calories from Protein (Average %) | Calories from Fat (Average %) | Considerations |
| Typical American Diet | | 2200 | 50 | 15 | 35 | |
| Low- and very low–fat diet | Dean Ornish's Eat More, Weigh Less | 1273 | 81 | 15 | 9 | May be deficient in zinc, vitamin $B_{12}$, and vitamin E. Eating fortified foods or taking a supplement maybe be necessary |
| Moderate Fat/high carbohydrate | Weight Watchers | 1462 | 56 | 20 | 25 | Usually balanced if dieter eats a variety of choices from all food groups |
| Low carbohydrate/high fat | Carbohydrate Addicts Diet | 1476 | 24 | 23 | 54 | May be deficient in vitamins A, E, $B_6$, folate, thiamin, calcium, magnesium, iron, zinc, potassium, and fiber (O'Neil & Nicklas, 2007) Contains high amounts of saturated fat and cholesterol. A nutritional supplement is highly recommended |

*Source:* Freedman, M., King, J., and Kennedy, E. (2001). Popular diets: A scientific review: High-fat, low-carbohydrate diets. *Journal of Obesity Research, 9*(Suppl. 1), 5S–17S.

| TABLE 14.3 | A Comparison of Sample Menus | | |
|---|---|---|---|
| | **Low- Fat/High-CHO Diet** | **Moderate-Fat/High-CHO Diet** | **Low-CHO/High-Fat Diet** |
| Total servings from each group per day | | | |
|   Milk or yogurt | 2 fat free | 2 fat free | 1 |
|   Fruit | 7 | 3 | 2 |
|   Vegetables | 5 | 2 | 2 |
|   Grains | 8 | 8 | 2 |
|   Meat and beans | 2 oz fat-free meat | 6 oz lean meat | 8 oz medium fat |
|   Fat | 3 | 4 | 11 |
| Breakfast | ½ cup orange juice<br>1 small banana<br>¼ cup scrambled egg beaters<br>2 slices whole wheat toast<br>2 tsp butter | ½ cup orange juice<br>1 oz shredded wheat<br>2 slices whole wheat toast<br>1 cup skim milk<br>2 tsp butter | ½ cup orange juice<br>2 scrambled eggs cooked in 2 tsp butter<br>1 oz pork sausage |
| Snack | ⅔ cup plain yogurt with ¾ cup blueberries<br>3 graham crackers | ⅔ cup artificially sweetened fat-free yogurt | ⅔ cup artificially sweetened yogurt |
| Lunch | 1 cup lentil soup<br><br>Grilled vegetable sandwich on 2 slices whole wheat bread<br>1 cup tossed salad<br><br>Fat-free dressing<br>1 slice watermelon | 1 hamburger bun<br><br>3 oz 95% ground round hamburger<br>1 cup salad made with greens, carrots, onions, and mushrooms<br>1 tbsp Italian dressing<br>1 small apple | 2 oz canned tuna mixed with 2 tsp mayonnaise<br>4 pieces melba toast<br><br>½ cup sliced tomatoes<br><br>1 tbsp Italian dressing |
| Snack | ½ cup fat-free pudding | ½ cup sugar-free, fat-free pudding | 20 peanuts |
| Dinner | ½ cup black beans with ⅓ cup rice and tomatoes<br>1 cup salad<br>1 tbsp Italian dressing<br>½ cup steamed broccoli<br>¾ cup canned mandarin oranges<br>1 cup skim milk<br>1 frozen 100% juice bar | 3 oz grilled skinless chicken breast<br>1 cup winter squash<br>⅓ cup rice<br>½ cup steamed broccoli<br>1 tsp butter<br><br>1¼ cup strawberries<br>1 cup skim milk | 3 oz steak<br>⅓ cup rice<br>1 cup salad topped with 8 large olives<br>1 tbsp Italian dressing<br>1¼ cup strawberries with 2 tbsp whipped cream<br>6 almonds |
| Snack | 1475 | 1482 | 1479 |
| Actual composition | 74 | 54 | 22 |
|   Total calories | 17 | 23 | 20 |
|   Calories from CHO (%) | 9 | 23 | 58 |
|   Calories from protein (%) | | | |
|   Calories from fat (%) | | | |

*The Practical Guide* (USDHHS et al., 2000) recommends weight loss diets to be composed of 55% or greater of total calories from carbohydrate, 30% or lesser of total calories from fat, and approximately 15% from protein, which could be achieved by following MyPyramid intake patterns, regardless of the total calorie count. However, the "best" type of diet is the one most easily followed. Some clients find that cutting down on bread, pasta,

**MyPyramid intake patterns for 1200-calorie and 1600-calorie plans**

| Group | Total cal/day 1200 | 1600 |
|---|---|---|
| Grains (oz-eq) | 4 | 5 |
| Vegetables (cups) | 1.5 | 2 |
| Fruits (cup/s) | 1 | 1.5 |
| Milk (cups) | 2 | 3 |
| Meat and Beans (oz-eq) | 3 | 5 |
| Oils (tsp) | 4 | 5 |

and rice is easiest for them, while others may prefer to curtail intake of margarine, mayonnaise, salad dressings, and fried foods. As long as total calories are reduced and healthy sources of fats and carbohydrates are chosen, the actual percentage of fat and carbohydrate consumed becomes moot.

**Micronutrient Composition.** Diets that are severely restricted in a given macronutrient or food group may be lacking in certain vitamins, minerals, fiber, or phytonutrients, increasing the risk of nutrient inadequacies or deficiencies (Table 14.2). Moderate-fat, high-carbohydrate diets are most likely to be nutritionally adequate, but a multivitamin and mineral supplement is recommended whenever calorie intake falls to 1200 calories or less.

**Nutrition Education.** Too often clients are told what not to eat but are left wondering what they should eat. Increasing a client's nutrition knowledge and skill may improve his or her food choices. Counseling the client to make healthier choices may include how to:

- *Eat smaller portions at meals and snacks.* Providing clients with common household equivalents to estimate portion sizes is a useful tool. While clients may not have any idea what 3 ounces of meat looks like, they can visualize the size of a deck of cards to estimate reasonable meat portions. Portion control is vital to staying within the prescribed calorie allowance.
- *Use "good" carbs in place of "bad" carbs.* "Good carbs" are fruits, vegetables, whole grain breads and cereals, and legumes; they are high in fiber and phytochemicals, provide high satiety, and have lower calorie density than refined carbohydrates. "Bad" carbs are generally refined products, such as white bread, refined cereals, soft drinks, and sweets.
- *Choose healthy fat—in moderation.* Unsaturated fats found in poultry, fish, nuts, salad dressings, and cooking oils are "good" fats because they do not raise serum LDL cholesterol (the "bad" cholesterol) levels. Saturated and trans fats found in red meats, dairy products, stick margarine, shortening, butter, and foods made with these items are "bad" because they raise LDL cholesterol, which increases the risk of coronary heart disease. Because all fats are calorically dense, neither healthy nor unhealthy fats should be eaten in unlimited quantities. Combining a high fiber intake with a low-fat diet causes a greater weight loss than diets with either of these attributes alone (Roberts et al., 2002).
- *Use cooking techniques that do not add additional calories.* Broiling, baking, roasting, and grilling are recommended over frying for meat, vegetables, and potatoes. Vegetables cooked without added butter, margarine, or cheese can be seasoned with herbs, spices, and butter sprays to lower calories.
- *Modify recipes to lower the calorie content.* In cooking, fat for sautéing can often be eliminated, especially if nonstick cookware is used. In baked goods, some of the fat can be replaced with applesauce or pureed prunes.
- *Read "Nutrition Facts" labels to comparison shop.* Because calories and nutrients differ among different brands of similar items, clients who know how to read a "Nutrition Facts" label can make informed decisions.
- *How to eat out without overeating.* Useful tips such as splitting an entrée with a companion, filling a doggie bag before beginning to eat, ordering regular size instead of "super size," and other eating out strategies are addressed in Chapter 10.

- *Distribute calories throughout the day.* The American Dietetic Association Evidence Library considers the strength of the evidence "fair" in recommending calories be distributed throughout the day in four to five meals and snacks, including breakfast (ADA Evidence Library, 2006). Regular, frequent meals and snacks may help clients avoid periods of hunger, increasing the likelihood of dietary adherence.
- *Use meal replacements to their advantage, if self-selecting or portion control is difficult.* Programs such as Jenny Craig and NutriSystem feature 1 to 2 meals per day of vitamin- and mineral-fortified, low-calorie "meals," which may be in the form of a shake, frozen entrée, or meal bar. Because choices are restricted and meals are portion controlled, the risk of poor food choices is reduced. A meta-analysis of six studies showed that people using meal replacement programs lost more weight over a period of 3 to 12 months than non–meal replacement users and fewer of them had dropped out of the program after a year compared to people in conventional low-calorie diet programs (Heymsfield et al., 2003).
- *Choose nutrient-dense foods to lower calorie density.* Feeling chronically hungry is a common complaint among dieters and usually leads to abandoning the weight loss plan. But hunger is not an obligatory component of a weight loss plan. Laboratory studies have shown that people tend to eat a consistent *weight* of food, not necessarily a consistent amount of calories (Kral & Rolls, 2004). By simply replacing high–**calorie density** foods with low–**calorie density** foods (which tend to be high in calorie-free water), the volume of food can remain high while the calorie content falls. Concentrating on minimally processed, high-satiety foods can enable clients to fill full *and* lose weight. Rolls and colleagues have shown that eating more water-rich fruits, vegetables, broth-based soups, and cooked whole grains allows clients to eat satisfying amounts of food while lowering calorie intake (Rolls et al., 2005). Adding vegetables to casseroles, soups, and sandwiches is a way to increase the volume of food eaten without significantly increasing the calorie content.

**Calorie Density:** the amount of calories in a given weight of food.

### QUICK BITE

**High-satiety (lowered calorie density) foods to help stave off hunger**

- Parfait made with low-fat vanilla yogurt layered with fresh strawberries and rolled oats
- A smoothie made with skim milk, vanilla yogurt, frozen blueberries, and a banana
- Oatmeal with strawberries and walnuts
- Vegetarian chili
- Minestrone soup
- Lentil soup
- Hummus with baby carrots
- Black beans and rice
- Salmon sushi roll with large green salad
- Lean meat or poultry stir-fried with vegetables

**Promoting Dietary Adherence.** Adding structure to a low-calorie diet improves adherence by limiting food choices, which reduces temptation and the potential for overeating (Fabricatore, 2007). Structure can be added by providing:

- Meal plans
- Grocery lists
- Menus
- Recipes

## Physical Activity

The benefits of exercise are numerous. Increasing activity during weight loss helps preserve or increase lean body mass. With or without weight loss, increasing activity lowers blood pressure and triglycerides, increases HDL cholesterol, improves cardiovascular fitness, and improves glucose tolerance. Subjectively, increased activity improves the sense of well-being, reduces tension, increases agility, and improves alertness. Unfortunately, most studies show that increasing physical activity, either alone or with a low calorie diet, is not effective in producing weight loss (Hill & Wyatt, 2005–2007; Catenacci & Wyatt, 2007). Exercise does play a major role in maintaining weight loss.

As stated in Chapter 7, the Dietary Guidelines recommend adults engage in approximately 60 minutes of moderate- to vigorous-intensity activity on most days of the week (while not exceeding caloric intake requirements) to *prevent* weight gain. Sixty to 90 minutes of daily moderate-intensity physical activity are recommended to sustain weight loss. *The Practical Guide* (USDHHS, 2000) recommends exercise be implemented gradually, beginning at 10 minutes/day to avoid fatigue, muscle soreness, strains, or more serious consequences.

**Promoting Exercise Adherence.** Unlike dietary adherence, exercise adherence seems to increase with less structure, possibly by eliminating the barriers of lack of time or financial expense (Fabricatore, 2007). Strategies that may promote exercise adherence include encouraging clients to:

- Exercise at home rather than on-site or supervised exercise sessions.
- Exercise in multiple short bouts (10 minutes each), instead of one long session.
- Adopt a more active lifestyle, such as taking the stairs instead of the elevator or pacing while on the phone instead of sitting down.

## Behavior Modification

Behavior modification focuses on changing the client's eating and exercise behaviors thought to contribute to obesity and closely monitoring those behaviors (Berkel et al., 2005). Box 14.2 lists behavior modification ideas that may help change eating behaviors. Key behavior modification strategies are discussed below.

---

**BOX 14.2** | **BEHAVIOR MODIFICATION IDEAS**

**Think Thin**
- Make a list of reasons why you want to lose weight.
- Set long-term goals; avoid crash dieting based on getting into a particular dress or weighing a certain weight for an upcoming event or occasion.
- Give yourself a nonfood reward (e.g., new clothes, a night of entertainment) for losing weight.
- Enlist the support of family and friends.
- Learn to distinguish hunger from cravings.

**Plan Ahead**
- Keep food only in the kitchen, not scattered around the house.
- Stay out of the kitchen except when preparing meals and cleaning up.
- Avoid tasting food while cooking; don't take extra portions to get rid of a food.
- Place the low-calorie foods in the front of the refrigerator; keep the high-calorie foods hidden.
- Remove temptation to better resist it: "Out of sight, out of mind."
- Plan meals, snacks, and grocery shopping to help eliminate hasty decisions and impulses that may sabotage dieting.

**Eat Wisely**
- Wait 10 minutes before eating when you feel the urge; hunger pangs may go away if you delay eating.
- Never skip meals.

*(box continues on page 336)*

| BOX 14.2 | **BEHAVIOR MODIFICATION IDEAS** (continued) |
|---|---|

- Eat before you're starving and stop when satisfied, not stuffed.
- Eat only in one designated place and devote all your attention to eating. Activities such as reading and watching television can be so distracting that you may not even realize you ate.
- Serve food directly from the stove to the plate instead of family style, which can lead to large portions and second helpings.
- Eat the low-calorie foods first.
- Drink water with meals.
- Use a small plate to give the appearance of eating a full plate of food.
- Chew food thoroughly and eat slowly.
- Put utensils down between mouthfuls.
- Leave some food on your plate to help you feel in control of food rather than feeling that food controls you.
- Eat before attending a social function that features food; while there, select low-calorie foods to nibble on.
- Eat satisfying foods and do not restrict particular foods.

**Shop Smart**
- Never shop while hungry.
- Shop only from a list; resist impulse buying.
- Buy food only in the quantity you need.
- Don't buy foods you find tempting.
- Stock upon fruits and vegetables for low-calorie snacking.

**Change Your Lifestyle**
- Keep busy with hobbies or projects that are incompatible with eating to take your mind off eating.
- Brush your teeth immediately after eating.
- Trim recipes of extra fat and sugar.
- Keep food and activity records.
- Keep hunger records.
- Give yourself permission to enjoy an occasional planned indulgence and do so without guilt; don't let disappointment lure you into a real eating binge.
- Exercise.
- Get more sleep if fatigue triggers eating.
- Weigh yourself regularly.

*Self-monitoring* involves keeping a detailed record of the time, amount, description, preparation, and calorie content of all foods and beverages consumed. Recording additional information such as the client's emotional state, intensity of hunger, and activities at the time of eating may help identify "problem" behaviors. The primary purpose of using food records is to increase awareness of how often and under what circumstances the client engages in behaviors that support or sabotage weight loss efforts (Berkel et al., 2005). The act of recording food eaten causes people to alter their intake. Self-monitoring of activity establishes a record of the type and amount (in minutes) of daily programmed activity. Lifestyle activity can be monitored with the use of a pedometer. Self-monitoring is often considered one of the most essential components of behavior modification.

*Goal setting* may involve specific calorie, fat gram, and physical activity goals designed to achieve a -1- to 2-pound weight loss per week or they may involve specific eating behaviors in need of improvement. Goals should be realistic, specific, and measurable so that success can be achieved to engender a sense of accomplishment and bolster motivation. Instead of a goal to "eat better" a goal may be to "eat oatmeal and fruit for breakfast 5 days/week."

*Stimulus control* involves restructuring the environment to avoid or change cues that trigger undesirable behaviors (e.g., keeping "problem" foods out of sight or out of the house) or instituting new cues to elicit positive behaviors (e.g., putting walking shoes by the front door as a reminder to go walking).

*Problem solving* involves identifying eating problems or high-risk situations, planning alternative behaviors, implementing the alternative behaviors, and evaluating the plan to determine whether it reduces problem eating behaviors.

*Cognitive restructuring* involves reducing negative self-talk, increasing positive self-talk, setting reasonable goals, and changing inaccurate beliefs.

*Relapse prevention* focuses on teaching clients how to prevent lapses from becoming relapses.

## Pharmacotherapy

In conjunction with lifestyle changes of diet, exercise, and behavior modification, pharmacotherapy is recommended for people with a BMI ≥30 or for people with a BMI ≥27 with comorbid conditions (Table 14.1). Clients whose waist circumference is greater than 35 in. (women) and 40 in. (men) are also candidates for pharmacotherapy if comorbidities are present.

Pharmacotherapy, specifically the two drugs approved by the FDA for long-term use (Table 14.4), has been shown effective in helping promote and maintain weight loss (Berkel et al., 2005). McTigue et al. (2003) demonstrated that clients using either of these two drugs, in conjunction with diet and lifestyle changes, lost significantly more weight compared

### TABLE 14.4 Drugs Approved for Long-Term Use in the Treatment of Obesity

| Drug | Effect | Common Side Effects | Contraindications | Nutritional Considerations |
|---|---|---|---|---|
| Sibutramine (Meridia) | Suppresses appetite and promotes satiety; lessens the decrease in metabolic rate that often occurs with weight loss. Associated with effective weight maintenance | Constipation, dry mouth, and headache are usually mild and transient. May ↑ heart rate and blood pressure | CVD; Uncontrolled HTN; Use of MAO inhibitors; Relative contraindication: use of other SSRI | May need ↑ fluid, ↑ fiber, ↓ Na, ↓ fat. Avoid ↑ tryptophan foods |
| Orlistat (Xenical) | ↓ Fat absorption from GI tract by inhibiting pancreatic lipase; ↓ LDL cholesterol independent of weight loss. Improves fasting glucose and glycohemoglobin in Type 2 diabetics | ↓ Absorption of fat-soluble vitamins; Significant GI side effects including diarrhea, flatulence, bloating, and abdominal pain; Oily anal leakage (initial side effects tend to ↓ over first several months) | Malabsorption syndromes; Caution with hyperoxaluria, calcium oxalate renal stones, and diabetes | Limit total fat to limit side effects; Distribute fat evenly throughout the day; Multivitamins may be needed; should not be taken within 2 hours of eating |

to those taking a placebo, and a greater percentage of clients using pharmacotherapy lost 5% to 10% of their initial weight than did nonusers. However, pharmacotherapy is not effective as a sole treatment and people usually regain the weight that was lost once the drug is stopped (Klein, 2004).

Alli is the only over-the-counter drug to gain FDA approval for the treatment of obesity. It is a reduced strength version of the prescription drug orlistat (Xenical). Expected weight loss is modest (perhaps half of the usual 6 lb/1 year credited to orlistat over diet and exercise alone) and side effects may be less intense but similar to orlistat. Long-term studies on its effectiveness are not available.

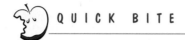 **Q U I C K   B I T E**

**Off-label drugs used for weight loss**

|  | *FDA Approved Use* |
| --- | --- |
| Topiramate (Topamax) | Antiseizure agent |
| Metformin (Glucophage) | Glycemic control in type 2 diabetes |
| Bupropion (Wellbutrin) | Treatment of depression and tobacco cessation |
| Acarbose (Precose) | Glycemic control in type 2 diabetes |
| Miglitol (Glyset) | Glycemic control in type 2 diabetes |
| Zonisamide (Zonegran) | Antiseizure agent |
| Fluoxetine (Prozac) | Treatment of depression |

Phentermine (Fastin), phentermine resin (Ionamin), phendimetrazine tartrate (Bontril), and diethylpropion hydrochloride (Tenuate) are approved for short-term use (≤3 months) in the treatment of obesity. All of these drugs are central nervous system (CNS) stimulants that work by causing loss of appetite. Tolerance may develop after only a few weeks and there is risk of abuse. Common side effects are generally increased heart rate and blood pressure, dry mouth, agitation, insomnia, nausea, diarrhea, and constipation. People with advanced cardiovascular disease, hypertension, hyperthyroidism, glaucoma, nervousness or agitation, a history of drug abuse, or use of CNS stimulants should not use these drugs (Moyers, 2005). Box 14.3 contains selected supplements that may be used for weight loss.

## Surgery

Bariatric surgery is the most effective treatment for severe obesity, defined as a BMI ≥40 (Blackburn, 2005). It is also appropriate for clients whose BMI is 35 to 39.9, who have major comorbidities (Blackburn, 2005). A meta-analysis shows that weight loss surgery is one of the most effective treatments for diabetes, hypertension, obstructive sleep apnea, and high cholesterol in patients with severe obesity (Buchwald et al., 2004).

Surgical procedures for obesity work by (1) restricting the stomach's capacity, (2) creating malabsorption of nutrients and calories, or (3) a combination of both. Intensive nutritional counseling is needed to help clients minimize GI distress after eating and optimize effectiveness of the surgery. Laparoscopic adjustable gastric banding (LAGB) and Roux-en-Y gastric bypass (RYGB) are discussed next.

**Laparoscopic Adjustable Gastric Banding.** In LAGB, an inflatable band is encircled around the uppermost stomach and buckled. A small pouch of approximately 15 to 30 mL

**SELECTED WEIGHT LOSS SUPPLEMENTS**

*Ephedra (Ma huang):* Shown to promote a modest but significant increase in weight loss when used 6 months or less; long-term efficacy untested. Associated with serious adverse events, such as seizures, stroke, and death. Sale banned in the United States since 2004.

*Bitter orange:* Claims state bitter orange is a substitute for ephedra. Little evidence of efficacy; more research is needed. Safety concerns have been raised.

*Chromium picolinate:* Little evidence that it increases lean body mass or decreases body fat; few or no adverse events.

*Conjugated linoleic acid:* Little evidence of benefit; few data available on safety.

*Chitosan:* Little evidence of benefit; there are no long-term safety trials in humans.

*Yohimbine:* Insufficient evidence on efficacy and safety to support its use in weight loss.

*L-Carnitine:* Studies are limited and do no support its use for weight loss.

*Calcium:* Diets rich in dairy products may lower the risk for obesity or promote weight loss in people who are overweight; to date, there is less evidence that calcium supplements have a similar effect on weight loss.

*Green tea extract:* A few, small studies suggest regular consumption of green tea/extract may promote weight control. More studies are needed.

**Source:** Dwyer, J., Allison, D., & Coates, P. (2005). Dietary supplements in weight reduction. *Journal of the American Dietetic Association, 105,* S80–S86.

Fragakis, A., & Thomson, C. (2006). *The health professional's guide to popular dietary supplements* (3rd ed.). Chicago: The American Dietetic Association.

capacity is created with a limited outlet between the pouch and the main section of the stomach (Fig. 14.1). The outlet diameter can be adjusted by inflating or deflating a small bladder inside the "belt" through a small subcutaneous reservoir. The size of the outlet can be repeatedly changed as needed. Clients must understand the importance of eating small

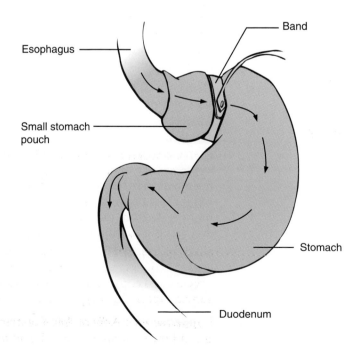

**FIGURE 14.1** Adjustable gastric banding.

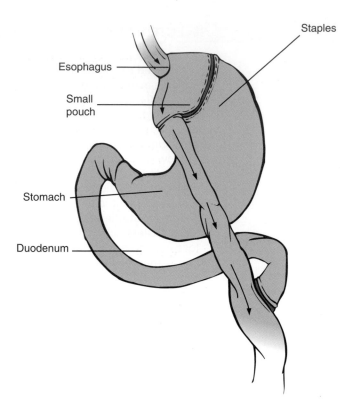

Staples

Esophagus

Small
pouch

Stomach

Duodenum

**FIGURE 14.2** Roux-en-Y
gastric bypass.

meals, eating slowly, chewing food thoroughly, and progressing the diet gradually from liquids, to pureed foods, to soft foods.

The mortality rate for gastric banding is the lowest of all bariatric procedures at 0.1% but
it yields a smaller weight loss and lower rate of cure of type 2 diabetes than RYGB (Sugerman
et al., 2007). Successful weight loss after LAGB requires frequent follow-up and band
adjustments. After 5 years, weight loss averages 44% to 68% of excess body weight
(Sugerman et al., 2007).

**Roux-en-Y Gastric Bypass.** Gastric bypass combines gastric restriction to limit food intake with the construction of bypasses of the duodenum and the first portion of the jejunum,
which creates malabsorption of calories and nutrients (Fig. 14.2). Rapid emptying of the
stomach pouch contents into the small intestine may produce the "dumping syndrome"
characterized by nausea, flushing, lightheadedness, diarrhea, and abdominal cramping that
improve over time. This procedure is superior to gastric resection in both promoting and
maintaining significant weight loss and has profound effects on type 2 diabetes, even before
weight loss occurs (Sugerman et al., 2007). The major complication with RYGB is anasto-
motic leak. Iron, calcium, and vitamin $B_{12}$ deficiencies may occur. After 5 years, weight loss
averages 68% to 80% of excess body weight (Sugerman et al., 2007).

**Post-Surgical Diet.** With both of these bariatric surgeries, the post-surgical diet progression begins with small quantities of sugar-free clear liquids. Within the first week the diet advances as tolerated to full liquids, followed by pureed foods and then a regular diet within 5
to 6 weeks after surgery. Nutrient deficiencies and dumping syndrome are a problem only
for gastric bypass, not for LAGB. Nutrition therapy guidelines for gastric bypass appear in
Box 14.4.

| BOX 14.4 | **NUTRITION THERAPY GUIDELINES AFTER GASTRIC BYPASS SURGERY** |

- Initially the diet consists of low-sugar/sugar-free liquids or semiliquids.
- Eat 5 times perday.
- Eat slowly; plan on 30 to 60 minutes per meal.
- Adequate protein is vital for healing. Begin each "meal" with protein. Liquid protein supplements may be used in place of a meal. Choose sugar-free varieties.
- Stop when you feel full.
- A multivitamin is necessary; an extra supplement containing folic acid, iron, vitamin $B_{12}$, and intrinsic factor may also be prescribed.
- A calcium supplement may be necessary if calcium intake is not adequate. Calcium supplements should be spread out over the day in doses of 500 mg or less.
- Nausea is common; diarrhea may occur, although some people experience constipation from a reduced food intake.

**Sample Meal Plan:**
*Breakfast:*

½ cup sugar-free instant breakfast made with fat-free milk
½ cup sugar-free gelatin

*Mid-Morning:*
½ cup diluted fruit juice

*Lunch:*
½ cup smooth, sugar-free low-fat yogurt, such as lemon or vanilla
½ cup broth

*Mid-Afternoon:*
Sugar-free popsicle

*Dinner:*
½ cup strained cream soup made with fat-free milk
½ cup low-sodium tomato juice

## Weight Maintenance after Loss

While losing weight may be difficult, keeping it off is even harder. Most evidence suggests that the majority of people who lose weight eventually regain the weight over subsequent months or years (Hill & Wyatt, 2005). Diets that lead to weight loss are not necessarily effective for maintaining weight loss. A negative calorie balance cannot be maintained indefinitely; learning how to achieve energy balance after weight loss is vital. Most people fail to maintain their new lower weight because they try to do so through calorie restriction alone (Hill & Wyatt, 2005). Data suggest that weight loss maintenance is most likely to succeed when physical activity increases significantly (Catenacci & Wyatt, 2007).

The National Weight Control Registry (NWCR) was founded in 1994 to identify and investigate characteristics of people who are successful in maintaining significant weight loss. To be eligible, participants must have lost a minimum of 30 pounds and kept it off for more than 1 year. There are currently 6000 people in the registry; the average participant has lost approximately 70 pounds and kept it off for 6 years. There is no "one" diet that participants used to lose weight; only 10% relied on diet alone, just 1% used exercise alone.

According to Rena Wing, cofounder of the NWCR and professor of psychiatry and human behavior at Brown University, the single best predictor of who will be successful

| BOX 14.5 | SUCCESSFUL WEIGHT MAINTENANCE |
|----------|-------------------------------|

Based on participants in the NWCR, people who are successful at maintaining weight loss:

- Eat a low-calorie diet. Most people eat a low-fat, high carbohydrate diet to maintain their loss.
- Eat 4 to 5 times/day.
- Eat a consistent diet from day to day. Eating a limited number of foods may make the diet boring, which helps limit eating.
- Seventy-eight percent eat breakfast every day, which may help control hunger later in the day.
- Are very physically active. Ninety percent of registrants exercise, on average, approximately 1 hour/day. Walking is the exercise of choice for most people.
- Seventy-five percent weigh themselves at least once a week.
- Sixty-two percent watch less than 10 hours of TV a week.

*Source:* NWCR Facts. (1994). Available at http://www.nwcr.ws/default.htm. Accessed on 1/15/08.
Schardt, D. (2008). Secrets of successful losers. *Nutrition Action Health Letter, 35*(1), 8.

at maintaining weight loss is how long someone has kept their weight off (Schardt, 2008). After maintaining weight loss for 2 years, the risk of regain is less than half. Weight regain is most likely to occur in people who ease up on physical activity, increase their fat intake, or start watching more television (Schardt, 2008). Once people start to regain weight, few are able to fully reverse it. The characteristics of successful weight maintainers appear in Box 14.5.

## Obesity Prevention

**Q U I C K   B I T E**

**What 100 calories looks like**
12 oz light beer
5 oz white wine
8 oz soft drink
3 buffalo wings
½ cup sweetened applesauce
1 medium size cookie
½ cup diet chocolate pudding
1 fun size Almond Joy
½ small McDonald's French fries
12 cashews

It is suggested that small changes in diet and exercise that total a mere 100 cal/day may be enough to prevent obesity in most of the population (Hill & Wyatt, 2005). Consider that for most people, obesity develops insidiously without a conscious change in food intake or activity. For instance, even a seemingly insignificant 1 ounce of cheddar cheese that supplies 100 calories will produce a 10-pound weight gain in a year if consumed daily and not offset by an increase in activity:

100 calories × 365 day/year
= 36,500 excess cal/year
= 36,500 cal/year divided by 3500 cal/lb
= slightly over 10 lb/year weight gain

Research suggests that it may take more behavior change to prevent weight regain after loss than to prevent weight gain in those who have never been obese, making prevention efforts imperative (Hill & Wyatt, 2005).

## NURSING PROCESS: Obesity

Rosa is 37 years old, 5 ft. 4 in. tall, and the mother of two children. Before her first child was born 10 years ago, her normal weight was 140 pounds. She gained 35 pounds during pregnancy and didn't regain her normal weight before her second pregnancy a year later. She is now at her heaviest weight of 168 pounds. She complains of fatigue and thinks her weight contributes to her asthma. She has tried several diets and has been unable to take weight off and keep it off. Her doctor told her she has prehypertension and encouraged her to lose weight to lower both her blood pressure and serum glucose levels. The fear of needing medication for hypertension or diabetes has made her motivated to lose weight.

### Assessment

| | |
|---|---|
| Medical–Psychosocial History | • Medical history and comorbidities such as hypertension, dyslipidemia, cardiovascular disease, diabetes, sleep apnea, osteoarthritis, esophageal reflux<br><br>• Medications that may promote weight gain or interfere with weight loss, such as insulin and other antidiabetes agents, steroid hormones, psychotropic drugs, mood stabilizers, antidepressants, and antiepileptic drugs<br><br>• Motivation to lose weight including previous history of successful and unsuccessful attempts to lose weight, social support, and perceived barriers to success |
| Anthropometric Assessment | Height, current weight, BMI<br><br>Weight history; heaviest adult weight, usual body weight<br><br>Waist circumference |
| Biochemical and Physical Assessment | • Lab values related to comorbidities, such as total cholesterol, LDL cholesterol, HDL cholesterol, triglycerides, glucose, HgBA1C<br><br>• Triiodothyronine ($T_3$), and thyroxine ($T_4$) for thyroid function<br><br>• Blood pressure |
| Dietary Assessment | • How many daily meals and snacks do you usually eat?<br><br>• What is a typical day's intake?<br><br>• How do you think your usual intake needs to be changed to be healthier or to help you lose weight?<br><br>• How often do you eat breakfast?<br><br>• How many servings of fruits and vegetables do you eat daily?<br><br>• How much sweetened soda do you drink daily?<br><br>• Do you watch your fat intake? If so, what do you do to limit fat?<br><br>• Do you watch your carbohydrate intake? If so, what do you do to limit carbohydrates?<br><br>• How many meals per week do you eat out?<br><br>• What is your "weakness?"<br><br>• Do you know if you eat for reasons other than hunger, such as when you are bored, sad, lonely, or anxious?<br><br>• Do you take vitamins, minerals, or supplements to help with weight loss? If so, what? |

*(nursing process continues on page 344)*

## *NURSING PROCESS: Obesity* (continued)

- What is your goal weight?
- How much moderate-intensity exercise do you do on a daily basis? How active is your lifestyle? How easy would it be for you to become more active?
- How much alcohol do you consume?
- Do you have any cultural, religious, or ethnic food preferences?
- Do you have any food allergies or intolerances?

### Diagnosis

Possible Nursing Diagnosis

Imbalanced nutrition: more than body requirements related to calorie intake in excess of calorie expenditure

### Planning

Client Outcomes

The client will

- Gradually increase physical activity to a total of 60 minutes of moderate-intensity activity on most days of the week.
- Explain the relationship between calorie intake, physical activity, and weight control.
- Consume a nutritionally adequate hypocaloric diet consisting of healthy carbohydrates, healthy fats, and lean protein.
- Eat at least 3 meals per day.
- Practice behavior modification techniques to change undesirable eating habits.
- Lose 1 to 2 lb/week on average until 10% of initial weight is lost.
- Improve health status as evidenced by a decrease in total cholesterol, LDL cholesterol, and glucose; an increase in HDL cholesterol; and improved blood pressure, as appropriate.

### Nursing Interventions

Nutrition Therapy

- Decrease calorie intake to 1200/day in three meals plus two to three snacks throughout the day to prevent intense hunger and subsequent overeating.
- Provide a 1200-calorie eating plan that specifies portion sizes and number of servings from each food group recommended for each meal and snack. The daily plan will include:

  1 cup of fruit

  1½ cups of vegetables

  4 grains, preferably all of them whole grains

  3 oz of meat and beans

  2 cups of skim milk

  4 tsp of oil
- Encourage ample fluid intake, preferably water and other noncalorie drinks, to promote excretion of metabolic wastes.

*(nursing process continues on page 345)*

## NURSING PROCESS: Obesity *(continued)*

| Client Teaching | Instruct the client on |
|---|---|
| | The interrelationship between a hypocaloric diet, increased physical activity, and behavior change in managing weight |
| | The eating plan essentials, including |
| | • Meal and snack timing and frequency |
| | • The emphasis on high-satiety foods, such as whole grains, fruit and vegetables, and lean protein |
| | • Tips for eating out (Chapter 10), food preparation techniques, and the basics of food purchasing and label reading |
| | Behavioral matters, including |
| | • Eating only in one place while sitting down |
| | • Putting utensils down between mouthfuls |
| | • Monitoring hunger on a scale of 1 to 10 with 1 corresponding to "famished" and 10 corresponding to "stuffed." Encourage clients to eat when the hunger scale is at about 3 and to stop when satisfied (not full) at about 6 or 7 |
| | • Weighing herself at least once a week |
| | • Periodic record keeping of food intake and activity |
| | • "Planned" splurges instead of eating on impulse. Planned splurges involve making a conscious decision to eat something, enjoying every mouthful of the food, then moving on from the experience without feelings of guilt or failure |
| | Changing eating attitudes, including |
| | • Replacing negative self-talk with positive talk |
| | • Replacing the attitude of "always being on a diet" with an acceptance of eating healthier and less as a way of life |
| | Consulting her physician or dietitian if questions concerning the eating plan or weight loss arise |

| **Evaluation** | |
|---|---|
| Evaluate and Monitor | • Monitor weight |
| | • Evaluate food and activity records to assess adherence. Suggest changes in the meal plan as needed |
| | • Provide periodic feedback and reinforcement |
| | • Monitor biochemical data for improvements attributable to weight loss |

## ▶ EATING DISORDERS: ANOREXIA NERVOSA, BULIMIA NERVOSA (BN), AND EATING DISORDERS NOT OTHERWISE SPECIFIED

Eating disorders are defined as psychiatric illnesses that can have a profound impact on nutritional status and health. They are generally characterized by abnormal eating patterns and distorted perceptions of food and body weight (Fig. 14.3). Eating disorders differ in how they are manifested, risk factors, nutritional complications, and medical complications (Table 14.5). Treatment approaches also differ.

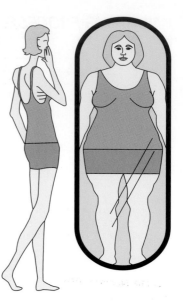

**FIGURE 14.3** A woman suffering from anorexia sees herself as overweight.

| TABLE 14.5 | A Comparison Between Anorexia Nervosa and Bulimia Nervosa | |
|---|---|---|
| | **Anorexia Nervosa** | **Bulimia Nervosa** |
| Major characteristic | Compulsive pursuit of thinness Intense fear of becoming fat; intense preoccupation with food<br>Self-worth based on size and shape | Lack of sense of control regarding eating Fear of being overweight |
| Onset and population | Usually develops during adolescence or young adulthood; 90–95% are female | Usually develops during adolescence or young adulthood; is more likely to occur in men than AN |
| Typical eating and exercise behaviors | Semistarvation with compulsive exercise; onset of disorder is usually preceded by dieting behavior | Gorging (e.g., 1200–11,500 calories in a short amount of time) followed by purging, such as self-induced vomiting, excessive exercise, abuse of laxatives, emetics, diuretics, or fasting; "dieting" is a way of life but bingeing may occur several times per day and may be planned |
| Weight | <85% of expected weight, which is a BMI ≤17.5 for adults | Fluctuations are normal; weight may be normal or slightly above normal |
| Emotional symptoms | Vicarious enjoyment of food; denial of the condition can be extreme; body image disturbance; pronounced emotional changes; low self-esteem | Displays mood swings; full recognition of the behavior as abnormal; ongoing feelings of isolation, self-deprecating thoughts, depression, and low self-esteem |
| Physical symptoms | Lanugo hair on the face and trunk; brittle, listless hair; dry skin, brittle nails, intolerance of cold | May appear normal<br>Swollen salivary glands in cheeks<br>Sore, scars, or calluses on knuckles or hands |
| Cardiovascular effects | Bradycardia, hypotension, orthostatic hypotension | Arrhythmias; palpitations; weakness |
| GI effects | Delayed gastric emptying, decreased motility, severe constipation | Bloating, constipation, flatulence; gastric dilation with rupture is a risk |

*(table continues on page 347)*

| TABLE 14.5 | A Comparison Between Anorexia Nervosa and Bulimia Nervosa (continued) | |
|---|---|---|
| | **Anorexia Nervosa** | **Bulimia Nervosa** |
| Endocrine/metabolic imbalances | Cold sensitivity; fatigue; hypercholesterolemia, hypoglycemia; amenorrhea or menstrual irregularities | Menstrual irregularities; dehydration, and electrolyte imbalances may occur secondary to vomiting and laxative abuse; rebound fluid retention with edema |
| Musculoskeletal | Osteopenia, osteoporosis, muscle wasting, and weakness | Dental erosion; muscular weakness |
| Growth status | Arrested growth and maturation | Usually not affected |
| Nutrient deficiencies | Protein–calorie malnutrition; various micronutrient deficiencies | Varies |

*Source:* American Dietetic Association. (2006). Position of the American Dietetic Association: Nutrition intervention in the treatment of anorexia nervosa, bulimia nervosa, and other eating disorders. *Journal of the American Dietetic Association, 106,* 2073–2082.

Laureate Eating Disorders Program available at http://eatingdisorders.laureate.com. Accessed on 1/27/08.

**Bulimia Nervosa (BN):** an eating disorder characterized by recurrent episodes of bingeing and purging.

**Anorexia Nervosa (AN):** a condition of self-imposed fasting or severe self-imposed dieting.

Over a lifetime, an individual may meet the diagnostic criteria for more than one of these disorders, suggesting a continuum of disordered eating. As many as 30% of clients with **bulimia nervosa (BN)** have a previous history of **anorexia nervosa (AN)**; however, BN in persons of normal weight rarely develops into AN.

## Etiology

Eating disorders are considered to be multifactorial in origin. Although numerous psychologic, physical, social, and cultural risk factors have been identified, it is not known how or why these factors interact to cause eating disorders. Risk factors that precede the diagnosis of an eating disorder include dieting, early childhood eating and GI problems, increased concern about weight and size, negative self-evaluation, and sexual abuse (ADA, 2006). Major stressors, such as the onset of puberty, parents' divorce, death of a family member, and ridicule of being or becoming fat are frequent precipitating factors. Athletes (e.g., dancers, gymnasts) may develop eating disorders to improve their performance. People with eating disorders often suffer from depression, anxiety, substance abuse, or **body dysmorphic disorder**.

**Body Dysmorphic Disorder:** excessive preoccupation with a real or imagined defect in physical appearance.

Each person's recovery process is unique; therefore, treatment plans are highly individualized. A multidisciplinary approach that includes nutrition counseling, behavior modification, psychotherapy, family counseling, and group therapy is most effective. Antidepressant drugs effectively reduce the frequency of problematic eating behaviors but do not eliminate them. Most eating disorders are treated on an outpatient basis; however, severe cases of anorexia nervosa may necessitate hospitalization. Bulimia tends to be easier to treat than anorexia because bulimics know their behavior is abnormal, and many are willing to cooperate with treatment. Nutritional intervention seeks to reestablish and maintain normal eating behaviors; correct signs, symptoms, and complications of the eating disorder; and promote long-term maintenance of reasonable weight. Treatment is often time consuming and frustrating.

## Nutrition Therapy for Anorexia Nervosa

Step-by-step goals of nutrition therapy are to (1) prevent further weight loss, (2) gradually reestablish normal eating behaviors, (3) gradually increase weight, and (4) maintain agreed-upon weight goals. Sometimes a lower-than-normal weight is selected as the initial weight goal (i.e., enough weight to regain normal physiologic function and menstruation). When

| BOX 14.6 | **NUTRITION THERAPY GUIDELINES FOR ANOREXIA NERVOSA** |

- Small, frequent meals help maximize intake and tolerance.
- The diet is advanced only when the client is able to complete a full meal. Calories may eventually be increased to 3000 or more per day.
- Because gastrointestinal intolerance may exist, limit gassy foods in the early stages of treatment, such as cruciferous vegetables (broccoli, cauliflower, cabbage), dried peas and beans, dried prunes and raisins, carbonated beverages, garlic, onions, melon, and products containing sorbitol. It may also be prudent to limit fatty and fried foods.
- Serve small, attractive meals based on individual food preferences. Foods that are nutritionally dense help minimize the volume of food needed. Finger foods served cold or at room temperature help minimize satiety sensations.
- Never force the client to eat and minimize the emphasis on food. Initially, clients may respond to nutritional therapy better if they are allowed to exclude high-risk binge foods from their diet. However, the binge foods should be reintroduced later so that the "feared food" (trigger food) idea is not promoted.
- A high-fiber or low-sodium diet may be helpful in controlling symptoms of constipation and fluid retention, respectively.
- A multivitamin and mineral supplement may be prescribed.
- Caffeine is avoided because it is both a stimulant and a mild diuretic.
- Tube feedings or parenteral nutrition is used only if necessary to stabilize the client medically. Overly aggressive nutritional repletion carries medical risks of fluid retention and refeeding syndrome; psychological risks may include a perceived loss of control, loss of identity, increased body distortion, and mistrust of the treatment team. Enteral support should never be used as punishment for difficult clients.

this has been achieved, the goal may be reevaluated. In reality, half of those who receive care are expected to recover, 21% experience partial recovery, and 26% display a poor response to treatment (ADA, 2006). The overall mortality rate is 9.8%.

Involving the client in formulating individualized goals and plans promotes compliance and feelings of trust. Offer rewards that are linked to the quantity of calories consumed, not to weight gain. Initially, it may be beneficial to have the client record food intake and exercise activity.

Even though calorie needs are high to restore body weight, the initial eating plan offered is low in calories to avoid overwhelming the client. Also, large amounts of food may not be well tolerated or accepted after prolonged semistarvation. Generally, initial intake may start at 1000 to 1200 calories with incremental increases to achieve a weekly weight gain of ½ to 1 pound. Nutrition therapy for AN appears in Box 14.6.

## Nutrition Therapy for Bulimia Nervosa

People with BN tend to have fewer serious medical complications than people with AN because their undernutrition is less severe. Nutritional counseling focuses on identifying and correcting food misinformation and fears and includes discussion on meal planning, establishing a normal pattern of eating, and the dangers of dieting. Bulimics must understand that gorging is only one aspect of a complex pattern of altered behavior; in fact, excessive dietary restriction is a major contributor to the disorder. Although most clients with BN want to lose weight, dieting and recovery from an eating disorder are incompatible. Normalization of eating behaviors is a primary goal.

Initially, nutrition therapy for bulimia is structured and relatively inflexible to promote the client's sense of control. Meal patterns similar to those used for people with diabetes can

---

BOX 14.7   **NUTRITION THERAPY GUIDELINES FOR BULIMIA NERVOSA**

- To increase awareness of eating and satiety, meals and snacks should be eaten while sitting down; finger foods and foods that are cold or at room temperature should be avoided; and the meal duration should be of appropriate length.
- Eating strategies that may help regulate intake include not skipping meals or snacks and using the appropriately sized utensils.
- Encourage clients to gradually introduce forbidden binge foods into their diets. This is a key step in changing the all-or-none behavior of bingeing/purging.
- Clients who are laxative dependent are at risk of bowel obstruction if the protocol for laxative withdrawal is not implemented. A high-fiber diet with plenty of fluids helps normalize bowel movements while the use of laxatives is gradually decreased. Stool softeners may be ordered.
- When relapse occurs, the structured meal plan should be resumed immediately.

be used to specify portion sizes, food groups to include with each meal and snack, and the frequency of eating. The initial meal plan provides adequate calories for weight maintenance so as to avoid hunger, which can precipitate a binge—usually not less than 1500 calories distributed among three balanced meals plus snacks. Adequate fat is provided to help delay gastric emptying and contribute to satiety. Calories are gradually increased as needed. Having the client record intake *before* eating adds to a sense of control. Nutrition therapy guidelines for BN appear in Box 14.7.

## Eating Disorders Not Otherwise Specified

Eating disorders not otherwise specified (EDNOS) are at least as common as AN and BN, but prevalence rates are unknown because there is no simple definition of EDNOS (ADA, 2006). This group represents subacute cases of AN or BN—clients who may meet all the criteria for anorexia except that they have not missed three consecutive menstrual periods, or clients of normal weight who purge without bingeing. Binge eating disorder, in which bingeing occurs without purging, is also classified as an EDNOS. Unlike AN and BN, binge eating disorder often precedes dieting, and incidence among men and women is similar. Bingeing must occur at least twice a week over at least 6 months. Most binge eating disorder clients are overweight and present with concerns about weight management, not disordered eating. Nutrition therapy for binge eating disorder is similar to that of BN, with normalization of eating behaviors as the primary goal. Weight loss may be a secondary or subsequent goal.

## ▶ How Do You Respond?

**Is it a good idea to substitute special low-carbohydrate products for regular foods?**
Choosing reduced carbohydrate versions of "empty calorie" foods ignores the big picture: to lose weight, calories have to be cut. Substituting reduced carbohydrate muffins or beer over their regular carbohydrate counterparts is likely to have little or no impact on calorie intake. In addition, specially prepared low-carbohydrate foods do not taste like the original food and may cost two to four times more. A better alternative to choosing low-carbohydrate items is to avoid foods made with white flour and sugar and switch to carbohydrates that provide satiety, namely, whole grain breads and cereals, fruits, vegetables, and dried peas and beans.

**What are "net carbs"?** Specially formulated low-carbohydrate products have starch and regular sweeteners removed and fiber and sugar alcohols added. Food manufacturers have created the "net carb" concept to show consumers that their products are carbohydrate savers. They reason that because fiber is not digested and, therefore, provides no calories, grams of fiber should not be counted as carbohydrates. While it is true that fiber is generally "calorie-free," it is common practice among diabetes educators to subtract fiber grams from total carbohydrate grams *only when* the fiber content is greater than 5 g/serving; for lesser amounts, no adjustment is needed. Food manufacturers also contend that the grams of sugar alcohols should be ignored even though they do provide calories, albeit about one-half the amount in regular sweeteners. Using their rationale, a product that has 10 g of total carbohydrates with 3 g of fiber and 4 g of maltitol would have a "net carb" content of only 3 g [10 g − (3 g + 4 g) = 3 g]. Unfortunately, the same math does not apply to calories available to the body. Advise clients to ignore "net carbs" and instead evaluate a product on the basis of calories, serving size, and taste.

**Do protein needs increase while on a weight loss diet?** During the process of weight loss, protein needs increase slightly depending on several metabolic factors and levels of physical activity (Melanson, 2007). In general, 65 to 70 g protein/day is recommended to reduce the loss of lean body mass and to promote satiety. Most Americans typically consume 25% more than the Recommended Dietary Allowance (RDA) for protein so an adjustment in intake may not be necessary.

▶ CASE STUDY

CC: "I hate being fat."

   Patient History: 43-year-old mother of three has experienced gradual weight gain after the birth of each of her children. Works full time; does not engage in regular exercise. She is considered "prediabetic" and has "prehypertension" and appears eager to make lifestyle changes to improve her health.

   Labs: Fasting glucose 118 mg/dL, total cholesterol 200 mg/dL, HDL cholesterol 38 mg/dL, triglycerides 220 mg/dL.

   Anthropometrics: Height 5 ft. 7in., weight 189 pounds, waist circumference 39 in., blood pressure 142/88.

   Diet History: Client does not eat breakfast. Snacks at vending machine 2 times per day. Eats fast food lunch, dinner with family is "normal" consisting of approximately 6 ounces of meat, potatoes, sometimes a vegetable, bread with butter, and dessert. Admits to a weakness for "sweets."

* Calculate BMI to determine her weight status. Assess her waist circumference. What are the treatment recommendations for her, based on her weight and comorbidities?
* What do her lab values indicate?
* According to MyPyramid recommendations, what are her estimated calorie needs based on her age and activity? How many calories should she consume to lose 1 to 2 pounds/week?
* Create a nursing care plan complete with nursing diagnosis, client goal, interventions, and monitoring recommendations.
* Devise a meal pattern with the calorie allowance you recommend; include three meals and 3 snacks per day. Prepare a sample menu.
* What additional information about her eating behaviors would be helpful?

1. The client asks if it is okay for her to follow a low-carbohydrate, Atkins-type diet in the short term to get her started on her weight loss efforts. Which of the following would be the nurse's best response?
   a. "No, low-carbohydrate diets are not healthy and would only sabotage your weight loss efforts."
   b. "A low-carbohydrate diet can help you lose weight initially but their long-term safety is not known. Use it for a couple of weeks but discontinue it if you experience any side effects."
   c. "A low carbohydrate is better than any other type of diet and is a good choice for you to use."
   d. "A low-fat diet is easier. Try that instead."

2. An example of a low calorie, nutrient-dense food is:
   a. Vegetable soup.
   b. Fruit roll-up.
   c. Diet soda.
   d. Low fat ice cream.

3. The client asks if meal replacements, such as Jenny Craig, are a good idea to help with weight loss. Which of the following would be the nurse's best response?
   a. "They are a great way to control portions and can help you adhere to your diet when used as suggested."
   b. "They are gimmicks that fail to teach you how to control your own intake. They are not recommended."
   c. "Most people gain weight while using them. You should stay away from them."
   d. "They are not nutritionally balanced, so you actually have to overeat to meet your nutritional requirements if you use them."

4. Which of the following strategies promotes adherence to exercise? Check all that apply.
   a. Promote structure by encouraging the client to exercise at on-site or supervised exercise sessions.
   b. Encourage the client to exercise in multiple short bouts (10 minutes each), instead of one long session.
   c. Encourage a more active lifestyle, such as parking far away from the door when going to the mall or work.
   d. Encourage the client to exercise at home.

5. Which of the following conditions is a complication of obesity? Check all that apply.
   a. Gall stones.
   b. Sleep apnea.
   c. Type 2 diabetes.
   d. Hypertension.
   e. Osteoporosis.

6. Which of the following should be given to a client to promote adherence to a hypocaloric diet?
   a. A meal plan and recipes.
   b. A list of forbidden foods.
   c. A calorie counter.
   d. A fat gram counter.

7. When instituting nutrition therapy for a client diagnosed with bulimia nervosa, the priority is to:
   a. Teach the client about nutrient and calorie requirements.
   b. Halt weight loss.
   c. Normalize eating behaviors.
   d. Provide sufficient calories for weight gain.

**8.** When instituting nutrition therapy for a client diagnosed with anorexia nervosa, the priority is to:
    **a.** Teach the client about nutrient and calorie requirements.
    **b.** Halt weight loss.
    **c.** Normalize eating behaviors.
    **d.** Provide sufficient calories for weight gain.

## KEY CONCEPTS

- Approximately 31% of American adults are obese. The prevalence of obesity has increased in both genders, all age groups, and among all races and ethnicities.

- Obesity is a chronic disease of multifactorial origin. It is likely that a combination of genetic and environmental factors is involved in its development.

- Obesity is resistant to treatment when success is measured by achieving healthy BMI alone. Rather than concentrating solely on weight loss to measure success, other health benefits, such as lowered blood pressure and lowered serum lipids, should also be considered.

- A modest weight loss of 5% to 10% of initial body weight usually effectively lowers disease risks.

- A hypocaloric intake, increased activity, and behavior therapy are the cornerstones to weight loss therapy. Pharmacotherapy and surgery are additional options for some people.

- Calorie intake should be lowered by 500 to 1000 cal/day to promote a gradual weight loss of 1 to 2 lb/week. For women, 1000 to 1200 cal/day are recommended; for men, 1200 to 1600 cal/day.

- As long as calories are reduced and healthy sources of fat and carbohydrates are used, the macronutrient composition of the diet does not impact weight loss. What matters is the relationship between calorie intake and calorie output, not the source of calories consumed.

- Nutrition education should cover the importance of portion sizes, sources of "good carbs" and "healthy fats," low-calorie cooking techniques, how to modify a recipe, label reading, how to eat out, meal frequency, and the concepts of nutrient- and calorie-density.

- An increase in activity helps to burn calories and has a favorable impact on body composition and weight distribution. Even without weight loss, exercise lowers blood pressure and improves glucose tolerance and blood lipid levels.

- The Dietary Guidelines for Americans recommends 60 minutes of moderate-intensity activity on most days of the week to prevent weight gain; 60 to 90 minutes/day are recommended to maintain weight loss.

- Behavior therapy promotes lifelong changes in eating and activity habits. It is a process that involves identifying behaviors that need improvement, setting specific behavioral goals, modifying "problem" behaviors, and reinforcing the positive changes.

- Pharmacotherapy is adjunctive therapy in the treatment of obesity. Drugs are not effective in all people, and they are only effective for as long as they are used.

- Surgery to promote weight loss therapy involves limiting the capacity of the stomach. Gastric bypass also circumvents a portion of the small intestine to cause malabsorption of calories. Both types effectively promote weight loss but have complications.

- Weight maintenance after loss may be more difficult to achieve than weight loss itself. Common characteristics of people who are able to maintain long-term weight loss are that they eat a low-calorie diet, eat consistently from day to day, eat breakfast, are very physically active, weigh themselves frequently, watch only a limited amount of television, and don't let a little weight gain become bigger.

- AN and BN are characterized by preoccupation with body weight and food and usually are preceded by prolonged dieting. Although their cause is unknown, they are considered to be multifactorial in origin.

- AN is a condition of severe self-imposed starvation, often accompanied by a frantic pursuit of exercise. Although they appear to be severely underweight, anorexics have a distorted self-perception of weight and see themselves as overweight. They may have numerous physical and mental symptoms. Anorexia can be fatal.

- Bulimia, which occurs more frequently than anorexia, is characterized by binge eating (consuming large amounts of food in a short period) and purging (e.g., self-induced vomiting, laxative abuse). Bulimics usually appear to be of normal or slightly above-normal weight, and they experience less severe physical symptoms than anorexics do. Bulimia is rarely fatal.

- Eating disorders are best treated by a team approach that includes nutritional intervention and counseling to restore normal eating behaviors and adequate nutritional status.

## ANSWER KEY

1. **FALSE** Calories eaten during the evening to not "count" more than calories eaten at any other time of day. It comes down to calories in versus calories out. The problem with eating in the evening is that it is frequently "mindless munching" in front of the TV and the calories seem to pile up unconsciously.

2. **FALSE** People who skip meals tend to feel hungrier later on and then eat more than they normally would.

3. **TRUE** Most people are able to lose weight through diet and exercise but most people eventually regain most or all of the weight they lost.

4. **FALSE** Although research suggests that calcium intakes lower than the DRI are associated with higher body weight, it is not clear if calcium intakes at or above the DRI impact body weight (ADA Evidence Library).

5. **FALSE** Obesity-related problems improve or are resolved with a modest weight loss of 5% to 10% of initial weight even if healthy weight is not achieved.

6. **TRUE** Most short-term weight loss occurs from a decrease in total calorie intake. Physical activity helps to maintain weight loss.

7. **TRUE** With or without weight loss, an increase in physical activity helps to lower blood pressure and improve glucose tolerance.

8. **TRUE** Eating plans that provide less than 1200 calories may not provide adequate amounts of essential nutrients.

9. **FALSE** Neither cutting carbohydrates nor cutting fat grams ensures weight loss unless total calories are reduced. There is no magic combination of nutrients that causes weight loss independent of reducing calories.

10. **TRUE** People affected by bulimia tend to have fewer medical complications than those affected by anorexia because the undernutrition is less severe.

## WEBSITES

*For reliable information on weight, dieting, physical fitness, and obesity*

American Obesity Association at **www.obesity.org/**
Calorie Control Council at **www.caloriecontrol.org**
Division of Nutrition and Physical Activity, National Center for Chronic Disease Prevention and Health Promotion at **www.cdc.gov/nccdphp/dnpa**
International Obesity Task Force at **www.iotf.org**
NHLBI Obesity Education Initiative at **www.nhlbi.nih.gov/about/oei/index.htm**

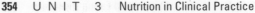

North American Association for the Study of Obesity at **www.naaso.org**
Partnership for Healthy Weight Management at **www.consumer.gov/weightloss**
Shape Up America at **www.shapeup.org**
Weight Control Information Network at **www.niddk.nih.gov/health/nutrit/win.htm**

*For free intake/diet analysis*

**www.fitday.com**
**www.dietsite.com**
**www.foodcount.com** (offers both free and fee-based subscriptions)
**www.nat.uiuc.edu/mynat**

*For eating disorders*

Anorexia Nervosa and Related Eating Disorders (ANRED) at **www.anred.com**
National Eating Disorders Organization at **www.laureate.com/aboutned.html**
The Renfrew Center at **www.renfrew.org**
Search "eating disorders" at **www.nal.usda.gov/fnic** for *Eating Disorders—A Food and Nutrition Resource List*
Something Fishy on Eating Disorders at **www.somethingfishy.org**
Overeaters Anonymous, Inc. at **www.oa.org**

## REFERENCES

American Dietetic Association. (2006). Position of the American Dietetic Association: Nutrition intervention in the treatment of anorexia nervosa, bulimia nervosa, and other eating disorders. *Journal of the American Dietetic Association, 106,* 2073–2082.

American Dietetic Association Evidence Library (2006). *Adult weight management guidelines.* Available at http://adaevidencelibrary.com. Accessed on 1/20/08.

Berkel, L. A., Poston, W. S., Reeves, R. S., et al. (2005). Behavioral interventions for obesity. *Journal of the American Dietetic Association, 105,* S35–S43.

Blackburn, G. (2005). Solutions in weight control: Lessons from gastric surgery. *The American Journal of Clinical Nutrition, 82*(Suppl.), 248S–252S.

Buchwald, H., Avidor, Y., Braunwald, E., et al. (2004). Bariatric surgery: A systematic review and meta-analysis. *The Journal of the American Medical Association, 292,* 1724–1737.

Catenacci, V., & Wyatt, H. (2007). The role of physical activity in producing and maintaining weight loss. *Nature Clinical Practice Endocrinology Metabolism, 3,* 518–529.

Chagnon, Y. C., Rankinen, T., Synder, E. E., et al. (2003). The human obesity gene map: The 2002 update. *Obesity Research, 11,* 313–367.

Cope, M., & Allison, D. (2006). Obesity: Person and population. *Obesity, 14,* 156S–159S.

Fabricatore, A. (2007). Behavior therapy and cognitive-behavioral therapy of obesity: Is there a difference? *Journal of the American Dietetic Association, 107,* 92–99.

Heymsfield, S. B., van Mierlo, C. A., van der Knaap, H. C., et al. (2003). Weight management using meal replacement strategy: Meta and pooling analysis from six studies. *International Journal of Obesity, 27,* 537–549.

Hill, J. O., & Wyatt, H. R. (2005). Role of physical activity in preventing and treating obesity. *Journal of Applied Physiology, 99,* 765–770.

Klein, S. (2004). Long-term pharmacotherapy for obesity. *Obesity Research, 12,* 163S–166S.

Knowler, W. C., Barrett-Connor, E., Fowler, S. E., et al. (2002). Reduction in the incidence of type 2 diabetes with lifestyle intervention or metformin. *The New England Journal of Medicine, 346,* 393–403.

Kral, T., & Rolls, B. (2004). Energy density and portion size: Their independent and combined effects on energy intake. *Physiology & Behavior, 82,* 131–138.

Loos, R., and Rankinen, T. (2005). Gene-diet interactions on body weight changes. *Journal of American Diet Association, 105*(Suppl), S29–S34.

McTigue, K. C., Harris, R., Hemphill, B., et al. (2003). Screening and interventions for obesity in adults: Summary of the evidence for the US Preventive Services Task Force. *Annals Internal Medicine, 139,* 933–949.

Melanson, K. (2007). Dietary considerations for obesity treatment. *American Journal of Lifestyle Medicine, 1,* 433–436.

Moyers, S. (2005). Medications as adjunct therapy for weight loss: Approved and off-label agents in use. *Journal of the American Dietetic Association, 105*, 948–959.

National Heart, Lung, and Blood Institute Expert Panel on the Identification, Evaluation, and Treatment of Overweight and Obesity in Adults. (1998). *Executive summary of the clinical guidelines on the identification, evaluation, and treatment of overweight and obesity in adults:* National Institutes of Health.

National Heart, Lung, and Blood Institute Obesity Education Initiative, North American Association for the Study of Obesity. U.S. Department of Health and Human Services, Public Health Service, National Institutes of Health (2000). *The practical guide: Identification, evaluation, and treatment of overweight and obesity in adults.* Available at http://www.nhlbi.nih.gov. Accessed on 1/20/08.

O'Neil, C., & Nicklas, T. (2007). Relationship between diet/physical activity and health. *American Journal of Lifestyle Medicine, 1*, 457–481.

Pi-Sunyer, F. (2002). The obesity epidemic: pathophysiology and consequences of obesity. *Obesity Research,* 10, suppl 2, 97S–104S.

Roberts, S., McCrory, M., & Saltzman, E. (2002). The influence of dietary composition on energy intake and body weight. *Journal of the American College of Nutrition, 21*, 140S–145S.

Rolls, B., Drewnowski, A., & Ledikwe, J. (2005). Changing the energy density of the diet as a strategy for weight management. *Journal of the American Dietetic Association, 105*, S98–S103.

Schardt, D. (2008). Secrets of successful losers. *Nutrition Action Health Letter, 35*(1), 8.

Schoeller, D., & Buchholz, A. (2005). Energetics of obesity and weight control: Does diet composition matter. *Journal of the American Dietetic Association, 105*, S24–S28.

Stevens, V. J., Obarzanek, E., Cook, N. R., et al. (2001). Long-term weight loss and changes in blood pressure: Results of the Trials of Hypertension Prevention, phase II. *Annals of Internal Medicine, 134*, 1–11.

Sugerman, H., Shikora, S., & Schauer, P. (2007). Bariatric surgery. *Obesity Management, 3*(6), 251–254.

USDHHS, NIH, NIDDK, Weight Control Information Network (WIN). (2007). *Statistics related to overweight and obesity.* Available at http://www.win.niddk.nih.gov/publications/PDFs/stat904z.pdf. Accessed on 1/28/08.

USDHHS, NIH, NIDDK, Weight Control Information Network (WIN). (2009). *Weight-loss and nutrition myths. How much do you really know?* Available at http://www.win.niddk.nih.gov/publications/PDFs/Myths.pdf. Accessed on 4/9/09.

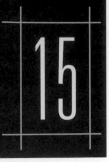

# Feeding Patients: Oral Diets and Enteral and Parenteral Nutrition

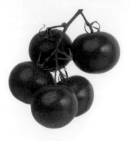

| TRUE | FALSE | |
|:---:|:---:|---|
| ☐ | ☐ | **1** Hospitalized patients are at risk for malnutrition. |
| ☐ | ☐ | **2** Patient tolerance is improved when oral intake progresses slowly after surgery from a clear liquid diet to regular food. |
| ☐ | ☐ | **3** Modular products provide a single nutrient and are used to increase the calorie or protein density of food or tube feedings. |
| ☐ | ☐ | **4** Osmolality is a primary consideration in selecting an appropriate enteral formula. |
| ☐ | ☐ | **5** The terms *fiber* and *residue* are synonymous. |
| ☐ | ☐ | **6** The patient's ability to digest nutrients is a primary consideration when deciding the type of enteral formula to use. |
| ☐ | ☐ | **7** A continuous drip delivered by a pump is recommended for administering tube feedings to patients who are critically ill. |
| ☐ | ☐ | **8** Parenteral nutrition can be infused through a peripheral or central vein. |
| ☐ | ☐ | **9** Hyperglycemia is a normal and harmless consequence of parenteral nutrition. |
| ☐ | ☐ | **10** Coloring tube-feeding formulas with food dye helps to prevent aspiration. |

### UPON COMPLETION OF THIS CHAPTER, YOU WILL BE ABLE TO

- Modify a menu to an altered consistency diet (e.g., clear liquid diet, blenderized diet, mechanically altered diet).
- Give examples of therapeutic diets and their uses.
- Compare intact enteral formulas with hydrolyzed formulas.
- Choose the most appropriate enteral formula for a given patient.
- Evaluate an enteral feeding schedule for appropriateness and adequacy.
- Propose interventions to combat various nutrition-related problems that may occur with enteral nutrition.
- Compare enteral nutrition to parenteral nutrition.
- Discuss the components of parenteral nutrition and the usual concentration of macronutrients provided.

U p to 25% to 40% of hospitalized patients have malnutrition, which is associated with post-operative complications, increased length of hospital stay, and death (Kruizenga et al., 2005). Patients may be malnourished upon admission due to the effects of chronic illness. Ironically, hospitalization may increase a person's risk of malnutrition. Appetite may be impaired by fear, pain, or anxiety. Hospital food may be refused because it is unfamiliar, tasteless (e.g., cooked without salt), inappropriate in texture (e.g., pureed meat), religiously

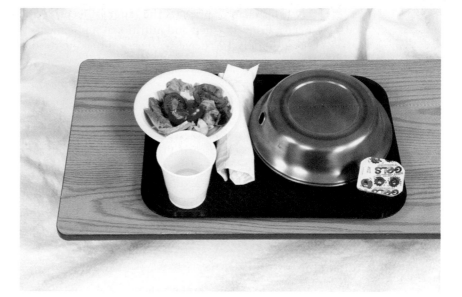

**FIGURE 15.1** Hospital meal.

or culturally unacceptable, or served at times when the patient is unaccustomed to eating (Fig. 15.1). Meals may be withheld or missed because of diagnostic procedures or medical treatments. Inadequate liquid diets may not be advanced to a solid food diet in a timely manner. Patients may underestimate the importance of nutrition in their recovery process. Giving the right food to the patient is one thing; getting the patient to eat (most of it) is another. See Box 15.1 for suggestions on how to promote an adequate intake.

| BOX 15.1 | PROMOTING AN ADEQUATE INTAKE |
| --- | --- |

Attention to details can make a big difference in the patient's acceptance of hospital food.

- Let the patient select his or her own menu whenever possible. This gives the patient a greater sense of control, increases the likelihood that the food will be consumed, and may prompt the patient to ask questions about the particular diet or provide information about his or her personal food and nutrition history.
- Offer patients who do not like menu selections the daily "standby" or choices as alternatives. Be aware that "hospital food" is frequently used as a vehicle for patients to vent anger and frustration over their loss of control.
- Be aggressive about diet progressions. Keep in mind that advancing the diet as quickly as possible allows the patient to meet nutritional requirements sooner and increases patient satisfaction.
- Set the stage for a pleasant meal. Be sure trays are delivered promptly to ensure foods are at the proper temperatures. Adjust the lighting and make sure the patient is in an appropriate sitting position. Screen the patient from offensive sights and remove unpleasant odors from the room. Encourage family to visit at mealtime, if appropriate. Offer mouth care to improve appetite, if appropriate.

- Be positive. Refrain from negative comments about the food. Also be aware of what your body language is saying to the patient. A frown or raised eyebrows can speak volumes.
- Provide assistance when necessary. Encourage the patient to self-feed to the greatest extent possible. Some patients may benefit from minor help such as opening milk cartons or buttering bread; others may need to be completely fed. Monitor the patient's ability to self-feed and adjust the intensity of help accordingly.
- Gently motivate the patient to eat. Sometimes encouragement is all that is needed to get the patient to eat. For other patients, motivation comes from being made aware of the importance of food in the recovery process. Thinking of food as part of treatment instead of a social function may improve intake even when appetite is compromised.
- Identify eating problems. Patients who feel full quickly should be encouraged to eat the most nutritious items first (meat, milk) and save the less dense items for last (juice, soup, coffee). Patients who have difficulty chewing benefit from a mechanical soft diet. Determine if the patient would accept between-meal supplements and a bedtime snack to help maximize intake.

This chapter presents the range of feeding options used to meet patients' nutritional needs, from oral diets and nutritional supplements to enteral nutrition and parenteral nutrition. Figure 15.2 depicts a decision-making model for choosing the appropriate type and method of feeding.

## ▶ ORAL DIETS

Oral diets are the easiest and most preferred method of providing nutrition. In most facilities, patients choose what they want to eat from a menu representing the diet ordered by the physician. Private and government regulatory agencies stipulate meal timing, frequency, and nutritional content and require that hospital menus be supervised by a qualified dietitian.

Oral diets may be categorized as "regular," modified consistency, or therapeutic. Often combination diets are ordered, such as a ground low-sodium diet or a high-protein, soft diet. The actual foods allowed on a diet vary among institutions and the diet manual used.

### Normal, Regular, and House Diets

Regular diets are used to achieve or maintain optimal nutritional status in patients who do not have altered nutritional needs. No foods are excluded, and portion sizes are not limited on a normal diet. The nutritional value of the diet varies significantly with the actual foods chosen by the patient.

Regular diets are adjusted to meet age-specific needs throughout the life cycle. For instance, a regular diet for a child differs from one for a pregnant woman or an elderly patient. Regular diets are also altered to meet specifications for vegetarian or kosher eating.

Sometimes physicians order a *diet as tolerated (DAT)* on admission or after surgery. This order is interpreted according to the patient's appetite and ability to eat and tolerate food. The nurse has the authority to advance the diet as tolerated.

### Modified Consistency Diets

Modified consistency diets include clear liquid and mechanically altered diets (Table 15.1). Clear liquid diets may be used after surgery, in preparation for bowel surgery or procedures, or when oral intake resumes after a prolonged period. Usually, clear liquids are ordered and progressed to a full liquid, soft, regular, or therapeutic diet as tolerated. Although a gradual progression from a clear liquid diet to a regular diet was once believed important for maximizing tolerance when eating resumes after surgery, there is little scientific evidence to support this practice. Most patients can tolerate a regular diet for their second postoperative meal, after their first meal of clear liquids.

**Viscosity:** resistance to flow.

Mechanically altered diets contain foods that are chopped, ground, pureed, or soft for patients who have difficulty chewing or swallowing. Blenderized diets provide food in liquid form for patients who are unable to tolerate solid foods; the **viscosity** of the blended food depends on the individual's tolerance. Dysphagia diets are another variation of modified consistency diets that are covered in Chapter 17.

### Therapeutic Diets

Therapeutic diets differ from a regular diet in the amount of one or more nutrients or food components for the purpose of preventing or treating disease or illness. The number or timing of meals may also be altered. Table 15.2 outlines the characteristics and indications of selected therapeutic diets.

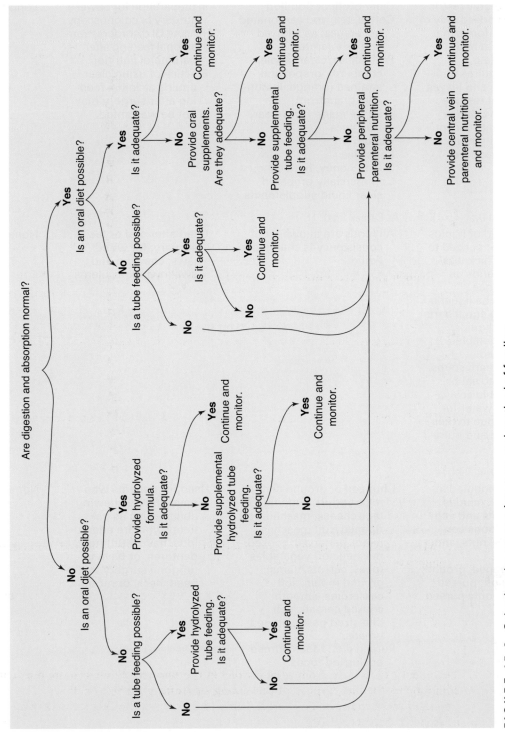

**FIGURE 15.2** Selecting the appropriate type and method of feeding.

| TABLE 15.1 | Characteristics, Indications, and Contraindications of Modified Consistency Diets | | |
|---|---|---|---|
| **Diet Characteristics** | **Foods Allowed** | **Indications** | **Contraindications** |
| **Clear Liquid** | | | |
| A short-term, highly restrictive diet composed only of clear fluids or foods that become fluid at body temperature (e.g., gelatin). It requires minimal digestion and leaves a minimum of residue. Inadequate in calories and all nutrients except vitamin C if vitamin C–fortified juices are used. | Clear broth or bouillon Coffee, tea, and carbonated beverages, as allowed and as tolerated Fruit juices; clear (apple, cranberry, grape) and strained (orange, lemonade, grapefruit) Fruit ice made from clear fruit juice Gelatin Popsicles Sugar, honey, hard candy Commercially prepared clear liquid supplements | In preparation for bowel surgery or colonoscopy; acute GI disorders; transitional feeding after parenteral nutrition. Practice of using clear liquids as initial feeding after surgery may not be warranted. | Long-term use |
| **Blenderized Liquid Diet (Also Known As Pureed Diet)** | | | |
| A diet composed of liquids and foods blenderized to liquid form. Thickness/viscosity depends on patient tolerance. Most foods can be liquefied by combining equal parts of solids and liquids; fruits and vegetables need less liquid. Broth, gravy, cream soups, cheese, tomato sauce, milk, and fruit juice are preferable to water for blenderizing due to their higher calorie and nutritional value. | All foods are allowed, but consistency is changed to liquid | Used after oral or facial surgery; for wired jaws; chewing and swallowing problems | None |
| **Mechanically Altered Diet** | | | |
| A regular diet modified in texture only. Excludes most raw fruits and vegetables and foods containing seeds, nuts, and dried fruit. Foods are chopped, ground, mashed or soft; pureed diet contains only pureed foods | Chopped or ground diet: milk, yogurt, pudding, cottage cheese; mashed, soft ripened fruit (peaches, pears, bananas); cooked, mashed soft vegetables (peas, carrots, yams); ground meats, soft casseroles, smooth cooked cereals, soft bite-sized pasta, pureed breads. Pureed diet: foods pureed or slurried foods | Used for patients who have limited chewing ability, such as patients who are edentulous, have ill-fitting dentures, or have undergone surgery to the head, neck, or mouth | None |

| TABLE 15.2 | Selected Therapeutic Diets: Characteristics and Indications | |
| --- | --- | --- |
| **Type of Diet** | **Characteristics** | **Indications** |
| "Diabetic" diet or consistent-carbohydrate diet | Total daily carbohydrate content is consistent with emphasis on general nutritional balance. Calories are based on attaining and maintaining healthy weight. A high fiber intake is encouraged, sodium may be limited, and heart healthy fats are encouraged over saturated fat. | Type 1 and type 2 diabetes, gestational diabetes; impaired glucose tolerance; impaired fasting glucose |
| Fat-restricted | Fat limited to <50 g or <25 g of fat per day | Malabsorption syndromes, liver disease, pancreatic disease, chronic cholecystitis, gastroesophageal reflux |
| High-fiber | A general diet with low-fiber foods replaced by foods high in fiber | To prevent or treat constipation, diabetes, irritable bowel syndrome, hypercholesterolemia, obesity |
| Low-fiber | Fiber limited to <10 g/day | Before surgery to minimize fecal residue; during acute phases of intestinal disorders such as ulcerative colitis, Crohn's disease, and diverticulitis |
| High-calorie, high-protein | A diet rich in calorie-dense and/or protein-dense foods | To meet increased nutritional requirements; also used in patients with poor intakes |
| Calcium-rich diet | Calcium-rich foods are emphasized in a regular diet | Used for patients with low calcium intake and those at risk for osteoporosis |
| Iron-rich diet | Iron-rich foods are emphasized in a regular diet | Used for patients with low iron intake and those with high iron requirements, such as pregnant women and endurance athletes |
| Potassium-modified | Potassium may be increased or restricted by manipulating potassium-rich foods, such as fruits, vegetables, whole grains, milk, and meats | Low-potassium diets may be used in the treatment of certain renal diseases, in conjunction with certain medications or in adrenal insufficiency; high potassium may be used in conjunction with certain medications and with certain renal diseases |
| Sodium-restricted | Sodium limit may be set at 500 mg/day, 1000 mg/day, 2000 mg/day, or 3000 mg/day | Hypertension, congestive heart failure, acute and chronic renal disease, liver disease |
| Gluten-free | Sources of gluten (a protein in wheat, rye, oats, and barley) are eliminated from the diet; gluten-free grains, such as corn, potato, rice, soy, and quinoa are encouraged as sources of complex carbohydrates | Celiac disease (celiac sprue, nontropical sprue, gluten-sensitive enteropathy) and dermatitis herpetiformis rash |
| Lactose-restricted | Limits foods with lactose ("milk sugar") to the amount tolerated by the individual | Lactose intolerance or lactase insufficiency, which may occur secondary to certain inflammatory GI disorders such as ulcerative colitis and Crohn's disease |

## Nutritional Supplements

Some patients are unable or unwilling to eat enough food to meet their requirements, either because intake is poor or because their nutritional needs are so high that it is difficult to meet requirements in a normal volume of food. For these patients, nutritional supplements with or between meals can significantly boost protein and calorie intakes.

Categories of supplements include clear liquid supplements, milk-based drinks, prepared liquid supplements, and specially prepared foods (Table 15.3). Liquid supplements are easy to consume, are generally well accepted, and tend to leave the stomach quickly, making them a good choice for between-meal snacks.

For nutritional supplements to effectively boost overall nutrient intake they must be consumed. If possible, allow the patient to taste test several options available and choose the most appealing. Explain the rationale for adding supplements and closely monitor acceptance. A rotation schedule of different types of supplements and various flavors may help forestall or prevent taste fatigue that tends to occur over time. To maximize acceptance, serve liquid supplements cold.

## Modular Products

A less frequently used option for maximizing a patient's oral intake is to add a modular product to foods or supplements the patient consumes. Modular products are generally composed of a single nutrient, either carbohydrate (e.g., hydrolyzed cornstarch), protein

| TABLE 15.3 | Nutritional Supplements | | |
|------------|-------------------------|---|---|
| **Type** | **Examples** | **Characteristics** | **Comments** |
| Clear Liquid | Enlive! <br> Forta Drink <br> Resource Fruit <br>   Beverage | Come ready-to-use or as a powder to be mixed with water <br> Provide protein or calories, or both for patients on clear liquid diets <br> Extremely low in fat | Although they come in flavors, they are not as well accepted as the other types of supplements |
| Milk-based | Forta Shake <br> Carnation Instant <br>   Breakfast <br> Boost Drink | May be "home made," such as a milkshake; commercially prepared; or in powdered form to be mixed with milk <br> Provide significant amounts of protein and calories; are relatively inexpensive and palatable | Not suitable for patients with lactose intolerance; are not nutritionally complete, so they cannot be used as the sole source of nutrition |
| Commercially prepared liquid | Ensure: Regular, Protein, Plus, and Fiber varieties <br> Boost: Drink High Protein, Plus, and Fiber varieties | Regular varieties: 8 g protein, 250 cal/8 oz <br> High protein: 12–15 g protein/8 oz <br> Plus: 14 g protein, 360 cal/8 oz <br> Fiber: regular formula with fiber added <br> Are lactose free | Generally sweet and flavored <br> Are quick, easy, varied in flavor, often available in grocery stores <br> Most provide complete nutrition, so they can be used as sole source of nutrition |
| Commercially prepared supplemental foods | Bars <br> Broth <br> Coffee <br> Coffee creamer <br> Gelatin <br> Pudding | Specially designed to provide a concentrated source of protein and calories | Offer an alternative to sweetened drinks |

(e.g., whey protein), or fat (e.g., medium-chain triglycerides [MCT oil]), and increase calorie or nutrient density of the diet without increasing volume. For instance, a patient with chronic renal failure may receive carbohydrate-fortified mashed potatoes to increase calorie intake without increasing protein or altering taste. Disadvantages of using modular products are ineffective quality control (calculation errors), bacterial contamination, and higher costs than standard formulas. Modular products added to tube feedings increase the risk of nutrient imbalances and clogged tubes.

## ▶ ENTERAL NUTRITION

**Enteral Nutrition (EN):** the delivery of nutrients by tube, catheter, or stoma into the gastrointestinal tract beyond the oral cavity; commonly known as tube feeding.

**Enteral nutrition (EN)** is a way of providing nutrition for patients who are unable to consume an adequate oral intake but have at least a partially functional gastrointestinal (GI) tract that is accessible and safe to use. EN may augment an oral diet or may be the sole source of nutrition. Patients who have problems chewing and swallowing; have a prolonged lack of appetite; have an obstruction, fistula, or altered motility in the upper GI tract; are in a coma; or have very high nutrient requirements are candidates for tube feeding. EN is contraindicated when the GI tract is nonfunctional as in diffuse peritonitis, gastric or intestinal obstruction, paralytic ileus, intractable vomiting, severe diarrhea, and GI ischemia.

According to the American Dietetic Association Evidence Library (2006), patients who receive enteral nutrition experience less septic morbidity and fewer infections complications than patients who receive parenteral nutrition. Enteral nutrition is also significantly less costly than parenteral nutrition. Administering nutrients enterally appears to help maintain the structure and function of the intestinal mucosa (ASPEN, 2002).

The benefit of EN over no treatment (e.g., a control group who did not receive EN) is less clear. Despite widespread belief, EN has not been proven to reduce length of hospital stay and improve mortality (ADA Evidence Library, 2006). A recent review of randomized controlled trials concluded that no high-quality data are available to prove enteral nutrition is of benefit (Koretz, 2007b). Opponents to this conclusion argue that not providing adequate nutrition contributes to poor patient outcomes and raises ethical concerns (Hopkins & Jonnalagadda, 2008). More high-quality trials are needed to determine if enteral and parenteral nutrition ultimately reduce morbidity and mortality or simply improve body weight.

Factors that influence how and what is used to feed patients enterally include the patient's calorie and protein requirements (Box 15.2), ability to digest nutrients, feeding route, characteristics of the formula, equipment available, and method of delivery.

**Transnasal Tubes:** feeding tubes that extend from the nose to either the stomach or the small intestine.

**Ostomy:** a surgically created opening (stoma) made to deliver feedings directly into the stomach or intestines.

**Percutaneous Endoscopic Gastrostomy (PEG) Tubes:** a feeding tube placed through an opening in the stomach made surgically or under local anesthesia with the aid of an endoscope.

### Feeding Route

The feeding route, or placement of the feeding tube, depends on the patient's medical status and the anticipated length of time tube feeding will be used. **Transnasal tubes**, of which the nasogastric (NG) tube is the most common, are generally used for tube feedings of relatively short duration (i.e., <3 to 4 weeks). **Ostomy** feedings are preferred for permanent or long-term feedings because they can be hidden under clothing and eliminate irritation to the mucous membranes. **Percutaneous endoscopic gastrostomy (PEG) tubes** are placed with the aid of an endoscope. The correct placement of any feeding tube should be determined by radiographs of the chest taken before the first feeding is initiated. Table 15.4 summarizes the advantages and disadvantages of various feeding routes.

BOX 15.2 **CALCULATING CALORIES**

To calculate calories needed to maintain body weight, a range of 25 to 30 cal/kg actual weight is used. Normal protein RDA is 0.8 g/kg; patients who have increased needs for healing need more, based on the extent of injury or surgery.

Example: Calculate the calorie and protein needs of a patient who weighs his or her healthy body weight of 165 pounds and has normal protein requirements.

1. 165 pounds ÷ 2.2 pounds/kg = 75 kg

2. 75 kg × 25 cal/kg = 1875 calories
   75 × 30 cal/kg = 2250 calories

Estimated calorie needs: 1875 − 2250

3. 75 kg × 0.8 g/kg = 60 g protein

If the patient's ability to digest and absorb nutrients is not impaired, a reasonable choice for an enteral formula (for short-term use) would be Isocal. It would supply adequate calories, protein, and vitamins and minerals when infused over 22 hours/day. Instead of 24 hours/day, 22 hours/day is used to allow "off" time to administer medications. Isocal is low in fiber so if the patient is to receive enteral nutrition for a prolonged period, a fiber-enriched formula may be more suitable.

A goal rate of 90 mL/hour × 22 hours = 1980 mL/day

1980 mL × 10.6 cal/mL = 2099 cal/day

1.980 L × 34 g protein/L = 67 g protein/day

Because the volume of Isocal needed to meet RDI for vitamins and minerals is 1890 mL, the patient's estimated nutritional needs would be met with this regimen.

## Formula Characteristics

Most institutions have a formulary of various enteral products available within major categories (Table 15.5). Formulas come in cans or sealed containers to which the tubing is attached for administration. Formulas are designed to provide complete nutrition with nutrient amounts similar to what a normal mixed diet supplies.

### Protein

**Standard Formulas:** tube-feeding formulas that contain whole molecules of protein; also known as intact or polymeric formulas.

**Protein Isolates:** semipurified, high-biologic-value proteins that have been extracted from milk, soybean, or eggs.

**Hydrolyzed:** broken down.

Enteral formulas are classified by the type of protein they contain. **Standard formulas**, also known as polymeric or intact formulas, are made from whole proteins found in foods. (e.g., milk, meat, eggs) or **protein isolates** (Table 15.5). Because they contain complex molecules of protein, carbohydrate, and fat, standard formulas are intended for patients who have normal digestive and absorptive capacity. Routine standard formulas provide 34 to 43 g protein per liter.

Variations of standard formulas include formulas that are high in protein, high in calories, and fiber-enriched, as well as disease-specific formulas designed for patients with diabetes, immune system dysfunction, renal failure, or respiratory insufficiency (Table 15.5). The other category of formulas is **hydrolyzed** protein formulas (Table 15.6). Completely hydrolyzed formulas contain only free amino acids as their source of protein; partially hydrolyzed formulas contain proteins that are broken down into small peptides and

| TABLE 15.4 | **Advantages and Disadvantages of Various Feeding Routes** | | |
|---|---|---|---|
| **Route** | **Indications** | **Advantages** | **Disadvantages** |
| Nasogastric (NG) | Inability to safely and adequately consume oral intake | Easy to place and remove tube. Uses stomach as reservoir | Contraindicated for clients at high risk for aspiration. Potentially irritating to the nose and esophagus |
| | Short-term feeding (<6 wk) with functional gastrointestinal tract | Can use intermittent feedings. Dumping syndrome less likely than with NI feedings | May be removed by uncooperative or confused patients. Not appropriate for long-term use. Unaesthetic for patient |
| Nasointestinal (NI) | Short-term feeding for patients at high risk of aspiration, delayed gastric emptying, or gastroesophageal reflux disease (GERD) | Less risk of aspiration, especially important for patients who have impaired gag or cough reflex, decreased consciousness, ventilator dependence, or a history of aspiration pneumonia | Increased risk of dumping syndrome. Not appropriate for intermittent or bolus feedings. Not appropriate for long-term use. Unaesthetic for patient |
| Gastrostomy | For long-term use in patients with a functional gastrointestinal tract. Frequently used for patients with impaired ability to swallow | Same advantages as NG, but more comfortable and aesthetic for patient. Confirmation of tube placement easier. Cannot be misplaced into the trachea | PEG insertion contraindicated for clients who cannot have an endoscopy. Risk of aspiration pneumonia in clients with GERD. Stoma care required. Danger of peritonitis. Potential for tube dislodgment |
| Jejunostomy | For long-term use in patients at high risk for aspiration pneumonia and in clients with altered gastrointestinal integrity above the jejunum | Low risk of aspiration. No risk of misplacing tube into the trachea. More comfortable and aesthetic for clients than transnasal tubes | Small-diameter tubes easily become clogged. Peritonitis can occur from tube dislodgment. Cannot be used for intermittent or bolus feedings |
| | For short-term use after gastrointestinal surgery | Because motility resumes more quickly in the intestines than in the stomach after gastrointestinal surgery, feedings can begin sooner than other feedings | Stoma care required |

free amino acids. Other nutrients in hydrolyzed formulas are also in simple forms that require little or no digestion, such as fat in the form of medium-chain triglycerides (MCT). Hydrolyzed formulas are intended for patients with impaired digestion or absorption, such as people with inflammatory bowel disease, short-gut syndrome, cystic fibrosis, and pancreatic disorders. Disease-specific formulas are available for liver failure, HIV/AIDS, and impaired immune system function. Hydrolyzed formulas are more expensive than intact formulas.

## Calorie and Nutrient Density

The calorie density of a product determines the volume of formula needed to meet the patient's estimated needs. Routine formulas provide 1.0 to 1.2 cal/mL, whereas high-calorie formulas provide 1.5 to 2.0 cal/mL. A patient who needs 2000 calories can meet her or his

| TABLE 15.5 | Selected Enteral Products | | | | |

| Product | cal/mL | Protein (g/L) | CHO (g/L) | Fat (g/L) | Volume Needed to Meet 100% RDI* (mL) |
|---|---|---|---|---|---|
| **Standard, Intact Formulas (lactose-free)** | | | | | |
| Isocal | 1.06 | 34 | 135 | 44 | 1890 |
| Isosource | 1.2 | 43 | 170 | 39 | 1165 |
| Osmolite | 1.06 | 37 | 151 | 35 | 2000 |
| **High Protein, Intact Formulas** | | | | | |
| Isocal HN | 1.06 | 44 | 124 | 45 | 1180 |
| Promote | 1.0 | 63 | 130 | 26 | 1000 |
| Ultracal HN Plus | 1.2 | 54 | 156 | 40 | 1000 |
| **High Calorie, Intact Formulas** | | | | | |
| Comply | 1.5 | 60 | 180 | 61 | 830 |
| Deliver 2.0 | 2.0 | 75 | 200 | 101 | 1000 |
| Nutren 1.5 | 1.5 | 60 | 169 | 68 | 1000 |
| **Fiber Enriched Intact Formulas** (each of the formulas below provide 14 g fiber per L) | | | | | |
| Jevity | 1.06 | 44 | 155 | 35 | 1321 |
| Nutren Fiber | 1.0 | 40 | 127 | 38 | 1500 |
| Promote with Fiber | 1.0 | 63 | 138 | 28 | 1000 |
| **Specialty Intact Formulas** | | | | | |
| For diabetes: Glucerna | 1.0 | 42 | 96 | 54 | 1420 |
| For immune system support: Impact | 1.0 | 56 | 130 | 28 | 1500 |
| For renal failure (after dialysis has been instituted): Magnacal Renal | 2.0 | 75 | 200 | 101 | 1000 |
| For respiratory insufficiency: Pulmocare | 1.5 | 63 | 106 | 93 | 1420 |

*RDI, Reference Daily Intakes, the labeling standard for vitamins, minerals, and protein.

| TABLE 15.6 | Selected Hydrolyzed Formulas | | | | |

| Product | cal/mL | Pro (g/L) | CHO (g/L) | Fat (g/L) | Volume Needed to Meet 100% RDI* (mL) |
|---|---|---|---|---|---|
| **Hydrolyzed Formulas for Malabsorption** | | | | | |
| Criticare HN | 1.06 | 38 | 220 | 5 | 1890 |
| Optimental | 1.0 | 51 | 139 | 28 | 1422 |
| Vivonex T.E.N. | 1.0 | 38 | 210 | 3 | 2000 |
| **Specialty Hydrolyzed Formulas** | | | | | |
| Liver Failure: Nutrihep | 1.5 | 40 | 290 | 21 | 1000 |
| HIV/AIDS: Advera | 1.28 | 60 | 216 | 23 | 1184 |
| Impaired immune function: Crucial | 1.5 | 94 | 135 | 68 | 1000 |

*RDI, Reference Daily Intakes, the labeling standard for vitamins, minerals, and protein.

calorie needs with 2000 mL of a 1.0 cal/mL formula. If that patient is volume- or fluid-restricted, a better option is 1000 mL of a 2.0 cal/mL formula.

Nutrient density, as indicated by the amount of formula needed to meet 100% of Reference Daily Intakes (RDIs) for vitamins and minerals, varies among formulas. Generally, the amount of formula needed to meet nutrient RDIs ranges from 1000 to 2000 mL/day.

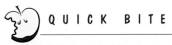 QUICK BITE

Periodic flushing of the tube with water helps meet water requirements and ensures patency (openness). The often-cited standard for maintaining patency is to flush with:

- 15 to 30 mL of water before and after medications
- 20 to 60 mL of water every 4 hours during continuous feedings
- 20 to 60 mL of water after each intermittent feeding
- 20 to 60 mL of water any time the feeding is interrupted

If the tube becomes clogged, a 60 mL syringe containing 30 to 60 mL of warm water is recommended.

When a tube feeding is the patient's sole source of nutrition, it is important to ensure nutritional adequacy within the volume of formula the patient receives.

## Water Content

The water content of tube feedings varies with the caloric concentration. Generally, formulas that provide 1.0 cal/mL provide 850 mL of water per liter. The water content of high-calorie formulas is lower at 690 to 720 mL/L. Adults generally need 30 to 40 mL/kg/day, so most patients who received EN need additional free water to meet fluid requirements. Free water is administered when water is used to flush the tube and as a bolus administration specifically for the purpose of meeting fluid requirement.

## Other Nutrients

Although the concentrations of fat and carbohydrate also vary among formulas, they are usually not a primary concern unless they are important because of disease. For instance, high-fat formulas are available for patients with respiratory disease, and modified-fat formulas are designed for patients with malabsorption. A number of diabetic formulas are available, as are electrolyte-modified formulas for renal disease.

## Fiber and Residue Content

**Fiber:** the group name for carbohydrates that are not digested in the human GI tract.

**Residue:** what remains in the GI tract after digestion, namely fiber, undigested food, intestinal secretions, bacterial cell bodies, and cells shed from the intestinal lining.

**Blenderized Formula:** a type of standard formula made from blenderized whole foods.

Although they are not synonymous, the terms **fiber** and **residue** are frequently used interchangeably. Fiber stimulates peristalsis, increases stool bulk, and is degraded by gastrointestinal bacteria to short-chain fatty acids that promote repair and maintenance of the intestinal lining. Fiber combines with undigested food, intestinal secretions, and other cells to make residue. Fiber is one component of residue, but residue encompasses other substances as well.

The residue content of enteral formulas varies greatly. Hydrolyzed formulas are essentially residue-free because they are completely absorbed. Most standard formulas are low in residue because low-residue formulas are not likely to cause gas or abdominal distention and are most suited as an initial feeding in patients who have been on bowel rest, in patients with certain GI disorders, or in patients who have had GI surgery.

Some standard formulas contain fiber. **Blenderized formulas** are a natural source of fiber because they are made whole foods. They generally provide approximately 4 g of fiber per liter. The fiber content of fiber-enriched formulas is generally 10 to 14 g/L. Fiber-enriched formulas may help to normalize bowel function in people with constipation or diarrhea but may cause gas and bloating. Because fiber helps to maintain GI integrity, formulas with added fiber should be considered when EN is to be used for a long period. Recommendations regarding the optimal amount of fiber for patients receiving EN have not been issued (ASPEN, 2002).

# Osmolality

**Osmolality:** the measure of the number of particles in solution; expressed as milliosmoles per kilogram (mOsm/kg).

In enteral formulas, **osmolality** is determined by the concentration of sugars, amino acids, and electrolytes. **Isotonic** formulas have approximately the same osmolality as blood and are well tolerated. Generally, the more digested the protein, the greater the osmolality; thus, hydrolyzed formulas are higher in osmolality than standard formulas.

For most people, osmolality does not impact tolerance. However, some patients develop diarrhea when a **hypertonic** formula is infused into the small intestine. Initiating the formula at a slow rate and advancing the rate gradually and slowly improves tolerance.

**Isotonic:** a formula that has approximately the same osmolality as blood, about 300 mOsm/kg.

**Hypertonic:** a formula with an osmolality greater than that of blood (>300 mOsm/kg).

# Equipment

Tubing size and pump availability impact formula selection. Generally, high-fiber formulas have a high viscosity and require a large bore tube (8 French or greater) to prevent clogging. Adding a modular product to a formula to increase the nutrient or calorie density may also necessitate the use of a larger tube. Hydrolyzed formulas have very low viscosity but should be delivered by pump to ensure controlled administration.

# Delivery Methods

Formulas may be given intermittently or continuously over a period of 8 to 24 hours. The rates may be regulated either by a pump or by gravity drip. The type of delivery method to be used depends on the type and location of the feeding tube, the type of formula being administered, and the patient's tolerance.

## Intermittent Tube Feedings

**Intermittent Feedings:** tube feedings administered in equal portions at selected intervals.

**Intermittent feedings** are administered throughout the day in equal portions of 250 to 300 mL of formula over 30 to 60 minutes every 4 to 6 hours, usually by gravity flow or an electronic pump. The number of feedings given per day depends on the total volume of feeding needed. Feedings may be spaced throughout an entire 24-hour period or may be scheduled only during waking hours to give patients time for uninterrupted sleep. Intermittent feedings are generally used for noncritical patients, home tube feedings, and patients in rehabilitation. They offer the advantage of resembling a more normal pattern of intake, and they allow the client more freedom of movement between feedings. Tolerance of intermittent feedings is optimized by infusing the formula at room temperature. To decrease the risk of aspiration, **gastric residuals** are checked before each feeding until tolerance is clearly established. Although there is no consensus on how much residual is too much, residual volumes of 200 mL or more on two successive assessments suggest poor tolerance (Palmer & Metheny, 2008).

**Gastric Residuals:** the volume of feeding that remains in the stomach from a previous feeding.

## Bolus Feedings

**Bolus Feedings:** rapid administration of a large volume of formula.

**Bolus feedings** are a variation of intermittent feedings. The formula is poured into the barrel of a large syringe attached to the feeding tube. A large volume of formula (500 mL maximum; usual volume is 250 to 400 mL) is delivered relatively quickly, usually in 15 to 30 minutes. These rapid feedings are given four to six times per day. They are used only for feedings into the stomach. Bolus feedings may be poorly tolerated and often cause *dumping syndrome:* nausea, diarrhea, glycosuria, distention, cramps, and vomiting. The risk of aspiration is increased.

## Continuous Drip Method

Continuous drip feedings are given at a constant rate over a 16- to 24-hour period to maximize tolerance and nutrient absorption. Infusion pumps are used to ensure consistent flow rates. This method is recommended for feeding of critically ill clients because it is associated with smaller residual volumes, lower risk for aspiration, and a decrease in the severity of diarrhea when compared to other delivery methods. Continuous feeding is also preferred for feedings delivered into the jejunum; it is frequently used to begin a feeding into the stomach (i.e., NG, gastrostomy, or PEG).

Continuous feedings should be interrupted every 4 hours so that water can be infused into the line to clear the tubing and hydrate the client. Gastric residuals are measured every 4 to 6 hours. If the volume of gastric residual exceeds the volume of formula given over the previous 2 hours, it may be necessary to reduce the rate of feeding.

## Cyclic Feedings

A variation of continuous drip feedings, cyclic feedings deliver a constant rate of formula over 8 to 12 hours, often during sleeping hours. Extra care must be taken to keep the head of the bed continuously elevated more than 30 degrees to avoid aspiration. Because there is "time off," the rate of infusion tends to be higher than for continuous feedings. Cyclic feedings are usually well tolerated and are often used to maintain a reliable source of nutrition while transitioning from total EN to an oral intake or in noncritical, undernourished patients unable to meet their nutritional needs orally.

## Initiating and Advancing the Feeding

Before initiating a feeding, tube placement is verified, ideally by radiography, and bowel sounds are confirmed to be present. Other common verification methods, such as aspirating gastric contents and pH testing, are less reliable and not recommended. Elevate the patient's upper body to at least a 30-degree angle during the feeding and for at least 30 minutes afterward to reduce the risk of aspiration.

Regardless of the access route, tube-feeding formulas are initiated at full strength. The previous practice of diluting hypertonic feedings has not been shown to improve tolerance, prolongs the period of inadequate nutrition support, and may increase the risk of bacterial contamination. Initiating feedings at full strength has not been found to cause tube feeding intolerance or diarrhea.

Although facility policies vary, initial feedings may begin at 25 to 50 mL/hour and advance by 10 to 25 mL/hour every 8 to 12 hours as tolerated until the desired rate is achieved. The commonly recommended maximum flow rate for gastric feedings is 125 mL/hour; higher volumes may increase the risk of aspiration. The maximum flow rate for small bowel feedings is determined by individual tolerance. Usually, rates of 140 to 160 mL/hour are well tolerated. Using a standard feeding progression schedule helps to ensure timely progression of feedings to the goal rate: the sooner the goal rate is achieved, the sooner the patient's nutritional needs are met.

Tolerance may be a problem for patients who are malnourished, who are under severe stress, or who have not eaten in a long time. Starting the feeding at the lower end of the recommended range and progressing slowly generally improves tolerance.

| BOX 15.3 | CRITERIA TO MONITOR IN HOSPITALIZED PATIENTS RECEIVING ENTERAL NUTRITION |
|---|---|

- Daily weight to detect fluid shifts.
- Daily intake and output.
- Gastric residuals every 4 to 6 hours in critically ill patients. Return all aspiration secretions to the stomach because they contain nutrients, electrolytes, and digestive enzymes.
- Character and frequency of bowel movements.
- Signs and symptoms of intolerance: vomiting, nausea, distention, constipation.
- Daily electrolyte levels, blood urea nitrogen (BUN), and creatinine until goal rate is achieved; thereafter two to three times per week. Minerals and a weekly blood count may be ordered.
- External length of the tube, to check for displacement
- Tube site for infection.

## Tube Feeding Complications

Enteral nutrition is generally considered safe, but GI, metabolic, and respiratory complications are possible (ASPEN, 2002). Monitoring ensures that the patient is tolerating the EN regimen and that it is adequately meeting the patient's needs (Box 15.3).

Aspiration is the most serious potential complication with enteral nutrition (Metheny, 2006). Patients with inhibited cough reflex related to debilitation, unconsciousness, or pulmonary complications are at high risk for aspiration as are those with delayed gastric emptying or gastroesophageal reflux. More common than large-volume aspirations is a series of clinically silent small aspirations. Aspiration increases the risk of aspiration-related pneumonia. Table 15.7 summarizes potential nutrition-related problems in tube-fed patients.

## Giving Medications by Tube

Although many medications are frequently given through feeding tubes to patients who are unable to swallow, they should never be given while a feeding is being infused. Some drugs become ineffective if added directly to the enteral formula; also, adding drugs to the formula may result in a clogged tube. It is important to stop the feeding before administering drugs and to make sure the tube is flushed with 15 to 30 mL of water before and after the drug is given. If more than one drug is given, flush the tube between doses with 5 mL of water. See Box 15.4 for other drug considerations.

## Transition to an Oral Diet

The goal of diet intervention during the transition period between EN and an oral diet is to ensure an adequate nutritional intake while promoting an oral diet. To begin the transition process, the tube feeding should be stopped for 1 hour before each meal. Gradually increase meal frequency until six small oral feedings are accepted. Actual intake should be recorded and evaluated daily. When oral calorie intake consistently reaches 500 to 750 cal/day, tube feedings may be given only during the night. When the patient consistently consumes two-thirds of protein and calorie needs orally for 3 to 5 days, the tube feeding may be totally discontinued.

| TABLE 15.7 | **Trouble-Shooting Nutrition-Related Problems in Tube-Fed Patients** | |
|---|---|---|
| **Potential Problem** | **Rationale** | **Nursing Interventions and Considerations** |
| Aspiration | Feeding infused into the lung | Confirm proper placement of the feeding tube by radiograph prior to initiating a feeding. |
| | Gastroesophageal reflux | Elevate the bed's headboard 30–45 degrees during feeding and for approximately 1 hour afterward |
| | Impaired cough reflex | Consider a nasointestinal or jejunostomy feeding |
| | Delayed gastric emptying | Monitor gastric residuals |
| | | Switch to a continuous drip delivery method |
| Diarrhea | Infusion of a formula that is too cold | Give canned formulas at room temperature |
| | | Warm refrigerated formulas to room temperature in a basin of warm water |
| | Bacterially contaminated formula | Follow handwashing and sanitation protocol |
| | | Refrigerate unused formula promptly |
| | | Discard opened cans within 24 hours |
| | | Flush the tubing as per protocol |
| | | Hang formulas less than 6 hours |
| | | Change extension tubing every 24 hours |
| | | Initiate and advance feedings as per protocol |
| | Feeding rate too rapid | For existing feedings, decrease the rate to the level tolerated then advance at half the original increment (e.g., 12 mL/hour instead of 25 mL/hour) |
| | | Feed smaller volumes more frequently or switch to continuous drip method |
| | Volume of formula too great | Consider a high-calorie formula if problem persists |
| | Side effect of antibiotics or other medications | Investigate drugs used for possible causes/possible alternatives |
| | | Administer antidiarrheals as ordered |
| | Malplacement of feeding tube | Check the position of the tube |
| | Feeding rate too rapid | Slow the rate of feeding; switch to a continuous drip method of delivery |
| Nausea (Discontinue the feeding. Administer antiemetics if ordered by the physician.) | Volume of formula too great → delayed gastric emptying | Check gastric residual and notify the physician if >100 mL |
| | | Reduce the volume, then increase gradually |
| | | If distention is contributing to nausea, encourage ambulation |
| | Feeding too soon after intubation | Explain the procedures to the client and encourage questions |
| | Anxiety | Allow approximately 1 hour between intubation and the first feeding |
| | | Allow client to verbalize his/her feelings; provide emotional support |
| | Intolerance to a specific formula, especially high-fat formulas | Switch to a different formula |

(table continues on page 372)

| TABLE 15.7 | Trouble-Shooting Nutrition-Related Problems in Tube-Fed Patients (continued) | |
|---|---|---|
| **Potential Problem** | **Rationale** | **Nursing Interventions and Considerations** |
| Distention and bloating | High fat content of formula | Switch to lower-fat formula |
| | Decrease in gastrointestinal function, especially among critically ill clients | Check for active bowel sounds; switch to a hydrolyzed formula if bowel sounds are hypoactive |
| Dehydration | Excessive protein intake → compensatory increase in urine output to excrete nitrogenous wastes | Switch to a formula with less protein. Increase water intake, if possible |
| | Inadequate fluid intake | Provide additional water |
| | Glycosuria (glucose in urine) | Test for glucose in the urine; notify physician of glycosuria of 3+ or 4+ |
| | | Administer insulin if ordered by physician |
| | | Switch to a continuous drip method to avoid giving a high-carbohydrate load with each feeding |
| Fluid overload | Excessive use of water to flush tube | Use only 30–50 mL of water to rinse tubing after each feeding |
| | Formula too dilute | Check formula preparation for proper dilution |
| Constipation | Low residue content of formula | Increase residue content if appropriate (i.e., change to a formula with added fiber or increase fruits and vegetables in a blenderized diet) |
| | Inactivity | Encourage ambulation as much as possible |
| | Dehydration | Monitor intake and output; add free water if intake is not greater than output by 500 to 1000 mL. |
| | Obstruction | Stop feeding and notify physician |
| Gastric rupture | Dangerous retention of feeding in the stomach related to gastric atony or obstruction | Check for residual before beginning each feeding; observe for signs of impending gastric rupture: distention, epigastric and upper quadrant pain, nausea, a large residual; if observed, discontinue feeding immediately and notify the physician |
| Clogged tube | Feeding heated formulas | Do not heat formula |
| | Improper cleaning of tube | Replace the feeding tube and bag every 12–24 hours |
| | | Flush the tube before and after each infusion (regardless of method) with 30–50 mL of water; if flushing fails to remove clog, the tube must be removed and replaced |
| | | High-viscosity formulas (i.e., blenderized tube feedings or commercial formulas that provide 1.5–2 cal/mL) should be infused by pump and possibly through a large-bore feeding tube to prevent clogging |
| | | If possible, consider switching to a less calorically dense formula |
| | | Because it is desirable to use the smallest size tube, viscous formulas may be delivered by a pump to help prevent clogging |

*(table continues on page 373)*

| TABLE 15.7 | **Trouble-Shooting Nutrition-Related Problems in Tube-Fed Patients** (continued) | |
|---|---|---|
| **Potential Problem** | **Rationale** | **Nursing Interventions and Considerations** |
| Anxiety | Deprivation of food → lack of sensory, social, and cultural satisfaction from eating | Allow oral intake of food that the client requests, if possible; if oral intake is contraindicated, allow the client to chew his/her favorite food without swallowing |
| | | If possible, liquefy and add the client's favorite food to the tube feeding |
| | | Encourage the client to leave the room when others are eating and find other enjoyable activities |
| | | Encourage client and family to view tube feeding as another way of eating, rather than a form of treatment |
| | Altered body image | Encourage client to verbalize his/her feelings |
| | | Stress positive aspects of tube feeding |
| | Loss of control; fear | Encourage client to become involved in preparation and administration of the formula, if possible |
| | | Inform client of problems that may occur and how to prevent or cope with them |
| | | Encourage socialization with other well-adapted tube-fed clients |
| | Limited mobility | Encourage normal activity |
| | Discomfort related to tube or formula intolerance | Control gastrointestinal symptoms, such as diarrhea, nausea, vomiting, and constipation, that interfere with normal activity |
| | | Observe for intolerances; alleviate with appropriate interventions |
| | | Be sure to inspect and properly care for the tube exit site to avoid potential complications |
| Dry mouth | Irritation of the mucous membranes related to lack of oral intake | Encourage good oral hygiene to alleviate soreness and dryness: mouthwash, warm water rinses, regular brushing |
| | | Apply petroleum jelly to the lips to prevent cracking |
| | | Allow ice chips, sugarless gum, and hard candies, if possible, to stimulate salivation |
| | Breathing through the mouth | Encourage client to breathe through the nose as much as possible |

| BOX 15.4 | **CONSIDERATIONS FOR GIVING MEDICATIONS THROUGH A FEEDING TUBE** |
|---|---|

- Drugs absorbed from the stomach should never be given through a nasointestinal tube.
- The liquid form of a medication diluted with 30 mL of water should be used for feeding tube administration. If there is no alternative, a drug can be crushed to a fine powder and mixed with water before it is administered. Slow-release drugs should never be crushed.
- Dilute highly viscous and hyperosmolar liquid medications with 10 to 30 mL of water before administering.
- Drugs should be given orally whenever possible.
- Tube feeding may need to be temporarily stopped to permit drug administration on an empty stomach or to avoid drug–nutrient interaction. Some experts recommend stopping a continuous feeding for 15 minutes before and after the delivery of the medication.

## NURSING PROCESS: Enteral Nutrition Support

Vince is 48 years old, 6 ft. tall, and has weighed 170 to 175 pounds throughout his adult life. Two weeks ago he was admitted to the ICU after an industrial accident caused first and second degree burns over 20% of his body. He was initially fed via a nasogastric tube and then started on an oral diet. Vince was only able to achieve 40% of the calorie goal set by the dietitian, so he has reluctantly agreed to be fed by tube for 8 hours during the night to supplement his daytime oral intake.

| **Assessment** | |
|---|---|
| Medical-Psychosocial History | • Medical history, such as diabetes or GI disorder |
| | • Medications that may affect nutrition |
| | • Current treatment plan |
| | • Level of tube feeding acceptance, including fears or apprehension about being tube-fed during the night |
| | • If Vince may need a tube feeding after discharge, assess living situation, such as availability of running water, electricity, refrigeration, cooking and storage facilities, employment, social support system, and financial status |
| Anthropometric Assessment | Height, current weight, BMI |
| | Percentage of usual body weight |
| Biochemical and Physical Assessment | • Check laboratory values—prealbumin (if available), hemoglobin, hematocrit, glucose, electrolytes; other abnormal values for their nutritional significance |
| | • Check tube for proper positioning; check external length of tube every 4 hours to ensure tube remains in proper position |
| | • Observe for signs of fluid overload |
| | • Ask if the client has any physical complaints associated with oral food intake or tube feeding, such as nausea or bloating |
| | • Observe abdomen for distention |
| | • Measure residual volumes |
| Dietary Assessment | • How many calories and how much protein is being provided via the tube feeding? |
| | • Do the nocturnal tube feedings affect the amount of food consumed orally during the day? |
| | • Is protocol being followed for administering the tube feeding and documenting administration and tolerance? |
| | • Is Vince able and willing to learn how to use tube feeding at home if necessary? |

| **Diagnosis** | |
|---|---|
| Possible Nursing Diagnoses | Risk for imbalanced nutrition: less than body requirements r/t inadequate calorie replacement to meet metabolic needs |

*(nursing process continues on page 375)*

## NURSING PROCESS: *Enteral Nutrition Support* (continued)

### Planning

| | |
|---|---|
| Client Outcomes | The client will<br>• Meet calorie and protein goals via combination of oral and tube feeding<br>• Be free of any signs or symptoms of aspiration and other complications<br>• Discontinue tube feedings when oral intake is >75% of calorie and protein goal |

### Nursing Interventions

| | |
|---|---|
| Nutrition Therapy | • Administer tube feeding as ordered<br>• Encourage oral intake |
| Client Teaching | Instruct the client<br>• On the importance of tube feedings for supplemental nutrition until oral intake meets 75% of goal<br>• On the signs and symptoms of intolerance of tube feeding and to alert the nurse if any problems arise<br>• Not to adjust the flow rate unless otherwise instructed<br>• On formula preparation, administration, and monitoring as well as the rationales and interventions for tube-feeding complications, if home enteral nutrition is indicated |

### Evaluation

| | |
|---|---|
| Evaluate and Monitor | • Monitor weight<br>• Monitor flow rate and administration<br>• Monitor for signs and symptoms of intolerance: aspiration, complaints of nausea, bloating, high gastric residuals, and diarrhea |

## ▶ PARENTERAL NUTRITION

**Parenteral Nutrition (PN):** the delivery of nutrients by vein; parenteral literally means "outside the intestinal tract."

**Parenteral nutrition (PN)** was developed in the 1960s when researchers from the University of Pennsylvania discovered how to deliver nutrients into the bloodstream via central venous access, thereby bypassing the GI tract (Koretz, 2007a). Using a large diameter central vein allows for the infusion of a nutritionally complete, hypertonic formula because it is quickly diluted; smaller veins are not able to handle such concentrated solutions. PN is a life-saving therapy in patients who have a nonfunctional GI tract, such as in the case of obstruction, intractable vomiting or diarrhea, short bowel syndrome, or paralytic ileus. In practice, PN is used for other clinical conditions such as critical illness, acute pancreatitis, liver transplantation, and AIDS, and in cancer patients receiving bone marrow transplants.

| BOX 15.5 | POTENTIAL COMPLICATIONS OF TOTAL PARENTERAL NUTRITION |
|---|---|

**Infection and Sepsis Related to**
Catheter contamination during insertion
Long-term indwelling catheter
Catheter seeding from bloodborne or distant
  infection
Contaminated solution

**Metabolic Complications**
Dehydration; hypovolemia
Bone demineralization
Hyperglycemia
Rebound hypoglycemia
Hyperosmolar, hyperglycemic, nonketotic coma
Azotemia
Electrolyte disturbances
  Hypocalcemia
  Hypophosphatemia, hyperphosphatemia
  Hypokalemia
  Hypomagnesemia
High serum ammonia levels
Deficiencies of
  Essential fatty acids
  Trace elements
  Vitamins and minerals

Altered acid–base balance
Elevated liver enzymes
Fluid overload

**Mechanical Complications Related to Catheterization**
Catheter misplacement
Hemothorax (blood in the chest)
Pneumothorax (air or gas in the chest)
Hydrothorax (fluid in the chest)
Hemomediastinum (blood in the mediastinal
  spaces)
Subcutaneous emphysema
Hematoma
Arterial puncture
Myocardial perforation
Catheter embolism
Cardiac dysrhythmia
Air embolism
Endocarditis
Nerve damage at the insertion site
Laceration of lymphatic duct
Chylothorax
Lymphatic fistula
Thrombosis

When PN was first introduced it was widely and enthusiastically embraced as state-of-the-art therapy. The prevailing school of thought was that "if some is good, more is better" and overfeeding was common practice (Koretz, 2007a). At that time parenteral nutrition was called "hyperalimentation"—literally excessive nourishment. It is now recognized that overfeeding, particularly overfeeding carbohydrates, in nutritionally debilitated patients, can lead to a life-threatening complication known as the **refeeding syndrome** (see Chapter 16). The practice of overfeeding has been replaced with a more conservative, lower-in-calories approach.

**Refeeding Syndrome:** a potentially fatal complication that occurs from an abrupt change from a catabolic state to an anabolic state and an increase in insulin caused by a dramatic increase in calories.

Because PN is expensive, requires constant monitoring, and has potential infectious, metabolic, and mechanical complications (Box 15.5), it should be used only when an enteral intake is inadequate or contraindicated and when prolonged nutritional support is needed. Current guidelines from the American Society for Parenteral and Enteral Nutrition state that specialized nutrition support (enteral and parenteral nutrition) should be initiated when oral intake has been or is expected to be inadequate over a 7- to 14-day period, with a preference to EN (ASPEN, 2002). In randomized controlled trials reported to date, untreated control groups have done at least as well as, if not better than, the treatment groups receiving PN (Koretz, 2007a). PN is never an emergency procedure, and it should be discontinued as soon as possible.

## Catheter Placement

**Central PN:** the infusion of nutrients into the bloodstream by way of a central vein. Central PN solutions are nutritionally complete.

The patient's anticipated length of need influences placement of the catheter. For short-term **central PN** in the hospital, a temporary central venous catheter is placed percutaneously into the subclavian vein by a physician at bedside. If PN is expected to be more than a few weeks, an operative procedure is performed to place a subcutaneously tunneled catheter with the tip at the superior vena cava. A Hickman catheter and Port-a-Cath are more permanent devices. Specially trained nurses can place a peripherally inserted central catheter (PICC) at bedside. The line is usually inserted on the inside of the elbow and threaded so the tip of the catheter rests at the superior vena cava. Peripheral parenteral nutrition (PPN) is not widely used because solutions infused into peripheral veins must be isotonic (i.e., they must have low concentrations of dextrose and amino acids) to prevent phlebitis and increased risk of thrombus formation.

**Dextrose:** another name for glucose.

## Composition of PN

Parenteral nutrition solutions provide protein, carbohydrate, fat, electrolytes, vitamins, and trace elements in sterile water. They are "compounded" or mixed in the hospital pharmacy, either manually by the pharmacist or through automated compounding equipment, which allows individualization of the solution based on the patient's fluid and nutrient requirements. Automated compounders can mix a 24-hour batch of PN solution into a single container that is either a two-in-one formula (dextrose and amino acids) or a three-in-one formula (dextrose, amino acids, and lipids). Most hospitals use a two-in-one system and deliver lipids separately.

### Protein

Protein is provided as a solution of crystalline essential and nonessential amino acids ranging in concentration from 3.5% to 20% of the solution, with the amounts of specific amino acids varying among manufacturers. Amino acid formulations are available with and without electrolytes. Although specially modified amino acid solutions are available for renal failure, liver failure, and high stress, they are not widely used because efficacy has not been proven (Miller, 2006).

Providing adequate protein is a primary concern when formulating PN. Typically, patients receiving PN are given 1 to 2 g protein/kg of body weight (Miller, 2006). Highly stressed patients may require more. In patients who weigh less than ideal body weight, actual weight is used to calculate protein and calorie requirements. For obese patients, adjusted weight is commonly used. A nitrogen balance study (see Chapter 3) can be used to determine adequacy of protein intake.

### Carbohydrate

The carbohydrate used in parenteral solutions in the United States is dextrose monohydrate, which provides 3.4 cal/g. It is available in 5%, 10%, 50%, and 70% concentrations. The minimal amount of carbohydrate needed to spare protein, that is to prevent protein from being used for energy, is generally accepted as 1 mg/kg/min (Nelms, Sucher, & Long, 2007). Although carbohydrate is an important energy source, giving a patient too much can have negative consequences. Hyperglycemia is associated with immune function impairments and increased risk of infectious complications (ASPEN, 2002). A high carbohydrate load may also lead to excessive carbon dioxide production, which may complicate weaning from mechanical ventilation. The trend toward less aggressive feeding has decreased the incidence of this complication.

### Fat

Lipid emulsions, made from soybean oil or safflower plus soybean oil with egg phospholipid as an emulsifier, are isotonic. They are available in 10%, 20%, and 30% concentrations, supplying 1.1, 2.0, and 2.9 cal/mL, respectively. Lipids are a significant source of calories and so are useful when volume must be restricted or when dextrose must be lowered because of persistent hyperglycemia. Lipids are also necessary to correct or prevent fatty acid deficiency. Calories from fat should not exceed 2.5 g/kg/day (ASPEN, 2002). Common clinical practice is to limit fat to 1.0 to 1.2 g/kg due to concerns about the proinflammatory properties of omega-6 fatty acids (Nelms et al., 2007).

## Electrolytes, Vitamins, and Trace Elements

The quantity of electrolytes provided is based on the patient's blood chemistry values and physical assessment findings. Generally, the requirements for intracellular electrolytes (potassium, magnesium, and phosphorus) increases as carbohydrate content increases.

Parenteral multivitamin preparations usually contain 12 to 13 essential vitamins. Commercial preparations have recently been reformulated based on FDA guidelines, with the most notable change that most adult formulations now contain a small amount of vitamin K (Miller, 2006).

Trace element preparations contain four to seven trace elements. Trace element preparations may be left out of PN if trace element toxicities are suspected. Individual trace elements may be given to meet increased needs related to illness (e.g., additional zinc may be needed in patients with diarrhea) or because they are not routinely added to PN solutions (e.g., iodine).

## Medications

Medications are sometimes added to intravenous solutions by the pharmacist or infused into them through a separate port. Patients receiving PN may have insulin ordered if glucose levels are greater than 150 to 200 mg/dL (levels higher than normal are considered acceptable because there is no fasting state with continuous infusions). Heparin may be added to reduce fibrin buildup on the catheter tip. In general, medications should not be added to PN solutions because of the potential incompatibilities of the medication and nutrients in the solution.

## Administration

PN is administered according to facility protocol. Although there is no one universally accepted "best" practice, PN is generally initiated slowly (i.e., 1 L in the first 24 hours) to give the body time to adapt to the high concentration of glucose and the hyperosmolality of the solution. Continuous drip by pump infusion is needed to maintain a slow, constant flow rate. After the first 24 hours, the rate of delivery is gradually increased by 1 L/day until the optimal volume is achieved.

Because rapid changes in the infusion rate can cause severe hyperglycemia or hypoglycemia and the potential for coma, convulsions, or death, rate changes must be made incrementally. If the rate of delivery falls behind or speeds up, the drip rate is adjusted to the correct hourly rate only; no attempts are made to "catch up" to the ordered volume. Other nursing management considerations appear in Box 15.6.

After the patient is stable, PN may be infused cyclically instead of continuously. **Cyclic PN** allows serum glucose and insulin levels to drop during the periods when PN is not infused, thus promoting fat and glycogen mobilization and a more normal pattern of intake. When it is given during the night, cyclic PN frees the patient to participate in normal activities during the day.

During the switch from continuous to cyclic PN, the infusion time is gradually decreased by several hours each day, as ordered, and assessment is ongoing for signs of glucose intolerance. To give the pancreas time to adjust to the decreasing glucose load, the infusion rate

**Cyclic PN:** infusing PN at a constant rate for 8 to 12 hours/day.

| BOX 15.6 | **NURSING MANAGEMENT CONSIDERATIONS FOR PN** |
|---|---|

- Once parenteral nutrition solutions are prepared, they must be used immediately or refrigerated. It is recommended that solutions be removed from the refrigerator 1 hour before infusion because they must reach approximately room temperature before they are hung. Once hung, the solution is infused or discarded within 24 hours.
- Inspect the solution for "cracking," (appearance of a layer of fat on top or oily globules in the solution) which may occur in 3-in-1 mixtures if the calcium or phosphorus content is relatively high or if salt-poor albumin has been added. A "cracked" solution cannot be infused; notify the pharmacy and the physician, who may need to adjust the original PN order to eliminate or reduce the offending component.
- Monitor the flow rate to avoid complications and ensure adequate intake.
- Observe for side effects of parenteral nutrition: weight gain greater than 1 kg/day (indicative of fluid overload), elevated temperature or sepsis, high blood glucose levels, shortness of breath, tightness of chest, anemia, nausea and vomiting, jaundice, allergy to protein content of the solutions, pneumothorax, or cardiac arrhythmias.
- Monitor laboratory data and clinical signs to prevent the development of nutrient deficiencies or toxicities.
- Some patients may feel hungry while receiving PN and should be allowed to eat, if possible. If oral intake is contraindicated, give mouth care.
- Begin weaning the client from PN to EN or oral intake as soon as possible. Gradual weaning is necessary to prevent rebound hypoglycemia. PN can be discontinued when enteral intake (an oral diet, tube feeding, or combination of the two) provides at least 60% of estimated calorie requirements.
- Patients who have permanently nonfunctional gastrointestinal tracts require PN indefinitely. For home PN to be successful, clients and their families must be physically and emotionally prepared. Intensive counseling focuses on preparation and administration of the solution, catheter and equipment care, and assessment skills as well as the psychological impact of permanent PN.

is tapered near the end of each cycle. For instance, during the last hour of infusion the rate may be reduced by one-half to prevent rebound hypoglycemia.

When the patient is able to begin consuming food orally or by EN, the amount of PN is gradually reduced to prevent metabolic complications and nutritional inadequacies.

## ▶ HOW DO YOU RESPOND?

**Why does it seem that "house" diets are not consistent with the *Dietary Guidelines for Americans* for healthy eating (e.g., low in saturated fat, high in fiber)?** The purpose of the *Dietary Guidelines for Americans* is to prevent chronic diseases associated with nutritional excesses, such as obesity, heart disease, and high blood pressure. The goal of feeding hospitalized patients is to prevent or treat acute malnutrition associated with illness or hospitalization. Therefore the focus is not on avoiding excess but on "getting enough."

**Is it good practice to color tube feedings?** The ADA Evidence Library 2006 states that blue dye should not be added to tube feedings for the detection of aspiration. The potential risks of using blue dye, such as skin discoloration, contamination of dye, allergic reactions, and association with mortality (exact method unknown), far outweigh any perceived benefit. Furthermore, the presence of blue dye in tracheal secretions is not a sensitive indicator for aspiration.

**My patient claims he can taste his tube feeding. Can he?** Except for patients who experience gastric reflux, patients cannot truly taste a tube feeding. However, the appearance and aroma of the formula may influence the patient's acceptance and perception of palatability. If the formula's appearance is offensive, cover the feeding reservoir or remove it from the patient's field of vision, if possible.

## ▶ CASE STUDY

Eugene is a 73-year-old man who weighs 168 pounds and is 5 ft.10 in. tall. He has had progressive difficulty swallowing related to supranuclear palsy. He has no other medical history other than hypertension, which is controlled by medication. He denies that the disease interferes with his ability to eat, even though he coughs frequently while eating and has lost 20 pounds over the last 6 months. He is currently hospitalized with pneumonia and a swallowing evaluation concluded that he should have nothing by mouth (NPO). He has agreed to an NG tube because he believes the "problem" will be short term and he will be able to resume a normal oral diet after he is discharged from the hospital.

- How many calories and how much protein does Eugene need? Is his weight loss classified as "significant"?
- What type of formula would be most appropriate for him? How much formula would he need to meet his calorie requirements? How much formula would he need to meet his vitamin and mineral requirements?
- What type of delivery would you recommend? What would the goal rate be?
- If the doctor convinces him to agree to having a PEG tube placed, what formula and feeding schedule would you recommend for use at home? What does his family need to be taught about tube feedings?

## STUDY QUESTIONS

1. Which of the following strategies may help promote an adequate oral intake in hospitalized patients? Select all that apply.
   a. Tell the patient that you wouldn't want to eat the food either but that it is important for their recovery.
   b. Encourage the patient to select his or her own menu.
   c. Offer standby alternatives when the patient cannot find anything on the menu he or she wants to eat.
   d. Advance the diet as quickly as possible, as appropriate.

2. For which of the following situations is a blenderized diet most appropriate?
   a. As an initial oral diet after surgery, to establish tolerance
   b. As a transition between a full liquid diet and a regular diet
   c. For patients who need a low-fiber diet
   d. For patients who have had their jaw wired

3. Which type of enteral formula would be most appropriate for a patient experiencing malabsorption related to inflammatory bowel disease?
   a. A standard intact formula
   b. A fiber-enriched intact formula
   c. A hydrolyzed formula for malabsorption
   d. A patient with malabsorption cannot receive enteral nutrition

4. Which type of formula may be most appropriate for patients who will need enteral nutrition for a long period?
   a. A fiber-enriched formula
   b. A formula intended for immune system support

c. A hydrolyzed formula
d. A standard, intact formula

5. Which tube-feeding delivery method is most likely to cause dumping syndrome?
a. Intermittent feedings
b. Bolus feedings
c. Continuous drip feedings
d. Cyclical feedings

6. Nausea in a tube-fed patient may be caused by: (Select all that apply.)
a. Malplacement of the feeding tube
b. A feeding rate that is too rapid
c. Providing an excessive volume of formula
d. Feeding too soon after intubation
e. Anxiety
f. Using a formula that is low in residue

7. Which of the following are indications for using parenteral nutrition? (Select all that apply.)
a. Paralytic ileus
b. Intractable vomiting
c. Dysphagia
d. Coma

8. It is recommended that parenteral nutrition not be used when the patient is adequately nourished and expected to resume oral intake within:
a. 2 to 3 days
b. 5 to 7 days
c. 7 to 14 days
d. 14 to 21 days

## KEY CONCEPTS

- Hospital food is intended to prevent malnutrition and nutrient deficiencies, not to prevent chronic disease. Regular diets may not be consistent with *Dietary Guidelines for Americans,* which recommends limiting intakes of fat, saturated fat, cholesterol, and sodium.

- Oral diets are classified as "regular," consistency modified, and therapeutic. Combination diets (e.g., a low-sodium, soft diet) are often ordered.

- Patients with altered appetites or increased needs may benefit from supplements given with or between meals. A variety of supplements are available (clear liquid, milk-based, routine, modified routine, puddings, and bars); they vary in nutritional composition, cost, and taste.

- Enteral nutrition commonly means tube feedings. Tube feedings are preferred to parenteral nutrition whenever the gastrointestinal tract is at least partially functional, accessible, and safe to use. Tube feedings may be delivered through transnasal tubes or through ostomy sites into the gastrointestinal tract.

- The choice of tube-feeding method depends on the patient's digestive and absorptive capacities, where the feeding is to be infused, the size of the feeding tube, the patient's nutritional needs, present and past medical history, and tolerance.

- Standard tube-feeding formulas require normal digestion; they contain intact molecules of protein, carbohydrate, and fat. Intact formulas come in several varieties: high-protein, high-calorie, fiber-added, and disease-specific.

- Hydrolyzed formulas are made from partially or totally predigested nutrients; they are higher in cost and osmolality; and they are used when digestion is impaired. Specially defined formulas are available for specific metabolic disorders (e.g., renal failure, hepatic failure).

● Routine formulas provide 1.0 to 1.2 cal/mL; high calorie or "plus" formulas range from 1.5 to 2.0 cal/mL.

● The volume of formula needed to meet RDIs for vitamins and minerals is available from the manufacturer.

● Most patients receiving enteral nutrition need additional free water to meet their estimated requirements. Free water includes water used to flush the tube and bolus infusions of water.

● Most hydrolyzed formulas are low residue or residue-free. Intact formulas range from low residue to fiber-enriched. Fiber-enriched formulas may be better than low-residue formulas for long-term use because fiber helps regulate bowel patterns.

● Osmolality, the concentration of particles in solution, does usually not affect tolerance in most people.

● Policies for initiating and advancing tube feedings vary among facilities. Generally, enteral feedings are started full strength at a rate of 25 to 50 mL/hour and are increased by 10 to 25 mL/hour every 8 to 12 hours as tolerated. A suggested maximum flow rate for gastric feedings is 125 mL/hour; feedings at 140 to 160 mL/hour are usually well tolerated when infused into the intestines.

● Continuous drip infusion with a pump is the preferred method for delivering tube feedings to critically ill patients and should be used whenever feedings are infused into the jejunum. Intermittent feedings may be preferable for long-term tube feeding and home enteral nutrition because they more closely resemble a normal intake and allow the client freedom between feedings. Bolus feedings are not recommended.

● Enteral nutrition is safe but not without the risk of various GI, metabolic, and respiratory complications. Aspiration is one of the most serious complications of enteral feedings and may be related to inhibited cough reflex, delayed gastric emptying, or gastroesophageal reflux. Ensuring the tube is properly placed and that it remains in position, as well as elevating the head of the bed at least 30 degrees, helps reduce the risk of aspiration.

● Parenteral nutrition delivers nutrients directly into the bloodstream when the gastrointestinal tract is nonfunctional or when oral or enteral intake is inadequate to meet the patient's needs.

● PN is usually infused into a central, large diameter vein, which quickly dilutes the hypertonic solution. Less frequently used is peripheral PN; it must be near-isotonic to avoid collapsing small diameter veins, so the amount of calories it supplies is limited.

● Various concentrations of amino acids, dextrose, lipid emulsions, electrolytes, multivitamins, and trace elements may be given by vein. Compounding is the process of combining the formula ingredients; it may be done manually by a hospital pharmacist or by automated compounding equipment.

● Because parenteral nutrition has numerous potential metabolic, infectious, and mechanical complications, it should be used only when necessary and discontinued as soon as feasible. It is never an emergency procedure.

## ANSWER KEY

1. **TRUE** Hospitalized patients are at risk of malnutrition. Some patients are admitted with malnutrition related to acute or chronic illness; others develop malnutrition over the course of hospitalization because intake is poor. Factors leading to poor intake may include fear, pain, or anxiety; culturally or religiously unacceptable food choices; altered meal schedule; inappropriate food texture; failure to advance a diet as tolerated; or tasteless food.

2. **FALSE** There is little evidence to support a slow diet progression after surgery. Most patients can tolerate a regular diet by the second postoperative meal. Dietary restrictions are not necessarily helpful in relieving flatulence, nausea, or vomiting that occurs secondary to anesthesia and decreased bowel motility.

3. **TRUE** Modular products, either singly or in combination, can increase the calorie or protein density of food or enteral formulas.

4. **FALSE** For most people, osmolality does not affect tolerance.

5. **FALSE** Although the terms *fiber* and *residue* are often used interchangeably, they are not synonymous. Fiber refers to carbohydrates not digested in the gastrointestinal tract. Residue is composed of fiber along with undigested food, intestinal secretions, bacterial cell bodies, and cells from the intestinal lining.

6. **TRUE** The individual's capability to digest food is a primary consideration when choosing a tube-feeding method for a patient. Intact formulas are appropriate when digestion is normal; hydrolyzed formulas are necessary when digestion is altered.

7. **TRUE** Continuous drip feedings are recommended for critically ill patients because there is a lower risk for aspiration, a decreased risk of diarrhea, and a decrease in the hypermetabolic response to stress when compared to other delivery methods.

8. **TRUE** Parenteral nutrition may be infused into a peripheral or central vein, but because smaller diameter veins cannot handle hypertonic formulas they are limited in the amount of calories they can provide. Most parenteral nutrition is infused through a central vein.

9. **FALSE** While hyperglycemia commonly occurs in patients receiving PN, it may not be solely related to PN nor is it harmless. An underlying disease state, such as sepsis, diabetes, trauma, or other physiological stress, may contribute to hyperglycemia. Hyperglycemia is associated with immune function impairments and increased risk of infectious complications, and may complicate weaning from a ventilator.

10. **FALSE** Coloring tube formulas with food dye does not prevent aspiration and is associated with potential complications, such as contamination of the dye, allergy to the dye, and increased mortality from unknown cause.

## WEBSITES

*Enteral Product Information*

Ross Products Division of Abbott Laboratories at **www.ross.com**
Mead Johnson at **www.meadjohnson.com**
Nestlé Nutrition at **www.nestle-nutrition.com**
Novartis Nutrition at **www.novartis.com**

## REFERENCES

American Dietetic Association Evidence Library. (2006). *Critical illness evidence-based nutrition practice guidelines.* Available at www.adaevidencelibrary.com/topic.cfm?cat=2799. Accessed on 2/18/08.

American Society of Parenteral and Enteral Nutrition Board of Directors. (2002). Guidelines for the use of parenteral and enteral nutrition in adult and pediatric patients. *Journal of Parenteral and Enteral Nutrition, 26*(1 suppl.), 1SA–138SA.

Hopkins, B., & Jonnalagadda, S. (2008). To the editor. *Journal of the American Dietetic Association, 108,* 220–222.

Koretz, R. (2007a). Do data support nutrition support? Part I: Intravenous nutrition. *Journal of the American Dietetic Association, 107,* 988–996.

Koretz, R. (2007b). Do data support nutrition support? Part II. Enteral artificial nutrition. *Journal of the American Dietetic Association, 107,* 1374–1380.

Kruizenga, H. M., Van Tilde, M. W., Slidell, J. C., et al. (2005). Effectiveness and cost-effectiveness of early screening and treatment of malnourished patients. *The American Journal of Clinical Nutrition, 82,* 1082–1089.

Metheny, N. (2006). Preventing respiratory complications of tube feedings: Evidence-based practice. *American Journal of Critical Care, 15,* 360–369.

Miller, S. (2006). *Parenteral nutrition.* US Pharm, 7, HS10-HS20. Available at www.uspharmacist .com/index.asp?show=article&page=8_1804.htm. Accessed on 2/20/08.

Nelms, M., Sucher, K., & Long, S. (2007). *Nutrition therapy and pathophysiology.* Belmont, CA: Thomson Wadsworth.

Palmer, J., & Metheny, N. (2008). How to try this: Preventing aspiration in older adults with dysphagia. *American Journal of Nursing, 108,* 40–48.

# 16

# Nutrition for Patients with Metabolic or Respiratory Stress

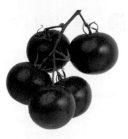

| TRUE | FALSE | |
|------|-------|---|
| ☐ | ☐ | **1** Aggressive nutrition therapy can reverse the metabolic derangements of severe stress. |
| ☐ | ☐ | **2** Stress hormones promote the breakdown of stored nutrients and lean body mass. |
| ☐ | ☐ | **3** The metabolic response to severe stress lasts 2 to 48 hours after injury. |
| ☐ | ☐ | **4** The acute-phase inflammatory response causes albumin levels to fall. |
| ☐ | ☐ | **5** After acute stress, the lower small intestine is less likely to have motility dysfunction than is the stomach. |
| ☐ | ☐ | **6** The Harris–Benedict equations accurately estimate energy requirements during critical illness. |
| ☐ | ☐ | **7** In patients with severe stress, overfeeding may be more detrimental than underfeeding. |
| ☐ | ☐ | **8** Stressed patients with low serum iron levels should be supplemented with iron to promote healing. |
| ☐ | ☐ | **9** Extensive burns are the greatest stress a person can experience. |
| ☐ | ☐ | **10** People with COPD generally need fewer calories than healthy people because they are less physically active. |

### UPON COMPLETION OF THIS CHAPTER, YOU WILL BE ABLE TO

- Explain how the hormonal response to severe acute stress impacts metabolism.
- Discuss why the Harris–Benedict equation to determine total energy expenditure is not accurate for patients with metabolic stress.
- Give examples of possible outcomes of an inadequate protein intake during metabolic stress.
- Teach a client how to increase protein and calorie intake.
- Devise a high-calorie, high-protein menu with small frequent meals.
- Counsel a patient with COPD on how to overcome symptoms that interfere with intake, such as anorexia, dyspnea, and early satiety.

Severe, acute stress—such as trauma (e.g., gunshot wounds, motor vehicle accidents, severe burns), certain diseases (e.g., pancreatitis, acute renal failure), extensive surgery, or infection (e.g., sepsis)—has a profound impact on metabolism and can eventually lead to organ failure and death. Nutrition support can improve some of the derangements of metabolic stress, but reversal occurs only when the underlying problem is resolved (Lowry & Perez, 2006).

This chapter discusses the stress response and nutrition therapy for metabolic stress. Nutrition therapy for burns and respiratory stress is presented.

# ▶ THE STRESS RESPONSE

**Stress Response:** a complex series of hormonal and metabolic changes that occur to enable the body to adapt to stressors.

**Metabolic Stress:** altered body chemistry related to the body's response to injury or disease.

**Shock:** a clinical syndrome characterized by varying degrees of decreased tissue oxygenation and impaired flow of blood to the heart.

**Counterregulatory Hormones:** hormones that have the opposite effect to that of insulin; they raise blood glucose levels.

**Hypercatabolism:** higher than normal breakdown of large molecules into smaller ones, such as muscle protein into amino acids.

**Hypermetabolism:** higher than normal metabolism.

The **stress response** is the body's attempt to promote healing and resolve inflammation when homeostasis is disrupted. The intensity of the stress response depends to some extent on the cause and/or severity of the initial injury (Lowry & Perez, 2006). Hormonal and inflammatory responses account for the changes in metabolic rate, heart rate, blood pressure, and nutrient metabolism that characterize **metabolic stress**.

## Hormonal Response to Stress

The immediate postinjury phase, known as the ebb phase, typically lasts 12 to 24 hours. It is characterized by **shock** with hypovolemia and diminished tissue oxygenation. Cardiac output, oxygen consumption, urinary output, and body temperature fall, and glucagon and catecholamine levels rise. Treatment goals are to restore blood flow to organs, maintain adequate oxygenation to all tissues, and stop bleeding. This initial phase ends when the patient is hemodynamically stable.

The flow phase follows, which is the metabolic response to stress. A spike in circulating levels of catecholamines, cortisol, and glucagon, known as **counterregulatory hormones**, promotes the breakdown of stored nutrients to make energy available to carry on essential bodily functions, such as preserving vital organs and repairing damaged tissue (Table 16.1). As body stores and tissues are catabolized, energy expenditure and metabolic rate increase, creating a state of **hypercatabolism** and **hypermetabolism**. Oxygen consumption, cardiac output, carbon dioxide ($CO_2$) production, and body temperature increase. The length of this phase depends on the severity of injury or infection and the development of complications (ADA, 2008).

Glycogen is depleted within the first 24 hours after the injury (Lowry & Perez, 2006). Thereafter, the body relies on lean body tissue, mostly muscle, to furnish amino acids that can be converted to glucose. Only certain amino acids can be converted to glucose, but whole proteins must be broken down to make them available. Stress hormones also stimulate

| TABLE 16.1 | Hormonal Effects of Metabolic Stress | |
|---|---|
| **Hormones** | **Impact on Metabolism** |
| Catecholamines (epinephrine, norepinephrine) | Breakdown of glycogen in the liver and muscles |
| | Synthesis of glucose from amino acids |
| | Release of fatty acids from adipose tissue |
| | Increase in metabolic rate |
| | Secretion of glucagon from the pancreas |
| Glucagon | Breakdown of liver glycogen |
| | Synthesis of glucose from amino acids |
| | Release of fatty acids from adipose tissue |
| Cortisol | Protein catabolism of skeletal muscle |
| | Impaired protein synthesis |
| | Synthesis of glucose from amino acids |
| | Release of fatty acids from adipose tissue |
| | Causes insulin resistance; contributes to hyperglycemia |
| Aldosterone | Sodium retention |
| Antidiuretic hormone | Water retention |

the breakdown of adipose tissue so that free fatty acids can be metabolized for energy. The overall effect is to break down body tissues to meet the metabolic demands of healing and recovery. An increase in the secretion of adolesterone and antidiuretic hormone helps maintain blood volume.

## Inflammatory Response

The **acute-phase response** is the body's attempt to destroy infectious agents and prevent further tissue damage. It is characterized by a change of at least 25% in the plasma concentration of certain proteins known as acute-phase proteins (Gabay & Kushner, 1999). Positive acute-phase proteins, such as **C-reactive protein**, increase in concentration. C-reactive protein is often used as a marker of metabolic stress. Negative acute-phase proteins decrease in response to inflammation; albumin is one example. **Cytokines** and other immune system molecules are responsible for regulating acute-phase proteins; they also produce changes in other cells that cause systemic symptoms of inflammation, such as anorexia, fever, lethargy, and weight loss (Charney, 2001).

Systemic inflammatory response syndrome (SIRS) is a life-threatening condition that may occur when severe inflammation lasts longer than a few days. Heart rate, respiratory rate, white blood cell count, and/or body temperature become critically elevated. When these symptoms are caused by infection, the result is **sepsis**. SIRS and sepsis cause excessive fluid accumulation, low blood pressure, and impaired blood flow. Inadequate oxygenation of tissues can lead to shock and **multiple organ failure**. The patient's prior nutritional status is an important predictor or morbidity and mortality (Biolo et al., 2003).

## Nutritional Needs

Nutritional needs are considered after the patient is hemodynamically stable, preferably within 24 hours after admission (Zaloga, 2008). The patient's age and prior nutritional status influence actual nutrient requirements. The overwhelming nutritional concern during metabolic stress is protein catabolism, as evidenced by a **negative nitrogen balance**. Protein catabolism can lead to impaired immune system functioning, increased risk of infection, impaired or delayed wound healing, and increased mortality. Therefore, the primary goal of nutrition therapy is to protect lean body mass and prevent or alleviate malnutrition, so immune system function is maintained and recovery can occur. Table 16.2 outlines the role of selected nutrients in wound healing and recovery, and possible outcomes of their deficiencies. The calorie and protein needs of people with critical illness are controversial and are still being studied.

## Calories

Indirect calorimetry is the most accurate method for measuring calorie expenditure (Compher et al., 2006). However, **indirect calorimetry** is not commonly done because the equipment is expensive, technical expertise is required to use the equipment and interpret the results, and it cannot be performed on all patients, such as on patients with a chest tube, those using supplemental oxygen, or patients who are uncooperative (Frankenfield et al., 2007).

---

**Acute-Phase Response:** trauma- or inflammation-induced release of inflammatory mediators that cause changes in the levels of plasma proteins and clinical symptoms of inflammation.

**C-Reactive Protein:** an acute-phase protein that is produced by the liver and released into circulation during acute inflammation.

**Cytokines:** a group name for more than 100 different proteins involved in immune responses. Prolonged production of proinflammatory cytokines promotes hypercatabolism.

**Systemic Inflammatory Response Syndrome (SIRS):** a whole-body response to inflammation characterized by elevated heart rate, increased respiratory rate, increased white blood cell counts, and fever.

**Sepsis:** systemic inflammatory response syndrome caused by infection.

**Multiple Organ Failure:** impaired organ function, usually of two or more organ systems, resulting from an uncontrolled inflammatory response. Also known as multiple organ dysfunction syndrome.

**Negative Nitrogen Balance:** a state that occurs when nitrogen excretion exceeds nitrogen (protein) intake.

**Indirect Calorimetry:** an indirect estimate of resting energy expenditure that measures the ratio of $CO_2$ expired to the amount of oxygen inspired and uses those values in a mathematical equation.

| TABLE 16.2 | Nutrients Important for Wound Healing and Recovery | |
|---|---|---|
| **Nutrient** | **Rationale for Increased Need** | **Possible Deficiency Outcome** |
| Protein | To replace lean body mass lost during the catabolic phase after stress | Significant weight loss |
| | | Impaired/delayed wound healing |
| | To restore blood volume and plasma proteins lost during exudates, bleeding from the wound, and possible hemorrhage | Shock related to decreased blood volume |
| | | Edema related to decreased serum albumin |
| | To replace losses resulting from immobility (increased excretion) | Diarrhea related to decreased albumin |
| | | Anemia |
| | To meet increased needs for tissue repair and resistance to infection | Increased risk of infection related to decreased antibodies, impaired tissue integrity |
| | | Increased mortality |
| Calories | To replace losses related to lack of oral intake and hypermetabolism during catabolic phase after stress | Signs and symptoms of protein deficiency due to use of protein to meet energy requirements |
| | To spare protein | Extensive weight loss |
| | To restore normal weight | |
| Water | To replace fluid lost through vomiting, hemorrhage, exudates, fever, drainage, diuresis | Signs, symptoms, and complications of dehydration such as poor skin turgor, dry mucous membranes, oliguria, anuria, weight loss, increased pulse rate, decreased central venous pressure |
| | To maintain homeostasis | |
| Vitamin C | Important for capillary formation, tissue synthesis, and wound healing through collagen formation | Impaired/delayed wound healing related to impaired collagen formation and increased capillary fragility and permeability |
| | Needed for antibody formation | Increased risk of infection related to decreased antibodies |
| Thiamin, niacin, riboflavin | Requirements increase with increased metabolic rate | Decreased enzymes available for energy metabolism |
| Folic acid, vitamin $B_{12}$ | Needed for cell proliferation and, therefore, tissue synthesis | Decreased or arrested cell division |
| | Important for maturation of red blood cells | Megaloblastic anemia |
| | Impaired folic acid synthesis related to some antibiotics; impaired vitamin $B_{12}$ absorption related to some antibiotics | |
| Vitamin A | Important for tissue synthesis, wound healing, and immune function | Impaired/delayed wound healing related to decreased collagen synthesis; impaired immune function |
| | Enhances resistance to infection | Increased risk of infection |
| Vitamin K | Important for normal blood clotting | Prolonged prothrombin time |
| | Impaired intestinal synthesis related to antibiotics | |
| Iron | To replace iron lost through blood loss | Signs, symptoms, and complications of iron deficiency anemia such as fatigue, weakness, pallor, anorexia, dizziness, headaches, stomatitis, glossitis, cardiovascular and respiratory changes, possible cardiac failure |
| Zinc | Needed for protein synthesis and wound healing | Impaired/delayed wound healing |
| | Needed for normal lymphocyte and phagocyte response | Impaired immune response |

| BOX 16.1 | **HARRIS–BENEDICT EQUATION FOR CALCULATING CALORIE NEEDS** |

**Total Energy Expenditure (TEE) = BEE × Stress Factor × Activity Factor**

*Basal Energy Expenditure (BEE)*

$$\text{Females} = 655.1 + 9.6(W) + 1.9(H) - 4.7(A)$$

$$\text{Males} = 66.5 + 13.8(W) + 5.0(H) - 6.8(A)$$

$$W = \text{weight in kilograms}$$

$$H = \text{height in centimeters}$$

$$A = \text{age in years}$$

*Stress Factors*

| | |
|---|---|
| Elective surgery | 1.05–1.15 |
| Sepsis | 1.2–1.4 |
| Closed head injury | 1.3 |
| Multiple trauma | 1.4 |
| Systemic inflammatory response syndrome | 1.5 |
| Major burn | 2.0 |

*Activity Factors*

| | |
|---|---|
| Confined to bed | 1.1 |
| Out of bed | 1.2 |

*Source:* Russell, M. & Malone, A. (2004). Nutrient Requirements. In P. Charney, A. Malone. (Eds.). *ADA Pocket guide to nutrition assessment.* Chicago: American Dietetic Association.

**Basal Energy Expenditure (BEE):** the calories expended maintaining basic, involuntary activities needed to sustain life such as beating the heart, inflating the lungs, and secreting enzymes. Commonly used interchangeably with resting energy expenditure (REE), except that REE is measured after a 12-hour fast.

Most often, calorie requirements are estimated using any one of a number of predictive equations, such as the Harris–Benedict equation (Box 16.1). Gender-specific mathematical equations based on the patient's age, height, and weight are used to predict **basal energy expenditure (BEE).** BEE is then adjusted for stress and possibly for activity to arrive at an estimate of total energy expenditure (TEE). The multiplication factors to adjust for stress and activity are not universally agreed upon, and ranges of values are often used because exact values are unknown.

A review of the evidence on the validity and accuracy of using the Harris–Benedict equation to calculate calorie needs concluded strongly that this equation should not be used for critically ill patients (Frankenfield et al., 2007). The equation was derived from well-nourished, healthy volunteers and is too unreliable to use in critically ill patients. The other predictive formulas also lack validity for use in critically ill patients or have limited and inconsistent data available to judge their validity (Frankenfield et al., 2007). More validation studies are needed to determine the usefulness of predictive equations among critically ill patients.

A simple alternative method for estimating calorie needs is to multiply the patient's weight in kilograms by a specified calorie level. Suggested standards for calorie goals are 25 cal/kg for most patients with critical illness and 20 cal/kg for patients with sepsis (Hise et al., 2007).

Regardless of the method or values used to estimate calorie needs, the initial calculation is considered a starting point that is adjusted upward or downward based on the patient's response.

**Underfeeding.** While it is important to provide enough calories to promote recovery and support immune function, an excessive calorie intake increases metabolism, oxygen consumption, and $CO_2$ production, which increase the burden already placed on the heart and lungs to regulate blood gases. An excess of calories taxes endocrine and thyroid functions and may precipitate dangerous shifts in serum phosphorus and other electrolytes that characterize the **refeeding syndrome**.

> **Refeeding Syndrome:** a potentially fatal complication that occurs from an abrupt change from a catabolic state to an anabolic state and increase in insulin caused by a dramatic increase in calories.

Experts have recently begun to suspect that feeding critically ill patients at 100% of calculated need is associated with worse, not better, clinical outcomes (Zaloga, 2008). A recent prospective cohort study showed that underfeeding during critical illness (e.g., 80% of goal calories) is associated with shorter ICU and hospital stays when compared to patients who received more nutrition (Heise et al., 2007). Several observational studies suggest that a calorie intake of approximately 60% of goal calories (or 9 to 18 cal/kg) creates less physiological burden on the patient and improves clinical outcomes in a variety of patient populations (Krishnan et al., 2003). A modest calorie intake is also associated with a higher chance of achieving ventilator independence before leaving the ICU compared to patients with the lowest calorie intake (0 to 9 cal/kg) (Kudsk & Sacks, 2006). Studies suggest that a modest calorie intake (33% to 65%) may be optimal; intakes either above or below the modest range are linked to increased risks to the patient (Zaloga, 2008). Proposed mechanisms by which underfeeding benefits patients are listed in Box 16.2.

When underfeeding is used, a hypocaloric intake is maintained for 3 to 5 days. As the patient improves, the feeding is advanced as tolerated over the next 3 to 5 days until 100% of the calculated needs are provided (Zaloga, 2008).

## Protein

As with calories, the recommendations for protein are not universally agreed upon. An appropriate starting level for metabolically stressed patients who have normal kidney function and are meeting their calorie needs may be 1.5 g protein/kg/day (Charney & Malone, 2004). Other recommendations cover a range from 1.0 to 2.0 g/kg (Charney & Malone, 2004). Patients with severe burns may need 2 to 2.5 g/kg because of excessive urinary losses and wound losses (Kudsk & Sacks, 2006). Even with a high-protein intake, protein catabolism cannot be halted during the metabolic response because of effects of stress hormones.

Besides the total quantity of protein provided, the specific types of amino acids given may influence the stress response and recovery. Arginine and glutamine, two nonessential amino acids, may become conditionally essential during periods of stress. Arginine synthesis

---

**BOX 16.2**     **PROPOSED MECHANISMS BY WHICH UNDERFEEDING BENEFITS PATIENTS**

- Lower intake of omega-6 fatty acids means less synthesis of the cytokines that promote inflammation
- Lower carbohydrate intake may decrease hyperglycemia
- Lower intakes of calcium, iron, and zinc may lower inflammatory response and cell injury
- Fewer free radicals generated from nutrient metabolism
- Less $CO_2$ production from less hypermetabolism

*Source:* Zaloga, G. Permissive underfeeding of crucially ill patients. *Nestle nutrition.* Available at www.nestle-nutrition.com/topics. Accessed on 2/18/08.

may be limited during illness; it plays a role in cellular immunity and promotes proliferation of T lymphocytes (Kudsk & Sacks, 2006). Glutamine appears to be rapidly depleted during stress; it provides fuel for cells of the immune system, especially T lymphocytes (Kudsk & Sacks, 2006). Although arginine and glutamine are constituents of enteral formulas designed to enhance immune system functioning, the use of these formulas is controversial and yields inconsistent results, especially in critical care populations (McCowen & Bistrian, 2003).

## Carbohydrates and Fat

Carbohydrates should provide 50% to 60% of total calorie needs (Kudsk & Sacks, 2006). Fat may provide up to 40% of total calories. When parenteral nutrition (PN) is used, fat may be increased and carbohydrate lowered in patients with severe hyperglycemia or high $CO_2$ production. Potential complications of a high intravenous lipid load include hyperlipidemia, suppression of the immune system, and increased risk of infection (Kudsk & Sacks, 2006).

## Fluid

During periods of acute stress, fluid requirements are highly individualized according to losses that occur through exudates, hemorrhage, emesis, diuresis, diarrhea, and fever. The physician determines the patient's fluid need based on intake and output, blood pressure, heart rate, respiratory rate, and body temperature. Care is taken to avoid overhydration; decreased renal output is a frequent complication of metabolic stress.

## Micronutrients

Vitamin and mineral requirements during stress are unclear. Fluid shifts that occur during the acute-phase response may be responsible for the apparent decrease in plasma concentrations of certain vitamins (Kudsh & Sacks, 2006). When the acute phase is resolved, plasma vitamin concentrations often return to normal. Supplemental vitamins may be needed only when low vitamin concentrations persist beyond the acute-phase response.

The low plasma concentrations of zinc and iron, characteristic of the acute-phase response, may be a protective mechanism by the body to make them unavailable to replicating bacteria (Lowry & Perez, 2006). Providing iron during infection may impair the body's ability to resist infection. However, zinc plays an important role in wound healing, and adequate levels are essential to ensure healing.

Trauma and burn patients have been documented to have high urinary and tissue losses of the trace elements selenium, zinc, and copper. When supplements of these three trace elements were given to severely burned patients, they experienced significantly fewer infections as a result of fewer pulmonary infections (Berger et al., 2007). Wound healing was also improved in the supplemented group, with fewer skin grafts required.

## Method of Feeding

Enteral nutrition (EN) is recommended over PN in critically ill patients who are hemodynamically stable and have a functional gastrointestinal (GI) tract. Patients who receive EN are less likely to experience sepsis and have fewer infectious complications than patients who receive PN (ADA, 2008). A common complication in critically ill patients is gastroparesis, which precludes early oral or gastric feedings. However, early EN feedings of isotonic formulas into the lower small bowel are reportedly well tolerated by ICU patients because the jejunum is less susceptible to motility dysfunction than the stomach and upper small bowel (ADA, 2008).

Parental nutrition is required when the GI tract is nonfunctional and may be used as supplemental nutrition in patients who are not able to obtain adequate nutrition via enteral feedings. Several studies that compared PN with EN in critically ill patients found no significant differences in mortality or morbidity between the two groups except for an increased rate of hyperglycemia in patients who received PN (Koretz et al., 2007).

### QUICK BITE

**Ways to increase protein density**
- Add skim milk powder to milk
- Substitute milk for water in recipes
- Melt cheese on sandwiches, casseroles, hot vegetables, or potatoes
- Spread peanut butter on apples or crackers or mix into hot cereals
- Sprinkle nuts on cereals, desserts, or salads; mix into casseroles or stir-fry
- Coat breaded meats with eggs first; add chopped hard-cooked eggs to casseroles
- Top fruit with yogurt

**Ways to increase calorie density**
- Spread cream cheese on hot bread
- Add butter or margarine to hot foods: potatoes, vegetables, cooked cereal, rice, pasta, pancakes, and soups
- Use gravy over potatoes, meat, or vegetables
- Use mayonnaise in place of salad dressing
- Use whipped cream on desserts and in coffee and tea
- Add honey to cooked cereals, fruit, coffee, or tea
- Add marshmallows to hot chocolate

Oral diets are provided as soon as possible. A high-calorie, high-protein diet with small frequent meals may help maximize intake (Box 16.3). Nutrition support—either complete or supplemental tube feedings—is necessary when calorie needs are not met through an oral intake.

## ▶ BURNS

Extensive burns are the most severe form of metabolic stress. The extensive inflammatory response causes rapid fluid shifts and large losses of fluid, electrolytes, protein, and other nutrients from the wound. Fluid and electrolyte replacement to maintain adequate blood volume and blood pressure are the priorities of the initial postburn period.

The degree of hypermetabolism and hypercatabolism in the metabolic response phase correlates to the extent of burn. It is estimated that within the first 2 weeks of a burn injury as much as 20% of body protein can be lost (Lee at al., 2005). Fluid and electrolyte imbalances, paralytic ileus, anorexia, pain, infection or other complications, emotional trauma, and medical–surgical procedures may complicate nutrition support.

| BOX 16.3 | A SAMPLE OF HIGH-CALORIE, HIGH-PROTEIN MENU |

**Breakfast**
Orange juice
Cheese and mushroom omelet
Wheat toast with butter and jelly
Milk
Coffee with whipped cream added

**Snack**
Smoothie made with yogurt, instant
    breakfast mix, whole milk, and strawberries

**Lunch**
New England clam chowder
Chicken salad sandwich on a croissant
Milk
Ice cream with chocolate sauce and
    whipped cream

**Snack**
Cottage cheese with fruit
Roll with butter

**Dinner**
Meat loaf with gravy
Baked potato with sour cream
Broccoli with cheese sauce
Spinach salad with hard cooked eggs,
    onions, walnuts, and vinaigrette dressing
Milk
Carrot cake with cream cheese frosting

**Snack**
Tuna salad sandwich
Melon topped with fruited yogurt

## Nutrition Therapy

As with metabolic stress caused by other stressors, the nutrition priority is to meet calorie and protein needs. Calorie requirements may be measured by indirect calorimetry or estimated by using a predictive formula. Notice in Box 16.1 that the largest injury factor listed is for severe burns. Protein needs are typically 2.0 to 2.5 g/kg, especially if burns are more than 10% of total body surface area (Kudsk & Sacks, 2006). Calorie and protein needs increase if complications develop and lessen as wound healing progresses.

Although it is generally agreed that vitamin needs increase in burn patients because of losses from wounds, healing, and changes in metabolism, the exact requirements are not known (ADA, 2008). Supplements of vitamin C, vitamin A, and zinc plus a multivitamin are recommended by the Shriners Burn Institute (ADA, 2008). Supplements of arginine, glutamine, fish oil, vitamin D, and vitamin K given to acutely burned patients may offer some benefit, but more research is needed before their use becomes mainstream (ADA, 2008). As previously stated, supplements of the trace elements selenium, zinc, and copper have been shown to promote healing and decrease the risk of infections in burn patients (Berger et al., 2007).

Unlike other patients with severe stress, burned patients develop less gastroparesis when they are given nasogastric or nasoduodenal tube feedings within 8 to 12 hours after admission (Kudsk & Sacks, 2006). Patients who are able to consume food orally are given small frequent feedings of a high-calorie, high-protein diet (Box 16.3). Daily calorie counts may be used to monitor intake. When intake is less than 75% of estimated need for more than 3 days, EN should be used for total or supplemental nutrition (ADA, 2008). Supplemental tube feedings given during the night are useful when nutritional needs are not met through food alone. Most patients with severe burns require nutrition support. Total PN is used with extreme caution because of the increased risks for infection and sepsis.

# ▶ RESPIRATORY STRESS

**Respiratory Stress:**
impaired gas exchange between the air and blood that leads to lower levels of oxygen in the blood and higher levels of $CO_2$.

Respiratory stress occurs when gas exchange between the air and blood is impaired, leading to lower levels of oxygen in the blood and higher levels of $CO_2$. Like metabolic stress, respiratory stress may cause hypermetabolism and a loss of muscle mass and function. When nutritional needs are not met—whether from increased needs related to hypermetabolism or inadequate intake related to anorexia and dyspnea—fewer nutrients are available to maintain respiratory muscle function. Gas exchange and exercise tolerance are further compromised, and a downhill spiral of malnutrition and worsening respiratory status may ensue. Chronic or acute respiratory stress can lead to respiratory failure, multiple organ failure, and death.

## Chronic Obstructive Pulmonary Disease

As many as 60% of patients with chronic obstructive pulmonary disease (COPD) have malnutrition, which is associated with poor outcomes (Suckling et al., 2006). Many patients with COPD are hypermetabolic from increased energy spent on labored breathing. Chronic inflammation also increases metabolism and impairs appetite. Anorexia may occur from fatigue, depression, anxiety, changes in taste, excess mucus production, dyspnea, or decreased peristalsis and digestion secondary to inadequate oxygen to GI cells. Early satiety may be related from flattening of the diaphragm and a decrease in abdominal volume or from bloating related to swallowed air. Steroid therapy increases the risk of GI upset and peptic ulcer disease. Improvements in nutritional status have been linked to improvements in survival (Suckling et al., 2006).

### Nutrition Therapy

Correcting or preventing malnutrition—namely, maintaining or restoring body weight, lean body mass, and respiratory muscle function—is a priority for patients with COPD. Generally a high-calorie, high-protein diet is used. Strategies for improving intake are tailored to the patient's symptoms (Table 16.3). Some patients may be overweight or may experience undesirable weight gain from chronic steroid use. Because excess weight poses an additional burden on the respiratory system, a healthy, calorie-restricted diet to promote gradual weight loss is recommended for these patients.

**QUICK BITE**

Enteral formulas designed for respiratory insufficiency

| | Calories from fat (%) |
|---|---|
| Novasource Pulmonary | 41 |
| NutriVent | 55 |
| Oxepa | 55 |
| Pulmocare | 55 |

For patients hospitalized with exacerbation of COPD, calorie needs may be 140% above BEE. If indirect calorimetry is not available, a reasonable starting point is to provide 25 to 30 cal/kg. Protein needs may be 1.2 g/kg of body weight (Thorsdottir & Gunnarsdottir, 2002). In patients who require mechanical ventilation, care is taken to avoid overfeeding because it increases $CO_2$ production, which can complicate ventilation. Specially formulated enteral products are available for patients with respiratory disease. They are lower in carbohydrate and higher in fat than routine formulas based on the assumption that lesser amounts of carbohydrate yield less $CO_2$, but these formulas have not been shown to improve clinical outcomes.

| TABLE 16.3 | Strategies to Promote Eating in Patients with COPD Based on Symptoms | |
|---|---|
| **Symptom** | **Strategies to Promote Eating** |
| Anorexia | Eat small frequent meals<br>Eat most nutritionally dense foods first<br>Drink high-protein, high-calorie nutrition formulas between meals |
| Shortness of breath | Eat small frequent meals<br>Eat a soft diet, avoiding foods that are difficult to chew or swallow<br>Rest before eating<br>Use bronchodilators before eating |
| Fatigue | Rest before eating |
| Early satiety | Limit "empty" liquids with meals (e.g., coffee, tea, water, carbonated beverages)<br>Eat small, frequent, nutritionally dense meals<br>Avoid "gassy" foods<br>Try high-calorie, high-protein nutrition formulas |
| Dry mouth | Add gravies and sauces to foods<br>Use artificial saliva before eating<br>Avoid dry and salty foods |
| Constipation/Straining at stool | Increase fiber intake, such as increasing intake of ready-to-eat bran or whole wheat cereals or drinking commercially prepared oral supplements with added fiber such as Promote with Fiber |
| Thick mucus | Increase fluid intake |

## NURSING PROCESS: *Metabolic Stress*

Vin is a frail, 74-year-old man admitted to the hospital with multiple, serious but non–life-threatening, injuries resulting from a car accident. He weighs 122 pounds and is 5 ft. 6 in. tall.

### Assessment

Medical–Psychosocial History

- Current diagnoses and medications
- Medical history, including hyperlipidemia, hypertension, cardiovascular disease, renal impairments, diabetes, GI complaints
- Medications that affect nutrition, such as lipid-lowering medications, cardiac drugs, antihypertensives
- Extent of injuries; significance of GI trauma, if appropriate
- Hemodynamic status; signs and symptoms of hemorrhaging
- Neurologic status (e.g., confusion, disorientation); ability to eat, ability to self-feed
- GI function such as hypoactive bowel sounds, distention, complaints of nausea, anorexia
- Psychosocial and economic issues prior to injury, such as if finances, loneliness, or isolation impaired his food intake. Determine who does food shopping and preparation and if the client is a candidate for the Meals on Wheels program

*(nursing process continues on page 396)*

# NURSING PROCESS: Metabolic Stress (continued)

| | |
|---|---|
| Anthropometric Assessment | • Height, current weight |
| | • Recent weight history; usual weight |
| | • Body mass index (BMI) |
| Biochemical and Physical Assessment | • Complete blood count |
| | • Blood chemistry, including major electrolytes |
| | • Serum glucose |
| | • I & O |
| | • Clinical symptoms of malnutrition such as wasted appearance |
| Dietary Assessment | • Do you have any difficulty chewing or swallowing? |
| | • Do you have nausea or any other symptoms that interfere with your ability to eat? |
| | • Are you able to feed yourself? |
| | • Do you follow a special diet at home? |
| | • Do you have enough food to eat at home? |
| | • Do you have any food intolerances or allergies? |
| | • Do you have any cultural, religious, or ethnic food preferences? |
| | • Do you take vitamins, minerals, or supplements? If so, what? |
| | • How much alcohol do you consume? |

## Diagnosis

| | |
|---|---|
| Possible Nursing Diagnosis | Imbalance nutrition: less than body requirements r/t low calorie intake and increased requirements related to injuries |

## Planning

| | |
|---|---|
| Client Outcomes | The client will |
| | • Maintain normal fluid and electrolyte balance |
| | • Meet 75% of his goal calories and protein via oral diet with supplements |
| | • Describe the principles and rationale of a high-calorie, high-protein diet |
| | • Avoid complications of undernutrition, such as weight loss, poor wound healing, infections |

## Nursing Interventions

| | |
|---|---|
| Nutrition Therapy | • Initially give intravenous fluid and electrolytes as ordered |
| | • When oral intake begins, encourage the intake of calorie- and protein-dense foods first; encourage intake of between meal supplements |
| Client Teaching | Instruct the client on |
| | The importance of protein and calories in promoting wound healing and recovery and overall health |
| | The eating plan essentials including: |
| | • How to increase calories and protein in the diet (Box 16.3) |
| | • To eat small frequent meals to maximize intake |

*(nursing process continues on page 397)*

*NURSING PROCESS: Metabolic Stress* (continued)

| Evaluation |
|---|

Evaluate and Monitor

- Monitor fluid and electrolyte balance and other biochemical values.
- Monitor intake and the need for total or supplemental EN.
- Monitor weight.
- Monitor for complications, such as delayed wound healing or infection.
- Observe for tolerance to oral diet.
- Suggest changes in the meal plan as needed.
- Provide periodic feedback and reinforcement.

## ▶ How Do You Respond?

**Do flavored waters marketed to improve immune function really work?** There are several flavored waters available on grocery store shelves that feature descriptive terms such as "defend," "protect," or "immunity" on the label. All of these products contain added vitamins and/or minerals, such as vitamins A, C, D, E, B vitamins, or zinc. Some provide calories from sweeteners, others are calorie free. While certain vitamins and minerals *are* important for normal immune system functioning, it is a huge leap to conclude that any of these products provide health benefits beyond those obtained from a normal mixed diet. Consuming more than required of any nutrients necessary for immune system functioning does not boost immune function—unless the immune system was impaired because of a nutrient deficiency. Manufacturers are free to put in whatever nutrients they desire in whatever amounts they choose; scientific evidence of benefit or need is not required to make a function claim.

## ▶ Case Study

Samuel was diagnosed with COPD 7 years ago and has had recurrent bronchitis over the past 40 years. He is 68 years old, 5 ft. 9 in. tall, and weighs 134 pounds. About 3 years ago he had a normal adult weight of 150 to 155 pounds. He has lost 7 pounds in the last month due to lack of appetite and early satiety. He complains of a dry mouth and that "food has lost its taste." He is currently on multiple medications, including a bronchodialator, an inhaler, and an antibiotic. He uses oxygen as needed. During his recent hospitalization for pneumonia, the dietitian told him he should be eating at least 2000 calories, but he doesn't have the energy to prepare or eat that much food.

His usual intake appears in the box to the left.

| | |
|---|---|
| **Breakfast:** | Coffee with creamer<br>2 Pieces of white toast with jelly |
| **Lunch:** | Cheese and crackers<br>Banana<br>Coffee with creamer |
| **Dinner:** | Canned soup with oyster crackers<br>Ice cream<br>Coffee with creamer |

- Evaluate Samuel's current BMI and normal adult weight. Calculate his percent weight loss over the past month. Is it significant?

• What factors contribute to Samuel's poor appetite and intake? What specific strategies would you recommend he implement to improve his intake?

• Is 2000 calories an appropriate amount of daily calories for him? How much protein should he consume in a day?

▶ Devise a sample menu for him that takes into account the calories and protein he needs and his symptoms of anorexia, early satiety, dry mouth, and fatigue.

STUDY QUESTIONS

1. Which of the following strategies would be most appropriate for a patient with COPD who is experiencing early satiety?
   a. Limiting "empty" beverages at meals
   b. Resting before eating
   c. Using bronchodilators before eating
   d. Limiting salt intake

2. When teaching a client diagnosed with COPD about nutritional needs, which of the following types of diet should the nurse discuss?
   a. A high-calorie, high-protein diet
   b. A low-residue diet
   c. A low-fat, low-cholesterol diet
   d. A low-sodium diet

3. In a burned patient with a functional GI tract, why is enteral nutrition preferred over parenteral nutrition?
   a. Because enteral nutrition can provide higher amounts of calories and protein.
   b. Because enteral nutrition is less likely to interfere with oral intake.
   c. Because enteral nutrition is less expensive.
   d. Because enteral nutrition has a lower risk of infectious complications.

4. Why may underfeeding critically ill patients be beneficial?
   a. Because it provides less work for the GI tract to do.
   b. Because all methods of measuring a person's energy expenditure overestimate their needs so a lower calorie load is a prudent approach.
   c. Because it provides fewer substrates for the body to make proinflammatory molecules and has a positive effect on hyperglycemia.
   d. Because it causes stress hormone levels to drop.

5. What does the patient require during the first 24 to 48 hours after a severe burn?
   a. Parenteral nutrition
   b. Supplements of trace elements
   c. Fluid and electrolytes
   d. A low-carbohydrate diet to decrease $CO_2$ production

6. What does a spike in C-reactive protein indicate in people with acute metabolic stress?
   a. Protein needs are not being met.
   b. Protein intake is adequate.
   c. An inflammatory response is occurring.
   d. The inflammatory response has ended.

7. How much daily protein may a 70-kilograms person with severe burns require?
   a. 56 grams
   b. 70 grams
   c. 105 grams
   d. 175 grams

8. If underfeeding is used for critically ill patients, when should the calories begin to be advanced toward 100% of need?
   a. After 3 to 5 days
   b. After 5 to 7 days
   c. After 7 to 10 days
   d. After 10 days

## KEY CONCEPTS

- The ebb phase following acute illness or injury lasts approximately 24 hours and is resolved when the patient is hemodynamically stable.

- The flow phase is a metabolic response to acute stress that is characterized by hormonal and inflammatory responses than change the body's chemistry. The duration of this phase varies with the severity of the stress and whether complications develop.

- Stress hormones, also known as counterregulatory hormones, increase blood glucose levels, metabolism, and body protein catabolism.

- The inflammatory response is mediated by immune system components that alter the concentration of certain plasma proteins. C-reactive protein is a positive acute-phase protein that is used as an indicator of inflammation in acute stress.

- Nutritional needs are considered after the patient is hemodynamically stable. The primary nutritional concern is the breakdown of body protein because protein deficiency increases the risks of infection, delayed or impaired wound healing, and mortality. Nutrition therapy focuses on preserving lean body mass and preventing or alleviating malnutrition.

- Recommendations regarding calorie and protein requirements during critical illness are imprecise. Indirect calorimetry is the gold standard for calculating calorie needs. Predictive equations are not recommended because they are unreliable. Calories per kilogram may be used when indirect calorimetry is not available.

- Providing 33% to 65% of actual calorie needs may be initially optimal in critically ill patients, possibly by several different mechanisms. If underfeeding is used, the calories are gradually increased after the first 3 to 5 days and eventually reach 100% over the next 3 to 5 days.

- Protein requirements are generally based on weight and range from 1.0 to 2.0 grams/ kilograms or higher depending on the type and severity of stressors as well as the patient's age and prior nutritional status.

- The intake of carbohydrates and fat are adjusted as needed, based on the patient's tolerance and method of feeding.

- Fluid needs during metabolic stress are highly variable and are determined by the physician.

- Micronutrient requirements during metabolic stress are not clear. Serum levels of vitamins may decrease because of fluid shifts, not necessarily because of deficiency. Low concentrations of iron and zinc in the blood may be a protective mechanism to make these nutrients unavailable for replicating bacteria.

- EN is preferred over PN whenever the GI tract is functional and the patient is hemodynamically stable. Gastroparesis is common but isotonic feedings infused into the lower small bowel are well tolerated by patients in ICU.

- PN is required when the GI tract is nonfunctional or when nutritional needs are so high they cannot be met by oral or EN alone. The risk of infection and complications is higher with PN than EN.

- Oral intake is resumed when possible. Small, frequent meals help achieve a high-calorie, high-protein intake.

● Extensive burns are the most severe form of stress that a person can experience. Nutritional support may be complicated by paralytic ileus, stress ulcers, anorexia, pain, and the consequences of medical–surgical treatments.

● Patients with severe burns need a high-calorie, high-protein diet. Nasogastric or nasoduodenal feedings infused within the first 8 to 12 hours are well tolerated among burn patients, unlike patients with other causes of metabolic stress. PN support is often needed because nutritional needs are so high.

● Patients with COPD are often underweight and malnourished. Shortness of breath can make eating difficult, and decreased oxygenation of the GI cells can impair peristalsis and digestion. Metabolism may be elevated from increased energy expenditure related to labored breathing and/or from chronic inflammation.

● Nutrition-dense, easy-to-consume foods are preferred for patients with chronic respiratory disorders. Patients on ventilator support may benefit from restricted carbohydrate enteral formulas to lower $CO_2$ production.

## ANSWER KEY

1. **FALSE** Aggressive nutrition therapy can improve some of the metabolic derangements of stress, but complete reversal only occurs after the underlying stressor is resolved.

2. **TRUE** Stress hormones have catabolic actions in the body; that is, they stimulate the break down of glycogen, adipose tissue, and lean body mass. They function opposite to the insulin, which lowers blood glucose levels.

3. **FALSE** The metabolic response to stress begins after the first 2 to 48 hours. Its duration is related to the severity of stress, the number of stressors, and the individual's ability to adapt to stress.

4. **TRUE** The acute-phase inflammatory response causes a decrease in serum albumin and other negative acute-phase proteins. C-reactive protein is a positive acute-phase protein that rises in response to inflammation.

5. **TRUE** After trauma, motility returns to the lower small intestine much sooner than to the stomach and upper small bowel.

6. **FALSE** Harris–Benedict equations are unreliable for use with critically ill patients. The formulas were derived from studies on healthy volunteers and do not accurately reflect calorie needs during metabolic stress.

7. **TRUE** Underfeeding is associated with lower risks than overfeeding, possibly because a lower nutrient and calorie load may lower hyperglycemia, decrease proinflammtory cytokine production, reduce $CO_2$ production, and lower nutrient oxidation.

8. **FALSE** The drop in serum iron that occurs during the acute-phase response may be a compensatory mechanism to remove iron, so it is not available for use by replicating bacteria. Supplemental iron may impair the body's ability to fight infection.

9. **TRUE** Extensive burns are the most severe form of stress and dramatically increase the need for calories, protein, nutrients, and fluid.

10. **FALSE** COPD actually increases REE through labored breathing and possibly through chronic inflammation. Weight loss may occur even when intake appears normal.

## WEBSITES

American Association of Critical Care Nurses at **www.aacn.org**
American Burn Association at **www.ameriburn.org**
American Lung Association at **www.lungusa.org**
Burn Survivor Resource Center at **www.burnsurvivor.com**
Society for Critical Care Medicine at **www.survivingsepsis.org**

# REFERENCES

American Dietetic Association (ADA). (2008). *Nutrition care manual.* (online). Available at www.nutritioncaremanual.org. Accessed on 8/25/08.

Berger, M. M., Baines, M., Falloul, W., et al. (2007). Trace element supplementation after major burns modulates antioxidant status and clinical course by way of increased tissue trace element concentrations. *The American Journal of Clinical Nutrition, 85,* 1293–1300.

Biolo, G., Grinble, G., & Preiser, J. (2003). Position paper of the ESICM Working Group on Nutrition and Metabolism. Metabolic basis of nutrition in intensive care unit patients: Ten critical questions. *Intensive Care Medicine, 28,* 1512–1520.

Charney, P. (2007). Nutrition assessment in the intensive care unit: Prealbumin, C-reactive protein, or none of the above? *Support Line, 29,* 13, 16–18.

Charney, P., & Malone, A. (Eds.). (2004). *ADA pocket guide to nutrition assessment.* Chicago, IL: American Dietetic Association.

Compher, C., Frankenfield, D., Keim, N., et al. (2006). Evidence Analysis Working Group. (2006). Best practice methods to apply to measurement of resting metabolic rate in adults: A systematic review. *Journal of the American Dietetic Association, 106,* 881–903.

Frankenfield, D., Hise, M., Malone, A., et al. (2007). Prediction of resting metabolic rate in critically ill adult patients: Results of a systematic review of the evidence. *Journal of the American Dietetic Association, 107,* 1552–1561.

Gabay, C., & Kushner, I. (1999). Acute phase proteins and other systemic responses to inflammation. *The New England Journal of Medicine, 340,* 448–454.

Heise, M. E., Halterman, K., Gajewski, B. J., et al. (2007). Feeding practices of severely ill intensive care unit patients: An evaluation of energy sources and clinical outcomes. *Journal of the American Dietetic Association, 107,* 458–465.

Koretz, R. L., Avenell, A., Lipman, T. O., et al. (2007). Does enteral nutrition affect outcome: A systematic review of the reandomized trials. *The American Journal of Gastroenterology, 102,* 412–429.

Krishnan, J., Parce, P., Martinez, A., et al. (2003). Caloric intake in medical ICU patients: Consistency of care with guidelines and relationship to clinical outcomes. *Chest, 124,* 297–305.

Kudsk, K., & Sacks, G. (2006). In M. Shils, M. Shike, A. Ross, et al. (Eds). *Modern nutrition in health and disease* (10th ed.). Philadelphia: Lippincott Williams & Wilkins.

Lee, J., Benjamin, D., & Herndon, D. (2005). Nutrition support strategies for severely burned patients. *Nutrition in Clinical Practice, 20,* 325–330.

Lowry, S., & Perez, M. (2006). In M. Shils, M. Shike, A. Ross, et al. (Eds.). *Modern nutrition in health and disease* (10th ed.). Philadelphia: Lippincott Williams & Wilkins.

McCowen, K., & Bistrian, B. (2003). Immunonutrition: Problematic or problem solving? *The American Journal of Clinical Nutrition, 77,* 764–770.

Russell, M., & Malone, A. (2004). Nutrient Requirements. In P. Charney, A. Malone. (Eds). *ADA pocket guide to nutrition assessment.* Chicago: American Dietetic Association.

Suckling, B., Johnson, M., & Chin, R. (2006). In M. Shiles, M. Shike, A. Ross, et al. (Eds.). *Modern nutrition in health and disease* (10th ed.). Philadelphia: Lippincott Williams & Wilkins.

Thorsdottir, I., & Gunnarsdottir, I. (2002). Energy intake must be increased among recently hospitalized patients with chronic obstructive pulmonary disease to improve nutritional status. *Journal of the American Dietetic Association, 102,* 247–249.

Zaloga, P. (2008). Permissive underfeeding of critically ill patients. *Nestle nutrition.* Available at www.nestle-nutrition.com/topics. Accessed 2/18/08.

# 17

## Nutrition for Patients with Upper Gastrointestinal Disorders

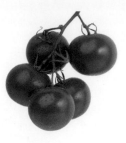

### UPON COMPLETION OF THIS CHAPTER, YOU WILL BE ABLE TO

- Give examples of ways to promote eating in people with anorexia.
- Describe nutrition interventions that may help maximize intake in people who have nausea.
- Compare the three levels of solid food textures included in the National Dysphagia Diet.
- Compare the four liquid consistencies included in the National Dysphagia Diet.
- Plan a menu appropriate for someone with GERD.
- Teach a patient about role of nutrition therapy in the treatment of peptic ulcer disease.
- Give examples of nutrition therapy recommendations for people experiencing dumping syndrome.

Nutrition therapy is used in the treatment of many digestive system disorders. For many disorders, diet merely plays a supportive role in alleviating symptoms rather than altering the course of the disease. For other gastrointestinal (GI) disorders, nutrition therapy is the cornerstone of treatment. Frequently nutrition therapy is needed to restore nutritional status that has been compromised by dysfunction or disease.

This chapter begins with disorders that affect eating and covers disorders of the upper GI tract (mouth, esophagus, and stomach) that have nutritional implications. Table 17.1 outlines the roles these sites play in the mechanical and chemical digestion of food. Problems with the upper GI tract impact nutrition mostly by affecting food intake and tolerance to

| TABLE 17.1 | The Role of the Upper GI Tract in the Mechanical and Chemical Digestion of Food | |
|---|---|---|
| **Site** | **Mechanical Digestion** | **Chemical Digestion** |
| Mouth | Chewing breaks down food into smaller particles<br>Food mixes with saliva for ease in swallowing | Saliva contains lingual lipase, which has a limited role in the digestion of fat, and salivary amylase, which digests starch. Food is not held in the mouth long enough for digestion to occur there; the majority of salivary amylase activity occurs in the stomach |
| Esophagus | Propels food downward into the stomach<br>Lower esophageal sphincter relaxes to move food into stomach | None |
| Stomach | Churns and mixes food with digestive enzymes to reduce it to a thin liquid called chyme<br>Forward and backward mixing motion at the pyloric sphincter pushes small amounts of chyme into the duodenum | Secretes pepsin which begins to break down protein into polypeptides<br>Secretes gastric lipase, which has a limited role in fat digestion<br>Secretes intrinsic factor, necessary for the absorption of vitamin B12<br>Absorbs some water, electrolytes, certain drugs, and alcohol |

| BOX 17.1 | DIET FOCUSED ASSESSMENT FOR UPPER GI DISORDERS |
|---|---|

- GI symptoms that interfere with intake such as anorexia, early satiety, difficulty chewing and swallowing; nausea and vomiting; heartburn
- Changes in eating made in response to symptoms
- Complications that impact nutritional status, such as weight loss, aspiration pneumonia, diarrhea
- Usual pattern of eating and frequency of meals and snacks
- Adequacy of intake according to MyPyramid recommendations, including fluid intake
- Use of tobacco, over-the-counter drugs for GI symptoms, alcohol, and caffeine
- Food allergies or intolerances, such as high-fat foods, citrus fruits, spicy food
- Use of nutritional supplements including vitamins, minerals, fiber, and herbs
- Client's willingness to change his or her eating habits

particular foods or textures. Diet-focused assessment criteria for upper GI tract disorders are listed in Box 17.1.

# ▶ DISORDERS THAT AFFECT EATING

## Anorexia

**Anorexia:** lack of appetite; it differs from anorexia nervosa, a psychological condition characterized by denial of appetite.

**Anorexia** is a common symptom of many physical conditions and a side effect of certain drugs. Emotional issues, such as fear, anxiety, and depression, frequently cause anorexia. The aim of nutrition therapy is to stimulate the appetite to maintain adequate nutritional intake. The following interventions may help:

- Serve food attractively and season according to individual taste. If decreased ability to taste is contributing to anorexia, enhance food flavors with tart seasonings (e.g., orange juice, lemonade, vinegar, lemon juice) or strong seasonings (e.g., basil, oregano, rosemary, tarragon, mint).

- Schedule procedures and medications when they are least likely to interfere with meals, if possible.
- Control pain, nausea, or depression with medications as ordered.
- Provide small, frequent meals.
- Withhold beverages for 30 minutes before and after meals to avoid displacing the intake of more nutrient-dense foods.
- Offer liquid supplements between meals for additional calories and protein if meal consumption is low.
- Limit fat intake if fat is contributing to early satiety.

## Nausea and Vomiting

Nausea and vomiting may be related to a decrease in gastric acid secretion, a decrease in digestive enzyme activity, a decrease in gastrointestinal motility, gastric irritation, or acidosis. Other causes include bacterial and viral infection; increased intracranial pressure; equilibrium imbalance; liver, pancreatic, and gallbladder disorders; and pyloric or intestinal obstruction. Drugs and certain medical treatments may also contribute to nausea.

The short term concern of nausea and vomiting is fluid and electrolyte balance. IVs can meet patient needs until an oral intake resumes. With prolonged or **intractable vomiting**, dehydration and weight loss are concerns.

Nutrition intervention for nausea is a common sense approach. Food is withheld until nausea subsides. When the patient is ready to eat, clear liquids are offered and progressed to a regular diet as tolerated. Small, frequent meals of low fat, readily digested carbohydrates are usually best tolerated. Other strategies that may help are to:

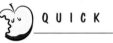

**QUICK BITE**

**High-fat foods**
- "Fats"—nuts, nut butters, oils, margarine, butter, salad dressings
- Fatty meats, such as many processed meats (bologna, pastrami, hard salami), bacon, sausage
- Milk and milk products containing whole or 2% milk
- Rich desserts, such as cakes, pies, cookies, pastries
- Many savory snacks, such as potato chips, cheese puffs, tortilla chips

**Intractable Vomiting:** vomiting that is difficult to manage or cure.

**QUICK BITE**

Readily digested carbohydrates that are low in fat:
Dry toast
Saltine crackers
Plain rolls
Pretzels
Angel food cake
Oatmeal
Soft and bland fruit like canned peaches, canned pears, and banana

- Encourage the patient to eat slowly and not to eat if he or she feels nauseated.
- Promote good oral hygiene with mouthwash and ice chips.
- Limit liquids with meals because they can cause a full, bloated feeling.
- Encourage a liberal fluid intake between meals with whatever liquids the patient can tolerate, such as clear soup, juice, gelatin, ginger ale, and popsicles.
- Serve foods at room temperature or chilled; hot foods may contribute to nausea.
- Avoid high-fat and spicy foods if they contribute to nausea.

# ▶ DISORDERS OF THE ESOPHAGUS

**Dysphagia:** impaired ability to swallow.

Symptoms of esophageal disorders range from difficulty swallowing and the sensation that something is stuck in the throat to heartburn and reflux. **Dysphagia** and gastroesophageal reflux disease are discussed next.

## Dysphagia

Swallowing is a complex series of events characterized by three basic phases (Fig. 17.1). Impairments in swallowing can have a profound impact on intake and nutritional status, and greatly increase the risk of aspiration and its complications of bacterial pneumonia and bronchial obstruction.

Many conditions cause swallowing impairments. Mechanical causes include obstruction, inflammation, edema, and surgery of the throat. Neurologic causes include amyotrophic lateral sclerosis (ALS), myasthenia gravis, cerebrovascular accident, traumatic brain injury,

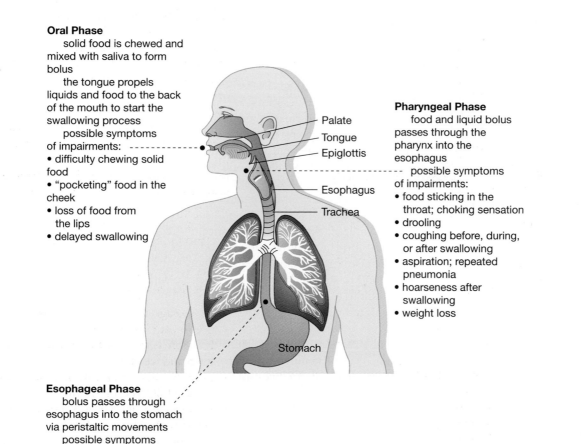

**Oral Phase**
  solid food is chewed and mixed with saliva to form bolus
  the tongue propels liquids and food to the back of the mouth to start the swallowing process
  possible symptoms of impairments:
- difficulty chewing solid food
- "pocketing" food in the cheek
- loss of food from the lips
- delayed swallowing

Palate
Tongue
Epiglottis
Esophagus
Trachea
Stomach

**Pharyngeal Phase**
  food and liquid bolus passes through the pharynx into the esophagus
  possible symptoms of impairments:
- food sticking in the throat; choking sensation
- drooling
- coughing before, during, or after swallowing
- aspiration; repeated pneumonia
- hoarseness after swallowing
- weight loss

**Esophageal Phase**
  bolus passes through esophagus into the stomach via peristaltic movements
  possible symptoms of impairments:
- difficulty with solid food (can handle pureed food)
- heartburn
- vomiting
- burping

**F I G U R E  1 7 . 1**  Swallowing phases and symptoms of impairments.

cerebral palsy, Parkinson's disease, and multiple sclerosis. Refer patients with actual or potential swallowing impairments to the speech pathology department for a thorough swallowing assessment.

## Nutrition Therapy

**Viscosity:** the condition of being resistant to flow; having a heavy, gluey quality.

The goal of nutrition therapy for dysphagia is to modify the texture of foods and/or **viscosity** of liquids to enable the patient to achieve adequate nutrition and hydration while decreasing the risk of aspiration. Solid foods may be minced, mashed, ground, or pureed and thin liquids may be thickened to facilitate swallowing, but these measures often dilute the nutritional value of the diet and make food and beverages less appealing (Germain et al., 2006). Emotionally, dysphagia can affect quality of life; patients with dysphagia may feel panic at mealtime and avoid eating with others (Ekberg et al., 2002). Meeting nutritional needs is a challenge and in some instances, enteral nutrition may be necessary.

The American Dietetic Association has published the National Dysphagia Diet, developed by a group of dietitians, speech and language therapists, and a food scientist for the purpose of standardizing dysphagia diets throughout the United States (The National Dysphagia Diet Task Force, 2002). It is composed of three levels of solid textures and four liquid consistencies (Table 17.2).

The levels of solid food and liquids are ordered separately to allow maximum flexibility and safety in meeting the patient's needs. The patient may start at any of the levels. The solid food consistencies include pureed, mechanically altered, and a more advanced consistency of mixed textures. The liquids are described as thin, nectarlike, honeylike, and spoon-thick.

Generally a speech or language pathologist (SLP) performs a swallowing evaluation on the patient to determine the appropriate consistency of food and liquids and recommends feeding techniques based on the patient's individual status. Changes to the diet prescription are made as the patient's ability to swallow improves or deteriorates.

Generally, moist, semisolid foods are easiest to swallow, such as pudding, custards, scrambled eggs, and yogurt because they form a cohesive bolus that is more easily controlled. Dry, crumbly, and sticky foods are avoided. Some foods, such as bread, are **slurried** to create a texture easily swallowed while retaining the appearance of "regular" bread. Commercial thickeners added to pureed foods can allow pureed foods to be molded into the appearance of "normal" food, which is more visually appealing than "baby food." (Fig. 17.2). In studies comparing molded food to standard pureed food, people with dysphagia found the molded food to be more difficult to eat, instead preferring pureed food (Ballou Stahlman et al., 2000). Flavor enhancers, colored plates, and attractive garnishes can improve the appearance of pureed food.

**Slurried:** a slurry is a thickener dissolved in liquid that is added to dry or pureed foods to produce a texture that is soft and cohesive.

Thickened liquids are more cohesive than thin liquids and are easier to control (Matta et al., 2006). Commercial thickening agents provide instructions on how to mix the product with liquids to achieve the desired consistency, yet wide variations in consistency occur depending on the beverage type, thickener brand, temperature of the liquid, and time between thickened fluid preparation and service to the patient (Adeleye & Rachal, 2007). Commercially prepared thickened beverages are available but viscosity varies among manufacturers and many product labels do not include viscosity. Thickened beverages are often poorly accepted making it difficult to maintain an adequate fluid intake.

Various feeding techniques may facilitate safe swallowing:

- Serve small, frequent meals to help maximize intake.
- Encourage patients with dysphagia to rest before mealtime. Postpone meals if the patient is fatigued.
- Give mouth care immediately before meals to enhance the sense of taste.

| TABLE 17.2 | **National Dysphagia Diet** | | |
|---|---|---|---|
| **Level of Diet** | **Description** | **Foods Allowed** | |
| **Three Levels of Solid Textures** | | | |
| Level 1: Dysphagia Pureed | Foods are totally pureed to a smooth, homogenous consistency. Eliminates sticky foods such as peanut butter and coarse-textured foods such as nuts and raw fruits and vegetables | Smooth cooked cereals; slurried or pureed bread products; milk; smooth desserts such as yogurt, pudding, custard, and applesauce; pureed fruits, vegetables, meats, scrambled eggs, and soups | |
| Level 2: Dysphagia Mechanically Altered | Soft-textured, moist foods that are easily chewed. Eliminates coarse textures, nuts, and raw fruits and vegetables (except banana) | Cooked cereals may have a little texture; some well-moistened ready-to-eat cereals; well-moistened pancakes with syrup; slurried bread; moist well-cooked potatoes, noodles, and dumplings; soft poached or scrambled egg; soft canned or cooked fruit; soft, well-cooked vegetables with $<\frac{1}{2}$ in. pieces (except no corn, peas, and other fibrous vegetables). Moist-ground or minced tender meat in pieces no larger than $\frac{1}{4}$ in., soft casseroles, cottage cheese, tofu; moist cobblers and moist soft cookies; soups with easy to chew meat or vegetables | |
| Level 3: Dysphagia Advanced | Near-normal textured foods; excludes crunchy, sticky, or very hard foods. Food is bite-sized and moist | All breads are allowed except for those that are crusty; moist cereals; most desserts except those with nuts, seeds, coconut, pineapple, or dried fruit; soft, peeled fruit without seeds; moist tender meats or casseroles with small pieces of meat; moist potatoes, rice, and stuffing; all soups except those with chewy meats or vegetables; most cooked, tender vegetables, except corn; shredded lettuce. No nuts, seeds, coconut, and chewy candy | |
| **Four Liquid Consistencies** | | | |
| Thin | All unthickened beverages and supplements | Clear juices, frozen yogurt, ice cream, milk, water, coffee, tea, soda, broth, plain gelatin, liquidy fruits such as watermelon | |
| Nectarlike | Liquids thicker than water but thin enough to sip through a straw | Nectars, vegetable juices, chocolate milk, buttermilk, thin milkshakes, cream soups, other properly thickened beverages | |
| Honeylike | Liquids that can be eaten with a spoon but do not hold their shape | Honey, tomato sauce, yogurt | |
| Spoon-thick | Liquids thickened to pudding consistency that need to be eaten with a spoon | Pudding, custard, hot cereal | |

*Source:* National Dysphagia Diet Task Force. (2002). *National dysphagia diet: Standardization for optimal care.* Chicago, IL: American Dietetic Association.

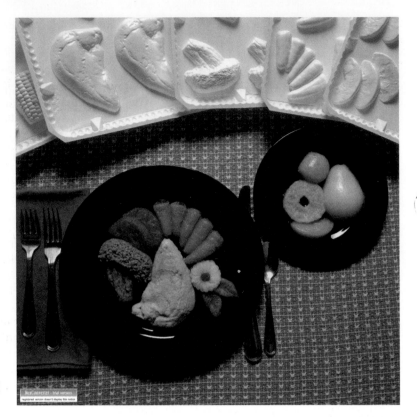

**FIGURE 17.2** Examples of pureed and molded foods.

- Instruct the patient to think of a specific food to stimulate salivation. A lemon slice, lemon hard candy, or dill pickles may also help to trigger salivation, as may moderately flavored foods.
- Reduce or eliminate distractions at mealtime so that the patient can focus his or her attention on swallowing. Limit disruptions, if possible, and do not rush the patient; allow at least 30 minutes for eating.
- Place the patient in an upright or high Fowler's position. If the patient has one-sided facial weakness, place the food on the other side of the mouth. Tilt the head forward to facilitate swallowing.
- Use adaptive eating devices such as built-up utensils and mugs with spouts, if indicated. Syringes should never be used to force liquids into the patient's mouth because this can trigger choking or aspiration. Unless otherwise directed, do not allow the patient to use a straw.
- Encourage small bites and thorough chewing.
- Discourage the patient from consuming alcohol because it reduces cough and gag reflexes.

## Gastroesophageal Reflux Disease

**Gastroesophageal Reflux Disease (GERD):** gastroesophageal reflux is the backflow of gastric acid into the esophagus; gastroesophageal reflux disease occurs when symptoms of reflux happen two or more times a week.

**Gastroesophageal reflux disease (GERD)** is caused by an abnormal reflux of gastric contents into the esophagus related to an abnormal relaxation of the lower esophageal sphincter (Vemulapalli, 2008). Other contributing factors are increased intra-abdominal pressure (e.g., related to hiatal hernia, obesity, or pregnancy) and decreased esophageal motility.

| BOX 17.2 | LIFESTYLE AND NUTRITION THERAPY RECOMMENDATIONS FOR THE TREATMENT OF GERD |
|---|---|

*Lifestyle Recommendations*

Exercise at moderate intensity for at least 30 minutes/day

Lose weight to keep BMI <25

Avoid lying down for 3 hours after meals

Elevate the head of the bed during sleep

*Nutrition Therapy Recommendations*

Avoid:

- Large and/or fatty meals within 3 hours of bed
- Eating too fast
- Drinking alcohol, caffeinated beverages, regular and decaffeinated coffee, soft drinks
- Eating high-fat foods, spicy foods, chocolate, mint, and citrus foods

*Source:* Vemulapalli, R. (2008). Diet and lifestyle modifications in the management of gastroesophageal reflux disease. *Nutrition in Clinical Practice, 23,* 293–298.

Although some people may be relatively asymptomatic, complaining only of a "lump" in their throat, indigestion, "heartburn," and regurgitation are common, especially after eating a large or fatty meal. Pain frequently worsens when the person lies down, bends over after eating, or wears tight-fitting clothing. Chronic untreated GERD may cause reflux esophagitis, dysphagia, adenocarcinoma, esophageal ulcers, and bleeding. The amount of acid refluxed, the severity of heartburn, and the damage to the esophagus do not always correlate: severe pain can occur in the absence of esophageal damage and severe damage may occur with minimal heartburn (Stenson, 2006).

## Nutrition Therapy

A three-pronged approach is used to treat GERD: lifestyle modification, including nutrition therapy; drug therapy; and surgical intervention, if necessary. Lifestyle and diet modifications focus on reducing or eliminating behaviors believed to contribute to GERD (Box 17.2), although proof that these approaches are effective is scarce (Holtmann et al., 2004; Vemulapalli, 2008). In an analysis of all published trials that looked at the impact of lifestyle and diet on GERD symptoms, Kaltenbach, et al. found that elevating the head of the bed, lying on the left side while sleeping, and weight loss were the only strategies that improved GERD somewhat in nonrandomized studies (Kaltenbach et al., 2006). Despite the lack of evidence, lifestyle and diet are considered important adjunct therapies in the treatment of GERD.

## ▶ DISORDERS OF THE STOMACH

Peptic ulcer disease and dumping syndrome from gastric surgery are disorders of the stomach that use nutrition therapy to help control symptoms.

**Peptic Ulcer:** erosion of the mucosal layer of the stomach (gastric ulcer) or duodenum (duodenal ulcer) caused by an excess secretion of, or decreased mucosal resistance to, hydrochloric acid.

### Peptic Ulcer Disease

Approximately 15% of ulcers occur in the stomach and the remaining 85% are in the duodenum; ulcers in either site are known as **peptic ulcer** disease. *Helicobacter pylori* infection is implicated in an estimated 70% of gastric ulcers and 92% of duodenal ulcers (Harbison & Dempsy, 2005), yet most people infected with *H. pylori* do not develop the disease, which suggests other factors may be involved (Ryan-Harshman & Aldoori, 2004). *H. pylori* appears to secrete an enzyme that depletes gastric mucus, making the mucosal layer more susceptible to erosion. For these patients, destroying the bacteria—with antibiotics—generally cures the ulcer. The second leading cause of peptic ulcers is the use of nonsteroidal antiinflammatory drugs (NSAIDs). Eating spicy food does not cause ulcers.

Some people who have peptic ulcers are asymptomatic, while others experience a burning or gnawing pain. Pain may be relieved by food, although gastric ulcers may sometimes be aggravated by eating. Pain, food intolerances, or loss of appetite may impair intake and lead to weight loss. Iron deficiency anemia can develop from blood loss.

Although dietary restrictions are commonly used for ulcers, there is no evidence that diet causes peptic ulcer disease or speeds ulcer healing (Shils et al., 2006). Patients may be told to avoid coffee, alcohol, and chocolate because they stimulate gastric acid secretion, yet consuming moderate amounts of these items has not been shown to impair ulcer healing (Stenson, 2006). Some evidence suggests that a high-fiber diet, especially soluble fiber, may reduce the risk of duodenal ulcer, but other dietary factors, including alcohol and caffeine, have little effect on ulcer risk (Ryan-Harshman & Aldoori, 2004). Nutrition intervention may play a supportive role in treatment by helping to control symptoms. Any of the following strategies may help:

> **QUICK BITE**
>
> **Foods high in soluble fiber**
> Dried peas and beans
> Lentils
> Oats
> Certain fruits and vegetables, such as oranges, potatoes, carrots, apples

- Avoid items that stimulate gastric acid secretion, namely coffee (decaffeinated and regular), alcohol, and pepper.
- Avoid eating 2 hours before bed.
- Avoid individual intolerances.

## Dumping Syndrome

Nutritional complications of gastric surgeries depend on the extent of gastric resection and the type of reconstruction performed. A common complication of gastrectomy and gastric bypass is dumping syndrome, a group of symptoms caused by rapid emptying of stomach contents into the intestine. As the hyperosmolar bolus enters the intestines, fluid shifts from the plasma and extracellular fluid into the intestines to dilute the high particle concentration. The large volume of hypertonic fluid into the jejunum and an increase in peristalsis leads to nausea, vomiting, diarrhea, and abdominal pain. Weakness, dizziness, and a rapid heartbeat occur as the volume of circulating blood decreases. These symptoms occur within 10 to 20 minutes after eating and characterize the early dumping syndrome.

An intermediate dumping reaction occurs 20 to 30 minutes after eating as digested food is fermented in the colon, producing gas, abdominal pain, cramping, and diarrhea (ADA Nutrition Care Manual, 2008). Late dumping syndrome occurs 1 to 3 hours after eating. The rapid absorption of carbohydrate causes a quick spike in blood glucose levels; the body compensates by over-secreting insulin. Blood glucose levels drop rapidly and symptoms of hypoglycemia develop, such as shakiness, sweating, confusion, and weakness.

A reduced stomach capacity, rapid gastric emptying, and rapid transit time increase the risk of maldigestion, malabsorption, and decreased oral intake. The excretion of calories and nutrients produces weight loss and increases the risk of malnutrition. Other potential nutritional complications are outlined in Table 17.3.

## Nutrition Therapy

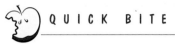

### QUICK BITE

**Sources of sugar alcohols**

- Dietetic foods, such as dietetic candies, sugarless gums, sugar-free cough drops, throat lozenges, and breath mints
- Some fruits and vegetables, such as cherries and berries

Nutrition intervention can control or prevent symptoms of dumping syndrome. Unlike most initial post-op feedings, clear liquids are not used. Patients are started on small frequent meals consisting of protein, fat, and complex carbohydrates, but only one or two items are given each meal. Liquids are provided between meals, not with meals, because they promote quick

| TABLE 17.3 | Potential Nutritional Complications of Dumping Syndrome | |
|---|---|---|
| **Potential Complication** | **Possible Contributing Factors** | **Possible Treatment** |
| Iron deficiency anemia | Decreased food intake<br>A decrease in HCL secretion impairs the conversion of iron to its absorbable form<br>If the duodenum is bypassed or food moves through it too quickly, iron absorption cannot occur (the duodenum is the site of iron absorption) | Iron supplementation is necessary |
| Steatorrhea (excess fat in the stools) | Rapid intestinal time does not allow enough time for fat to be exposed to digestive enzymes<br>If the duodenum is bypassed, less pancreatic lipase mixes is available to digest fat<br>Bacterial overgrowth (excessive growth of intestinal bacteria) can develop from low-gastric acidity or altered motility; it interferes with the action of bile which is important for the emulsification of fat | Supplemental pancreatic enzymes may be necessary<br>Medium chain triglycerides may be used for additional calories (but lack the essential fatty acids)<br>Supplements of fat soluble vitamins may be prescribed; their absorption is dependent upon the absorption of fat |
| Pernicious anemia | Intrinsic factor, necessary for the absorption of vitamin B12 from the intestine, is produced by the stomach. It may be absent after gastric surgery. It may take years for a deficiency to develop | Injections of vitamin B12 may be necessary |
| Osteomalacia (softening of the bones) | Calcium is normally absorbed in the duodenum; if it is bypassed or the transit time is too rapid, calcium malabsorption can occur<br>Fat malabsorption causes calcium and vitamin D to be malabsorbed<br>Lower calcium intake related to lactose intolerance | Supplements of calcium and vitamin D may be necessary |

**Functional Fiber:** fiber that has been isolated from food that has beneficial physiological effects.

movement through the GI tract. Simple sugars and sugar alcohols are avoided to limit the hypertonicity of the mass as it reaches the jejunum. Lactose may be restricted because lactose intolerance is common. Patients are advised to lie down after eating and **functional fibers**, such as pectin and guar gum, may be used to delay gastric emptying and treat diarrhea (ADA Nutrition Care Manual, 2008). Over time the diet is liberalized as the remaining portion of the stomach or duodenum hypertrophies to hold more food and allow for more normal digestion. Box 17.3 features antidumping syndrome diet guidelines (see Chapter 14 for more on bariatric surgery).

---

| BOX 17.3 | ANTIDUMPING SYNDROME DIET GUIDELINES |
|---|---|

Eating strategies:

- Eat small, frequent meals
- Consume beverages between, not with, meals
- Avoid sugar, honey, syrup, sorbitol, and xylitol and all food and beverages that have any of those listed as one of the first 3 ingredients on the label
- Eat a source of protein at each meal because it helps slow gastric emptying
- Choose low-fiber grains; mostly canned, not fresh fruit; nongassy, well-cooked vegetables without seeds or skins

Recommended foods:

- Breads and cereals: refined plain breads, crackers, rolls, unsweetened cereal, rice, and pasta that provide less than 2 g fiber/serving
- Vegetables: well-cooked or raw vegetables without seeds or skins, vegetable juice Avoid "gassy" vegetables such as broccoli, cauliflower, cabbage, and corn
- Fruits: banana, soft melons, unsweetened canned fruit, unsweetened fruit juices
- Milk and milk products: any milk (if not lactose intolerant); choose yogurt, soy milk, and ice cream without sugar added
- Meat and meat alternatives: avoid all of the following: *except* fried meats, fish, and poultry; high-fat luncheon meats, sausage, hot dogs, and bacon; tough or chewy meats; dried peas and beans; nuts and nut butters
- Fats: oils, butter, margarine, cream cheese, mayonnaise
- Beverages: decaffeinated tea, artificially sweetened soft drinks; diluted fruit juice. Avoid caffeinated beverages, alcohol

**Sample Menu**

*Breakfast:*
1 poached egg
1 slice white toast with butter
1 hour later: 6 oz apricot nectar

*Mid-Morning Snack:*
Firm banana
Butter crackers

*Lunch:*
½ cup cottage cheese with two unsweetened,
  canned peach halves
Dinner roll with butter
1 hour later: 8 oz artificially sweetened ginger ale

*Mid-Afternoon Snack:*
2 oz cheddar cheese
4 saltine crackers

*Dinner:*
3 oz baked chicken
½ cup white rice with butter
½ cup cooked carrots with butter
1 hour later: hot tea

*Bedtime Snack:*
1 cup yogurt without sugar added

*Source:* American Dietetic Association. *Nutrition care manual* (online). Copyright 2008. Accessed on 5/30/08.

## *NURSING PROCESS: GERD*

Jason is 28 years old and complains of frequent painful heartburn. He takes antacids on a daily basis and has lost 14 pounds over the last few months. His strategy to avoid pain is to avoid eating. He smokes 2 packs of cigarettes/day. He is 5 ft. 8 in. tall, weighs 170 pounds, and has an appointment to see his doctor. In the meantime he has come to you, the corporate nurse on staff where he works, to see what he can do to help control his heartburn.

| Assessment | |
|---|---|
| Medical–Psychosocial History | • Medical history that would contribute to GERD, such as hiatal hernia |
| | • Symptoms that may affect nutrition, such as difficulty swallowing or nausea and vomiting |
| | • Use of medications that may lower LES pressure, such as anticholinergic agents, diazepam, or theophylline |
| | • Use of medications that may damage the mucosa, such as NSAIDs or aspirin |
| | • History of smoking |
| | • Level of activity |
| Anthropometric Assessment | BMI, % weight loss |
| Biochemical and Physical Assessment | Abnormal lab values, if available, especially hemoglogin and hematocrit because low values may indicate bleeding, |
| | • How many meals do you eat daily? |
| Dietary Assessment | • Would you say your meals are small, medium, or large in size? |
| | • Are there any particular foods that cause indigestion, especially alcohol, coffee, tea, caffeine, pepper, mint, chocolate, or fatty foods? |
| | • What foods do you avoid? |
| | • Can you correlate your symptoms to: <br> • Lying down after eating? <br> • Wearing tight clothes? <br> • Eating right before bed? |
| | • Do you take vitamins, minerals, herbs, or other supplements? |
| | • Do you have ethnic, religious, or cultural food preferences? |

| Diagnosis | |
|---|---|
| Possible Nursing Diagnosis | Imbalanced nutrition: less than body requirements as evidenced by weight loss related to inadequate intake secondary to heartburn |

| Planning | |
|---|---|
| Client Outcomes | The client will: |
| | • Report relief from symptoms |
| | • Consume adequate calories and nutrients |
| | • Use less medication to control symptoms |
| | • Explain the role of diet in controlling GERD symptoms |
| | • Exhibit normal laboratory values |

*(nursing process continues on page 414)*

## *NURSING PROCESS: GERD* (continued)

### Nursing Interventions

| | |
|---|---|
| Nutrition Therapy | • Avoid items that increase gastric acid secretion and/or lower LES pressure<br> • Alcohol<br> • Black and red pepper<br> • Coffee<br> • Chocolate<br> • Fatty foods<br> • Mint<br>• Eat small frequent meals to avoid increasing intra-abdominal pressure but avoid eating within 3 hours of bedtime<br>• Consume liquids between meals instead of with meals to limit distention of the stomach<br>• Avoid spicy, acidic, or tomato-based foods that may irritate the esophagus<br>• Eliminate any foods not tolerated |
| Client Teaching | Instruct the client:<br>• That nutrition interventions may help control symptoms but do not treat the underlying problem<br>• On lifestyle modifications that may help improve symptoms, such as losing weight, smoking cessation, and regular exercise<br>• To avoid pressure on the abdomen and LES<br> • Raise the head of the bed<br> • Do not bend over or lie down after eating<br> • Do not wear tight-fitting clothes |

### Evaluation

| | |
|---|---|
| Evaluate and Monitor | • Monitor for improvement in symptoms<br>• Monitor weight<br>• Monitor for medication usage |

### ▶ HOW DO YOU RESPOND?

**If over-the-counter drugs to combat heartburn are as good as advertised, why should I worry about what to eat if taking a pill can allow me to eat what I want without any pain?** Although they work well, relying on medications to stave off pain after eating whatever, whenever, and in any amount is foolhardy. All medications have the potential to cause side effects, and pain is a signal that something is wrong. Encourage clients to implement eating and lifestyle changes to see if they alone can prevent symptoms.

### ▶ CASE STUDY

Barbara is a 72-year-old, "Type A" personality who was diagnosed with a peptic ulcer more than 40 years ago. At that time her doctor told her to follow a bland diet and eat 3 meals/day with 3 snacks/day of whole milk to "quiet" her stomach. She meticulously complied with the diet to the point of becoming obsessive about eating anything that may not be "allowed." She lost 15 pounds by following the bland diet because her intake was so restricted. She recently began experiencing ulcer symptoms and has put herself back on the bland diet, convinced it is necessary in order to recover from her ulcer.

Yesterday she ate:

| | |
|---|---|
| **Breakfast:** | 1 poached egg<br>2 slices dry white toast<br>1 cup whole milk |
| **Morning Snack:** | 1 cup whole milk |
| **Lunch:** | ¾ cup cottage cheese with ½ cup canned peaches |
| **Afternoon snack:** | 1 cup whole milk |
| **Dinner:** | 3 oz boiled chicken<br>½ cup boiled plain potatoes<br>½ cup boiled green beans<br>½ cup gelatin |
| **Evening snack:** | 1 cup whole milk |

- Barbara's 1600 calorie MyPyramid plan calls for 1.5 cups of fruit, 2 cups of vegetables, 5 grains, 5 ounces of meat/beans, 3 cups of milk, and 5 teaspoons of oils. How does her intake compare? What food groups is she undereating? Overeating? What are the potential nutritional consequences of her current diet?
- What other information would be helpful for you to know in dealing with Barbara?
- Barbara clearly wants to be on a bland diet; what would you tell her about diet recommendations for peptic ulcer disease? What recommendations would you make to improve her symptoms and meet her nutritional requirements while respecting her need to follow a "diet"?

1. The patient asks if coffee is bad for his peptic ulcer. Which of the following would be the nurse's best response?
   a. "Coffee does not cause ulcers and drinking it probably does not interfere with ulcer healing. You may try eliminating it from your diet to see what impact it has on your symptoms and then decide whether or not to avoid it."
   b. "Both caffeinated and decaffeinated coffee can cause ulcers and interfere with ulcer healing. You should eliminate both from your diet."
   c. "You need to eliminate caffeinated coffee from your diet but it is safe to drink decaffeinated coffee."
   d. "You can drink all the coffee you want; it does not affect ulcers."

2. Which statement indicates the patient needs further instruction about GERD?
   a. "I know a bland diet will help prevent the heartburn I get after eating."
   b. "Lying down after eating can make GERD symptoms worse."
   c. "High-fat meals can make GERD symptoms worse."
   d. "Losing excess weight can help prevent symptoms of GERD."

3. Which of the following snacks would be best for a patient who wants to eat who has nausea?
   a. Cheese
   b. Peanuts
   c. Fat-free pudding
   d. A milkshake

4. The nurse knows her instructions have been effective when the patient with dumping syndrome verbalizes she should:
    a. Avoid lying down after eating.
    b. Drink liquids between, not with, meals.
    c. Eat easily digested carbohydrates.
    d. Avoid protein.

5. A patient with dumping syndrome asks why it is so important to avoid sugars and sweets. Which of the following is the nurse's best response?
    a. "Sugars and sweets provide empty calories, so they should be limited in everyone's diet."
    b. "Sugars draw water into the intestines and cause cramping and diarrhea."
    c. "Sugar makes blood glucose levels increase; hyperglycemia is a complication of dumping syndrome."
    d. "Avoiding sugars and sweets helps ensure that they will not displace the intake of protein, which you need for healing."

6. Which of the following is an appropriate breakfast for a patient on a level 1 dysphagia diet?
    a. Poached egg
    b. Cream of wheat
    c. Granola with milk
    d. Toast cut into small pieces

7. A patient who develops pernicious anemia after gastric surgery needs supplemental:
    a. Protein
    b. Iron
    c. Calcium
    d. Vitamin B12

8. The best dessert for a patient with GERD is:
    a. Chocolate cake
    b. Peppermint ice cream
    c. Fresh orange sections
    d. Pineapple sherbet

## KEY CONCEPTS

- Nutrition therapy for GI disorders may help minimize or prevent symptoms. For some GI disorders, nutrition therapy is the cornerstone of treatment.

- Small, frequent meals may help to maximize intake in patients who have anorexia. Avoiding high-fat foods may lessen the feeling of fullness.

- After nausea and vomiting subside, low-fat, easily digested carbohydrate foods, such as crackers, toast, oatmeal, and bland fruit, usually are well tolerated. Patients should avoid liquids with meals because liquids can promote the feeling of fullness.

- The National Dysphagia Diet has three different solid food textures and four different liquid consistencies. A speech and language pathologist recommends the appropriate level for solids and liquids based on a swallowing evaluation.

- Pureed foods are less calorically dense than normal textured foods. They are also less visually appealing. Patients with dysphagia are monitored for poor intakes and weight loss.

- People with GERD should lose weight if overweight, avoid large meals and bedtime snacks, eliminate individual intolerances, and avoid alcohol, caffeine, decaffeinated coffee, chocolate, fatty foods, peppermint and spearmint flavors, and cigarette smoke.

- There is no evidence that diet causes ulcers or promotes their healing. Patients are commonly advised to avoid items that stimulate gastric acid secretion and any foods not tolerated.

- Nutrition therapy for dumping syndrome consists of eating small, frequent meals; eating protein at each meal; and avoiding concentrated sugars and sugar alcohols. Liquids should be consumed 1 hour before or after eating instead of with meals.

## ANSWER KEY

1. **TRUE** Drinking liquids with meals may promote a bloated feeling and contribute to nausea. Encourage patients to drink fluids between meals, especially clear liquids such as water, clear juices, gelatin, ginger ale, and Popsicles.

2. **FALSE** Thin liquids are the most difficult consistency to control for people who have swallowing difficulties. Thickened liquids have a more cohesive consistency that is easier to manage.

3. **FALSE** The degree of texture modification for dysphagia is determined by the individual's ability to chew and swallow. There are three levels of solid textures: pureed, mechanically altered, and an advanced consistency of mixed textures.

4. **FALSE** The severity of the pain is not correlated to the extent of esophageal damage. Some people have severe damage with only minor symptoms.

5. **TRUE** Fat lowers LES pressure so high-fat meals may cause symptoms of GERD.

6. **TRUE** Spicy or acidic foods may irritate the esophagus when it is inflamed. Patients should avoid any foods not tolerated.

7. **TRUE** Alcohol stimulates gastric acid secretion and, in theory, should be avoided by people with peptic ulcer disease.

8. **FALSE** A bland diet is considered obsolete. It does not promote ulcer healing and eating moderate amounts of nonbland foods has not been shown to irritate peptic ulcers.

9. **TRUE** People with dumping syndrome should avoid sugars and sweets because they contribute to a high osmolar load when the gastric contents enter the intestine. Over time the diet is liberalized to allow sugars and sweets as the remaining stomach and intestine accommodate to the change in the stomach's holding capacity.

10. **TRUE** Because intrinsic factor is produced in the stomach and is necessary for the intestinal absorption of vitamin B12, people who have had a gastrectomy are at risk of developing pernicious anemia. The symptoms may take years to develop because the body stores vitamin B12.

## WEBSITES

American College of Gastroenterology at **www.acg.gi.org**
American Gastroenterological Association at **www.gastro.org**

## REFERENCES

Adeleye, B., & Rachal, C. (2007). Comparison of the rheological properties of ready-to-serve and powdered instant food-thickened beverages at different temperatures for dysphagic patients. *Journal of the American Dietetic Association, 107,* 1176–1182.

American Dietetic Association (ADA) Nutrition Care Manual (2008). Retrieved <5/30/08 from http://www.nutritioncaremanual.org.

Ballou Stahlman, L., Mertz Garcia, J., Hakel, M., et al. (2000). Comparison ratings of pureed versus molded fruits: Preliminary results. *Dysphagia, 15,* 2–5.

Ekberg, O., Hamdy, S., Woisard, V., et al. (2002). Social and psychological burden of dysphagia: Its impact on diagnosis and treatment. *Dysphagia, 17,* 139–146.

Germain, S., Dufresne, T., & Gray-Donald, K. (2006). A novel dysphagia diet improves the nutrient intake of institutionalized elders. *Journal of the American Dietetic Association, 106,* 1614–1623.

Harbison, S., & Dempsey, D. (2005). Peptic ulcer disease. *Current Problems in Surgery, 42,* 346–454.

Holtmann, D., Adam, B., & Liebregts, T. (2004). Review article: The patient with gastro-esophageal reflux disease. *Alimentary Pharmacology & Therapeutics, 20,* 24–27.

Kaltenbach, T., Crockett, S., & Gerson, L. (2006). Are lifestyle measures effective in patients with gastroesophageal reflux disease? An evidence-based approach. *Archives of Internal Medicine, 166,* 965–971.

Matta, Z., Chambers, E., IV, Garcia, J., et al. (2006). Sensory characteristics of beverages prepared with commercial thickeners used for dysphagia diets. *Journal of the American Dietetic Association, 106,* 1049–1054.

National Dysphagia Diet Task Force (2002). *The national dysphagia diet: Standardization for optimal care.* Chicago, IL: American Dietetic Association.

Ryan-Harshman, M., & Aldoori, W. (2004). How diet and lifestyle affect duodenal ulcers. *Canadian Family Physician, 50,* 727–732.

Stenson, W. (2006). In: Shils, M. E., Shike, M., Ross, A. C., et al. (Eds.). *Modern nutrition in health and disease* (10th ed.). Philadelphia: Lippincott Williams & Wilkins.

Vemulapalli, R. (2008). Diet and lifestyle modifications in the management of gastroesophageal reflux disease. *Nutrition in Clinical Practice, 23,* 293–298.

# 18

# Nutrition for Patients with Disorders of the Lower GI Tract and Accessory Organs

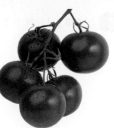

| TRUE | FALSE | |
|:---:|:---:|---|
| ☐ | ☐ | **1** A high-fiber diet can prevent or alleviate constipation in most people. |
| ☐ | ☐ | **2** A clear liquid diet is the best oral diet for a patient with acute diarrhea. |
| ☐ | ☐ | **3** Medium chain triglyceride (MCT) oil is used to provide essential fatty acids to people who have fat malabsorption. |
| ☐ | ☐ | **4** Many people with lactose intolerance can tolerate cheddar cheese. |
| ☐ | ☐ | **5** People with inflammatory bowel disease (IBD) should follow a low-fiber diet to prevent exacerbation of their disease. |
| ☐ | ☐ | **6** People with celiac disease need a gluten-free diet even when they are asymptomatic. |
| ☐ | ☐ | **7** A high-fiber diet has been proven to control symptoms of irritable bowel syndrome. |
| ☐ | ☐ | **8** A high-fiber diet may prevent diverticulosis and diverticulitis. |
| ☐ | ☐ | **9** Fat is the nutrient most problematic for people with chronic pancreatitis. |
| ☐ | ☐ | **10** Most people with gallstones benefit from a low-fat diet. |

## UPON COMPLETION OF THIS CHAPTER, YOU WILL BE ABLE TO

- Modify a regular diet to be high in fiber.
- Instruct a patient on the nutrition therapy recommendations for diarrhea.
- Give examples of appropriate nutrition interventions for various symptoms and complications of malabsorption syndrome.
- Modify a regular diet to be low in residue.
- Identify sources of gluten.
- Instruct a patient with an ileostomy on appropriate diet modifications.
- Compare a low-fat diet to a regular diet.

The lower gastrointestinal (GI) tract consists of the small and large intestines, rectum, and anus. Ninety to ninety-five percent of nutrient absorption occurs in the first half of the small intestine (Fig. 18.1). The large intestine absorbs water and electrolytes and promotes the elimination of solid wastes. The accessory organs—liver, gallbladder, and pancreas—play vital roles in nutrient digestion. With many disorders of the lower GI tract and accessory organs, nutrition therapy is used to improve or control symptoms, replenish losses, and promote healing, if applicable. For one GI disorder, celiac disease, nutrition therapy is the sole mode of treatment. This chapter presents nutrition therapy for altered bowel elimination, malabsorption syndromes, disorders of the large intestine, and disorders of the accessory organs. Box 18.1 lists diet-focused assessment criteria for lower GI disorders.

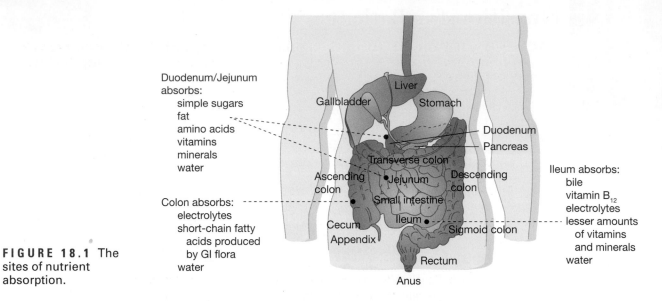

**FIGURE 18.1** The sites of nutrient absorption.

Duodenum/Jejunum absorbs:
  simple sugars
  fat
  amino acids
  vitamins
  minerals
  water

Colon absorbs:
  electrolytes
  short-chain fatty
    acids produced
    by GI flora
  water

Liver
Gallbladder
Stomach
Duodenum
Pancreas
Transverse colon
Ascending colon
Jejunum
Descending colon
Small intestine
Cecum
Ileum
Appendix
Sigmoid colon
Rectum
Anus

Ileum absorbs:
  bile
  vitamin B$_{12}$
  electrolytes
  lesser amounts
    of vitamins
    and minerals
  water

---

| BOX 18.1 | DIET-FOCUSED ASSESSMENT FOR LOWER GI DISORDERS |
|---|---|

- GI symptoms that interfere with intake, such as anorexia, early satiety, pain, abdominal distention
- Changes in eating made in response to symptoms
- Complications that impact nutritional status, such as weight loss, diarrhea, blood loss
- Usual pattern of eating and frequency of meals and snacks
- Adequacy of intake according to MyPyramid recommendations, including fluid intake
- Use of tobacco, over-the-counter drugs for GI symptoms, alcohol, and caffeine
- Food allergies or intolerances, such as high-fat foods, milk, high-fiber foods
- Use of nutritional supplements including vitamins, minerals, fiber, and herbs
- Client's willingness to change his or her eating habits

## ▶ ALTERED BOWEL ELIMINATION

### Constipation

Constipation is the difficult or infrequent passage of stools that are hard and dry. It can occur secondary to irregular bowel habits, psychogenic factors, lack of activity, chronic laxative use, inadequate intake of fluid and fiber, metabolic and endocrine disorders, and bowel abnormalities (e.g., tumors, hernias, strictures). Certain medications, such as codeine, aluminum hydroxide, iron supplements, and morphine, cause constipation. Contrary to popular belief, daily bowel movements are not necessary provided the stools are not hard and dry.

#### Nutrition Therapy

Constipation is treated by treating the underlying cause. For most people, increasing fiber and fluid intake effectively relieves and prevents constipation. Fiber, particularly insoluble fiber found in wheat bran and fruit and vegetable skins, increases stool bulk and stimulates peristalsis. Soluble fiber, such as psyllium and inulin, absorbs water to produce softer, bulkier stools that are more easily passed.

A high-fiber diet substitutes high-fiber grains for refined grains and increases the intake of other food sources of fiber, namely fresh fruits, vegetables, and dried peas and beans (Box 18.2). Exactly how much fiber is needed to alleviate constipation varies among

| BOX 18.2 | **HIGH-FIBER DIET** |

- A high-fiber diet is a regular diet that substitutes whole grains for refined grains and is high in other fiber-rich foods, namely fresh fruits, vegetables, and dried peas and beans
- Unprocessed bran may be added as tolerated
- At least eight 8-ounce glasses of fluid are recommended daily
- A high-fiber diet is used for constipation, diverticulosis, and irritable bowel syndrome. It may also promote weight loss and helps lower serum cholesterol levels and improve glucose tolerance in diabetes. All healthy Americans are urged to increase their intake of fiber
- The diet should not be used in cases of intestinal inflammation or stenosis, gastroparesis, postgastrectomy, or pseudo-obstruction

### Guidelines to Achieve a High-Fiber Diet
- Substitute whole grains for refined grains:

| *Use* | *In place of* |
|---|---|
| Whole wheat bread | White bread |
| Brown rice | White rice |
| Whole wheat pasta | White pasta |
| Bran or whole grain cereal | Refined cereals |
| Whole-wheat flour | White flour |

- Eat one serving of dried peas or beans daily
- Eat more fresh fruit; leave the skin on whenever possible. Apples, blackberries, blueberries, figs, dates, kiwifruit, mango, oranges, pears, prunes, strawberries, and raspberries are high in fiber
- Eat more vegetables. Cooked asparagus, green beans, broccoli, Brussels sprouts, cabbage, carrots, celery, corn, eggplant, parsnips, peas, snowpeas, Swiss chard, and turnips are good choices
- Other foods with fiber include popcorn, nuts, sunflower seeds, and sesame seeds

### Sample Menu

| Breakfast | Lunch | Dinner | Snacks |
|---|---|---|---|
| Prune juice | Split pea soup | Roast chicken | Low-fat popcorn |
| Bran flakes with milk | Ham sandwich on whole-wheat bread with lettuce and tomato | Brown rice | Dried fruit and nuts |
| Whole-wheat toast with jelly | Fresh strawberries | Tossed salad with fresh vegetables | Raw carrots and celery with dip |
| Fresh orange sections | Date cookie | Steamed broccoli | |
| | Milk | Whole-wheat roll with butter | |
| | | Milk | |
| | | Blueberries over ice cream | |

### Potential Problems

Flatus, distention, cramping, and osmotic diarrhea related to increasing fiber content of the diet too much or too quickly

Possible malabsorption of calcium, zinc, and iron from increased GI motility (which allows less time for absorption to occur) or from the binding of these minerals with fiber to form compounds the body cannot absorb

### Recommended Interventions

Initiate a high-fiber diet gradually to develop the patient's tolerance. If symptoms of intolerance persist, reduce fiber content to maximum amount tolerated by the patient

Actual fiber-induced deficiencies are unlikely because the body adapts to a high-fiber diet. However, foods rich in calcium, zinc, and iron should be encouraged

*(box continues on page 422)*

| BOX 18.2 | HIGH-FIBER DIET (continued) |
| --- | --- |

**Patient Teaching**

Instruct the patient that

- A high-fiber diet increases stool bulk and speeds passage of food through intestines
- Fiber intake may be increased by making subtle changes in eating and cooking habits such as eating more fresh fruits and vegetables, especially with the skin on
- Switching to high-fiber breads and cereals can significantly increase fiber intake. The first ingredient on the label should be "whole wheat" or "100% whole wheat," not just "wheat"
- A variety of foods high in fiber should be eaten; numerous forms of fiber exist and each performs a different action in the body (see Chapter 2)
- A meatless main dish made with dried peas and beans is a high-fiber alternative to traditional entrées
- Fresh or dried fruit make high-fiber snacks
- Although nuts and seeds are high in fiber, they are also high in fat and should be used sparingly
- Coarse, unprocessed wheat bran is most effective as a laxative. It can be incorporated into the diet by mixing it with juice or milk; by adding it to muffins, quick breads, casseroles, and meat loaves before baking; or by sprinkling it over cereal, applesauce, eggs, or other foods
- Bran should be added to the diet slowly (up to 3 tbsp/day) to decrease the likelihood of developing flatus and distention
- Certain foods (in addition to being high in fiber) have laxative effects: prunes and prune juice, figs, and dates
- At least eight 8-ounce glasses of fluid should be consumed daily

**QUICK BITE**

**Fiber supplements**

*Promoted for regularity*

Metamucil

Ready fiber

Citrucel

*Promoted for lowering LDL cholesterol*

Fibersure          Metamucil

Benefiber          Ready Fiber

individuals. The adequate intake (AI) set for fiber is 25 g/day for women and 38 g/day for men, approximately double the average American adult intake of approximately 12 to 18 g of fiber per day (IOM, 2005). Most fruits, vegetables, and whole-wheat breads provide only 1 to 3 g of fiber per serving; without a high-fiber cereal or daily intake of dried peas and beans, many people may require a fiber supplement to meet the *Dietary Reference Intake* (DRI) for fiber (Timm & Slavin, 2008).

It is common practice to recommend that fiber intake be gradually increased to avoid symptoms of intolerance such as gas, cramping, and diarrhea. If these side effects do occur, they are usually temporary and subside within several days. To achieve maximum benefit, fiber intake should be spread throughout the day. In some people, a high-fiber diet makes constipation worse (Muller-Lissner et al., 2005).

Lifestyle changes to promote bowel regularity include drinking more fluid and increasing exercise. Without adequate fluid, a high-fiber diet can lead to more constipation, abdominal pain, bloating, and gas (ADA Nutrition Care Manual, 2006). Aerobic exercise helps promote muscle tone and stimulates bowel activity.

# Diarrhea

Diarrhea is characterized by more than three bowel movements a day of large amounts of liquid or semiliquid stool. A shortened transit time decreases the time available for water, sodium, and potassium to be absorbed through the colon; the result is more water and electrolytes in the stools and the potential for dehydration, hyponatremia, hypokalemia, acid–base imbalance, and metabolic acidosis. Chronic diarrhea can lead to malnutrition related to impaired digestion, absorption, and intake.

Osmotic diarrhea occurs when there is an increase in particles in the intestine, which draws water in to dilute the high concentration. The causes of osmotic diarrhea include maldigestion of nutrients (e.g., lactose intolerance), excessive intake of sorbitol or fructose, dumping syndrome, tube feedings, and some laxatives. It is cured by treating the underlying cause.

Secretory diarrhea is related to an excessive secretion of fluid and electrolytes into the intestines. Bacterial, viral, protozoan, and other infections cause secretory diarrhea, as do some medications, and some GI disorders, such as Crohn's disease and celiac disease. An excessive amount of bile acids or unabsorbed fatty acids in the colon can also cause secretory diarrhea (ADA, 2006). If the cause is infectious, antibiotics are the primary component of treatment. Symptoms may be treated with medications that decrease GI motility or thicken the consistency of stools, such as the soluble fiber psyllium (Metamucil).

## Nutrition Therapy

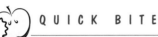

**QUICK BITE**

**The World Health Organization's recipe for an oral rehydration solution**

⅓–⅔ tsp table salt
¾ tsp baking soda
⅓ tsp potassium chloride (salt substitute)
1⅓ tbsp sugar or rice powder
1 L bottled or sterile water

*Source:* ADA. Nutrition Care Manual. 2006; (Available at: www.nutritioncare manual.org. Accessed in 2008).

**QUICK BITE**

High-potassium foods include

| | |
|---|---|
| Apricot nectar | Orange juice |
| Avocado | Papaya |
| Banana | Potatoes |
| Canned apricots and peaches | Tomato juice |
| Cantaloupe | Yogurt |

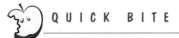

**QUICK BITE**

**Items that stimulate GI motility**

• Alcohol
• Caffeine
• Clear liquids and other foods high in simple sugars, such as milk (lactose) and fruit (fructose)
• High-fiber and gas-producing foods, such as nuts, beans, corn, broccoli, and cabbage
• Sugar alcohols (e.g., sorbitol in "dietetic" products)

*Source:* ADA Nutrition Care Manual, 2006. (Available at: www.nutritioncare manual.org. Accessed in 2008).

**Probiotics:** "live organisms which when administered in adequate amounts confer a health benefit on the host" (FAO/WHO, 2002)

The primary nutritional concern with diarrhea is maintaining or restoring fluid and electrolyte balance. Mild diarrhea lasting 24 to 48 hours usually requires no nutrition intervention other than encouraging a liberal fluid intake to replace losses. High-potassium foods are encouraged. Clear liquids are avoided because they have high osmolality related to their high sugar content, which may promote osmotic diarrhea. For more serious cases, commercial (e.g., Pedialyte, Rehydralyte) or homemade oral rehydration solutions or IV therapy is used to replace fluid and electrolytes.

Diarrhea may improve by avoiding foods that stimulate GI motility. **Probiotics** may

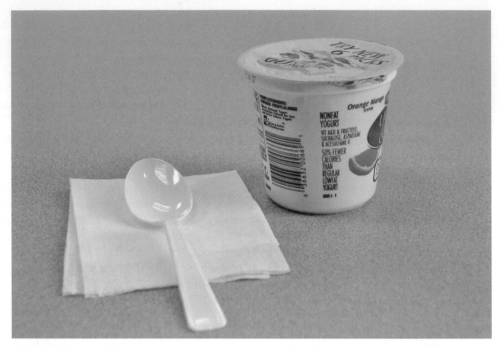

**FIGURE 18.2** Many yogurts now contain beneficial microorganisms called "probiotics."

**Lactose:** the disaccharide (double sugar) in milk composed of glucose and galactose

help lessen diarrhea related to intolerance to antibiotics or **lactose** (Douglas & Sanders, 2008) (Fig. 18.2). On a short-term basis, a low-fiber diet (Box 18.3) that is also low in fat and lactose may help decrease bowel stimulation. This diet may be inadequate in all nutrients depending on the specific foods chosen (ADA, 2006). Patients with intractable diarrhea may need complete bowel rest (i.e., total parenteral nutrition, or TPN).

## ▶ MALABSORPTION DISORDERS

**Malabsorption:** a broad term that describes altered or inadequate nutrient absorption from the GI tract

**Malabsorption** occurs secondary to nutrient maldigestion or from alterations to the absorptive surface of the intestinal mucosa. Generally malabsorption related to maldigestion involves one or few nutrients, whereas malabsorption that stems from an altered mucosa is more generalized, resulting in multiple nutrient deficiencies and weight loss.

Symptoms of malabsorption vary with the underlying disorder, ranging from minimal to widespread and serious. Malabsorption may be suspected in patients who have weight loss, growth failure, bloating, and flatulence (Kelly, 2006). Watery diarrhea and distention are symptoms of malabsorption from carbohydrate maldigestion (e.g., lactose intolerance), whereas the passage of less frequent stools that are oily, bulky, and foul-smelling is a symptom of malabsorption related to fat maldigestion (e.g., pancreatitis). The excretion of fat in the stools means that essential fatty acids, fat-soluble vitamins, calcium, and magnesium are also lost through the stools. Deficiencies of these nutrients can cause metabolic complications (Table 18.1). Appetite may be poor and nutrient needs may be elevated for healing. The risk for malnutrition is high.

**Steatorrhea:** excess fat in the stools that are loose, foamy, and foul-smelling

The goal of nutrition therapy for malabsorption syndromes is to control **steatorrhea**, promote normal bowel elimination, restore optimal nutritional status, and promote healing, when applicable. Nutrition therapy is individualized according to symptoms and complications;

| BOX 18.3 | LOW-FIBER DIET |

- This diet restricts insoluble fiber because it increases stool bulk, which decreases transit time and stimulates peristalsis. Soluble fiber has less of an effect on stool bulk and is not restricted
- This diet is a short-term diet to be used when the bowel is inflamed, such as in the acute stages of diverticulitis, ulcerative colitis, and regional enteritis. It may also be used for esophageal and intestinal stenosis and in preparation for bowel surgery

**General Guidelines to Achieve a Low-Fiber Diet**
- Use refined breads and cereals that provide 0–1 g fiber/serving, such as white bread and rolls, white pasta, white rice, low-fiber cereals
- Eat only vegetables that do not have skins or seeds and are well-cooked
- Choose canned or cooked fruit and fruit juices without pulp (except prune juice); ripe bananas, citrus sections without membranes
- Eat plain desserts made without nuts or coconut, such as plain cakes, puddings (rice, bread, plain), cookies, and ice cream
- Avoid foods high in fiber
  - Whole-grain breads and cereals
  - Most raw vegetables, vegetables with seeds, gassy vegetables
  - Fresh fruit with skins or seeds, dried fruits, prune juice
  - Dried peas and beans
  - Anything containing nuts, seeds, or coconut; popcorn

**Sample Menu**

| Breakfast | Lunch | Dinner | Snacks |
|---|---|---|---|
| Strained orange juice | Tomato juice | Roast chicken | Saltine crackers |
| Cream of rice | Ham sandwich on white bread with mayonnaise | White rice | Rice cakes |
| Poached egg | | Cooked carrots | Tomato juice |
| White toast with jelly | Canned peach halves | Italian bread with olive oil | Fresh banana |
| Milk | Sponge cake | Gelatin made with ripe bananas | |
| | Milk | Milk | |

| Potential Problems | Recommended Interventions |
|---|---|
| Constipation related to low-fiber content of diet: insufficient fiber intake causes decrease in stool bulk and slowing of intestinal transit time | Liberalize diet to allow more fiber. This diet is intended to be short-term |
| Persistent diarrhea related to poor tolerance of even small amounts of fiber contained in a low-residue diet. Tolerance of fiber varies among patients and conditions | Further reduce fiber content by eliminating all fruits and vegetables except strained fruit juice |

**Patient Teaching**
Instruct the patient that

- Fiber is a component of plants and, therefore, is found in fruits, vegetables, grains, and nuts
- Insoluble fiber, the fiber restricted in this diet, is most abundant in bran, whole-wheat breads and cereals, and skins and seeds of fruits and vegetables
- Reducing insoluble fiber slows passage of food through the bowel
- Diet is intended to be short-term
- Food preparation techniques to reduce fiber include removing skins, seeds, and membranes of fruits and vegetables that are high in fiber and cooking allowed vegetables until they are very tender

| TABLE 18.1 | Potential Secondary Nutrient Deficiencies and Metabolic Disturbances of Malabsorption Syndrome |
|---|---|

| Nutrient | Potential Problems |
|---|---|
| **Potential Secondary Nutrient Deficiencies** | |
| Potassium | Muscle weakness |
| Protein | Hypoalbuminemia, edema, muscle weakness, increased risk of infection, poor wound healing |
| Iron, folic acid, vitamin B$_{12}$ | Anemia, fatigue, pallor, weakness, palpitations, anorexia, indigestion, sore mouth |
| Vitamin K | Purpura and easy bleeding |
| Vitamin A | Roughening of skin, impaired night vision, increased risk of infections |
| Calcium, magnesium, vitamin D | Osteomalacia and bone pain |
| Calcium, magnesium | Tetany |
| B-complex vitamins | Stomatitis, cheilosis, glossitis, and dermatitis |
| **Potential Metabolic Disturbances** | |
| Impaired absorption of bile salts | Cholesterol gallstone formation (cholesterol from cholesterol-saturated bile may precipitate out into gallstones) |
| Increased urinary excretion of oxalate related to increased oxalate absorption secondary to the loss of calcium in the stools | Increased risk of oxalate kidney stone formation |
| Lactose intolerance | Cramping, distention, flatus, and diarrhea after milk ingestion related to secondary lactose deficiency |

possible diet modifications appear in Table 18.2. Specific malabsorption syndromes are discussed below, namely lactose intolerance, inflammatory bowel disease (IBD), celiac disease, and short bowel syndrome.

## Lactose Intolerance

Lactose intolerance occurs when the levels of lactase, the enzyme that splits lactose into its component simple sugars glucose and galactose, is absent or deficient. Without adequate lactase, lactose digestion is impaired; particles of undigested lactose increase the osmolality of intestinal contents, which may lead to osmotic diarrhea. Lactose is fermented in the colon, which produces bloating, cramping, and flatulence. Symptoms occur between 15 minutes and 2 hours after eating and range from mild to severe depending on the amount of lactase actually produced and the amount of lactose consumed.

Primary lactose intolerance occurs in "well" people who simply do not secrete adequate lactase. Eighty percent or more of Asians, Native Americans, and Africans are lactose intolerant; lactose intolerance is least common in people of northern European descent (NIDDK, 2006). People with primary lactose intolerance may be asymptomatic when they consume doses less than 4 to 12 g of lactose (e.g., ⅓ to 1 cup of milk) or when lactose is consumed as part of a meal. Chocolate milk is usually better tolerated than plain milk, and because much

| TABLE 18.2 | **Nutrition Therapy for Malabsorption Symptoms** | |
|---|---|---|
| **Symptoms** | **Dietary Interventions** | **Rationale** |
| Anorexia | Small, frequent meals | To maximize intake |
| | Commercial supplements | Liquid supplements are easy to consume, are nutritionally dense, and leave the stomach quickly |
| | Enteral nutrition if anorexia is severe and/or prolonged | To meet calorie and nutrient needs until the patient is able to consume an adequate oral intake |
| Diarrhea | Low-fiber diet | To minimize stimulation to the bowel |
| | Ensure adequate fluid and electrolytes | Increased losses of fluid and electrolytes in the stool |
| Lactose intolerance | Avoid lactose | Lactase activity may be lost during acute episodes of malabsorption due to altered integrity and function of intestinal villi cells; lactase deficiency may persist into remission |
| Nutrient deficiencies | Nutrient-dense diet | To replenish losses, facilitate healing, and meet increased needs related to the metabolism of a high-calorie, high-protein diet |
| | Vitamin supplements; may need water-soluble forms of the fat-soluble vitamins | Dietary sources may not be adequate to meet need. Water-soluble forms do not require normal fat absorption to be absorbed, as do fat-soluble vitamins in their natural form |
| | Oral or parenteral vitamin $B_{12}$ | Bacterial overgrowth, pancreatic insufficiency, and ileal disease or resection impair $B_{12}$ absorption |
| | Calcium supplements | Serum calcium may be low related to low serum albumin or calcium malabsorption related to poor vitamin D absorption or the binding of calcium with unabsorbed fats to form unabsorbable soaps |
| | Other mineral supplements | Magnesium levels are often low in some malabsorption syndromes; losses of zinc are high in patients with fistulas |
| Steatorrhea | Limit fat | To avoid aggravating fat malabsorption |
| | MCT oil may be used for calories | MCT oil is absorbed without undergoing digestion |
| Tissue damage (e.g., resulting from inflammation or surgery) and/or weight loss | Increase calories (2000–3500 cal/day). Increase protein (1.0–1.5g/kg/day) | Calories and protein are needed to facilitate healing and restore weight |
| Calcium oxalate kidney stones related to binding of calcium to fat instead of oxalate, leaving increased amount of oxalate available for absorption into the blood | Increase fluids | To dilute the urine |
| | Avoid high-oxalate foods, such as green leafy vegetables, chocolate milk, dried peas and beans, potatoes, and whole-wheat products | To limit oxalate available for absorption |

of the lactose in yogurt is digested by its bacteria, it is also usually well tolerated unless milk is added. Simply knowing individual limits (e.g., 8 ounces of milk with dinner is tolerated but 8 ounces of milk between meals is not) is enough to prevent symptoms. For people who want to consume milk or lactose-containing foods beyond their limit, lactose-reduced milk and lactase enzyme tablets or liquid may be used.

A more problematic lactose intolerance occurs secondary to GI disorders that alter the integrity and function of intestinal villi cells, where lactase is secreted. For instance, people with IBD lose lactase activity when the disease is active and sometimes for a prolonged period afterward. The loss of lactase may also develop secondary to malnutrition because the rapidly growing intestinal cells that produce lactase are reduced in number and function. Secondary lactose intolerance tends to be more severe than primary lactose intolerance and symptoms occur more quickly after eating lactose.

## Nutrition Therapy

Nutrition therapy for lactose intolerance is to reduce lactose to the maximum amount tolerated by the individual (Box 18.4). For patients with GI disorders, a lactose-restricted diet is indicated at least until the disorder is resolved and sometimes for a prolonged period thereafter. Because lactose is used as an ingredient in many foods and drugs, a lactose-free diet is not realistic.

## Inflammatory Bowel Disease

Inflammatory bowel disease primarily refers to two chronic inflammatory GI diseases: Crohn's disease and ulcerative colitis. IBD is believed to be caused by an abnormal immune

---

| BOX 18.4 | **LOW-LACTOSE DIET** |
| --- | --- |

- Lactose is the sugar in milk; limit or avoid milk and foods made with milk
- Individual tolerance varies; eat dairy foods as tolerance allows
- Choose nondairy sources of calcium to ensure an adequate intake, such as canned salmon with bones, calcium-fortified tofu, orange juice, and soy milk; shellfish; "greens" such as turnip, collard, and kale; dried peas and beans; broccoli; almonds
- Read labels to identify lactose
  - Lactate, lactalbumin, and calcium compounds are lactic acid salts and are lactose free
  - Kosher foods labeled *pareve* are made without milk
  - Avoid products whose ingredient list contains butter, cream, milk, milk solids, or whey

| Lactose-free milk and nondairy foods | Low-lactose dairy foods | Possible hidden sources of lactose |
| --- | --- | --- |
| Lactose-free milk | Aged cheese, such as | Bread |
| Almond, rice, or soy milk | cheddar, Swiss, | Baked goods |
| Soy yogurt, soy cheese | and parmesan | Breakfast cereals |
| Soy sour cream | Cream cheese | Instant potatoes and soups |
| | Ricotta cheese | Margarine |
| | Cottage cheese | Lunch meats |
| | Yogurt | Salad dressings |
| | | Mixes for pancakes, biscuits, and cookies |
| | | Powdered meal-replacement supplements |

response to a complex interaction between environmental and genetic factors (Hanauer, 2006). Crohn's disease and ulcerative colitis are characterized by periods of exacerbation and remission; they share common symptoms and treatments (Table 18.3).

## Nutrition Therapy

Nutrition therapy for IBD depends on the presence and severity of symptoms, the presence of complications, and the nutritional status of the patient. Diet restrictions are kept to a minimum to encourage an adequate intake, and the diet is liberalized during periods of

| TABLE 18.3 | Comparison Between Crohn's Disease and Ulcerative Colitis | |
|---|---|---|
| | **Crohn's Disease** | **Ulcerative Colitis** |
| Area affected | Can occur anywhere along the GI tract but most commonly occurs in the ileum and colon | Confined to the rectum and colon |
| Disease pattern | Inflammation is discontinuous, with normal tissue between patches of inflamed tissue | Inflammation is continuous, beginning at rectum and usually extending into the colon |
| | All layers of the bowel are affected | Affects only the mucosal layer |
| Main symptoms | Diarrhea, abdominal pain, weight loss | Diarrhea, abdominal pain, rectal bleeding<br>Weight loss, fever, and weakness are common when most of the colon is involved |
| Complications | Fistulas, abscesses<br>Stricture of the ileum<br>Bowel perforation<br>Bowel obstructions may occur from scar tissue formation<br>Toxic megacolon<br>Increased risk of intestinal cancer | Tissue erosion and ulceration<br>Toxic megacolon<br>Greatly increased risk of cancer |
| Nutritional complications | Impaired bile acid reabsorption may cause malabsorption of fat, fat-soluble vitamins, calcium, magnesium, and zinc<br>Malnutrition may occur from nutrient malabsorption, decreased intake, or intestinal resections<br>Anemia related to blood loss or malabsorption<br>Vitamin $B_{12}$ deficiency related to $B_{12}$ malabsorption from the ileum due to inflammation | Anemia related to blood loss<br>Dehydration and electrolyte imbalances related to diarrhea<br>Protein depletion from losses through inflamed tissue |
| Medical treatment | Antidiarrheals, immunosuppressants, immunomodulators, biologic therapies, and antiinflammatory agents | Antidiarrheals, immunosuppressants, and antiinflammatory agents |
| Surgical intervention | Most common procedure is ileostomy; disease often recurs in the remaining intestine | Most common procedure is total colectomy; surgery prevents recurrence |

remission. Patients are often reluctant to eat because they associate eating with pain and diarrhea. In general, Crohn's disease is more likely to cause nutritional complications than ulcerative colitis.

**Glutamine:** a nonessential amino acid that maintains the integrity of the intestinal mucosa and helps prevent pathogenic bacteria from crossing the intestinal barrier into the bloodstream, thereby reducing the risk of GI-derived septicemia

The focus of therapy for acute exacerbation of IBD is to correct deficiencies by providing nutrients in a form the patient can tolerate. In some cases, a hydrolyzed enteral feeding, possibly one fortified with **glutamine**, may be used to minimize fecal volume. TPN is used for patients who need complete bowel rest or who are unable to meet their nutritional requirements through an oral diet or enteral feeding.

For patients consuming an oral diet, a low fiber one is recommended to minimize bowel stimulation (Box 18.3). Lactose is avoided if lactose intolerance is suspected. Protein and calorie needs are elevated to facilitate healing. Other diet modifications are made according to symptoms (Table 18.2). The diet is liberalized as soon as possible, and a diet as near normal as tolerated is recommended during remission.

## Celiac Disease

Celiac disease is a genetic autoimmune disorder characterized by chronic inflammation of the proximal small intestine mucosa related to a permanent intolerance to certain proteins found in wheat, barley, and rye. When ingested, these proteins trigger an immune response that damages the mucosa of the small intestine. Malabsorption of carbohydrates, protein, fat, vitamins, and minerals may occur, resulting in diarrhea, flatulence, weight loss, vitamin and mineral deficiencies (e.g., folate, calcium, and fat-soluble vitamins), iron deficiency anemia, and loss of bone (Thompson, 2005).

Symptoms and their severity vary widely among individuals depending on the patient's age and the duration and extent of the disease (Chand & Mihas, 2006). Classic symptoms in children are diarrhea, abdominal distention, and failure to thrive (Green & Jabri, 2003). Typically adults present with diarrhea, constipation, weight loss, weakness, flatus, abdominal pain, and vomiting (Green, 2005). Atypical presentations may include iron deficiency anemia, chronic fatigue, irritable bowel syndrome, dyspepsia, infertility, and unexplained neurological disorders (Green, 2005). In 10% to 20% of people with celiac disease, **dermatitis herpetiformis** is the presenting symptom (Reunala, 1998). Although these patients do not usually have GI symptoms, results of serology and biopsies are identical to those of people with celiac disease. Symptoms of dermatitis herpetiformis respond to a gluten-free diet (Niewinski, 2008).

**Dermatitis Herpetiformis:** a chronic inflammatory disease characterized by groups of red, raised blisters that itch and burn

People with subclinical celiac disease have no symptoms yet they have positive serological test results, and biopsy of the intestinal villi shows atrophy (NIH, 2005). These people are identified through screening of at-risk groups or from biopsies obtained for other reasons, such as dyspepsia. People who have a first-degree relative with celiac disease, people with Down syndrome, and those with an autoimmune disease are at risk for celiac disease. Untreated celiac disease is associated with an increased incidence of small bowel cancers and enteropathy-associated T-cell lymphoma (Card et al., 2004).

### Nutrition Therapy

**Gluten:** a general name for the storage proteins gliadin (in wheat), secalin (in rye), and hordein (in barley)

The only scientifically proven treatment for celiac disease is to completely and permanently eliminate **gluten** from the diet (Niewinski, 2008). A gluten-free diet (Box 18.5) allows the villi to return toward normal, usually within a few weeks, although complete regeneration may never occur. Lactose intolerance secondary to celiac disease may be temporary or permanent.

Gluten is found in wheat, rye, and barley—grains that form the foundation of a healthy diet in most cultures. Pure oats are gluten free and, therefore, not harmful to people with celiac disease. However, there is worldwide concern that the risk of oats being contaminated with

| BOX 18.5 | **GLUTEN-FREE DIET** |
|---|---|

- Gluten, a protein fraction found in wheat, rye, and barley, is eliminated. Oats are also eliminated due to the high risk of gluten contamination. All products made from these grains or their flours are eliminated
- Many foods are naturally gluten free: milk, butter, cheese; fresh, frozen, and canned fruits and vegetables; fresh meat, fish, poultry, eggs; dried peas and beans; nuts; corn; and rice

**Allowed Grains and Related Foods**
Almond flour
Amaranth
Arrowroot
Buckwheat
Cassava
Channa flour
  (a type of chickpea)
Corn
Cornstarch
Flax seed
Indian rice grass
Job's tears
Legumes
Millet
Nuts
Oats (uncontaminated)
Potatoes
Potato flour
Quinoa
Rice (all plain forms)
Sago
Seeds
Soy
Sorghum
Tapioca
Taro flour
Teff
White rice flour
Wild rice
Yucca

**Grains to Eliminate**
Wheat
- Wheat flours, such as bromated flour, durum flour, enriched flour, graham flour, phosphated flour, plain flour, self-rising flour, semolina, white flour
- Wheat starch, wheat bran, wheat germ, cracked wheat, hydrolyzed wheat protein, farina
- Einkorn, emmer, spelt, kamut
Barley
Rye
Triticale (a cross between wheat and rye)
Bouillon cubes

**Questionable Foods (may contain wheat, barely, or rye)**
Brown rice syrup
Chips/potato chips
Candy
Cold cuts, hot dogs, salami, sausage
Communion wafer
French fries
Gravy
Imitation fish
Matzo
Rice mixes
Sauces
Seasoned tortilla chips
Self-basting turkey
Soups
Soy sauce
Vegetables in sauce

**Sample Menu**

| **Breakfast** | **Lunch** | **Dinner** | **Snacks** |
|---|---|---|---|
| Orange juice | Cuban black beans with rice | Tomato juice | Yogurt |
| Cornflakes | Pure corn tortilla | Roast chicken | Rice cake |
| Milk | Milk | Baked potato with margarine | Banana |
| Coffee | Tapioca pudding | Tossed salad with olive oil and cider vinegar dressing | Apple slices with peanut butter |
| | Coffee/tea | Steamed broccoli | |
| | | Corn bread made without wheat flour | |
| | | Blueberries over ice cream made without gluten stabilizers | |

*(box continues on page 432)*

| BOX 18.5 | **GLUTEN-FREE DIET** (continued) |

**Additional Considerations**
- Patients may be discouraged and overwhelmed when faced with a lifelong restricted diet. Provide support, encouragement, and thorough diet instructions
- The patient may be temporarily lactose-intolerant and may require a lactose-restricted diet

**Potential Problems**

Difficulty obtaining a variety of allowed foods from grocery stores related to the highly restrictive nature of the diet

Inadequate intake of several nutrients (thiamin, riboflavin, niacin, folate, and iron) related to the lower content of these nutrients in gluten-free products compared to the enriched and fortified grains and cereals they replace

Inadequate intake of fiber related to the absence of whole-wheat products

**Recommended Interventions**

Encourage the patient to use as many "normal" items as possible such as corn cereals, grits, rice, and rice cereals They are easy to obtain and less expensive than special products
Encourage the patient to shop in health-food stores to obtain hard-to-find items such as potato and soybean flours

Encourage a varied diet; consider vitamin supplements

Encourage fiber from legumes, nuts, fruit, vegetables, and gluten-free whole grains such as flax seed, millet, unconta-minated oats, quinoa, brown rice, and amaranth

**Patient Teaching**
Instruct the patient on the importance of adhering to the diet even when no symptoms are present. "Cheating" on the diet can damage intestinal villi even if no symptoms develop. To eliminate all wheat, oat, rye, and barley flours and products permanently, the patient should

- Read labels. As per the Food Allergen Labeling and Consumer Protection Act of 2004, all food products must be clearly labeled to indicate the presence of wheat. This Act simplifies label reading to identify wheat gluten, but less obvious sources of gluten from barley (e.g., malt flavorings and extracts) require more careful reading. Patients should check with the manufacturer *before* using products of questionable composition
- Use corn, potato, rice, arrowroot, and soybean flours and their products
- Use the following as thickening agents: arrowroot starch, cornstarch, tapioca starch, rice starch, sweet rice flour
- Eat an otherwise normal, well-balanced diet adequate in nutrients and calories. Lactose is restricted only if not tolerated. Weight gain may be slowly achieved

Provide the patient with the following aids:

- A detailed list of foods allowed and not allowed
- Information regarding support groups; see websites at the end of this chapter
- Gluten-free recipes

gluten is unacceptably high. Celiac organizations in the United States do not endorse the use of oats.

A gluten-free diet requires a major lifestyle change, so compliance is a major challenge. Gluten-free products (e.g., breads, pastry) made with rice, corn, or potato flour have different textures and tastes than "normal" products and are not well accepted. They are also expensive. Even patients who are willing to comply have difficulty following the diet because of the pervasiveness of gluten in prepared foods and medications and confusion over identifying sources of gluten on food labels. The diet is very restrictive, requires conscientious label reading, and is difficult to adhere to while eating out.

Many patients with celiac disease eat gluten occasionally or in normal amounts and do not complain of symptoms. Yet even without symptoms, the intestinal mucosa is abnormal in most patients, and the risk of cancer is increased. Conversely, strict adherence to a gluten-free diet usually allows the mucosa to heal, resolves GI symptoms, and helps prevent complications associated with long-term untreated celiac disease, such as non-Hodgkin's lymphoma (Thompson, 2005). A gluten-free diet can restore body weight and nutritional status, although it may take at least 12 months of dietary compliance (AGA, 2006). Patients need to understand that the long-term effects of eating even small amounts of gluten are harmful, even in asymptomatic patients.

## Short Bowel Syndrome

**Short bowel syndrome (SBS):** a complex condition resulting from extensive surgical resection of the intestinal tract usually because of inflammatory bowel disease, cancer, or obstruction

**Short bowel syndrome (SBS)** occurs when the bowel is surgically shortened to the extent that the remaining bowel is unable to absorb adequate levels of nutrients to meet the individual's needs. Crohn's disease, traumatic abdominal injuries, malignant tumors, and mesenteric infarction are the most common reasons for extensive intestinal resections that result in SBS.

Nutrition complications experienced by people with SBS depend on the amount and location of resected and remaining bowel. Patients who have 150 cm or more of remaining small bowel without a colon, or 60 to 90 cm of remaining small bowel with a colon, initially require TPN and may progress to an oral diet over a 1- to 2-year period (Matarese et al., 2005). Adaptation depends on the length of remaining jejunum and/or ileum and whether the colon is present. Other factors that influence adaptation include the patient's age, whether the ileocecal value remains, the health of the remaining bowel, and the health of the stomach, liver, and pancreas (Fessler, 2007). Patients with less than 100 to 140 cm of small bowel and no colon will likely need either intestinal transplantation or permanent TPN.

### Nutrition Therapy

In the early months after bowel surgery, TPN is the major source of nutrition and hydration until the remaining bowel adapts. When the patient is able to consume oral nutrition without excessive stool or ostomy output and can maintain or gain weight, the amount of TPN is gradually decreased (Fessler, 2007). During the weaning process, TPN may be infused every other day.

Consuming intact nutrients promotes bowel adaptation because they stimulate blood flow to the intestine and the secretion of pancreatic enzymes and bile acids (Fessler, 2007). It is important to get the patient to eat as soon as possible and reduce reliance on specialized enteral formulas or parenteral nutrition. Six to eight small meals per day are recommended. Simple sugars are avoided to limit the osmolar load to the intestine and osmotic diarrhea. The patient may be intolerant of lactose. If the patient's colon is intact, fat intake is restricted to avoid steatorrhea and increased fluid losses; the intake of complex carbohydrates is

| BOX 18.6 | SAMPLE MENU FOR PATIENT WITH SHORT-BOWEL SYNDROME: VERY LOW FAT, LOW LACTOSE, LOW FIBER, LOW SUGAR IN EIGHT SMALL MEALS |

**Breakfast**
Diluted orange juice
Poached egg
White toast with diet jelly

**Snack**
6 oz Artificially sweetened low-fat yogurt

**Snack**
8 oz Promote (low-fat, lactose-free,
   high-protein oral formula)

**Lunch**
Fat-free deli turkey on white bread
Banana
Artificially sweetened low-fat yogurt

**Snack**
8 oz Promote

**Snack**
Low-fat cheddar cheese on saltines

**Dinner**
Lean roast beef
Boiled potatoes
Green beans
Unsweetened applesauce

**Snack**
8 oz Promote

encouraged because colonic bacteria ferment them to short-chain fatty acids, an important source of energy. When the colon is absent, fat intake is not restricted (Matarese et al., 2005). Other diet modifications are made according to the patient's symptoms/complications (Table 18.2). A sample menu appears in Box 18.6.

# ▶ CONDITIONS OF THE LARGE INTESTINE

## Irritable Bowel Syndrome

Irritable bowel syndrome (IBS), the most frequently diagnosed digestive disorder in the United States (Cremonini & Taylor, 2005) affects as many as 20% of American adults (Wald & Rakel, 2008). Although it is commonly categorized as a motility disorder, there are likely many factors involved in its etiology, including genetics, environmental factors, alterations in gut flora, nervous system alterations, and psychosocial stressors (Clark & DeLegge, 2008). Symptoms include lower abdominal pain, constipation, diarrhea, alternating periods of constipation and diarrhea, bloating, and mucus in the stools. IBS can significantly impair quality of life.

**Elimination Diet:** a diet that eliminates foods suspected of producing symptoms of intolerance or allergies; suspected foods are added back to the diet individually to identify offending foods

**Probiotics:** live organisms that provide health benefits to the host, e.g., yogurt with active cultures

**Grade A Level Evidence:** indicates that a recommendation is based on consistent and good-quality patient-oriented evidence

### Nutrition Therapy

There is inconclusive evidence for any of the current treatments used for IBS (Quartero et al., 2005). Antidiarrheals, antispasmodics, and antidepressants are pharmacologic treatment options that meet with limited success. Complementary therapies include cognitive behavior therapy, hypnosis, and various dietary inventions, including avoiding caffeine, moderating fat intake, and an **elimination diet** to identify potential food intolerances or allergies (Box 18.7). A high-fiber diet has been studied extensively with IBS with mixed results (Wald & Rakel, 2008).

Emerging, but promising, evidence suggests that **probiotics** such as yogurt may improve IBS symptoms by altering intestinal flora (Guslandi, 2007). In addition, **Grade A level evidence** exists for the use of 5 g of guar gum daily to reduce IBS symptoms and improve overall quality of life (Ebell et al., 2004). Guar gum is a soluble, nongelling fiber that acts as

| BOX 18.7 | **FOODS TO CONSIDER ELIMINATING ON A TRIAL BASIS TO TEST FOR SYMPTOMATIC IMPROVEMENT IN IBS** |
|---|---|

| | |
|---|---|
| Milk and dairy foods containing lactose | Shellfish |
| Wheat and other sources of gluten | Soybeans |
| High-fructose corn syrup | Beef |
| Sorbitol | Pork |
| Eggs | Lamb |
| Nuts | |

**Prebiotic:** a nondigestible food ingredient, e.g., fiber, that benefits the host by stimulating the growth of colonic bacteria

a **prebiotic** to increase certain beneficial gut flora. When compared to bran fiber, both guar and bran improved IBS symptoms but patients preferred guar gum over bran (Parisi et al., 2002). Benefits of guar gum ceased when the therapy was over, suggesting the need for on-going use.

## Diverticular Disease

**Diverticula:** pouches that protrude outward from the muscular wall of the intestine usually in the sigmoid colon

**Diverticulitis:** inflammation and infection that occurs when fecal matter gets trapped in the diverticula

**Bacterial Overgrowth:** excessive bacterial growth in the stomach or small intestine that impairs digestion and absorption; may be caused by low gastric acidity, altered GI motility, mucosal damage, or contamination

**Diverticulosis:** an asymptomatic condition characterized by diverticula

**Diverticula** are caused by increased pressure within the intestinal lumen; they are usually asymptomatic. **Diverticulitis** occurs when diverticula become inflamed, possibly from trapped stool or bacteria. Symptoms of diverticulitis include cramping, alternating periods of diarrhea and constipation, flatus, abdominal distention, and low-grade fever. Potential complications include occult blood loss and acute rectal bleeding leading to iron deficiency anemia; abscesses and bowel perforation leading to peritonitis; fistula formation causing bowel obstruction; and **bacterial overgrowth** (in small bowel diverticula) that leads to malabsorption of fat and vitamin $B_{12}$.

Although not proven, the dominant theory is that diverticular disease is caused by a low-fiber diet (NIDDK, 2008). Chronic constipation, obesity, and low physical activity are also implicated (Beitz, 2004).

### Nutrition Therapy

A high fiber intake may prevent and improve symptoms of **diverticulosis** and prevent diverticulitis by producing soft, bulky stools that are easily passed, resulting in decreased pressure within the colon and shortened transit time. Once the diverticula develop, a high-fiber diet cannot make them disappear. It is common practice for patients to be told to avoid nuts, seeds, and popcorn because these can become trapped in diverticula and cause inflammation; yet there is no scientific evidence to support this practice (NIDDK, 2008).

During an acute phase of diverticulitis, patients are given nothing by mouth (NPO) until bleeding and diarrhea subside. Oral intake resumes with clear liquids and progresses to a low-fiber diet until inflammation and bleeding are no longer a risk (ADA, 2006). A high-fiber diet is recommended unless symptoms of diverticulitis recur. Patients who are treated with a low-fiber diet in the hospital may be reluctant to switch to a high-fiber diet on discharge. Diet compliance depends on the patient's understanding of the rationale and benefits of a high-fiber diet for long-term treatment of diverticulosis and prevention of diverticulitis.

**Ileostomy:** a surgically created opening (stoma) on the surface of the abdomen from the ileum

**Colostomy:** a surgically created opening on the surface of the abdomen from the colon

## Ileostomies and Colostomies

An **ileostomy** and a **colostomy** are performed after part or all of the colon, anus, and rectum are removed, usually for treatment of severe IBD, intestinal lesions, obstructions, or colon cancer.

Potential nutritional problems arise because large amounts of fluid, sodium, and potassium are normally absorbed in the colon. The smaller the length of remaining colon, the greater the potential for nutritional problems. For that reason ileostomies create more problems than colostomies, in which some of the colon is retained. In addition to fluid and electrolyte losses, ileostomies cause a decrease in fat, bile acid, and vitamin $B_{12}$ absorption. **Effluent** from an ileostomy is liquidy, and fluid and electrolyte losses are considerable. Effluent through a colostomy varies from liquid to formed stools, depending on the length of colon that remains. Over time, adaptation occurs.

**Effluent:** flowing discharge

## Nutrition Therapy

The goals of nutrition therapy for ileostomies and colostomies are to minimize symptoms (Box 18.8) and replenish losses. Initially only clear liquids that are low in simple sugars (e.g., diluted fruit juice, broth, tea) are given to reduce the risk of osmotic diarrhea. The diet is advanced slowly, based on individual tolerance. Patients need extra protein and calories to promote healing and may have experienced weight loss prior to surgery related to diarrhea or the underlying disease. Fear of eating is common. Within 6 to 8 weeks after surgery, the patient should be consuming a near-regular diet. Foods not tolerated initially can be reintroduced in a few months.

| BOX 18.8 | NUTRITION THERAPY GUIDELINES FOR COLOSTOMIES AND ILEOSTOMIES |

**Colostomies**
- Chew food thoroughly because improperly chewed food can cause a stomal blockage
- Limit fiber
  If the patient has a high output, insoluble fiber intake (e.g., whole-grain breads and cereals) is minimized because it reduces intestinal transit time
- Avoid odor-causing foods
  Asparagus, dried peas and beans, eggs, fish, garlic, onions, some spicy foods
- Avoid gas-producing foods
  Alcohol, beer, carbonated beverages, chewing gum, cucumbers, dried peas and beans, melon, onion, peppers, pickles, sauerkraut, cabbage, broccoli, Brussels sprouts, cauliflower
- Avoid foods that may cause blockage
  Cabbage, raw carrots, celery, coconut, corn, cucumbers, dried fruit, lettuce, mushrooms, nuts, olives, peas, pickles, pineapple, popcorn, seeds, skins and seeds from fruits and vegetables
- Add foods that may thicken stool
  Banana flakes, applesauce, pectin, pasta, potatoes, rice, barley, cheese, and oatmeal

**Ileostomies: All of the Above Plus**
- Eat meals on a schedule to help promote a regular bowel pattern. A small evening meal helps to reduce nighttime stool output
- Eat small, frequent meals
- Avoid beverages with meals; consume before or after eating
- Encourage higher salt intake to replenish losses
- Use oral rehydration beverages to help maintain fluid and electrolyte balance
- Limit fat if the patient has steatorrhea or diarrhea from a significant ileal resection. MCT oil may be used for calories because it is absorbed without the aid of bile salts
- Provide supplemental nutrients as needed. Because vitamin $B_{12}$ is normally absorbed in the distal ileum, anemia related to vitamin $B_{12}$ malabsorption can occur in patients with ileostomies, necessitating lifelong parenteral injections or nasal sprays of vitamin $B_{12}$

Obtaining adequate fluid and electrolytes is a major concern. A high fluid intake (8 to 10 cups daily) is needed to replenish losses. A high fluid intake is especially important for ileostomy patients to maintain a normal urine output and minimize the risk of renal calculi. Many patients inaccurately assume that a high fluid intake contributes to diarrhea. Reassure the patient that excess fluid is excreted through the kidneys, not the stoma.

# ▶ DISORDERS OF THE ACCESSORY GI ORGANS

The liver, pancreas, and gallbladder are known as accessory organs of the GI tract. Although food does not come in direct contact with these organs, they play vital roles in the digestion of macronutrients. Liver disease, pancreatitis, and gallbladder disease are discussed next.

## Liver Disease

**Hepatitis:** inflammation of the liver, which may be caused by viral infections, alcohol abuse, and hepatotoxic chemicals such as chloroform and carbon tetrachloride

**Cirrhosis:** liver disease that occurs when damaged liver cells are replaced by functionless scar tissue, seriously impairing liver function and disrupting normal blood circulation through the liver

**Hepatic Encephalopathy:** the central nervous system (CNS) manifestations of advanced liver disease characterized by irritability, short-term memory loss, and impaired ability to concentrate

**Hepatic Coma:** unconsciousness caused by severe liver disease

The liver is a highly active organ involved in the metabolism of almost all nutrients. After absorption, almost all nutrients are transported to the liver, where they are "processed" before being distributed to other tissues. The liver synthesizes plasma proteins, blood clotting factors, and nonessential amino acids and forms urea from the nitrogenous wastes of protein. Triglycerides, phospholipids, and cholesterol are synthesized in the liver, as is bile, an important factor in the digestion of fat. Glucose is synthesized and glycogen is formed, stored, and broken down as needed. Vitamins and minerals are metabolized, and many are stored in the liver. Finally the liver is vital for detoxifying drugs, alcohol, ammonia, and other poisonous substances.

Liver damage can have profound and devastating effects on the metabolism of almost all nutrients. It can range from mild and reversible (e.g., fatty liver) to severe and terminal (e.g., hepatic coma). Liver failure can occur from chronic liver disease or secondary to critical illnesses.

Early symptoms of **hepatitis** include anorexia, nausea and vomiting, fever, fatigue, headache, and weight loss. Later, symptoms such as dark-colored urine, jaundice, liver tenderness, and possibly liver enlargement may develop. In many cases, liver cell damage that occurs from acute hepatitis is reversible with proper rest and nutrition.

Sometimes acute hepatitis advances to chronic hepatitis, which may lead to **cirrhosis**, liver cancer, and liver failure. Early symptoms include fever, anorexia, weight loss, and fatigue. Glucose intolerance is common. Later, portal hypertension, dyspepsia, diarrhea or constipation, jaundice, esophageal varices, hemorrhoids, ascites, edema, bleeding tendencies, anemia, hepatomegaly, and splenomegaly may develop. Cirrhosis can progress to **hepatic encephalopathy** and **hepatic coma**.

The liver "fails" when liver cell loss is extensive. Ominous changes in mental function, such as impaired memory and concentration, slow response time, drowsiness, irritability, flapping tremor, and fecal odor of the breath, signal hepatic encephalopathy, which may progress to hepatic coma. Although the exact cause of these CNS changes are unknown, altered blood amino acid patterns and high serum ammonia levels may be involved.

### Nutrition Therapy

The objectives of nutrition therapy for liver disease are to avoid or minimize permanent liver damage, promote liver cell regeneration, restore optimal nutritional status, alleviate symptoms, and avoid complications. Depending on the extent of liver damage, regeneration may not be possible.

| TABLE 18.4 | Nutrition Therapy Guidelines for Liver Disorders | | |
|---|---|---|---|
| **Nutrient** | **Guideline** | | **Rationale** |
| Calories | 20–70% above basal energy expenditure (BEE) based on the individual's status | | Malnutrition, fever, infection, and weight loss influence calorie needs |
| Protein | 0.8–1.2 g/kg | | An adequate protein intake is vital to prevent body protein catabolism and worsening of nutritional status |
| Carbohydrates | No restriction unless diabetes is present | | If hyperglycemia is a problem, carbohydrates should be mostly in the form of complex carbohydrates, and meal timings should be consistent |
| Fat | Limit if patient experiences steatorrhea | | Fat aggravates malabsorption in people with steatorrhea |
| | MCT oil may be used for additional calories | | MCT oil is absorbed without undergoing digestion |
| Sodium | Limit to 2000 mg if the patient has ascites | | Limiting sodium helps control fluid accumulation |
| Fluid | 1200–1500 mL/day if serum sodium <128 mEq/L | | To limit fluid accumulation |
| Supplements | As needed to correct for deficiencies | | Supplements of B vitamins, vitamin C, and vitamin K may be needed to compensate for alterations in metabolism |
| | | | Zinc supplements may help to improve appetite |
| | | | Impaired liver function increases the risk of vitamin A toxicity, so excess amounts are avoided |

Generally, patients with acute hepatitis have difficulty consuming an adequate diet because of anorexia, early satiety, and fatigue. A balanced diet with between-meal feedings of commercial supplements may help ensure an adequate intake. For people with chronic hepatitis, dietary restrictions are usually not necessary unless symptoms interfere with nutrient intake or utilization.

Malnutrition is common among patients with cirrhosis and may be related to altered nutrient metabolism, anorexia, nausea, vomiting, maldigestion, and malabsorption. Metabolic rate may be increased or decreased. Glucose intolerance may develop but hyperinsulinism is common. Impaired or reduced bile flow, drug therapy, or alcohol-induced changes in the GI tract may lead to fat intolerance. Deficiencies of fat-soluble vitamins may arise secondary to steatorrhea. If a regular diet irritates the esophageal mucosa, a soft, low-fiber, or full liquid diet may be warranted. Spices, pepper, caffeine, and coarse foods may also irritate esophageal varices. Meeting nutrient and calorie needs is difficult and enteral nutrition support may be necessary. Nutrition therapy guidelines are outlined in Table 18.4.

## Nutrition Therapy for Liver Transplantation

Liver transplantation is a treatment option for patients with severe and irreversible liver disease. Many patients awaiting a transplant are malnourished (Stephenson et al., 2001).

| TABLE 18.5 | Posttransplant Nutrient Recommendations | |
|---|---|---|
| **Nutrient** | **Short-Term Recommendations (e.g., 20 Months Following Surgery)** | **Long-Term Recommendations (Lifetime Maintenance)** |
| Calories | 130% of BEE; 100–120% for obese patients | 120–130% of BEE; 100–120% for weight loss |
| Protein | 1.5–2.0 g/kg | 0.8–1.0 g/kg; may need more during antirejection treatment with corticosteroids |
| Carbohydrate | 50–70% of total calories<br><br>Limit sugars if hyperglycemia is a problem | 50–60% of total calories as complex carbohydrates<br>25 g fiber per day |
| Fat | 30% of total calories | 25–35% of total calories with an emphasis on monounsaturated and omega-3 fats |
| Fluid | 30–35 mL/kg | 30–35 mL/kg |
| Vitamins and minerals | Recommended dietary allowances (RDA) amounts unless individual adjustments are needed | RDA amounts unless individual adjustments are needed |
| Electrolytes | Individualized<br><br>Monitor sodium, potassium, phosphorus, and magnesium; dramatic shifts may signal refeeding syndrome in severely malnourished patients | Limit sodium to <2–3 g/day; individualize other electrolytes<br>Monitor serum levels |

*Source:* ADA. *Nutrition Care Manual.* Chicago, IL: American Dietetic Association; 2007.

Moderate to severe malnutrition increases the risk of complications and death after transplantation. Whenever possible, nutrient deficiencies and imbalances are corrected before the transplantation to promote a positive outcome.

There is not one specific posttransplant diet. Nutrient recommendations vary with the post transplant stage and are individualized according to the patient's nutritional status, weight, tolerance, and laboratory values (Table 18.5). Eating resumes as soon as possible after surgery, usually within 2 to 4 days. Small, frequent meals and commercial supplements may help maximize intake. Although oral nutrition is the preferred route, enteral nutrition support is used if the patient is unable to consume adequate nutrition for 5 to 7 days.

After the initial hypermetabolic period, the patient's calorie and protein needs return toward normal. Patients may have difficulty transitioning from a high-calorie, high-protein diet to a healthy maintenance diet that is low in fat, lower in calories, high in fiber, with good quality protein (ADA, 2006). Long-term complications associated with immunosuppressive therapy, such as excessive weight gain, hypertension, hyperlipidemia, osteopenic bone disease, and diabetes, may require nutrition therapy. The use of immunosuppressant drugs elevates the importance of safe food handling practices to avoid foodborne illness.

## Pancreatitis

The pancreas is responsible for secreting enzymes needed to digest dietary carbohydrates, protein, and fat. Until they are needed, these enzymes are held in the pancreas in their inactive form. Inflammation of the pancreas causes digestive enzymes to be retained in the pancreas and converted to their active form so they literally begin to digest the pancreas. Because the pancreas also produces insulin, people with **pancreatitis** may also develop hyperglycemia related to insufficient insulin secretion.

**Pancreatitis:** inflammation of the pancreas

**Amylase:** a class of enzymes that split starch molecules

**Lipase:** an enzyme that splits fat molecules

Alcohol abuse and gallstones account for 75% to 85% of cases of acute pancreatitis (Raimonda & Scholapio, 2006). Patients present with acute abdominal pain in the upper quadrant and have elevated levels of serum **amylase** and **lipase**. Mild acute pancreatitis usually resolves in a few days; moderate to severe forms often require prolonged hospitalization that may preclude patients from eating.

Acute pancreatitis that is not resolved or recurs frequently can lead to chronic pancreatitis characterized by scarring, fibrosis, and loss of organ function. Seventy percent of cases are caused by alcohol abuse, 20% are idiopathic. Acute pancreatitis is characterized by intermittent pain that is made worse by eating. Because the pancreas normally secretes enzymes in amounts that exceed physiologic need, malabsorption does not occur until pancreatic enzyme secretion is less than 10% of normal (Raimonda & Scholapio, 2006). Steatorrhea occurs late in the disease, and weight loss is gradual. Symptoms of diabetes, such as increased thirst and urination, may develop.

## Nutrition Therapy

Acute pancreatitis is treated by reducing pancreatic stimulation. In mild cases, the patient is given pain medications, IV therapy, and NPO. How and when an oral intake resumes is based on anecdotal experience and physiologic studies in healthy people, not from controlled studies on patients with acute pancreatitis. Generally, when pain subsides, amylase levels fall to near-normal levels, and there are no complications, patients are given a clear liquid diet and advanced to a low-fat diet as tolerated. Small, frequent meals may be better tolerated initially because they help to reduce the amount of pancreatic stimulation at each meal. A prospective, randomized trial by Jacobson et al. showed that initiating a solid low-fat diet after mild acute pancreatitis was safe and provided more calories than a clear liquid diet, although the length of hospitalization did not improve (Jacobson et al., 2008).

For patients with moderate to severe acute pancreatitis, patients are ordered NPO, and a nasogastric tube is inserted to suction gastric contents. Appropriate measures are taken to correct fluid and electrolyte imbalance, to control pain, and to treat or prevent symptoms. The preferred route of delivering nutrition to patients with moderate to severe pancreatitis has shifted away from TPN to enteral nutrition (Raimonda & Scholapio, 2006). Enteral nutrition, particularly jejunal feedings, offer the advantage of being well tolerated and less likely to cause septic and other complications (Raimonda & Scholapio, 2006), and feeding into the jejunum does not stimulate pancreatic secretions.

The goals of nutrition therapy for chronic pancreatitis are to maintain weight, reduce steatorrhea, minimize pain, and avoid acute attacks while meeting the patient's nutrient needs. A mildly low-fat diet (Box 18.9) that is high in protein is recommended. Fat is restricted further for patients with steatorrhea. Patients whose insulin secretion is impaired may need a diabetic diet to help control hyperglycemia. Supplements of antioxidants may help reduce pancreatic inflammation and pain in patients with either acute or chronic pancreatitis (Raimonda & Scholapio, 2006). Taking pancreatic enzyme replacement pills at the beginning, end, and during each meal is crucial for maximum effectiveness.

## Gallbladder Disease

The gallbladder's role in digestion is to store and release bile, which prepares fat for digestion. Bile, which is made in the liver, consists of cholesterol, bile salts, bile pigments, and water. As it is held in the gallbladder, water is slowly removed from bile, making it more concentrated and increasing the likelihood that solids (either cholesterol crystals or pigment material) will precipitate out into clumps known as gallstones. Incomplete emptying of the gallbladder may also be involved in gallstone formation.

---

**BOX 18.9**      **LOW-FAT DIET**

- Total fat is limited to reduce symptoms of steatorrhea and pain in patients who are intolerant to fat, such as for people with chronic pancreatitis, Crohn's disease, radiation enteritis, and short bowel syndrome

**Guidelines to Achieve a Low-Fat Diet**
- Eat nonfat or low-fat food to meet appropriate MyPyramid amounts
- Select only very lean meats, fish, and skinless poultry; egg whites; and low-fat egg substitutes
- Bake, broil, or boil foods instead of frying
- Use milk and dairy products that provide less than 1 g fat per serving and use low-fat cheese with 3 g or less of fat per serving.
- Enjoy all fruits and vegetables that are prepared without added fat except avocado and coconut
- Choose grain products that are prepared without added fat (e.g., avoid muffins, waffles, biscuits, pastries, other baked goods)
- Choose low-fat desserts: sherbet, fruit ices, gelatin, angel food cake, vanilla wafers, graham crackers, nonfat ice cream and frozen yogurt; fruit whips with gelatin
- Limit fats to less than 8 equivalents per day. Each of the following constitutes one serving (one "equivalent"):

| | |
|---|---|
| 1 tsp butter, margarine, shortening, oil, or mayonnaise | 1 tbsp heavy cream<br>2 tsp regular creamy salad dressing |
| 1 tbsp diet margarine, diet mayonnaise, or reduced-calorie cream salad dressing | 2 tsp peanut butter<br>2 tsp light cream |
| 1 strip crisp bacon | 6 small nuts |
| 1 tbsp sesame, sunflower, or pumpkin seeds | 8–10 olives |
| 2 tbsp sour cream, cream cheese, half-and-half, or coffee whitener | ⅛ medium avocado |

**Sample Menu**

| Breakfast | Lunch | Dinner | Snacks |
|---|---|---|---|
| Orange juice | Fat-free vegetable soup | 2 oz broiled lean chicken | Fat-free popcorn |
| Oatmeal with fat-free milk | 2 oz of fat-free ham on whole-wheat bread with lettuce and fat-free mayonnaise | Brown rice | Carrots and celery with fat-free dressing |
| Whole-wheat toast with jelly | Fresh strawberries | Tossed salad with vegetables and fat-free dressing | Tomato juice |
| | Fat-free milk | Steamed broccoli | |
| | | Whole-wheat roll with 1 tsp butter | |
| | | Blueberries | |
| | | Fat-free milk | |

*(box continues on page 442)*

**BOX 18.9**     **LOW-FAT DIET** (continued)

| **Potential Problems** | **Recommended Interventions** |
|---|---|
| Noncompliance related to decreased palatability and satiety from the reduction in fat intake | Encourage the patient to eat a variety of foods and to use nonfat and fat-free versions of familiar foods. Encourage use of butter-flavored sprinkles and sprays to season hot vegetables and potatoes |
| Persistent symptoms of steatorrhea or pain after eating that are related to fat intolerance | Decrease fat content by eliminating fat equivalents and limiting the amount of low-fat meat allowed |
| Inadequate intake of iron related to the limited allowance of meat (red meat is the best absorbed source of iron in the diet) | Monitor hemoglobin and hematocrit; recommend iron supplements as needed |
| | Encourage a liberal intake of high-iron foods such as fortified cereals and grains and dried peas and beans. Advise the patient to consume a rich source of vitamin C at each meal to maximize iron absorption |

**Patient Teaching**

Ensure the patient understands that
• The total amount of dietary fat must be reduced regardless of the source
• Sources of fat may be visible (e.g., butter, margarine, shortening, fat on meat, salad dressings) or invisible (e.g., marbled meat, whole milk and whole-milk products, egg yolks, nuts)
• Substitutions can be made to individualize the diet
• Oil-packed tuna and salmon may be used if thoroughly rinsed
• Fat-free salad dressings may be used as desired

• Tips for reducing fat content when eating out:
  • Choose juice or broth-based soup instead of cream soup as an appetizer
  • Use lemon, vinegar, low-calorie dressing (if available), or fresh ground pepper on salad, or request that the dressing be brought on the side
  • Order plain baked or broiled foods
  • Avoid warm bread and rolls, which absorb more butter than those at room temperature
  • Order fresh fruit, gelatin, or sherbet for dessert
  • Request milk for coffee or tea in place of cream and nondairy creamers

Food preparation techniques to reduce fat content:
• Trim fat from meat and remove skin from chicken before cooking
• Place meats to be baked or roasted on a rack to allow the fat to drain
• Bake, broil, steam, or sauté foods in a vegetable cooking spray or allowed fats
• Cook with bouillon, lemon, vinegar, wine, herbs, and spices instead of adding fat
• Make fat-free soup stock by preparing the stock a day ahead and refrigerating it overnight. The fat will harden and can easily be removed from the surface. Make fat-free gravies also by this method
• Purchase "select" grade meats because they are lower in fat than "choice" and "prime" grades

**Cholelithiasis:**
formation of gallstones

A large majority of people with **cholelithiasis** are asymptomatic, but some experience episodic, upper GI pain that spreads to the chest and shoulders in a manner similar to the symptoms of a heart attack. For some people, eating a fatty meal precipitates symptoms; for others, symptoms develop during sleep. Gallstones that obstruct the cystic duct can lead to **cholecystitis**, causing abdominal pain, nausea and vomiting, jaundice, fever, fat intolerance, and flatulence. Surgical removal of the gallbladder may be used to treat symptomatic gallstones. After the gallbladder is removed, the common bile duct collects and holds bile until mealtime when it is released into the duodenum.

**Cholecystitis:**
inflammation of the gallbladder

No diet modifications are necessary for healthy people with asymptomatic gallstones. Patients with symptomatic gallstones may be told to limit their intake of fat based on the rationale that limiting fat intake reduces stimulation to the gallbladder and minimizes pain. However, it is not known if patients with gallstones are any more intolerant of fat than the general population. Other practices, based more on popular belief than on scientific data, include limiting spicy foods, high-fiber foods, and foods that cause gas. Most patients do not experience problems after recovery from surgery.

## NURSING PROCESS: Crohn's Disease

A ndrew is a 20-year-old man who is admitted to the hospital for suspected Crohn's disease. His chief complaints are crampy abdominal pain, diarrhea, weight loss, fatigue, and anorexia. He has lost 15 pounds since his symptoms began 2 weeks ago. He is prescribed intravenous fluids, sulfasalazine, prednisone, an antidiarrheal medication, and a diet as tolerated.

| Assessment | |
| --- | --- |
| Medical–Psychosocial History | • Medical and surgical history |
| | • Use of prescribed and OTC medications |
| | • Support system |
| Anthropometric Assessment | • Height, current weight, usual weight; % weight loss; BMI |
| Biochemical and Physical Assessment | • Hemoglobin (Hgb), hematocrit (Hct) |
| | • Serum electrolyte levels |
| | • Prealbumin, if available |
| | • Blood pressure |
| | • Signs of dehydration (poor skin turgor, dry mucous membranes, etc.) |
| Dietary Assessment | • How has your intake changed since you began experiencing symptoms? |
| | • Do you know if any particular foods cause problems? Did you have any food intolerances or allergies before your symptoms began? |
| | • How many meals per day are you eating? |
| | • How much fluid are you drinking in a day? |
| | • Have you ever followed any kind of diet before? |
| | • Do you take vitamins, minerals, or other supplements? |
| | • Do you use alcohol? |
| | • Who prepares your meals? |

*(nursing process continues on page 444)*

## NURSING PROCESS: Crohn's Disease (continued)

### Diagnosis

**Possible Nursing Diagnosis**

Imbalanced nutrition less than body requirements related to diarrhea, and altered ability to digest and absorb food.

### Planning

**Client Outcomes**

The client will
- Consume adequate calories and protein to restore normal weight.
- Experience improvement in symptoms (diarrhea, abdominal pain, fatigue, anorexia).
- Restore normal fluid balance.
- Describe the principles and rationale of nutrition therapy for Crohn's disease and implement the appropriate interventions.

### Nursing Interventions

**Nutrition Therapy**

- Provide a low-fat, low-fiber, high-protein lactose-restricted diet as tolerated
- Provide lactose-free commercial supplements between meals to enhance protein and calorie intake
- Encourage high fluid intake, especially of fluids high in potassium such as tomato juice, apricot nectar, and orange juice
- Promote gradual return to normal diet as tolerated

**Client Teaching**

Instruct the client:
- On the purpose and rationale of a low-fat, low-fiber, lactose-restricted diet. Advise the patient that he may be able to tolerate fiber and milk after the disease goes into remission
- On the importance of consuming adequate protein, calories, and fluid to promote healing and recovery
- To maximize intake by eating small, frequent meals
- To avoid colas and other sources of caffeine because they stimulate peristalsis
- To eliminate individual intolerances
- To chew food thoroughly and avoid swallowing air
- On the importance of consuming adequate fluid while taking sulfasalazine
- That prednisone should improve his appetite but may cause fluid retention and gastrointestinal upset
- To communicate any side effects he experiences from the medications

### Evaluation

**Evaluate and Monitor**

- Intake and output; fluid and electrolyte status
- Appetite
- Tolerance to fat (may need to reduce fat level)
- Diarrhea (if patient does not tolerate an oral diet, determine whether a defined formula feeding or TPN is appropriate) and other symptoms
- Weight changes and BMI

## ▶ HOW DO YOU RESPOND?

**Are probiotics safe?** Probiotics that contain *Lactobacillus, Bifidobacterium, Streptococcus thermaophilus,* and *Saccharomyces* strains are safe for use in generally healthy people (Douglas & Sanders, 2008). Other types of probiotics (e.g., *Enterococcus*) should be reserved for specific individuals. People who are immunocompromised, recovering from surgery, or who have altered GI integrity are at increased risk for infection from any source and should not take probiotics without their physician's approval.

**Are "live active cultures" the same thing as probiotics?** Live cultures are associated with foods; they are often added to ferment foods. Probiotics are live microorganisms that have been shown to benefit health. Some probiotics are not normally found in foods, such as *Escherichia coli,* and so they are not synonymous with "live culture."

## ▶ CASE STUDY

Brittany is a 33-year-old woman who has recently been diagnosed with IBS. She alternates between episodes of diarrhea and constipation and complains of distention and abdominal pain. Her doctor suggested she eat more fiber and take Metamucil. She dislikes whole-wheat bread. She is reluctant to take a fiber supplement; she knows fiber helps people with constipation, and because she also has diarrhea, she believes it will only make her problem worse. She is thinking about adding yogurt to her usual diet to see if that helps. She drinks an "irritable bowel syndrome–friendly tea" that is supposed to help, but she hasn't noticed any improvement.

Her usual intake is as follows:

| | |
|---|---|
| **Breakfast:** | Orange juice <br> White toast with peanut butter <br> Coffee |
| **Snacks:** | Small bag of chips from the vending machine |
| **Lunch:** | Fast-food hamburger on a bun <br> Small French fries <br> Diet coke |
| **Snacks:** | Cheese and crackers <br> Glass of wine |
| **Dinner:** | Beef or chicken <br> Mashed potatoes with sour cream <br> Tossed salad with Italian dressing <br> Ice cream <br> Coffee |
| **Snacks:** | Milk and cookies, usually peanut butter |

- What does Brittany need to know about fiber and bowel function? What would you say to her about eating more fiber? About taking a fiber supplement? About yogurt? And "irritable bowel syndrome–friendly tea"?
- What else do you need to know about Brittany to help relieve her symptoms?
- Modify Brittany's diet to be high in fiber despite her refusal to eat whole-wheat bread.
- What other diet interventions could she implement to try to improve her symptoms?
- What elimination diet items is she consuming? What alternatives to those foods would you suggest?

STUDY QUESTIONS

1. When developing a teaching plan for a patient who has chronic diarrhea, which of the following foods would the nurse suggest as an appropriate source of potassium?
   a. Tomato juice
   b. Pinto beans
   c. Milk
   d. Broccoli

2. Which statement indicates the patient with an ileostomy needs further instruction about what to eat?
   a. "Drinking lots of water increases the output from my ileostomy."
   b. "It is best to eat a small evening meal."
   c. "Oatmeal and bananas may help control diarrhea."
   d. "A regular eating schedule will help regulate my bowel pattern."

3. The client asks if yogurt with probiotics will relieve her symptoms of irritable bowel syndrome. Which of the following would be the nurse's best response?
   a. "Unfortunately there isn't anything that will help relieve irritable bowel syndrome."
   b. "Although it is not guaranteed to help, probiotics may help and do not pose a health risk in healthy people."
   c. "Because little is known about the effects of probiotics on health, you should avoid consuming them."
   d. "Probiotics are the only dietary intervention known to help irritable bowel syndrome."

4. The nurse knows his or her instructions have been effective when the client with celiac disease verbalizes that an appropriate breakfast is
   a. Eggs and toast
   b. Cornflakes with milk
   c. Bran flakes cereal with milk
   d. Buttermilk pancakes with syrup

5. Which of the following would be most appropriate in modifying a regular diet to a high-fiber diet?
   a. Ice cream in place of gelatin
   b. Apple in place of apple juice
   c. Rice in place of mashed potatoes
   d. Cream of wheat in place of cream of rice

6. Which of the following would be an appropriate source of calcium for a client who is lactose intolerant?
   a. Green leafy vegetables
   b. Pudding
   c. Lean meats
   d. Refined breads and cereals

7. A client with fat malabsorption is at risk for which of the following?
   a. Oxalate kidney stones
   b. Constipation
   c. Deficiencies of essential amino acids
   d. Type 2 diabetes

8. Which of the following strategies would help a client achieve a low-fat diet?
   a. Substitute margarine for butter
   b. Limit portion sizes of meat
   c. Substitute whole-wheat bread for white bread
   d. Eat more fruit in place of vegetables

**KEY CONCEPTS**

- The first half of the small intestine is the site where most nutrients are absorbed. Conditions that affect the small intestine can impair the absorption of one or many nutrients.

- The large intestine absorbs water, electrolytes, vitamin $B_{12}$, and bile salts. Disorders of the colon can cause major problems with fluid and electrolyte balance and vitamin $B_{12}$ deficiency.

- Most cases of constipation can be alleviated or prevented by increasing fiber and fluid intake. Most Americans consume approximately half the amount of fiber recommended daily.

- To achieve a high-fiber diet, high-fiber foods are eaten in place of those low in fiber, such as whole-wheat bread for white bread, high-fiber cereal for refined cereal, and whole fruits for fruit juices. High-fiber foods to add to a usual diet include dried peas and beans, more vegetables, nuts, and seeds.

- Other than encouraging fluids and foods high in potassium, nutrition therapy usually is not necessary for acute diarrhea of short-term duration. Because many clear liquids are hyperosmolar and may contribute to osmotic diarrhea, they should be avoided until diarrhea subsides. Foods that help thicken stools, such as bananas and oatmeal, are encouraged. Patients should avoid items that stimulate peristalsis, such as caffeine, alcohol, and high-fiber, gassy foods.

- A low-fiber diet is appropriate only for short-term use. Its effect is to decrease stimulation to the bowel and slow intestinal transit time.

- Primary lactose intolerance is common in much of the world's adult population; tolerance varies considerably among individuals. Some people tolerate milk with food; others tolerate only lactose-reduced milk. Lactose intolerance that occurs secondary to intestinal disorders is usually more symptomatic than primary lactose intolerance and requires a more restrictive intake.

- During exacerbation of inflammatory bowel diseases, patients need increased amounts of calories and protein and may not tolerate fiber and lactose. Patients are often reluctant to eat, fearing that food will cause pain and diarrhea. Some patients require enteral or parenteral nutrition for bowel rest. During remission, the diet is liberalized as tolerated.

- A gluten-free diet prevents intestinal villi changes, steatorrhea, and other symptoms in patients with celiac disease. All forms and sources of wheat, oats, rye, and barley must be permanently eliminated from the diet, even in patients who are asymptomatic. A gluten-free diet requires major lifestyle changes and is difficult to follow.

- Short bowel syndrome occurs in patients who have had more than 50% of the small intestine removed. Maldigestion and malabsorption may lead to malnutrition. TPN is usually used until adaptation begins. Calorie and protein requirements increase. Tolerance to fat, lactose, and fiber is impaired.

- Irritable bowel syndrome is a common but not serious disorder. A high-fiber diet may help relieve symptoms in some people, and fiber supplements may also be beneficial. Research on the benefits of probiotics and prebiotics is encouraging but not conclusive.

- A high-fiber diet alleviates and prevents diverticulosis and diverticulitis. During acute diverticulitis, however, patients may be given a low-fiber diet to reduce bowel stimulation. Patients are often confused about the apparent inconsistency in nutrition therapy.

- Fluid and electrolytes are of primary concern for patients with ileostomies and colostomies. Low-fiber foods may help to reduce stoma discharge and irritation. Additional calories and protein are needed to promote healing.

- Adequate calories and protein promote liver cell regeneration in patients with hepatitis and cirrhosis. Sodium and fluid may be restricted if ascites develop. A liquid or soft diet is recommended if regular textured foods irritate esophageal varices.

- People who have undergone liver transplantation have high protein and calorie needs. Glucose intolerance may occur, and sodium and potassium intakes may be restricted depending on the individual's profile. Immunosuppressant drugs may interfere with intake and appetite.

- Chronic pancreatitis is treated with a low-fat diet. Patients who develop glucose intolerance may benefit from a diabetic diet.

- A common practice is to recommend a low-fat diet for patients with symptomatic gallstones and for people who have had a cholecystectomy. Evidence is lacking on the benefits of restricting fat.

## ANSWER KEY

1. **TRUE** For most people, consuming more fiber and fluid prevents or alleviates constipation.

2. **FALSE** A clear liquid diet contains items that are hyperosmolar, such as sweetened carbonated beverages, fruit juice, and flavored ices; consuming them may contribute to osmotic diarrhea.

3. **FALSE** Although MCT oil is a good source of calories for people who have fat malabsorption, it does not provide essential fatty acids.

4. **TRUE** Because most of the lactose in cheddar and other natural, aged cheeses has been converted to lactic acid in the cheese-making process, most people who are lactose intolerant can tolerate cheddar cheese.

5. **FALSE** Eating a low-residue/low-fiber diet is not necessary for people with IBD except during acute exacerbation or if there are strictures. A low-residue diet does not prevent exacerbation of the disease.

6. **TRUE** For a patient with celiac disease, the long-term effects of eating even small amounts of gluten are harmful, even when patients are asymptomatic.

7. **FALSE** Although a high-fiber diet may help relieve symptoms of IBS in some people, it is not guaranteed to help all people with IBS.

8. **TRUE** A high-fiber diet may help prevent both diverticulosis and diverticulitis by decreasing pressure within the bowel.

9. **TRUE** Extensive pancreatic damage impairs digestion, especially fat digestion. A low-fat diet is used when pancreatitis causes steatorrhea.

10. **FALSE** Dietary intervention is not necessary for cholelithiasis or cholecystitis.

## WEBSITES

Celiac Disease Foundation at **www.celiac.org**
Celiac Sprue Association/USA at **http://csaceliacs.org**
Crohn's and Colitis Foundation of America at **www.ccfa.org**
Gluten Intolerance Group at **www.gluten.net**
Information on prebiotics and probiotics is available at **www.usprobiotics.org**, a nonprofit research and educational website made possible by the California Dairy Research Foundation and Dairy & Food Culture Technologies.
National Digestive Disease Information Clearinghouse at **http://digestive.niddk.nih.gov**

# REFERENCES

American Dietetic Association (ADA) Nutrition Care Manual (2008). Retrieved 5/30/08 from www.nutritioncaremanual.org.

American Gastroenterological Association (AGA), Clinical Practice and Economics Committee. (2006). AGA institute medical position statement on the diagnosis and management of celiac disease. *Gastroenterology, 131,* 1977–1980.

Beitz, J. (2004). Diverticulosis and diverticulitis spectrum of a modern malady. *Journal of Wound, Ostomy, and Continence Nursing, 31,* 75–82.

Card, T., West, J., & Holmes, G. (2004). Risk of malignancy in diagnosed coeliac disease: A 24-year prospective, population-based, cohort study. *Alimentary Pharmacology & Therapeutics, 20,* 769–775.

Chand, N., & Mihas, A. (2006). Celiac disease: Current concepts in diagnosis and treatment. *Journal of Clinical Gastroenterology, 40,* 3–14.

Clark, C., & DeLegge, M. (2008). Irritable bowel syndrome: A practical approach. *Nutrition in Clinical Practice, 23,* 263–267.

Cremonini, F., & Talley, N. (2005). Irritable bowel syndrome: Epidemiology, natural history, heatlh care seeking and emerging risk factors. *Gastroenterol Clinics North America, 34,* 189–204.

Douglas, L., & Sanders, M. (2008). Probiotics and prebiotics in dietetics practice. *Journal of the American Dietetic Association, 108,* 510–521.

Ebell, M. H., Siwek, J., Weiss, B. D., et al. (2004). Strength of Recommendation Taxonomy (SORT): A patient-centered approach to grading evidence in the medical literature. *The Journal of the American Board of Family Practice, 17,* 59–67.

FAO/WHO. (2002). *Guidelines for the evaluation of probiotics in food.* Available at http://www.who.int/foodsafety/fs_management/en/probiotic_guidelines.pdf. Accessed on June 18, 2008.

Fessler, T. (2007). A dietary challenge: Maximizing bowel adaptation in short bowel syndrome. *Today's Dietitian, 9*(10), 40–45.

Green, P. (2005). The many faces of celiac disease: Clinical presentation of celiac disease in the adult population. *Gastroenterology, 128*(suppl. 1), S74–S78.

Green, P., & Jabri, B. (2003). Coeliac disease. *Lancet, 362,* 383–391.

Guslandi, M. (2007). Probiotic agents in the treatment of irritable bowel syndrome. *The Journal of International Medical Research, 35,* 583–589.

Hanauer, S. (2006). Inflammatory bowel disease: Epidemiology, pathogenesis, and therapeutic opportunities. *Inflammatory Bowel Diseases, 12,* S3–S9.

Institute of Medicine (IOM). (2005). *Dietary reference intakes for energy, carbohydrates, fiber, fat, fatty acids, cholesterol, protein, and amino acids.* Washington, DC: National Academies Press.

Jacobson, B. C., VanderVliet, M. B., Hughes, M. D., et al. (2008). A prospective, randomized trial of clear liquids versus low-fat solid diet as the initial meal in mild acute pancreatitis. *Nutrition in Clinical Practice, 23,* 341–342.

Kelly, D. (2006). Assessment of malabsorption. In M. Shils, M. Shike, A. Ross, et al. (Eds.), *Modern Nutrition in Health and Disease* (10th ed.). Philadelphia: Lippincott Williams & Wilkins.

Matarese, L. E., O'Keefe, S. J., Kandil, H. M., et al. (2005). Short bowel syndrome: Clinical guidelines for nutrition management. *Nutrition in Clinical Practice, 20,* 493–502.

Muller-Lissner, S. A., Kamm, M. A., Scarpignato, C., et al. (2005). Myths and misconceptions about chronic constipation. *The American Journal of Gastroenterology, 100,* 123–129.

National Institute of Diabetes and Digestive and Kidney Diseases (NIDDK). (2006). *Lactose intolerance.* Available at http://www.digestive.niddk.nih.gov/ddiseases/pubs/lactoseintolerance/ Accessed on 6/12/08.

National Institute of Diabetes and Digestive and Kidney Diseases (NIDDK). (2008). *Diverticulosis and diverticulitis.* Available at http://digestive.niddk.nih.gov/ddiseases/pubs/diverticulosis/index.htm. Accessed on 6/16/08.

National Institutes of Health (NIH). (2005). NIH consensus development conference statement on celiac disease. *Gastroenterology, 128*(suppl. 1), S1–S9.

Niewinski, M. (2008). Advances in celiac disease and gluten-free diet. *Journal of the American Dietetic Association, 108,* 661–672.

Parisi, G. C., Zilli, M., Miani, M. P., et al. (2002). High-fiber diet supplementation in patients with irritable bowel syndrome (IBS): A multicenter, randomized, open trial comparison between wheat bran diet and partially hydrolyzed guar gum (PHGG). *Digestive Diseases and Sciences, 47,* 1697–1704.

Quartero, A. O., Meineche-Schmidt, V., Muris, J., et al. (2005). Bulking agents, antispasmodic and antidepressant medication for the treatment of irritable bowel syndrome. *Cochrane Database of Systematic Reviews, 18*(2), CD003460.

Reunala, T. (1998). Dermatitis herpetiformis: Celiac disease of the skin. *Annals of Medicine, 5,* 416–418.

Stephenson, G. R., Moretti, E. W., El-Moalem, H., et al. (2001). Malnutrition in liver transplant patients: Preoperative subjective global assessment is predictive of outcome after liver transplantation. *Transplantation, 72*(4), 666–670.

Thompson, T. (2005). National Institutes of Health consensus statement on celiac disease. *Journal of the American Dietetic Association, 105,* 194–195.

Timm, D., & Slavin, J. (2008). Dietary fiber and the relationship to chronic disease. *American Journal of Lifestyle Medicine, 2,* 233–240.

Wald, A., & Rakel, D. (2008). Behavioral and complementary approaches for the treatment of irritable bowel syndrome. *Nutrition in Clinical Practice, 23,* 284–292.

# 19

# Nutrition for Patients with Diabetes Mellitus

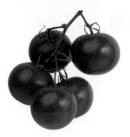

| TRUE | FALSE | |
|:---:|:---:|:---|
| ☐ | ☐ | **1** The progression of prediabetes to diabetes is inevitable. |
| ☐ | ☐ | **2** The cornerstone of nutrition therapy for diabetes is to eat a low-carbohydrate diet. |
| ☐ | ☐ | **3** Weight loss lowers the risk of type 2 diabetes only when it achieves a weight within an individual's healthy BMI range. |
| ☐ | ☐ | **4** Alcohol is more likely to cause hypoglycemia when consumed without food rather than with food. |
| ☐ | ☐ | **5** People with diabetes should avoid fruit because fructose produces a higher postprandial rise in glucose than sucrose. |
| ☐ | ☐ | **6** People with diabetes should eat more fiber than the general population. |
| ☐ | ☐ | **7** All people with diabetes should consume a bedtime snack to avoid hypoglycemia. |
| ☐ | ☐ | **8** People who practice carbohydrate counting do not have to pay attention to protein or fat intake. |
| ☐ | ☐ | **9** A chocolate candy bar is a good choice for treating mild hypoglycemia. |
| ☐ | ☐ | **10** People with diabetes should limit their intake of saturated fat and cholesterol. |

### UPON COMPLETION OF THIS CHAPTER, YOU WILL BE ABLE TO

- Summarize nutrition recommendations for the primary prevention of diabetes.
- Describe the nutrition recommendations for managing diabetes.
- Explain nutrition recommendations for managing the complications of diabetes.
- Compare the use of exchange lists to carbohydrate counting as a means of tracking carbohydrate intake.
- Compose a 2000-calorie diet using the carbohydrate counting method of meal planning.
- Determine the number of carbohydrate choices a serving of food provides by using the Nutrition Facts label.
- Discuss diabetes nutrition therapy in childhood, pregnancy, and older adults.

Glucose circulating in the blood is a source of ready fuel for body cells. It comes primarily from recently absorbed dietary carbohydrates and liver glycogen, although glucose is available from some amino acids and the glycerol portion of fatty acids. All body cells use glucose for energy to some extent; under normal conditions, cells of the brain and the rest of the nervous system rely solely on glucose for energy.

The amount of carbohydrate and to a lesser extent the type of carbohydrate consumed are the primary determinants of how quickly and how high blood glucose levels rise after eating. A rise in postprandial blood glucose levels stimulates the pancreas to secrete insulin. As an anabolic hormone, insulin promotes the formation of glycogen, the storage of fat, and protein synthesis; conversely, it inhibits the breakdown of stored macronutrients. Its most well-known role is facilitating glucose uptake from the blood into the cells. The amount and effectiveness of circulating insulin determines how quickly blood glucose levels return to normal after eating.

When insulin secretion is absent or deficient, or circulating insulin is ineffective, glucose levels remain high after eating. Fasting blood glucose levels ≥126 mg/dL indicate diabetes. This chapter presents nutrition therapy aimed at preventing diabetes, managing existing diabetes, and preventing or forestalling diabetes complications.

## ▶ DIABETES

Diabetes is one of the most costly and burdensome chronic diseases of our time and is increasing in epidemic proportions. From 1990 to 2005, the prevalence of diabetes increased from 26.4 to 54.5 cases per 1000 adults (Geiss et al., 2007). The statistics are staggering:

- In 2007, an estimated 23.6 million Americans, or 7.8% of the population, had diabetes (CDC, 2007). Of those cases, 5.7 million were undiagnosed (CDC, 2007).
- In 2003–2004, an estimated 57 million American adults (25.9% of the adult population) had impaired fasting glucose, a prediabetic condition (CDC, 2007).
- Over the next 45 years, diagnosed diabetes is projected to increase by 165% in the United States (Daly, 2007).
- The CDC estimates that one in three children born in the United States in 2000 will have diabetes in his or her lifetime; for Hispanics, the estimate is one out of two (Narayan et al., 2003).
- The estimated direct and indirect cost associated with diabetes in 2007 was $174 billion (CDC, 2007).

### Type 1 Diabetes

**Type 1 diabetes**, formerly known as insulin-dependent **diabetes mellitus**, is characterized by the absence of insulin. It occurs from an autoimmune response that damages or destroys pancreatic beta cells, leaving them unable to produce insulin. Risk factors for type 1 diabetes may be autoimmune, genetic, or environmental. There is no known way to prevent type 1 diabetes. All people with type 1 diabetes require exogenous insulin to control blood glucose levels.

Although it can occur at any age, type 1 diabetes is most often detected in children, adolescents, and young adults. The classic symptoms of **polyuria, polydipsia**, and **polyphagia** appear abruptly. Sometimes the first sign of the disease is **ketoacidosis**. Type 1 diabetes accounts for 5% to 10% of all diagnosed diabetes cases.

### Type 2 Diabetes

Type 2 diabetes occurs most often after the age of 45 and accounts for 90% to 95% of diagnosed cases of diabetes. It is largely responsible for the increasing prevalence of diabetes (CDC, 2007). Unlike type 1 diabetes in which there is a relatively abrupt end to insulin production, type 2 diabetes is a slowly progressive disease that usually begins as a problem

**Type 1 Diabetes:** diabetes characterized by the absence of insulin secretion.

**Diabetes Mellitus:** a chronic heterogeneous disorder characterized by elevated blood glucose levels (hyperglycemia) related to a relative or absolute deficiency of insulin.

**Polyuria:** excessive urine excretion.

**Polydipsia:** excessive thirst.

**Polyphagia:** excessive appetite.

**Ketoacidosis:** the accumulation of ketone bodies leading to acidosis related to incomplete breakdown of fatty acids from carbohydrate deficiency or inadequate carbohydrate utilization.

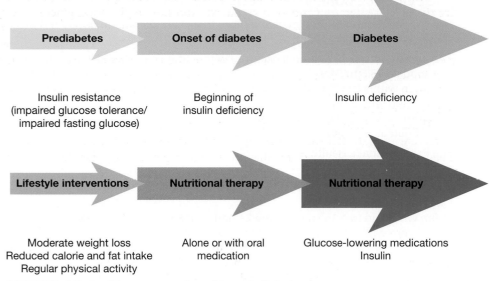

**FIGURE 19.1**   The progression of type 2 diabetes.

**Insulin Resistance:** decreased cellular response to insulin.

**Impaired Glucose Tolerance:** a condition in which blood glucose levels are elevated, but not high enough to be classified as diabetes. Also known as prediabetes.

**Hyperinsulinemia:** elevated blood levels of insulin.

of **insulin resistance** (Fig. 19.1). Cells do not respond to insulin as they should, which causes the pancreas to compensate by secreting higher than normal levels of insulin. During this period of **impaired glucose tolerance**, glucose levels are relatively normal but insulin levels are high. Over time, chronic **hyperinsulinemia** leads to a decrease in the number of insulin receptors on the cells and a further reduction in tissue sensitivity to insulin. Eventually and progressively, insulin sensitivity and insulin secretion deteriorate, and frank type 2 diabetes develops. Type 2 diabetes is often asymptomatic.

Insulin resistance, the precursor condition of type 2 diabetes, is strongly linked to obesity. Epidemiological studies clearly show that the risk of type 2 diabetes increases as body weight increases (Cummings et al., 2008) (Box 19.1). Other risk factors for type 2 diabetes appear in Box 19.2.

Many of the risks for type 2 diabetes are characteristics of metabolic syndrome (MetS), a group of interrelated risk factors including central obesity, hypertension, altered blood lipid levels (especially low high-density lipoprotein [HDL] cholesterol and high triglycerides), and altered glucose/insulin metabolism (NCEP, 2001). People with MetS are twice as likely to develop heart disease and five times as likely to develop diabetes compared to those without MetS (Grundy et al., 2005). Definitions and threshold values used to diagnose MetS differ, so the prevalence depends on the diagnostic criteria used. It is estimated that more than two-thirds of people with type 2 diabetes have MetS (Smith, 2007).

Modifiable risk factors for MetS include excess body fat, a sedentary lifestyle, and a high saturated fat diet. Weight loss through a combination of diet and exercise is recommended as the initial therapy for MetS (Grundy et al., 2005). Even modest weight loss can lessen the risks associated with MetS.

## Gestational Diabetes

Gestational diabetes is hyperglycemia that develops during pregnancy, usually between 24 and 28 weeks of gestation. Risk factors for gestational diabetes include a family history of gestational diabetes, obesity, being a member of a certain ethnic population (native Americans, Hispanic Americans, Mexican Americans, African Americans, Asian Americans,

| BOX 19.1 | THE EVIDENCE CORRELATING BODY WEIGHT TO TYPE 2 DIABETES |

The Nurse's Health Study, involving more than 121,000 female registered nurses, showed (Colditz et al., 1995):

- An *increased* risk of diabetes occurred with a BMI as low as 22 ("healthy" BMI is defined as 18.5 to 24.9).
- Women with a healthy BMI of 24.0 to 24.9 had *up to a fivefold increased* risk compared to women with a BMI of <22.
- In women with a BMI >31, the risk of diabetes increased by *more than 40-fold* (BMI >30 is defined as obesity).

The Professional's Health Study, involving more than 51,000 male health professionals, showed (Chan et al., 1994):

- Relative risk of diabetes in men with a BMI of 35 was *42 times higher* than that in men with a BMI <23.
- Men who gained ≥15 kg after age 21 had an *8.9 times higher* risk of diabetes than those who were within 2 kg of their weight at 21 years of age.

| BOX 19.2 | RISK FACTORS FOR TYPE 2 DIABETES |

- ≥45 years of age
- Overweight (BMI ≥25 kg/m$^2$)
- First-degree relative with diabetes
- Physically inactive or exercises fewer than 3 times/week
- Member of high-risk ethnic group: African American, Latino, Native American, Asian American, Pacific Islander
- Previously identified with prediabetes such as impaired fasting glucose or impaired glucose tolerance
- History of gestational diabetes or giving birth to a baby weighing >9 pounds
- Hypertensive
- HDL <35 mg/dL and/or triglyceride level ≥250 mg/dL

*Source:* National Institute of Diabetes and Digestive and Kidney Diseases, National Institutes of Health, Diabetes Information Clearinghouse. *Diabetes prevention program.* Available at diabetes.niddk.nih.gov/dm/pubs/preventionprogram. Accessed on 6/23/08.

and Pacific Islanders), or a history of giving birth to an infant weighing more than 9 pounds. Because even mild hyperglycemia can cause fetal problems and complications during delivery, all women are routinely screened between 24 and 28 weeks of gestation. High-risk women are screened before or shortly after conception. Immediately after pregnancy, 5% to 10% of women with gestational diabetes are diagnosed with diabetes, usually type 2 (CDC, 2007). For more on gestational diabetes, see Chapter 11.

## ▶ ACUTE DIABETES COMPLICATIONS

Untreated or poorly controlled diabetes can lead to acute life-threatening complications related to high blood glucose concentrations. Conversely, hypoglycemia caused by overuse of medication, too little food, or too much exercise can also be life-threatening. Diabetic ketoacidosis (DKA), hyperosmolar hyperglycemic nonketotic syndrome (HHNS), and hypoglycemia are presented next.

## Diabetic Ketoacidosis (DKA)

People with type 1 diabetes are susceptible to DKA, characterized by hyperglycemia (glucose levels >250 mg/dL) and ketonemia. It is caused by a severe deficiency of insulin or from physiologic stress, such as illness or infection. Without insulin, fat catabolism proceeds unchecked, leading to a dangerous accumulation of acidic ketone bodies in the blood (ketoacidosis), which spills over into the urine (ketonuria). Polyuria may lead to dehydration, electrolyte depletion, and hypotension. Hyperventilation occurs in an attempt to correct acidosis by increasing expiration of carbon dioxide. Fatigue, nausea, vomiting, and confusion develop; diabetic coma and death are possible.

DKA is sometimes the presenting symptom when type 1 diabetes is diagnosed. Incorrect or missed insulin injections can lead to DKA. DKA rarely develops in people with type 2 diabetes because only very little insulin is needed to prevent ketosis. If DKA does occur in people with type 2 diabetes, infection or illness is usually to blame. DKA is treated with electrolytes, fluid, and insulin.

## Hyperosmolar Hyperglycemic Nonketotic Syndrome

HHNS is characterized by hyperglycemia (>600 mg/dL) without significant ketonemia. It occurs most commonly in people with type 2 diabetes because they have enough insulin to prevent ketosis. Dehydration and heat exposure increase the risk; illness or infection is usually the precipitating factor. Older people may be particularly vulnerable because they have a diminished sense of thirst or may be unable to replenish fluid losses due to illness or physical impairments. HHNS develops relatively slowly over a period of days to weeks. Symptoms include dehydration, hypotension, decreased mental acuity, confusion, seizures, and coma. The best protection against HHNS is regular glucose monitoring. Treatment includes insulin and fluid and electrolyte replacement.

## Hypoglycemia

Hypoglycemia (blood glucose level <70 mg/dL) is often referred to as insulin reaction. It occurs from taking too much insulin (or sulfonylureas, but less frequently), inadequate food intake, delayed or skipped meals, extra physical activity, or consumption of alcohol without food. Symptoms include shakiness, dizziness, sweating, hunger, headache, pale skin, confusion, and seizure.

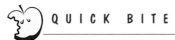

**QUICK BITE**

To counter mild hypoglycemia:
Each of the following contains approximately
   15 g of readily absorbable sugar:

- 3 to 4 glucose tablets
- 1 individual tube of glucose gel
- 8 to 10 lifesavers
- 4 to 6 oz regular soft drink
- 4 to 6 oz fruit juice

Mild hypoglycemia is treated with 15 to 20 g of glucose, although any carbohydrate that contains glucose may be used (ADA, 2008). Pure sugars are better than items like candy bars, which contain fat that slows the gastric emptying time and delays the rise in blood glucose. After eating a dose of sugar, symptoms normally improve in 10 to 20 minutes. A blood glucose test is repeated in 10 to 15 minutes, and another dose of fast-acting sugar is consumed if the glucose level is still low. All clients should carry a readily absorbable source of carbohydrate with them at all times to treat hypoglycemia. Frequent bouts of hypoglycemia may mean the care plan needs to be revised or the client needs to be counseled to ensure better compliance.

Patients with long-standing diabetes may develop hypoglycemic unawareness. This occurs because the body no longer signals hypoglycemia. Consistent monitoring of blood glucose is especially important for people who are not cognizant of hypoglycemic symptoms.

## ▶ LONG-TERM COMPLICATIONS

Diabetes significantly increases morbidity and mortality and is the seventh leading cause of death by disease in the United States, although it is likely to be underreported as a cause of death (CDC, 2007). The pathogenesis of long-term diabetes complications is poorly understood (Anderson, 2006). What is known is that sustained hyperglycemia alters glucose metabolism in virtually every tissue. Among other metabolic abnormalities, excess glucose and glucose fragments combine with proteins to form compounds that accumulate and damage cells and small and large blood vessels (Anderson, 2006). Complications are listed in Box 19.3. The occurrence of long-term complications can be lowered by controlling blood glucose levels, blood pressure, and blood lipid levels (CDC, 2007).

## ▶ DIABETES MANAGEMENT

Type 1 diabetes is managed by a coordinated regimen of nutrition therapy and insulin. Lifestyle interventions—namely diet and exercise—are standard approaches for the treatment of type 2 diabetes. If lifestyle interventions fail to achieve glycemic control, oral medications and/or insulin are added to the regimen. Regardless of the type of diabetes, nutrient recommendations are the same; only issues of body weight and meal timing may differ between the two types of diabetes.

In the American Diabetes Association's position statement on nutrition recommendations and interventions for diabetes, calories, overweight, and obesity are addressed before

---

| BOX 19.3 | LONG-TERM COMPLICATIONS OF DIABETES |
| --- | --- |

Microvascular complications: closely linked to the duration and severity of hyperglycemia.

• Retinopathy

Diabetes is the leading cause of new blindness.

• Nephropathy

Diabetes is the leading cause of kidney failure.

• Neuropathy

Almost 30% of people over the age of 40 who have diabetes have impaired sensation in the feet.

• Sixty to 70% of people with diabetes have mild to severe forms of nervous system damage, which can lead to gastroparesis, carpel tunnel syndrome, and impotence in men.

Macrovascular complications: may occur with only minimal elevation of blood glucose levels.

• Myocardial infarction

Diabetes increases the risk of heart disease death two to four times above that of people who do not have diabetes.

More than half of adults with diabetes have coronary heart disease and more than two-thirds die from CVD.

• Stroke

The risk for stroke is two to four times higher in people with diabetes.

Other complications include

• Impaired wound healing, which can lead to gangrene

Diabetes is the major cause of lower extremity amputations.

• Periodontal disease
• Pregnancy complications
• Increased susceptibility to other illnesses

***Source:*** Center for Disease Control (CDC). (2007). *National diabetes fact sheet, 2007.* Available at www.cdc.gov/diabaetes/pubs/pdf/ndfs_2007.pdf. Accessed on 6/25/08.

nutrient recommendations are made to highlight the importance of body weight in type 2 diabetes prevention and management. Goals and interventions are specified for three levels of prevention: the primary prevention of diabetes among people with prediabetes or at high risk of diabetes; the secondary prevention of managing existing diabetes; and tertiary prevention of preventing or slowing the rate of diabetes complications (ADA, 2008). These recommendations are discussed below.

## Calories, Overweight, and Obesity

Weight loss has traditionally been the focus of nutrition intervention for overweight and obese people with prediabetes or type 2 diabetes. Short-term studies show that moderate weight loss (5% of body weight) in people with type 2 diabetes improves insulin resistance, glycemic control, lipid levels, and blood pressure (Klein et al., 2004).

There is no one proven strategy that can be uniformly recommended to promote weight loss in all clients. Although standard weight loss diets that provide 500 to 1000 fewer calories than usual daily intake can promote a weight loss of as much as 10% in 6 months, most people regain weight without continued support and follow-up (ADA, 2008). Very low calorie diets (≤800 cal/day) produce substantial weight loss and rapid improvements in blood glucose and lipid levels in people with type 2 diabetes, but weight gain is common after the diet stops. Weight loss medications may be useful for people with prediabetes or type 2 diabetes; combined with lifestyle changes, they can promote a 5% to 10% weight loss. Drug labels state that the medications should only be used in people with diabetes who have a body mass index (BMI) >27 (ADA, 2008). Bariatric surgery can lead to substantial weight loss, complete resolution of type 2 diabetes, and improvement in cardiovascular risk factors (except hypercholesterolemia) (ADA, 2008). It is reserved for people with a BMI ≥35. An individualized approach takes into account the client's treatment goals and his or her ability and willingness to change.

## Preventing Diabetes

Because of the strong link between excess weight and insulin resistance/type 2 diabetes, weight loss through a combination of healthy eating and exercise is the primary focus of diabetes prevention (Box 19.4). A major, multicenter clinical trial called the Diabetes Prevention Program (DPP) found that in a diverse group of overweight people with impaired glucose tolerance, diet, exercise, and behavior modification decreased the incidence of diabetes by 58% (Diabetes Prevention Research Group, 2002). Study participants walked at moderate intensity, an average of 150 minutes/week, and decreased their intake of fat and calories. Average weight loss was a modest 5% to 7% of initial weight, or about 15 pounds. Participants also benefited from improvements in their lipid profiles, blood pressure, and markers of inflammation (Haffner et al., 2005; Ratner et al., 2005). The DPP results were so quick and convincing that the program was halted a year early. Clearly, millions of overweight Americans at high risk for type 2 diabetes can delay and possibly prevent the disease with a modest weight loss brought about by a moderate diet and regular exercise.

The type of fat consumed may also influence diabetes risk (ADA, 2008). Specifically, a low saturated fat intake may reduce the risk for diabetes by improving insulin resistance and promoting weight loss. Beyond its potential beneficial effects on diabetes risk, a low saturated fat diet is well established as a strategy to lower the risk of heart disease (NCEP, 2001).

Several studies show that an increased intake of whole grains and fiber lowers the risk of diabetes (ADA, 2008). Whole grains correlate to improved insulin sensitivity, regardless of body weight. Fiber has been associated with improved insulin sensitivity and improved ability to secrete insulin to overcome insulin resistance (Liese et al., 2003).

| BOX 19.4 | **PRIMARY PREVENTION: NUTRITION RECOMMENDATIONS TO PREVENT TYPE 2 DIABETES BASED ON GRADES "A" AND "B" EVIDENCE** |
|---|---|

- Make lifestyle changes to produce a moderate weight loss (7% of body weight). A structured program that includes regular physical activity (150 min/week) and a healthy diet that is lower in calories and fat is recommended.
- Consume the Dietary Reference Intakes for fiber, which is 14 g/1000 cal or approximately 21 to 25 g/day for women and 30 to 38 g/day for men. At least ½ of all grains consumed should be whole grains.
- Observational studies show that moderate alcohol intake may lower the risk for diabetes but data do not support a recommendation to consume alcohol.

*There is insufficient (grade "E") evidence to recommend:*

- *Low glycemic index foods*
- *Specific recommendations to prevent type 2 diabetes in youth*
- *Any nutrition recommendations to prevent type 1 diabetes*

## Secondary Prevention: Managing Diabetes

The primary goal of diabetes management is to keep blood glucose levels as near normal as possible. Additional goals are to

- Attain and maintain control of blood lipid levels and blood pressure
- Prevent or delay the development of complications
- Meet the individual's cultural and personal needs while respecting preferences and willingness to change
- Maintain the pleasure of eating by not limiting any foods unless indicated by scientific evidence

Nutrition therapy is an essential component of diabetes management regardless of the client's weight, blood glucose levels, or use of medication. People with diabetes generally have the same nutritional requirements as the general population; therefore, dietary recommendations to promote health and well-being in the general public—lose weight if overweight; eat less saturated fat and cholesterol; eat more fiber and less sodium—are also appropriate for people with diabetes. Because coronary heart disease (CHD) is the leading cause of death among people with diabetes, it makes sense that nutrition recommendations issued by the ADA to prevent and treat diabetes are remarkably similar to recommendations put forth by the American Heart Association (AHA) for the primary and secondary prevention of CHD (Chapter 20). Nutrition recommendations for diabetes management are summarized in Table 19.1.

| TABLE 19.1 | **Secondary Prevention: Nutrition Recommendations for the Management of Diabetes (Grades A and B Evidence Except Where Noted)** |
|---|---|
| Calories | Weight loss is recommended for all overweight and obese people who have or are at risk of diabetes. Modest weight loss improves insulin resistance. |
| | For periods of up to 1 year, either a low-carbohydrate or low-fat diet that is restricted in calories may be effective. |
| | Physical activity and behavior modification are integral components of weight loss programs and are essential for weight loss maintenance. |
| | Weight loss medications combined with lifestyle changes can help produce a 5–10% weight loss. |

*(table continues on page 459)*

| TABLE 19.1 | Secondary Prevention: Nutrition Recommendations for the Management of Diabetes (Grades A and B Evidence Except Where Noted (continued) |
|---|---|
| | Bariatric surgery can greatly improve glycemic control in people with type 2 diabetes who have a BMI ≥35. |
| | *Grade "E" evidence:* |
| | • *Monitor lipid levels, renal function, protein intake (in patients with nephropathy) and adjust hypoglycemic therapy, as needed, in patients on low-carbohydrate diets.* |
| Carbohydrates | Carbohydrates from fruits, vegetables, whole grains, legumes, and low-fat milk are part of a healthy diet. |
| | Monitoring carbohydrate intake is essential to achieve glycemic control. |
| | Attention to glycemic index may provide some benefit above simply consuming a consistent carbohydrate intake. |
| Sweeteners | Foods containing sucrose can be substituted for other carbohydrate foods. If they are added to the meal plan, they should be covered with insulin or other glucose-lowering medications. Be mindful of the "empty calories" provided by high-sugar foods. |
| | Sugar alternatives, such as sugar alcohols and nonnutritive sweeteners, are safe when used within daily intake levels set by the FDA. |
| Fiber | An adequate intake of fiber from a wide variety of sources is recommended. People with diabetes do not need more fiber than the general population. |
| Fat | Limit saturated fat to <7% of total calories. |
| | Consume 2 or more servings of fatty fish per week (excluding commercially fried fish fillets). |
| | *Grade "E" evidence:* |
| | • *Minimize trans fat intake.* |
| | • *Limit dietary cholesterol to <200 mg/day.* |
| Protein | In people with type 2 diabetes, protein does not increase plasma glucose levels, so it should not be used to treat acute or prevent nighttime hypoglycemia. |
| | *Grade "E" evidence:* |
| | • *There is not enough evidence to recommend protein intake should differ from the usual intake of 15–20% of total calories consumed for people with type 2 diabetes and normal renal function.* |
| | • *High-protein diets (>20% of total calories) are not recommended for weight loss because the long-term effects on diabetes management and complications are unknown.* |
| Alcohol | Moderate alcohol intake (when consumed alone) has no short-term effect on glucose and insulin in people with diabetes. Alcoholic beverages that contain carbohydrates may raise blood glucose levels. |
| | *Grade "E" evidence:* |
| | • *People with diabetes who choose to drink should limit their intake to one drink per day or less for women and two drinks per day or less for men.* |
| | • *Alcohol should be consumed with food to reduce the risk of nighttime hypoglycemia in people who use insulin or drugs that stimulate insulin secretion.* |
| Micronutrients | In the absence of underlying deficiencies, vitamin and mineral supplements do not provide any benefit. |
| | Routine supplements of antioxidants (vitamins C, E, and beta-carotene) are not recommended due to lack of evidence that they are effective or safe for long-term use. |
| | *Grade "E" evidence:* |
| | • *Chromium supplements are not recommended because no clear benefit has been observed.* |

Grade is based on the American Diabetes Association evidence-grading system of a scale of A to E with an "A" representing evidence from large well-designed multicenter or multiple randomized clinical trials or well-done meta-analyses. An "E" grade is used when evidence is lacking, findings are conflicting, or research is limited.

*Source:* American Diabetes Association. (2008). Nutrition recommendations and interventions for diabetes. A position statement of the American Diabetes Association. *Diabetes Care, 31*(Suppl. 1), S61–S78.

## Total Carbohydrates

The RDA for carbohydrate is 130 g/day, based on the minimum amount of glucose used by the brain (IOM, 2005). For most Americans, carbohydrates provide approximately 50% of total calories consumed, a figure safely within the Acceptable Macronutrient Distribution Range (AMDR) of 45% to 65% of total calories. At intakes below 45% of total calories, intake of fat is too high and the intake of fiber and vitamins and minerals may be inadequate. At intakes above 65% of total calories, protein needs may not be met. It is reasonable that people with diabetes follow these guidelines.

Glycemic control is dependent on matching carbohydrate intake with the action of insulin or other medication. Although carbohydrate intake monitoring is essential in managing diabetes, no single method of estimating carbohydrate intake has been proven superior to the others (ADA, 2008).

**Glycemic Index:** the incremental rise in blood glucose (above baseline) compared to that induced by a standard, usually 50 g glucose or a white bread challenge.

Several randomized clinical trials have shown that low **glycemic index** diets improve glycemic control but other trials have not confirmed this (Sheard et al., 2004). The ADA states that a low glycemic index diet may provide a modest benefit in controlling postprandial hyperglycemia when used in place of a high glycemic index diet (ADA, 2008). For more on glycemic index, see Chapter 2.

## Sweeteners

**Isocalorically:** of the same calorie level.

Substantial evidence from clinical studies demonstrates that when sucrose is **isocalorically** substituted for starch, there is no difference in glycemic control in either type 1 or type 2 diabetes (Franz et al., 2002). Sucrose and sucrose-containing foods are not restricted but should be substituted for other carbohydrates in the meal plan, not eaten as "extras." Many people with long-standing diabetes resist accepting this shift in thinking because sugar was once taboo. Others find the freedom to choose sweetened foods difficult not to abuse. Even though foods high in sugar do not aggravate glycemic control, they are usually nutrient poor and may be high in fat. Care should be taken to avoid an excess calorie intake.

**Sugar Alcohols:** natural sweeteners derived from monosaccharides; these are considered low-calorie sweeteners because they are incompletely absorbed. They produce a smaller rise in postprandial glucose levels and insulin secretion than sucrose.

The use of fructose as an added sweetener is not recommended because even though it produces a lower postprandial response than sucrose, it may adversely affect serum lipid levels by raising low-density lipoprotein (LDL) and triglyceride levels (ADA, 2008). There is no reason for people with diabetes to avoid naturally occurring fructose in fruit and vegetables.

**Sugar alcohols** (sorbitol, mannitol, and xylitol) provide fewer calories and cause a smaller increase in glucose than sucrose or glucose. They do not contribute to dental cavities, yet using them is not likely to produce weight loss or improve glycemic control (ADA, 2008). They appear safe to use but may cause diarrhea when consumed in large amounts, especially in children.

**Nonnutritive Sweeteners:** synthetically made sweeteners that do not provide calories.

The **nonnutritive sweeteners**, saccharin, aspartame, acesulfame-K, sucralose, and neotame, are approved for use by the U.S. Food and Drug Administration (FDA) and may safely be used by people with diabetes. There is no indication that these will promote weight loss or gain (ADA, 2008).

## Fiber

The recommendations for fiber are the same as for the general population—that is, 14 g/1000 cal consumed, or approximately 25 g/day for women and 38 g/day for men. Evidence is lacking that amounts greater than this are beneficial for people with diabetes (Wheeler & Pi-Sunyer, 2008). However, foods rich in fiber provide other benefits such as increasing satiety (a plus for weight management); providing vitamins, minerals, and phytochemicals; and lowering serum cholesterol levels (Wheeler & Pi-Sunyer, 2008). People with diabetes are encouraged to eat more fiber than the typical American consumes, but they do not need to eat more than what is recommended for the general population. A variety of sources is recommended.

## Fat

> ### QUICK BITE
>
> To achieve a low saturated fat, low trans fat, low-cholesterol diet:
> - Limit meat and meat substitute intake to 4 to 6 oz/day of lean choices
> - Use only nonfat or low-fat milk, cheese, and yogurt
> - Use a soft, trans fat–free spread in place of margarine
> - Avoid processed foods such as frozen French fries, frozen chicken fingers, potato chips
> - Avoid fried fast food
> - Avoid commercially baked products such as cakes, cookies, crackers, and doughnuts
> - Limit egg yolks to 2 to 3/week
> - Avoid organ meats

**Plant Sterols/Stanols:** naturally occurring substances in plants that help block the absorption of cholesterol from the GI tract. Some margarines have plant sterols added for therapeutic benefit.

People with diabetes appear to have the same cardiovascular risk as people with pre-existing cardiovascular disease (CVD), so recommendations concerning fat intake are the same for both groups (ADA, 2008). Specifically, people with diabetes are advised to limit their intake of saturated fat to less than 7% of total calories, minimize their intake of trans fat, and consume less than 200 mg of cholesterol daily. Two or more servings of fish per week are recommended for their omega-3 fatty acid content; omega-3 fatty acids have been shown to lower adverse CVD outcomes (ADA, 2008). **Plant sterols/stanols** lower LDL cholesterol by up to 15% with maximum effects at ~2 g/day and are another option for lowering CVD risk (Lichtenstein et al., 2006). The difference between these recommendations and those made by the AHA for people with or at risk for CVD is slight; the AHA recommends trans fat be limited to less than 1% of total calories and suggests cholesterol be restricted to less than 300 mg/day (Lichtenstein et al., 2006).

## Protein

In the typical American diet, including the diets of people with diabetes, protein provides 15% of total calories, a value within the AMDR of 10% to 35% of total calories. There is insufficient evidence to suggest that people with diabetes who have normal renal function should alter their usual intake of protein.

## Alcohol

Moderate use of alcohol (1 drink/day or less in women and 2 drinks/day or less in men) by people who have well-controlled diabetes has minimal effects on blood glucose and insulin levels, as long as it is not mixed with another liquid that provides carbohydrates (e.g., mixed drinks). For people who take insulin, alcohol should be consumed with food to avoid hypoglycemia. People with type 1 diabetes should not reduce their food intake to compensate for alcohol calories. Light to moderate use of alcohol by people with diabetes is associated with a lower risk of CVD regardless of the type of beverage consumed (ADA, 2008).

## Vitamins and Minerals

The vitamin and mineral requirements of people with diabetes are not different from those of the general population. Supplements provide no proven benefit in managing diabetes unless underlying nutrient deficiencies exist. Uncontrolled diabetes is often associated with micronutrient

QUICK BITE

Sources of chromium:

| | |
|---|---|
| Whole grains | Some dried peas |
| Nuts | and beans |
| Mushrooms | Yeast |
| Broccoli | Organ meats |
| Egg yolks | Pork |

*Source:* Melanson, K. (2007). Diet and nutrients in the prevention and treatment of type 2 diabetes. *American Journal of Lifestyle Medicine, 1,* 339–343.

deficiencies; when deficiencies are diagnosed, the approach should be a balanced diet that supplies natural sources of nutrients.

The essential mineral chromium has been studied for its possible role in the prevention and treatment of diabetes. It promotes glucose uptake by cells, possibly by increasing the number and activity of insulin receptors on the cells (Melanson, 2007). Some studies show that chromium supplementation improves glucose tolerance (Anderson, 2000). Although the ADA states that there is currently insufficient evidence to recommend chromium supplementation, an ample dietary intake is advised. Studies are also needed to determine if magnesium and antioxidant supplements are beneficial to type 2 diabetes management (ADA, 2008).

## Tertiary Prevention: Controlling Diabetes Complications

The progression of microvascular diabetes complications may be modified by improving glycemic control and lowering blood pressure (ADA, 2008). The EDIC (Epidemiology of Diabetes Interventions and Complications) study showed that people with type 1 diabetes were able to significantly reduce their risk of cardiovascular death, myocardial infarction, and stroke through improved glycemic control (Nathan et al., 2005). Table 19.2 highlights the ADA's recommendations for treating and controlling microvascular and cardiovascular complications.

| TABLE 19.2 | Tertiary Prevention: Nutrition Recommendations for Controlling Diabetes Complications (Grades A and B Evidence Except Where Noted) |
|---|---|
| For Microvascular Complications | Reduce protein intake to 0.8 to 1.0 g/kg for people with early stage chronic kidney disease; lower to 0.8 g/kg for later stages of diabetic kidney disease. |
| | *Grade "C" evidence:* |
| | • *Nutrition therapy used for cardiovascular disease risk factors may benefit microvascular complications, such as retinopathy and nephropathy.* |
| Treatment and Management of CVD | Control A1c as close to normal as possible without significant hypoglycemia. |
| Risk | Whether normotensive or hypertensive, lower sodium intake to 2300 mg/day and eat a diet rich in fruits, vegetables, and low-fat dairy products to lower blood pressure. |
| | *Grade "C" evidence:* |
| | • *For people at risk of CVD, a diet rich in fruits, vegetables, whole grains, and nuts may lower risk.* |
| | • *For people with symptomatic heart failure, a sodium intake of <2000 mg/day may improve symptoms.* |
| | • *In most people, modest weight loss improves blood pressure.* |

*Source:* American Diabetes Association. (2008). Nutrition recommendations and interventions for diabetes. A position statement of the American Diabetes Association. *Diabetes Care, 31*(Suppl. 1), S61–S78.

# Meal-Planning Approaches

Monitoring carbohydrate intake, either by exchange lists, carbohydrate counting, or experience-based estimation, is key to controlling blood glucose levels (Wheeler et al., 2008). Regardless of the strategy used, the meal plan should reflect the individual's lifestyle, preferences, and willingness/ability to make dietary changes. While snacks are necessary for some people depending on their calorie needs and insulin/medication regime, they are not necessary for obese people with type 2 diabetes who are diet controlled or who take insulin sensitizer oral medications. The exchange list system and carbohydrate counting are presented below.

## Exchange Lists for Meal Planning

Devised by the American Diabetes Association and the American Dietetic Association, the *Choose Your Foods: Exchange Lists for Meal Planning* is a framework for choosing a healthy diet that groups foods into lists that, per serving size given, are similar in carbohydrate, protein, fat, and calories based on rounded averages (ADA and ADA, 2008). Its three major categories are carbohydrates, meat and meat substitutes, and fats. Supplemental lists provide guidance on free foods, combination foods, fast foods, and alcohol. Within each of the major groupings are subgroups that form the exchange lists (Box 19.5). Any food (in the serving size specified) can be exchanged for any other within each list. With a few caveats, any carbohydrate choices can be exchanged for any others.

A sample meal pattern is designed for clients, based on their usual pattern of eating. For each meal and snack, the number of exchanges from each list is specified; clients simply refer

---

| BOX 19.5 | **EXCHANGE LISTS FOR DIABETES** |

**Carbohydrate Group**

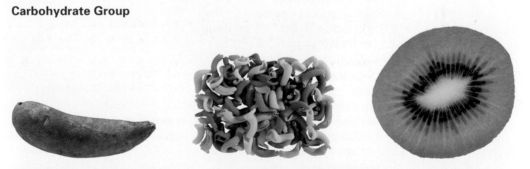

The carbohydrate group is divided into five different lists: starch; fruit; milk; sweets, desserts, and other carbohydrates; and nonstarchy vegetables.

- One choice from the starch, fruit, or milk list provides approximately 15 g carbohydrate; any item from any of these lists can be substituted for another.
- A dairy-like category (e.g., soy milk, chocolate milk, smoothies) is contained in the milk list; a serving from this category may count as more than just one carbohydrate choice because it has sugar or is high in fat.
- Generally, one choice from the sweets, desserts, and other carbohydrate list also provides 15 g of carbohydrate and is one carbohydrate choice. Many items also provide fat. They lack the vitamins, minerals, and fiber that other carbohydrates provide, so they should be used less frequently.
- Three choices from the nonstarchy vegetables list count as one carbohydrate choice.

*(box continues on page 464)*

| BOX 19.5 | **EXCHANGE LISTS FOR DIABETES** (continued) | | | |
|---|---|---|---|---|
| **List and Representative Foods** | **Serving Sizes** | **CHO (g)** | **Protein (g)** | **Fat (g)** |
| **Starch** | | 15 | 0–3 | 0–1 |
| Bread | 1 slice | | | |
| Cereals and grains | ½ cup cooked cereal or grain; 1 oz ready-to-eat cereal ⅓ cup cooked rice or pasta | | | |
| Starchy vegetables | ½ cup cooked | | | |
| Crackers and snacks | ¾ to 1 oz of most snack foods (may have extra fat) | | | |
| Beans, peas, and lentils | ½ cup | | | |
| **Fruit** | | 15 | 0 | 0 |
| Canned fruit, fresh fruit, or unsweetened fruit juice | ½ cup | | | |
| Fresh fruit | 1 small fruit | | | |
| Dried fruit | 2 tbsp | | | |
| **Milk** | | | | |
| Fat-free and low-fat milk and yogurt | 1 cup milk; ⅔ cup plain or artificially sweetened yogurt | 12 | 8 | 0–3 |
| Reduced-fat milk and yogurt | 1 cup milk; ⅔ cup plain yogurt | 12 | 8 | 5 |
| Whole milk and yogurt | 1 cup milk; 8 oz yogurt | 12 | 8 | 8 |
| **Sweets, Desserts, and Other Carbohydrates** | | 15 | Varies | Varies |
| Cranberry juice cocktail | ½ cup | | | |
| Gingersnap cookies | 3 | | | |
| Regular pancake syrup | 1 tbsp | | | |
| Ice cream, sherbet, or frozen yogurt | ½ cup | | | |
| **Nonstarchy Vegetables** | | 5 | 2 | 0 |
| Cooked vegetables (fresh, canned, or frozen) | ½ cup | | | |
| Vegetable juice | ½ cup | | | |
| Raw vegetables (excludes salad greens, which are on the Free Food List) | 1 cup | | | |

**Meat and Meat Substitutes Group**

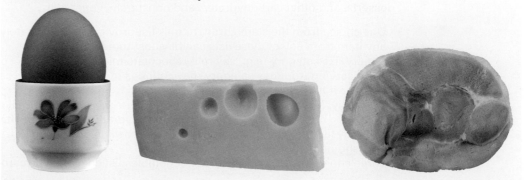

BOX 19.5  **EXCHANGE LISTS FOR DIABETES** (continued)

Meat and meat substitutes are divided into four lists based on the amount of fat: lean meat and meat substitutes; medium-fat meat and meat substitutes; high-fat meat and meat substitutes; and plant-based proteins.

- All meat and meat substitutes provide 7 g of protein per serving.
- Clients are encouraged to choose items with 5 g of fat or less per ounce.
- Items in the plant-based protein list vary in carbohydrate and fat content and so each has a citing as to how it is to be "counted" (e.g., soy nuts are counted as ½ carbohydrate choice + 1 medium-fat meat).

| List and Representative Foods | Serving Sizes | CHO (g) | Protein (g) | Fat (g) |
|---|---|---|---|---|
| **Lean meat and meat substitutes** | | — | 7 | 0–3 |
| Lean meat, poultry, pork, veal; fish, shellfish, game | 1 oz | | | |
| Egg whites | 2 | | | |
| Cottage cheese | ¼ cup | | | |
| **Medium-Fat Meat and Meat Substitutes** | | — | 7 | 4–7 |
| Cheese with 4–7 g fat per ounce | 1 oz | | | |
| Egg | 1 | | | |
| Fried fish | 1 oz | | | |
| Prime grades of beef, chicken with skin, veal cutlet | 1 oz | | | |
| **High-Fat Meat and Meat Substitutes** | | — | 7 | 8+ |
| Pork bacon | 2 slices | | | |
| Regular cheese | 1 oz | | | |
| Hot dogs | 1 | | | |
| Processed sandwich meats and sausage with 8 g of fat or more per ounce | 1 oz | | | |
| **Plant-Based Proteins** | | Varies | 7 | Varies |
| Soy bacon | 3 strips | | | |
| Nut butters (e.g., almond butter, cashew butter, peanut butter) | 1 tbsp | | | |
| Refried beans, canned | ½ cup | | | |
| Hummus | ⅓ cup | | | |

**Fats**

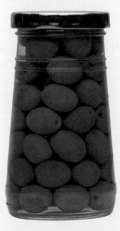
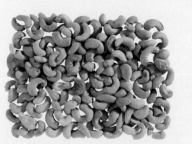
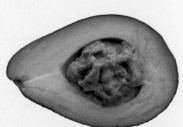

(box continues on page 466)

| BOX 19.5 | **EXCHANGE LISTS FOR DIABETES** (continued) |
|---|---|

Fats are divided into three lists based on the type of fat they contain: monosaturated, polyunsaturated, and saturated.

• All items on the fats list provide 5 g of fat per serving.

| List and Representative Foods | Serving Sizes | CHO (g) | Protein (g) | Fat (g) |
|---|---|---|---|---|
| **Monounsaturated Fats** | | — | — | 5 |
| Avocado | 2 tbsp | | | |
| Nut butters | 1½ tsp | | | |
| Nuts | 2–16, depending on the type | | | |
| Canola, olive, and peanut oil | 1 tsp | | | |
| Olives | 8–10 | | | |
| **Polyunsaturated Fats** | | — | — | 5 |
| Low-fat margarine | 1 tbsp | | | |
| Regular mayonnaise | 1 tsp | | | |
| Corn, soybean, sunflower oil | 1 tsp | | | |
| Reduced-fat salad dressing | 2 tbsp | | | |
| **Saturated Fats** | | — | — | 5 |
| Bacon | 1 slice | | | |
| Chitterlings, boiled | 2 tbsp | | | |
| Half and half cream | 2 tbsp | | | |
| Salt pork | ¼ oz | | | |
| Regular sour cream | 2 tbsp | | | |

to the list to choose the appropriate types and amounts of food allowed. They are encouraged to eat a variety of foods within each list and to make healthy choices, such as whole grains over refined products, low-fat dairy items, lean meats or plant-based proteins, and heart-healthy fats. Because accurate portion sizes are vital to maintaining a consistent carbohydrate intake, food should be weighed or measured until portion sizes can be accurately estimated (Fig. 19.2).

The advantages of using the exchange list system is that it eliminates the need for daily calculations, ensures a relatively consistent intake, and emphasizes important nutrition principles such as limiting and modifying fat, increasing fiber, and controlling sodium intake. Yet there are several drawbacks. The terminology may be confusing, such as carbohydrate choice versus grams of carbohydrates. Some items on some lists are counted as more than just one choice or one exchange, such as black-eyed peas, which are counted as one starch plus one lean meat. Some items appear on more than one list and in different amounts, such as 1 tablespoon of peanut butter on the plant-based protein list and 1½ teaspoon of peanut butter on the monounsaturated fat list. In addition, the exchange system is less flexible than carbohydrate counting and may not be appropriate or acceptable for all age, ethnic, and cultural groups. The exchange list approach is best suited to people who want or need structured meal-planning guidance and are able to understand complex details.

## Carbohydrate Counting

Carbohydrate counting is gaining in popularity as an easier and more flexible alternative to using the exchange system. Based on their usual pattern of eating and daily calorie allowance,

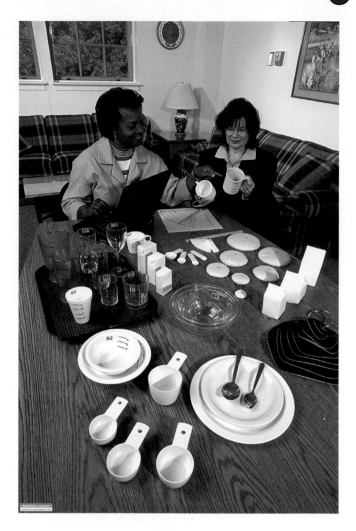

**FIGURE 19.2** Serving size aids help clients learn appropriate serving sizes. (Photo by Stephen Ausmus. United States Department of Agriculture, Agricultural Research Service.)

clients are given an individualized meal pattern that specifies the number of carbohydrate "choices" (1 choice = 15 g carbohydrate) for each meal and snack (Box 19.6). Most adults are allowed three to five carbohydrate choices per meal and one to two for each snack, depending on their calorie needs. Sample 1800-calorie menus using carbohydrate counting are featured in Box 19.7. To assist people with identifying sources of carbohydrates and the appropriate portion sizes, clients are given carbohydrate choice lists, similar to the exchange lists but generally focused specifically on carbohydrates. Clients also need to know how to read the Nutrition Facts label to accurately count carbohydrates (Fig. 19.3).

Although carbohydrate counting has the advantage of focusing on a single nutrient (carbohydrates) rather than all the energy-yielding nutrients, protein and fat cannot be disregarded, especially if weight is a concern. Generally, clients are advised to eat 4 to 6 ounces of lean meat or meat substitute, some healthy fats, and little to no saturated and trans fat. The goals of weight control and healthful eating may be forgotten or forsaken when the emphasis is placed solely on carbohydrate.

Basic carbohydrate counting is appropriate for people who understand the importance of consuming a consistent carbohydrate intake to match insulin or medication peaks. Some people progress to a more advanced level of carbohydrate counting that allows clients to adjust their mealtime insulin dosage based on the grams of carbohydrate they want to eat

| BOX 19.6 | THE NUMBER OF CARBOHYDRATE CHOICES AT VARIOUS CALORIE LEVELS |

One carbohydrate choice equals (15 g carbohydrate):

- 1 serving from the bread, cereal, rice, and pasta group
- 1 serving of fruit
- 1 serving from the Milk group
- 1 serving from the sweets and desserts
- 3 servings of nonstarchy vegetables (because they are so low in carbohydrates and are "healthy," oftentimes people are encouraged to eat these as desired)

The diet should also include

- 4 to 6 oz of lean meat or meat substitutes per day
- Healthy fats

| Total Calories | Carbohydrate Choices for Each Meal | Carbohydrate Choices for Snacks/Day |
|---|---|---|
| 1200–1500 | 3 | 1 |
| 1600–2000 | 4 | 2–3 |
| 2100–2400 | 5 | 4–6 |

| BOX 19.7 | CARBOHYDRATE COUNTING: SAMPLE 1800-CALORIE MENUS |

| Sample Menu | Carbohydrate Choices | Sample Menu | Carbohydrate Choices |
|---|---|---|---|
| **Breakfast** | | | |
| ½ cup orange juice | 1 | A parfait consisting of: | |
| 1 low-fat waffle topped with | 1 | 1¼ cup strawberries | 1 |
| ¾ cup blueberries | | ½ cup low-fat granola | 2 |
| 1 cup nonfat milk | 1 | 6 oz plain yogurt | 1 |
| 1 tsp light margarine | 1 | Coffee | |
| **Lunch** | | | |
| 6-in. submarine with 2 oz | 3 | Hamburger on a bun | 2 |
| meat and light mayonnaise | | 1 cup oven-baked French fries | 1 |
| 1 apple | 1 | Lettuce and tomato | |
| Diet soft drink | | Light mayonnaise | |
| | | 1 cup nonfat milk | 1 |
| **Dinner** | | | |
| 1 taco shell | 2 | 1 cup spaghetti noodles | 3 |
| 3 oz taco meat | | 2 meatballs | |
| 1½ cups combined lettuce, | 1 | 1 cup spaghetti sauce | 1 |
| tomato, onion | | Tossed salad | |
| ⅓ cup rice | 1 | 1 slice Italian bread | 1 |
| 1 cup cubed papaya | 1 | 1 tsp butter | |
| | | Diet soft drink | |
| **Bedtime Snack** | | | |
| ½ cup shredded wheat | 1 | 3 cups no fat added popcorn | 1 |
| 1 cup nonfat milk | 1 | 1 cup nonfat milk | 1 |
| Total carbohydrate choices/day | 15 | | 15 |

Step 1: Identify the serving size. The nutrition content is based on this serving size.

**Example: 1 serving = 3/4 c**

Step 2: Find the grams of total carbohydrates. 1 carbohydrate choice = 15 g CHO, with a range of 11–20 counted as 1 choice.

| g total carbohydrate | # CHO choices |
|---|---|
| 6–10 | 1/2 |
| 11–20 | 1 |
| 21–25 | 1 1/2 |
| 26–35 | 2 |
| 36–40 | 2 1/2 |
| 41–50 | 3 |

The grams of sugar are part of the total carbohydrate and do not require special attention.

**Example: 1 serving = 1 1/2 carbohydrate choices**

Step 3: Check on the grams of total fiber per serving. If a serving provides >5 g total fiber, subtract 1/2 the total grams of fiber from the grams of carbohydrates (because fiber is relatively nondigestable and provides less than 4 cal/g) to get the total carbohydrate grams.

Example: 1 serving has 10 g fiber
10 g ÷ 2 = 5 g fiber
25 g total carbohydrate − 5 g fiber =
20 g carbohydrate
This counts as 1 carbohydrate choice.

Step 4: If a serving provides more than 5 g of sugar alcohols, subtract 1/2 the grams of sugar alcohol from the carbohydrate grams to get the total carbohydrate grams.

**Example: Sugar alcohols are not listed on this nutrition facts label therefore this product does not contain any. No further adjustment in total carbohydrate grams is needed.**

## Nutrition Facts

Serving Size          3/4 cup (33 g/1.2 oz.)
Servings Per Container          About 11

**Amount Per Serving**

**Calories** 110          Calories from Fat 15

|  | % Daily Value** |
|---|---|
| **Total Fat** 1.5 g* | **2**% |
| Saturated Fat 0 g | **0**% |
| *Trans* Fat 0 g | |
| **Cholesterol** 0 mg | **0**% |
| **Sodium** 90 mg | **4**% |
| **Potassium** 100 mg | **3**% |
| **Total Carbohydrate** 25 g | **8**% |
| Dietary Fiber 10 g | **18**% |
| Soluble Fiber 2 g | |
| Insoluble Fiber 5 g | |
| Sugars 5 g | |
| Other Carbohydrate 10 g | |
| **Protein** 4 g | |

| | | |
|---|---|---|
| Vitamin A 25% (25% DV as beta carotene) | | |
| Vitamin C 50% | * | Calcium 0% |
| Iron 10% | * | Vitamin E 100% |
| Vitamin B$_6$ 100% | * | Folic Acid 100% |
| Vitamin B$_{12}$ 100% | * | Zinc 10% |

* Amount in cereal. One half cup of fat free milk contributes and additional 40 calories, 65 mg sodium, 6 g total carbohydrates (6 g sugars), and 4 g protein.
** Percent Daily Values are based on a 2,000 calorie diet. Your daily values may be higher or lower depending on your calorie needs.

| | Calories: | 2,000 | 2,500 |
|---|---|---|---|
| Total Fat | Less than | 65 g | 65 g |
| Sat.Fat | Less than | 20 g | 20 g |
| Cholesterol | Less than | 300 mg | 300 mg |
| Sodium | Less than | 2,400 mg | 2,400 mg |
| Potassium | | 3,500 mg | 3,500 mg |
| Total Carbohydrate | | 300 g | 300 g |
| Dietary Fiber | | 25 g | 25 g |
| Protein | | 50 g | 50 g |

Calories per gram:
Fat 9      *      Carbohydrate 4      *      Protein 4

**FIGURE 19.3**   Label reading for carbohydrate counting.

and their premeal blood glucose level. Clients feel more in control and benefit from improved glucose control. On the minus side, carbohydrate counting requires clients to be diligent to the plan and prudent in their food choices. Keeping records of blood glucose tests and food intake helps to identify sources of problems.

## Changing Behaviors

The diagnosis of diabetes often triggers anxiety and uncertainty. People often see "diet" as the most difficult part of treatment. Even people with healthy eating styles may need to make changes in their intake to improve glycemic control. Giving someone a preprinted list of do's and don'ts can add to a resentful client's frustration. Before recommending dietary changes, it may be useful to ask:

• What are your goals for nutrition counseling?
• What behaviors do you want to change?
• What changes can you make in your present lifestyle?
• What obstacles may prevent you from making changes?
• What changes are you willing to make right now?
• What changes would be difficult for you to make?

Mastering the intricacies of eating for diabetes—what, when, and why—occurs over a continuum from learning basic facts to assimilating and implementing information. Individuals differ in how much information they want or need to know and in how motivated they are to improve their eating behaviors. Ideally, positive changes occur progressively over time in stepwise fashion with the client actively involved in goal setting, self-monitoring, and record keeping (Fig. 19.4). In reality, motivation to follow a meal

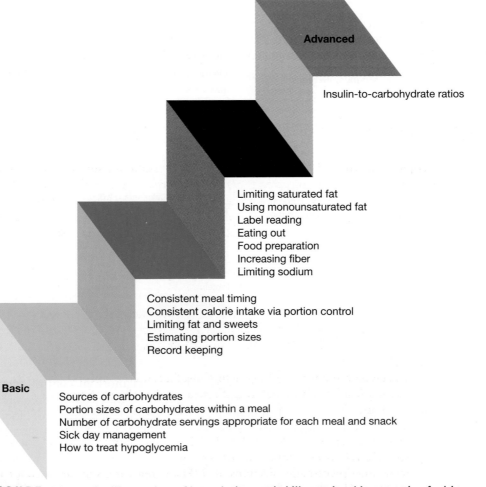

**Advanced**

Insulin-to-carbohydrate ratios

Limiting saturated fat
Using monounsaturated fat
Label reading
Eating out
Food preparation
Increasing fiber
Limiting sodium

Consistent meal timing
Consistent calorie intake via portion control
Limiting fat and sweets
Estimating portion sizes
Record keeping

**Basic**

Sources of carbohydrates
Portion sizes of carbohydrates within a meal
Number of carbohydrate servings appropriate for each meal and snack
Sick day management
How to treat hypoglycemia

**FIGURE 19.4** An illustration of knowledge and skills attained in stepwise fashion. Actual progression and concepts learned vary among individuals.

| BOX 19.8 | **TIPS FOR EATING OUT** |
|---|---|

- Eat the same size portion you would at home. Order only what you need and want.
- Select a restaurant with a variety of choices.
- Eat slowly.
- Choose tomato juice, unsweetened fruit juice, clear broth, bouillon, consommé, or shrimp cocktail as an appetizer instead of sweetened juices, fried vegetables, or creamed or thick soups.
- Choose fresh vegetable salads and use oil and vinegar or fresh lemon instead of regular salad dressings, or request that the dressing be put on the side. Avoid coleslaw and other salads with the dressing already added.
- Order plain (without gravy or sauce) roasted, baked, or broiled meat, fish, and poultry instead of fried, sautéed, or breaded entrées. Avoid stews and casseroles. Request a doggie bag if the portion exceeds the meal plan allowance.
- Order steamed, boiled, or broiled vegetables.
- Choose plain, baked, mashed, boiled, or steamed potatoes, rice, or noodles.
- Select fresh fruit for dessert.
- Request a sugar substitute for coffee or tea, if desired.

plan may be initially high, but commitment and diligence may dwindle when clients realize that "cheating" does not cause immediate illness. Periodic and ongoing follow-up improves compliance. Arming the client with behavior skills, such as tips for eating out (Box 19.8), provides them with the tools to make better choices. Basic label reading skills are vital (see Chapter 9).

# ▶ PHARMACOLOGICAL MANAGEMENT OF DIABETES

People with type 1 diabetes rely on exogenous insulin for survival—delivered by injection or pump. In contrast, nutrition therapy and exercise are capable of controlling glucose levels for the majority of people with type 2 diabetes. However, because of the progressive nature of the disease most people with type 2 diabetes eventually require oral agents, insulin, or a combination of both to manage blood glucose levels (Fonseca & Kulkarni, 2008).

## Insulin Therapy for People with Type 1 Diabetes

Insulin preparations vary in how quickly they act, when their peak action occurs, and how long their effects last. They are classified as rapid acting, short acting, intermediate acting, and long acting (Table 19.3). Varying ratios of insulin mixtures may be used to achieve glycemic control.

Usually intermediate- or long-acting insulin is used to meet basal needs, and a rapid- or short-acting insulin is used before each meal so that the total number of daily injections is three to four. This regimen most closely resembles how insulin is normally secreted, does not require a rigid eating schedule, and decreases the risk of hypoglycemia. Although multiple injections allow for a more flexible lifestyle and better glycemic control, they require frequent and consistent blood glucose testing.

Sometimes twice-daily injections of NPH and regular insulin are used for a simplified insulin regimen. This approach requires that meals and snacks be consumed at specified times and in consistent amounts to prevent hypoglycemia. For optimum effect, regular insulin

| TABLE 19.3 | **Insulin: Types, Onset of Action, Peak Activity, and Duration of Activity** | | | |
|---|---|---|---|---|
| **Insulin** | **Onset of Action** | **Peak Activity** | **Duration of Activity** | |
| Rapid Acting: lispro aspart | 15 minutes | 30 minutes to 2 hours | 4–5 hours | |
| Short Acting: regular | 30 minutes | 3–4 hours | 6–8 hours | |
| Intermediate Acting: lente NPH | 1–1.5 hours | 5–12 hours | 10–16 hours | |
| Very Long Acting: Glargine | 2–4 hours | Flat | 24 hours | |

should be injected 30 minutes prior to eating, which can be inconvenient. Nighttime hypoglycemia can be a problem with NPH peaking during the night.

## Intensive Insulin Therapy for People with Type 1 Diabetes

Intensive insulin therapy is a popular and dynamic insulin regimen for type 1 diabetes. Clients vary their mealtime insulin dose based on the carbohydrate content and timing of the food; they are also able to change their insulin dose for stress or exercise and to change their bolus insulin dose as needed. The regimen may use a long-acting insulin once or twice a day (usually at bedtime) and an injection of rapid-acting insulin before meals and snacks and to correct for high glucose readings. Another option is to have rapid-acting insulin delivered through an insulin pump. An algorithm gives formulas for clients to calculate the **carbohydrate-to-insulin ratio** for the anticipated carbohydrate content of a meal/snack, to correct for a high blood glucose reading, and to determine the amount of basal insulin needed.

**Carbohydrate-to-Insulin Ratio:** the amount of carbohydrate that can be handled per unit of insulin, usually 15 g CHO requires about one unit of rapid- or short-acting insulin.

Intensive insulin therapy requires more calculations at each meal but allows greater flexibility in when meals are eaten and how much carbohydrate is consumed. An accurate insulin dose also helps clients achieve better glycemic control in that corrections can be made as needed.

## Insulin Therapy for People with Type 2 Diabetes

Approximately 30% of people with type 2 diabetes eventually require insulin—either alone or in combination with glucose-lowering medications. Insulin therapy for people with type 2 diabetes often begins with a single injection of intermediate- or long-acting insulin at bedtime when fasting glucose levels are high; oral agents are taken during the day. Another regimen uses a morning injection of rapid and intermediate-acting insulin with an intermediate- or long-acting insulin at dinner or before bedtime. Self-monitoring of blood glucose levels is needed to optimize doses and timing.

## Glucose-Lowering Medications

Oral glucose-lowering medications vary in their mechanism of action and food concerns (Box 19.9). Medications may be used singly or in combination. They are considered adjunct to nutrition therapy and exercise, not a sole mode of therapy.

| BOX 19.9 | ORAL GLUCOSE-LOWERING AGENTS |
|---|---|

| **Drug** | **Food Concerns** |
|---|---|
| Secretagogues: stimulate the pancreas to secrete insulin | |
| **Sulfonylureas**<br>Brand names in this class include<br>  Diabinese, Amaryl, Glucotrol, Glucotrol<br>  XL, DiaBeta, Micronase, Glynase<br>  PresTab, Tolinase, and Orinase | Snacks may be needed, especially at bedtime<br>Missing meals or snacks can cause hypoglycemia<br>Clients should consume the same number of carbohydrate servings per meal |
| **Nonsulfonylurea secretagogues:** stimulate rapid insulin production; these have a quicker onset than sulfonylureas and carry a lower risk of hypoglycemia and weight gain | |
| Repaglinide (brand name Prandin),<br>  Nateglinide (Starlix) | May be preferred by clients with erratic eating schedules and those concerned about weight gain<br>These drugs should only be taken before meals or large snacks that contain substantial amounts of carbohydrate to avoid hypoglycemia |
| **Sensitizers:** enhance insulin action through a variety of mechanisms | |
| Alpha-glycosidase inhibitors [acarbose (Precose) and miglitol (Glyset)]: work by delaying the absorption of carbohydrates | These drugs should be taken with the first bite of each meal; these should not be taken when meals are missed<br>Side effects include bloating, abdominal cramps, flatulence, and diarrhea. Clients should be advised to avoid foods that cause gas, such as cauliflower, broccoli, cabbage, legumes, and lentils |
| Biguanide (metformin; brand name Glucophage): inhibits liver glucose production and liver glycogen breakdown | Does not cause hypoglycemia when used as monotherapy, and can cause weight loss<br>Side effects include abdominal cramping, nausea, diarrhea, and a metallic taste<br>Clients should avoid gassy foods (see above) to minimize side effects |
| Thiazolidinediones [rosiglitazone (Avandia) and pioglitazone (Actos)]: increase efficiency of glucose transporters | These are taken once or twice daily with food and may cause weight gain and mild edema; calorie and sodium restrictions are recommended |

*Source:* Fonseca, V., & Kulkarni, K. (2008). Management of type 2 diabetes: Oral agents, insulin, and injectables. *Journal of the American Dietetic Association, 108,* S29–S33.

## ▶ EXERCISE

Exercise is an important aspect of treatment for both types of diabetes regardless of weight status unless it is contraindicated for other medical reasons.

## Exercise in Insulin Users

Exercise has not been shown to improve glycemic control among people with type 1 diabetes, but it imparts other important benefits such as improving cardiovascular fitness, promoting bone strength, and enhancing the sense of well-being. When diabetes is poorly controlled, exercise may worsen hyperglycemia; without sufficient insulin, the muscle cannot adequately use glucose, so the liver compensates by producing or releasing stored glucose.

Exercise lowers blood glucose levels both during and after the activity, so care must be taken to avoid hypoglycemia. Reducing the insulin dose before planned exercise may be the best way to prevent hypoglycemia. Another option is to eat a carbohydrate snack if the blood glucose level is less than 100 mg/dL before exercise begins. If possible, exercise should occur within 2 hours of eating because beyond that time hypoglycemia is more likely. A carbohydrate snack may be necessary during prolonged exercise and during the hours following exercising. If exercise is unplanned, an additional 10 to 15 g carbohydrate per hour of moderate activity is recommended. More intense exercise requires more carbohydrate.

## Exercise in Type 2 Diabetes

Among people with type 2 diabetes, exercise offers substantial benefits. Regular exercise improves blood glucose control independent of weight loss. It also reduces insulin resistance, improves blood lipid levels, improves blood pressure, and enhances sense of well-being and quality of life. Exercise helps to maintain long-term weight reduction. Because people with type 2 diabetes who are treated with oral glucose-lowering medications or insulin may experience exercise-induced hypoglycemia, they should monitor their blood glucose levels, exercise within 2 hours after eating, and stop activity if signs and symptoms of hypoglycemia develop.

## ▶ SICK-DAY MANAGEMENT

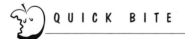 **Q U I C K   B I T E**

Sick-day management of carbohydrates:
  Each is approximately one carbohydrate
    choice (15 g carbohydrate)
  6 oz regular ginger ale
  ½ cup ice cream
  ½ cup apple juice
  1 frozen juice bar
  ½ cup sherbet
  ½ cup regular gelatin
  ½ cup orange juice
  1 cup creamed soup

Acute illnesses, even mild ones such as a cold or flu, can significantly raise blood glucose levels. Unless otherwise instructed by the physician, clients should maintain their normal medication schedule, monitor their blood glucose levels every 2 to 4 hours, and maintain an adequate fluid intake. Urine or blood should be checked for ketones at least twice a day. Unless blood glucose levels are higher than 250 mg/dL, clients should eat the usual amount of carbohydrate, divided into smaller meals and snacks if necessary. Sweetened liquids are generally a well-tolerated source of carbohydrates and fluid. A daily intake of 150 to 200 g of carbohydrates, approximately 45 to 50 g every 3 to 4 hours, is recommended.

## ▶ LIFE CYCLE CONSIDERATIONS

Diabetes nutrition therapy can influence growth and development in children and adolescents and the quality of life in older adults. Special considerations for these groups are presented below; diabetes in pregnancy is covered in Chapter 11.

## Children and Adolescents

Children with diabetes appear to have the same nutrient needs as their age-matched peers. However, managing diabetes in children and adolescents is complicated by the impact of growth on nutrient needs, irregular eating patterns, and erratic activity levels. More frequent adjustments in insulin and food intake are necessary to compensate for growth and activity needs. Failure to provide adequate calories and nutrients results in poor growth, as does poor glycemic control and inadequate insulin administration. Conversely, excessive weight gain occurs from excessive calorie intake, overtreatment of hypoglycemia, or excess insulin administration. Neither withholding food nor having a child eat when not hungry is an appropriate strategy to manage glucose levels. Rather, individualized meal plans and intensive insulin regimens can provide flexibility for erratic eating, activity, and growth. Box 19.10 lists questions to consider when dealing with children with diabetes.

Although type 2 is most often diagnosed after 45 years of age, 2002–2003 data show that 3700 American youth are diagnosed with type 2 diabetes annually. For Asian, Pacific Islander, and American Indian youth 10 to 19 years old, the rate of new cases of type 2 diabetes exceeds that of type 1 (CDC, 2007). Weight control is key to preventing type 2 diabetes in children.

## Diabetes in Later Life

There are unique considerations related to aging that affect glycemic control. First, blood glucose levels rise with age for reasons that are unclear. Treatment may not be instituted for glucose elevations that are considered "high" in younger populations but may be "normal" for the elderly. Cognitive impairments, such as memory loss, impaired concentration, dementia, and depression, may preclude self-management. Physical impairments may impede exercise. Sensory impairments, such as decreased hearing, poor eyesight, and decreased senses of taste and smell, may complicate teaching and self-management. For instance, older clients who could clinically benefit from insulin may be treated instead with oral agents if

---

| BOX 19.10 | **QUESTIONS TO CONSIDER WHEN DEALING WITH CHILDREN WITH DIABETES** |

Is the child responsible for any or all of his or her diabetes management?
Does the child feed himself or herself?
Do the child's routine and activity expenditure differ on weekdays and on the weekend?
What is the child's school schedule?
What is the child's social life?
Are school lunches eaten?
Does the child have food jags or use food to manipulate parents?
If the child does not attend school, who is the primary caretaker during the day?

poor eyesight or decreased manual dexterity precludes self-injection. Older adults may be at greater nutritional risk for a variety of reasons, including poor dentition, physical impairments that make shopping or cooking difficult, poor appetite related to lack of socialization, and an inadequate food budget. For many, a strict calorie-controlled diet is more harmful than beneficial. Because older adults are more susceptible to severe hypoglycemia, a fasting target level of 120 to 150 mg/dL may be considered appropriate.

## ▶ DIABETIC DIETS IN THE HOSPITAL

Traditionally, standardized calorie-level meal plans based on the exchange lists were used to provide "diabetic" diets to hospitalized diabetics. The physician would order a specific calorie-level "ADA diet" that was composed of specific percentages of carbohydrate, protein, and fat. Because the ADA no longer endorses any single meal plan or specified nutrient composition, it is recommended that this term and approach no longer be used.

Also considered obsolete are "no concentrated sweets," "no sugar added," "low sugar," and "liberal diabetic" diets. They do not reflect the diabetes nutrient recommendations and are unnecessarily restrictive in sugar. These diets may give patients the false impression that glycemic control is achieved by limiting sugar.

An alternative to the traditional "ADA diet" is a consistent carbohydrate diet. In this approach, calories are not specified but carbohydrate intake is consistent, such as four carbohydrates for every meal with one to two for an evening snack. A typical day's intake from meals and snacks may range from 1500 to 2000 calories, with adjustments made for individual patients as needed. Appropriate modifications in fat intake are made, and consistent timing of meals and snacks is stressed. However, just as there is no longer one diabetic diet, neither is there one correct way to provide nutrition therapy to hospitalized people with diabetes. See Box 19.11 for additional considerations when people with diabetes are hospitalized.

| BOX 19.11 | **ADDITIONAL CONSIDERATIONS WHEN PEOPLE WITH DIABETES ARE HOSPITALIZED** |
| --- | --- |

- Patients given clear or full liquid diets should receive approximately 200 g of carbohydrate per day in equally divided amounts at meals and snacks. Sugar-free items should not be used. Adjustments in diabetes medication may be needed to achieve glycemic control.
- Sometimes people with diabetes are given a regular diet based on the rationale that a sliding scale insulin regimen will take care of hyperglycemia related to the stress of hospitalization, acute illness, and changes in diet. While that is true, the risk is that patients may not understand a "regular" diet is not appropriate after discharge.
- The diet should be progressed as soon as possible after surgery with the goal of providing adequate carbohydrates and calories.
- Continuous monitoring is needed during catabolic illnesses to ensure that nutritional needs are met and hyperglycemia is prevented. Overfeeding exacerbates hyperglycemia.
- For tube feedings, standard enteral formulas (~50% of calories from carbohydrate) or a lower-carbohydrate content formula (33–40% carbohydrate) may be used. Medication adjustments are made according to the results of blood glucose monitoring.

# NURSING PROCESS: Type 2 Diabetes

Mark is 52 years old and is sedentary. His doctor monitored his fasting blood glucose and cholesterol levels for several years, urging Mark to eat better and exercise or he would eventually need medications to bring down both his glucose and cholesterol levels. Mark was unmotivated to change and so he is now taking metformin and Lipitor. He feels great, his glucose and cholesterol are "fine," and he sees no need to change anything when the pills work so good alone. He is 5 ft. 9 in. tall and weighs 190 pounds.

## Assessment

| | |
|---|---|
| Medical-Psychosocial History | • Medical history and comorbidities, including hyperlipidemia, hypertension, CVD, renal impairments, neuropathy, and gastrointestinal complaints |
| | • Use of prescribed and over-the-counter medications |
| | • Psychosocial and economic issues such as the living situation, cooking facilities, adequacy of food budget, education, need for food assistance, and level of family and social support |
| | • Usual activity patterns |
| Anthropometric Assessment | • Height, current weight, usual weight; recent weight history |
| | • BMI |
| | • Waist circumference to identify abdominal obesity |
| Biochemical and Physical Assessment | • A1c, fasting glucose levels |
| | • Lipid profile |
| | • Measures of renal function, if available |
| | • Blood pressure |
| | • Record of self-monitored blood glucose (SMBG) levels |
| Dietary Assessment | • How many meals and snacks do you usually eat in a day? Do you ever skip meals? Do you eat at regular intervals? When do you eat snacks? |
| | • What is a typical day's intake? |
| | • Have you ever tried to follow a diet or improve your eating habits? |
| | • What do you know about nutrition for diabetes? |
| | • How is your appetite? |
| | • Do you have any food intolerances or allergies? Do you ever have GI symptoms that impact what you eat? |
| | • Do you ever experience symptoms of low blood glucose? What do you do to raise your blood glucose when you are feeling low? |
| | • What do you know about how your medication and exercise impacts blood glucose levels? |
| | • Are you willing/able to change your eating habits if necessary? |
| | • How do you feel about your weight? |
| | • Do you have any cultural, religious, or ethnic food preferences? |
| | • Who prepares your meals? |
| | • Do you take vitamins, minerals, or other supplements? |
| | • Do you use alcohol? |

*(nursing process continues on page 478)*

## NURSING PROCESS: *Type 2 Diabetes* (continued)

| Diagnosis | |
|---|---|
| Possible Nursing Diagnosis | Ineffective health maintenance, related to the lack of knowledge of nutrition therapy for diabetes mellitus |

| Planning | |
|---|---|
| Client Outcomes | **Short term** |

**Short term**

The client will

- State three signs/symptoms of hypoglycemia
- Eat three meals plus a bedtime snack at approximately the same times every day
- Begin strategies to shift toward a nutritionally adequate, balanced, and varied diet that has

    4 carbohydrate choices at each meal and 2 at a bedtime snack

    5 servings of fruits and vegetables

    3 servings of whole grains

    3 cups of milk

    4–6 oz of protein

    Healthy fats

    Little saturated fat and minimal trans fats

- Monitor his blood glucose level daily
- Keep periodic food records that include the timing of meals and snacks and type and amount of food eaten
- State 3 emergency foods to use during hypoglycemic episodes
- Walk 10 minutes 3 times/day at least 3 days/week

**Long term**

The client will

- Lose 9 pounds in 6 months (5% of initial weight)
- Achieve A1c and pre- and postprandial blood glucose levels within target levels established by his physician
- Avoid hypoglycemia
- Improve lipid profile
- Prevent or delay chronic complications
- Increase physical activity to 30 minutes daily 5 times/week

| Nursing Interventions | |
|---|---|
| Nutrition Therapy | Introduce basic concepts: which foods contain carbohydrates, appropriate serving sizes for carbohydrates, and how many carbohydrate choices are appropriate for each meal and snack |

*(nursing process continues on page 479)*

## NURSING PROCESS: Type 2 Diabetes (continued)

| | |
|---|---|
| Client Teaching | Instruct the client |

On the role of nutrition therapy in managing blood glucose levels, including that

- Nutrition therapy is essential and that nutrition is important even when no symptoms are apparent
- Medication is used in addition to nutrition therapy not as a substitute
- Ongoing or follow-up counseling is necessary to make adjustments and expand skills and knowledge to optimize diabetes management

On eating plan essentials, including the importance of

- Eating meals and snacks at regular times every day
- Eating approximately the same amount of food every day especially the same amount of carbohydrates
- Eating enough high-fiber foods such as oats, oat bran, other whole grains, and dried peas and beans
- Using less fat, sugar, and salt

On behavioral matters, including

- How to read labels to determine the amount of carbohydrate choices a serving of food provides
- Making healthy choices overall, such as lean meats, fat-free milk, soft spread margarines
- Not skipping meals or snacks
- Physical activity goals
- Having a source of glucose handy at all times
- The importance of monitoring food intake and blood glucose levels
- Where to get additional information

## Evaluation

| | |
|---|---|
| Evaluate and Monitor | - Food intake records for consistency in meal timing, the number of carbohydrate choices per meals and snacks, and overall quality and adequacy of food choices made |

- Appetite/satiety
- Self-monitoring blood glucose records to determine if 50% are within target range
- Lab data as available
- Weight
- Need for nutritional counseling
- Progress toward physical activity goals

## ▶ HOW DO YOU RESPOND?

**How can I follow a diabetic diet with my relentless "sweet tooth"?** Small amounts of sweet foods are permitted, especially if weight is not a problem, as long as they are counted as part of the meal plan, not added as "extras." Diabetic cookbooks are helpful in incorporating sweet foods into the eating pattern. Calorie-free foods sweetened with non-nutritive sweeteners (e.g., saccharin, aspartame) add sweetness and interest without calories. Encourage the client to use artificially sweetened soft drinks and gelatin.

**Are "dietetic" products like candy and cookies worth the added expense?** Dietetic products are not necessarily calorie-free or specifically intended for diabetics. Foods that are labeled "dietetic" may be made without sugar, without salt, with a particular type of fat, or for special food allergies. Read the ingredient label and check with a diet counselor before adding a dietetic food to the diet—or avoid dietetic foods altogether because they are expensive and usually do not taste as good as the foods they are intended to replace.

## ▶ CASE STUDY

Keisha is a 42-year-old Black female with a BMI of 29. She was recently diagnosed with diabetes and hypertension. Her mother and two sisters also have type 2 diabetes. She is the mother of three children, who each weighed more than 10 pounds at birth. Although she knows she should exercise, she doesn't have time in her busy schedule.

The doctor gave her a 1500-calorie diet and told her if her glucose does not improve, she will have to go on medication and possibly insulin. She has tried the "diet" but finds it too restrictive: it tells her to eat things she doesn't like (such as milk) and won't let her eat the things she loves (like sweet tea and fried foods). She is scared of the potential for needing insulin and the complications associated with diabetes.

- What risk factors does Keisha have for type 2 diabetes?
- Is a 1500-calorie diet appropriate for her? Should it promote weight loss or maintain her current weight?
- What would you tell Keisha about weight and diabetes management?
- What would you tell her about drinking milk? What about sweet tea and fried foods?
- What approaches would you take to improve compliance yet increase her satisfaction with eating?

## STUDY QUESTIONS

What other lifestyle changes would you propose to Keisha to manage diabetes and reduce the risk of complications?

1. Which statement indicates the patient understands nutrition recommendations regarding carbohydrate intake?
   a. "People with diabetes should avoid sugars and foods that contain sugars."
   b. "It is important to consume the proper balance of starch, sugar, and fiber at each meal."
   c. "It is important to consume the correct amount of carbohydrate at each meal and snack."
   d. "Carbohydrates must be balanced in relation to the amount of protein and fat consumed."

2. The client with type 1 diabetes asks if she can have a glass of wine with dinner on the weekends. Which of the following would be the nurse's best response?
   a. "It is better to have wine between meals than with meals so that it doesn't interfere with your normal food intake."

    **b.** "People with diabetes cannot have alcohol because it raises blood glucose levels very quickly."

    **c.** "A mixed drink would be better than wine because the mixer will help slow the absorption of the alcohol."

    **d.** "An occasional glass of wine with dinner will not cause any problems. Be sure to limit yourself to 1 serving."

**3.** When developing a teaching plan for a client who is taking insulin, which of the following foods would the nurse suggest the client carry with him to treat mild hypoglycemia?

    **a.** Crackers       **b.** Peanuts       **c.** Chocolate drops       **d.** Lifesavers

**4.** The best approach for monitoring carbohydrate intake is to use:

    **a.** The exchange system

    **b.** Carbohydrate counting

    **c.** Sample menus

    **d.** The approach that best helps the individual control blood glucose levels

**5.** How many carbohydrate choices are provided in a serving of food that supplies 19 grams of carbohydrate?

    **a.** 1       **b.** 2       **c.** 3       **d.** 4

**6.** The nurse knows her instructions about label reading have been effective when the client verbalizes that to determine the amount of carbohydrate choices, you must:

    **a.** Add the grams of total carbohydrate and grams of sugars together to determine total carbohydrates provided

    **b.** Adjust total carbohydrates for foods that provide more than 5 grams of fiber or more than 5 grams of sugar alcohols per serving

    **c.** Add grams of total carbohydrate fiber and sugars to determine total carbohydrate grams

    **d.** Use only the grams of total carbohydrate to determine carbohydrate choices

**7.** What is the priority for preventing diabetes in people who are at high risk?

    **a.** Eat a low-carbohydrate diet

    **b.** Consume a consistent amount of carbohydrate at every meal

    **c.** Achieve moderate weight loss through increased activity and lowered calorie and fat intake

    **d.** Eat a heart-healthy diet

**8.** Which food groups provide carbohydrates? Select all that apply.

    **a.** Vegetables       **b.** Fruit       **c.** Milk       **d.** Meat

## KEY CONCEPTS

- Diabetes is a group of diseases characterized by hyperglycemia. It is increasing in epidemic proportions, largely due to the increase in type 2 diabetes.

- Type 1 diabetes is characterized by the lack of insulin secretion. It is usually diagnosed before the age of 30 years in people who are of normal or below normal weight.

- Ninety percent to 95% of diabetes cases are type 2 diabetes. It begins with prediabetes that is characterized by hyperinsulinemia and insulin resistance. Hyperglycemia provides constant stimulation for insulin secretion, further aggravating hyperinsulinemia.

- Acute diabetes complications include DKA, HHNS, and hypoglycemia. Acute complications are more likely during illness. Frequent blood glucose monitoring can help avoid acute complications.

- Long-term diabetes complications include damage to both small and large vessels in the body. Tight glycemic control delays or prevents the onset of long-term microvascular complications and probably macrovascular complications as well.

● Nutrition therapy is the cornerstone of treatment for all people with diabetes, regardless of weight status, use of medication, blood glucose levels, and presence or absence of symptoms. The goals of nutrition therapy are to achieve optimal blood glucose and lipid levels, attain or maintain reasonable weight, and avoid acute and chronic complications.

● Lifestyle changes that include moderate weight loss, regular physical activity, and a lowered calorie and fat intake can reduce the risk of developing diabetes.

● Nutrient needs of people with diabetes are not different than the general population. Dietary recommendations to promote health and well-being, such as eating less saturated fat, trans fat, and cholesterol and more fiber and whole grains, are also appropriate for people with diabetes.

● The ADA recommends that people with diabetes limit saturated fat intake to less than 7% of total calories and minimize their intake of trans fat. Cholesterol should be limited to less than 200 mg/day, and 2 servings of fatty fish are recommended per week. These suggestions are relatively consistent with the AHA's dietary recommendations for people at high risk of heart disease.

● Sucrose ("sugar") is no longer considered detrimental to glucose control so long as it is eaten as part of the meal plan and not as an "extra." However, if weight loss is a goal, high-sugar foods should be limited.

● Diets for people with diabetes are not "one size fits all." Dietary changes should be made sequentially and restrictions kept to a minimum to maximize compliance.

● There is not one superior method of monitoring carbohydrate intake. The method used should be determined by the individual's lifestyle, preferences, and willingness/ability to make dietary changes.

● Exchange lists for diabetes group foods into lists based on their macronutrient content. A meal plan shows the client how many exchanges from each list he or she should have for every meal and snack. Any item in a list can be exchanged for any other. The exchange lists are complex and very structured.

● Carbohydrate counting focuses mainly on the carbohydrate content of foods; protein and fat are not tightly controlled. Clients select foods for each meal based on how many grams of carbohydrate or carbohydrate choices their meal plan allows. It provides more flexibility than the exchange system and is easier to use.

● People with type 1 diabetes must take exogenous insulin. Intensive insulin therapy allows clients to determine their premeal insulin dosage based on their glucose level and the amount of carbohydrate they anticipate eating.

● Although most people with type 2 diabetes have the potential to achieve glycemic control through diet and exercise, the progressive nature of the disease causes most people to eventually need oral medications and/or insulin. Oral medications vary in their mode of action, side effects, and food concerns.

● Children and adolescents have a greater variation in their daily calorie needs than do adults because of their nutritional needs for growth and their more erratic activity and eating patterns. Managing diabetes is more challenging in young people.

● Diabetes during pregnancy can cause problems in the fetus and complications at delivery. Frequent glucose monitoring and three meals and two to three snacks daily are recommended.

● Older people with diabetes may need to be treated more conservatively than younger people because they are more susceptible to severe hypoglycemia, are at greater nutritional risk, and may have physical or sensory impairments that complicate self-management.

● Diabetic diets in the hospital were traditionally identified as "ADA diets." Because there is no one diabetic diet recommended for all people with diabetes, this term should be discontinued. Consistent carbohydrate diets are recommended.

## ANSWER KEY

1. **FALSE** Diabetes is not an inevitable consequence of prediabetes. Weight loss and exercise can prevent or delay diabetes and normalize blood glucose levels.

2. **FALSE** People with diabetes should consume a "normal" carbohydrate intake of 45% to 65% of total calories (within the Acceptable Macronutrient Distribution range), just like the general population. Low-carbohydrate diets tend to be high in fat; high saturated fat diets increase the risk of cardiovascular disease.

3. **FALSE** Modest weight loss, such as 5% to 7%, has been shown to dramatically reduce the risk of type 2 diabetes even when healthy BMI is not attained.

4. **TRUE** Alcohol is more likely to cause hypoglycemia when consumed without food rather than with food.

5. **FALSE** People with diabetes should avoid the use of fructose as an added sweetener because it causes adverse effects on serum triglycerides and LDL cholesterol, but do not need to avoid natural fructose found in fruit.

6. **FALSE** People with diabetes do not need more fiber than the general population.

7. **FALSE** Hypoglycemia is a risk with insulin and certain oral medications, but not with all medications, so the use of snacks should be tailored to the individual's insulin and/or medication regime. People with type 2 diabetes who are controlled by diet alone do not need snacks, and snacks may be counterproductive in people trying to lose weight.

8. **FALSE** People who practice carbohydrate counting cannot ignore protein and fat intake; they are urged to eat 4–6 oz of lean protein/day and choose healthy fats.

9. **FALSE** Although a chocolate candy bar does provide ample sugar, it also provides substantial amounts of fat that delay the absorption of glucose. The best choice for treating mild hypoglycemia is readily absorbable pure sugars, such as glucose tablets, fruit juice, soft drinks, or lifesavers.

10. **TRUE** People with diabetes should limit their intake of saturated fat and cholesterol because their risk of CHD is very high.

## WEBSITES

American Diabetes Association at **www.diabetes.org**
Joslin Diabetes Center at **www.joslin.org**
National Institute of Diabetes and Digestive and Kidney Diseases at **www.niddk.nih.gov**

## REFERENCES

American Diabetes Association. (2008). Nutrition recommendations and interventions for diabetes. A position statement of the American Diabetes Association. *Diabetes Care, 31*(Suppl. 1), S61–S78.

American Diabetes Association and American Dietetic Association. (2008). *Choose your foods: Exchange lists for diabetes.* Alexandria, VA: American Diabetes Association; Chicago: American Dietetic Association.

Anderson, F. (2000). Chromium in the prevention and control of diabetes. *Diabetes & Metabolism, 26,* 22–27.

Anderson, J. (2006). Diabetes mellitus: Medical nutrition therapy. In: M. Shils, M. Shike, R. Ross, et al. (Eds.), *Modern nutrition in health and disease* (10th ed.). Philadelphia: Lippincott Williams & Wilkins.

Center for Disease Control (CDC). (2007). *National diabetes fact sheet, 2007.* Available at www.cdc.gov/diabaetes/pubs/pdf/ndfs_2007.pdf. Accessed on 6/25/08.

Chan, J. M., Rimm, E. B., Colditz, G. A., et al. (1994). Obesity, fat distribution, and weight gain as risk factors for clinical diabetes in men. *Diabetes Care, 17,* 961–969.

Colditz, G. A., Willett, W. C., Rotnitzky, A., et al. (1995). Weight gain as a risk factor for clinical diabetes mellitus in women. *Annals of Internal Medicine, 122,* 481–486.

Cummings, S., Apovian, C., & Khaodhiar, L. (2008). Obesity surgery: Evidence for diabetes prevention/management. *Journal of the American Dietetic Association, 108,* S40–S44.

Daly, A. (2007). Use of insulin and weight gain: Optimizing diabetes nutrition therapy. *Journal of the American Dietetic Association, 107,* 1386–1393.

Diabetes Prevention Research Group. (2002). Reduction in the evidence of T2DM with life-style intervention or metformin. *The New England Journal of Medicine, 346,* 393–403.

Fonseca, V., & Kulkarni, K. (2008). Management of type 2 diabetes: Oral agents, insulin, and injectables. *Journal of the American Dietetic Association, 108,* S29–S33.

Franz, M. J., Bantle, J. P., Beebe, C. A., et al. (2002). Evidence-based nutrition principles and recommendations for the treatment and prevention of diabetes and related complications. *Diabetes Care, 25,* 148–198.

Geiss, L., Wang, J., & Gregg, E. (2007). Long-term trends in the prevalence and incidence of diagnosed diabetes. *Diabetes Care, 56*(Suppl. 1), A33.

Grundy, S. M., Cleeman, J. I., Daniels, S. R., et al. (2005). *Diagnosis and management of the metabolic syndrome. An American Heart Association/National Heart, Lung, and Blood Institute Scientific Statement. Executive summary.* Available at circ.ahajournals.org. Accessed on 2/8/08.

Haffner, S., Temprosa, M., Crandall, J., et al. (2005). Intensive lifestyle intervention or metformin on inflammation and coagulation in participants with impaired glucose tolerance. *Diabetes, 54,* 1566–1572.

Institute of Medicine (IOM). (2005). *Dietary reference intakes for energy, carbohydrates, fiber, fat, fatty acids, cholesterol, protein, and amino acids (macronutrients).* Washington, DC: National Academies Press.

Klein, S., Sheard, N. F., Pi-Sunyer, X., et al. (2004). Weight management through lifestyle modification for the prevention and management of type 2 diabetes: Rationale and strategies: A statement of the American Diabetes, the North American Association for the Study of Obesity, and the American Society for Clinical Nutrition. *Diabetes Care, 27,* 2067–2073.

Lichtenstein, A. H., Appel, L. J., Brands, M., et al. (2006). Diet and lifestyle recommendations revision 2006. A scientific statement from the American Heart Association Nutrition Committee. *Circulation, 114,* 82–96.

Liese, A. D., Roach, A. K., Sparks, K. C., et al. (2003). Whole-grain intake and insulin sensitivity: The Insulin Resistance Atherosclerosis Study. *The American Journal of Clinical Nutrition, 78,* 965–971.

Melanson, K. (2007). Diet and nutrients in the prevention and treatment of type 2 diabetes. *American Journal of Lifestyle Medicine, 1,* 339–343.

Narayan, K., Boyle, J., & Thompson, T. (2003). Lifetime risk for diabetes mellitus in the United States. *The Journal of the American Medical Association, 290,* 1884–1890.

Nathan, D. M., Cleary, P. A., Backlund, J. Y., et al. (2005). Intensive diabetes treatment and cardiovascular disease in patients with type 1 diabetes. *The New England Journal of Medicine, 353,* 2643–2653.

National Cholesterol Education Program. (2001). *Third report of the expert panel on detection, evaluation, and treatment of high blood cholesterol in adults (Adult Treatment Panel III). Executive Summary.* (NIH Publication No. 01-3670). Bethesda, MD: U.S. Department of Health and Human Services, Public Health Service, National Institutes of Health.

National Institute of Diabetes and Digestive and Kidney Diseases, National Institutes of Health, Diabetes Information Clearinghouse. *Diabetes prevention program.* Available at diabetes.niddk.nih.gov/dm/pubs/preventionprogram/. Accessed on 6/23/08.

Ratner, R., Goldberg, R., Haffner, S., et al. (2005). Impact of intensive lifestyle and metformin therapy on cardiovascular disease risk factors in the Diabetes Prevention Program. *Diabetes Care, 28,* 888–894.

Sheard, N. F., Clark, N. G., Brand-Miller, J. C., et al. (2004). Dietary carbohydrate (amount and type) in the prevention and management of diabetes: A statement of the American Diabetes Association. *Diabetes Care, 27,* 2266–2271.

Smith, S. (2007). Multiple risk factors for cardiovascular disease and diabetes mellitus. *The American Journal of Medicine, 120,* S3–S11.

Wheeler, M., Daly, A., Evert, A., et al. (2008). Choose your foods: Exchange lists for diabetes (6th ed.). Description and guidelines for use. *Journal of the American Dietetic Association, 108,* 883–888.

Wheeler, M., & Pi-Sunyer, X. (2008). Carbohydrate issues: type and amount. *Journal of the American Dietetic Association, 108*(suppl 1), S34–S39.

# 20

# Nutrition for Patients with Cardiovascular Disorders

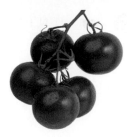

| TRUE | FALSE | |
|------|-------|---|
| ☐ | ☐ | **1** The DASH diet for preventing and controlling high blood pressure is simply low in sodium. |
| ☐ | ☐ | **2** The majority of sodium in the typical American diet comes from salt added during cooking and at the table. |
| ☐ | ☐ | **3** Weight loss lowers high blood pressure. |
| ☐ | ☐ | **4** The focus of preventing and treating CHD is to raise HDL cholesterol. |
| ☐ | ☐ | **5** The most effective dietary intervention to lower LDL cholesterol is to limit the percentage of calories consumed as fat. |
| ☐ | ☐ | **6** A heart healthy diet recommends most grain choices be whole grains. |
| ☐ | ☐ | **7** It is not known whether the cardioprotective benefits of eating fish are due solely to the omega-3 fatty acids or if the benefits are derived from something else in the fish. |
| ☐ | ☐ | **8** Alcohol may be good for heart health. |
| ☐ | ☐ | **9** For plant sterols to effectively lower cholesterol levels, they must be consumed daily. |
| ☐ | ☐ | **10** A heart healthy diet is intended only for adults hoping to avoid heart disease and for those who are diagnosed with heart disease. |

## UPON COMPLETION OF THIS CHAPTER, YOU WILL BE ABLE TO

- Determine whether a sample 2000-calorie menu complies with the DASH-sodium eating plan.
- Compare the DASH-sodium diet with the TLC diet.
- Give examples of foods that are limited in a heart healthy diet.
- Give examples of foods that are encouraged in a heart healthy diet.
- Create a 2000-calorie heart healthy menu.
- Counsel a client on how to read a Nutrition Facts label to determine whether a food is appropriate for a 2000-mg sodium diet.

ardiovascular disease (CVD) is an umbrella term for diseases that affect the heart and blood vessels. Atherosclerotic CVD are caused by atherosclerosis, a progressive narrowing and hardening of blood vessels that may lead to blocked blood flow to the heart (myocardial infarction), brain (cerebrovascular accident), or legs (peripheral arterial disease). Atherosclerosis can also cause a ballooning out of blood vessel walls (aneurysm). CVD accounted for 36.3% of all American deaths in 2004—more than any other single cause or

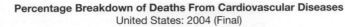

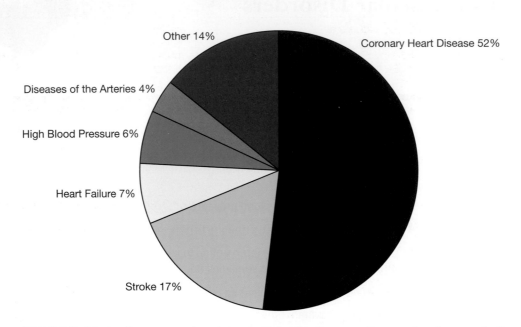

**FIGURE 20.1**   Percentage breakdown of deaths from cardiovascular diseases in the United States in 2004. (**Source:** CDC/NCHS.)

group of causes of death in the United States (AHA, 2008). More American men and women die from coronary heart disease (CHD) than from any other CVD (Fig. 20.1).

This chapter addresses nutrition for the prevention and treatment of hypertension, atherosclerotic CVD, and heart failure.

## ▶ HYPERTENSION

Hypertension is a symptom, not a disease, arbitrarily defined as sustained elevated blood pressure greater than or equal to 140/90 mmHg (Table 20.1)—"arbitrarily defined" because problems associated with high blood pressure occur on a continuum with no obvious threshold of where risk begins (Lichtenstein et al., 2006). Hypertension is a major risk factor for heart disease, stroke, kidney failure, and peripheral arterial disease. Even people with prehypertension are urged to take measures to lower their blood pressure.

Hypertension is one of the most common chronic conditions in the United States. An estimated 27% of American adults have hypertension and another 31% have prehypertension (Appel, 2006). For Americans over the age of 50, the lifetime risk of developing hypertension is estimated to be 90% (Vasan et al., 2002). Compared to nonblacks, blacks have a higher prevalence of hypertension, develop hypertension earlier in life, and have higher risks of hypertension-related complications, especially stroke and kidney failure (Appel et al., 2006).

Dietary factors play a prominent role in blood pressure regulation (Appel et al., 2006). In people who are normotensive or prehypertensive, dietary changes have the potential

| TABLE 20.1 | Blood Pressure Classifications | | |
|---|---|---|---|
| | | **Systolic** | **Diastolic** |
| Normal blood pressure | | <120 | and <80 |
| Prehypertension | | 120–139 | or 80–89 |
| Stage 1 hypertension | | 140–159 | or 90–99 |
| Stage 2 hypertension | | ≥160 | ≥100 |

*Source:* USDHHS, NIH, NHLBI. (2004). *The seventh report of the Joint National Committee on prevention, detection, evaluation, and treatment of high blood pressure* (NIH Publication No. 04-5230). Bethesda, MD: NHLBI Health Information Center.

| TABLE 20.2 | Diet and Lifestyle Recommendations to Lower Blood Pressure and Reduce the Risk of CVD | | |
|---|---|---|---|
| | | **Diet-Related Lifestyle Modifications that Effectively Lower Blood Pressure*** | **AHA Diet and Lifestyle Recommendations to Reduce the Risk of CVD[†]** |
| Attain/maintain healthy body weight. | | ✓ | ✓ |
| Consume a diet rich in vegetables and fruit. | | ✓ | ✓ |
| Consume a diet rich in low-fat dairy products. | | ✓ | |
| Choose whole grains. | | ✓** | ✓ |
| Consume 2 servings of fish/week, preferably fatty fish. | | | ✓ |
| Limit saturated fat and cholesterol intake. | | ✓ | ✓ |
| Limit added sugars. | | ✓ | ✓ |
| Limit salt. | | ✓ | ✓ |
| Increase potassium intake. | | ✓** | |
| Follow recommendations when food is eaten outside the home. | | | ✓ |
| Drink alcohol in moderation, if at all. | | ✓ | ✓ |

*Appel, L. J., Brands, M. W., Daniels, S. R., Karanja, N., Elmer, P. J., Sacks, F. M., et al. (2006). Dietary approaches to prevent and treat hypertension: A scientific statement from the American Heart Association. *Hypertension, 47*, 296–308.

[†]Lichtenstein A. H., Appel, L. J., Brands, M., Carnethon, M., Daniels, S., Franch, H. A., et al. (2006). Diet and lifestyle recommendations revision 2006. A scientific statement from the American Heart Association Nutrition Committee. *Circulation, 114*, 82–96.

**As part of the DASH diet

to reduce blood pressure and prevent hypertension and its complications. In people with stage 1 hypertension, diet is the initial treatment before drug therapy is introduced and may eliminate the need for medication. In people who have hypertension and are treated with medication, diet can lower blood pressure and reduce the dose of medication needed. Diet-related lifestyle recommendations to lower blood pressure are highlighted in Table 20.2.

| TABLE 20.3 | "Heart Healthy" Eating Plans: Dash-Sodium and TLC Diet for a 2000-Calorie Intake | | |
|---|---|---|---|
| **Food Group/Representative Serving Sizes** | **DASH-Sodium*** | **TLC†** | **Types of Foods Recommended** |
| Grains<br>1 slice bread; ½ cup cooked rice, pasta, or cereal | 6–8 servings/day | 7 servings/day | Whole grains are recommended for most grain servings, such as whole-wheat bread, whole-grain cereals, whole-wheat pasta, and brown rice<br>Commercial products, such as crackers, cookies, chips, and cakes, should be trans fat free and low in fat |
| Vegetables<br>1 cup raw leafy vegetable<br>½ cup cut-up raw or cooked vegetable<br>½ cup vegetable juice | 4–5 servings/day | 5 servings/day | All fresh, plain frozen, and low-sodium canned vegetables<br>Use preparation methods to retain the fiber content, such as leaving skins on potatoes |
| Fruit<br>1 medium fruit<br>¼ cup dried fruit<br>½ cup fresh, frozen, or canned fruit;<br>½ cup fruit juice | 4–5 servings/day | 4 servings/day | All; eat skins and seeds for fiber whenever possible<br>Whole fruits are better choices than fruit juice |
| Milk and dairy products<br>1 cup milk or yogurt<br>1 ½ oz natural cheese | 2–3 servings/day | 2–3 servings/day | Nonfat or low-fat milk, yogurt, and cheese |
| Lean meats, poultry, and fish<br>1 oz lean meat, poultry, or fish<br>1 egg | ≤6 oz/day | ≤5 oz/day | Lean cuts of beef (sirloin tip, round steak, arm roast), lean cuts of pork (center-cut ham, loin chops, tenderloin)<br>Ground beef that is at least "90% lean"<br>Skinless poultry (chicken breast and turkey cutlets are the leanest poultry choices)<br>Fish and seafood that are not fried<br>Limit egg yolks to 2/week; egg whites or egg substitutes as desired |
| Nuts, seeds, and legumes<br>¼ to ½ cup beans<br>½ oz seeds<br>1–2 tbsp peanut butter | 4–5 servings/week | Counted in vegetable servings | Any unsalted nuts and seeds<br>Any dried peas and beans (drain and rinse canned varieties) |
| Fats and oils<br>1 tsp soft margarine<br>1 tsp oil | 2–3 servings/day | Amount varies with calories | Canola, olive, peanut, corn, soybean, and sunflower oils<br>Soft trans fat–free margarines in tubs of liquid form<br>Margarine with plant sterols/stanols added |
| Sweets and added sugars<br>1 tbsp sugar<br>1 tbsp jelly or jam<br>½ cup sorbet and ices | 5 or fewer servings/week | No recommendations | Sweets that are low in fat, such as low-fat ice cream, low-fat pudding, sherbet, ices, fruit bars, angel food cake, fig bars |

*Dietary Approaches to Stop Hypertension. Available at http://www.nhlbi.nih.gov/health/public/heart/hbp/dash.

†Therapeutic Lifestyle Changes (TLC). Available at http://www.nhlbi.nih.gov/cgi-bin/chd/step2intro.cgi

## The DASH Diet

Dietary approaches to stop hypertension (DASH) was a multicenter feeding study funded by the National Heart, Lung and Blood Institute that set out to test if eating whole "real" foods rather than individual nutrients would lower blood pressure as a result of some combination of nutrients, interactions among individual nutrients, or other food factors. The results clearly showed that eating a diet rich in fruit, vegetables, low-fat dairy products, and nuts and legumes (a high intake of potassium, magnesium, calcium, protein, and fiber) with reduced amounts of fat, red meat, sweets, and sugar-sweetened beverages (a low intake of saturated fat, cholesterol, total fat, and extra sugars) significantly lowers both systolic and diastolic blood pressures as well as cholesterol (USDHHS, NIH, NHLBI, 2006). Table 20.3 shows a DASH eating plan for a 2000-calorie diet.

A second study, DASH-sodium, was designed to test if limiting sodium on a DASH diet would yield even better results. The results showed that

- Lowering sodium with either the control diet or DASH diet lowers blood pressure; the lower the sodium intake, the lower the blood pressure.
- At each sodium level, blood pressure was lower on the DASH diet than on the control diet.
- The greatest reduction in blood pressure occurred at 1500 mg of sodium.
- The greatest blood pressure reductions occurred in blacks; middle aged and older people; and people with hypertension, diabetes, or chronic kidney disease.

Although 1500 mg sodium may be an optimal intake for blood pressure control and is the AI set by the Institute of Medicine (IOM, 2004), it is not easily achieved, given our grab-and-go style of eating. Approximately 77% of sodium in the typical American diet comes from processed foods (Box 20.1). Tips for lowering sodium intake while eating out appear in Box 20.2. The DASH diet recommends that sodium intake initially be lowered to 2300 mg and gradually decreased to 1500 mg for maximum benefit. Table 20.4 shows a DASH diet menu at two different sodium levels.

## Weight Loss

Observational and clinical studies consistently show that weight is directly related to blood pressure and weight loss lowers blood pressure, even if healthy weight is not attained (Appel et al., 2006). The greater the weight loss, the greater the reduction in blood pressure in both hypertensive and nonhypertensive people (Stevens et al., 2001). Modest weight loss, with or without sodium restriction, can prevent hypertension by approximately 20% in overweight people who have prehypertension (The Trials of Hypertension Prevention Collaborative Research Group, 1997). Achieving a healthy weight (BMI <25) is an effective intervention to prevent and treat hypertension (Appel et al., 2006). Preventing weight gain is critical in people of normal weight. Although only a 2000-calorie DASH eating plan is shown, the DASH diet can be achieved at any calorie level.

## Potassium

As potassium intake increases, blood pressure decreases in hypertensive and nonhypertensive people (Appel, 2006). The effect is greater in blacks than in whites (Whelton et al., 1997). The impact potassium has on blood pressure depends on sodium intake: potassium is more effective in lowering blood pressure when sodium intake is high, and conversely, a high

| BOX 20.1 | THE EFFECT OF FOOD PROCESSING ON SODIUM CONTENT | |
|---|---|---|
| **Food Groups** | | **Sodium (mg)** |
| **Whole and other grains and grain products*** | | |
| Cooked cereal, rice, pasta, unsalted, ½ cup | | 0–5 |
| Ready-to-eat cereal, 1 cup | | 0–360 |
| Bread, 1 slice | | 110–175 |
| **Vegetables** | | |
| Fresh or frozen, cooked without salt, ½ cup | | 1–70 |
| Canned or frozen with sauce, ½ cup | | 140–460 |
| Tomato juice, canned, ½ cup | | 330 |
| **Fruit** | | |
| Fresh, frozen, canned, ½ cup | | 0–5 |
| **Low-fat or fat-free milk and milk products** | | |
| Milk, 1 cup | | 107 |
| Yogurt, 1 cup | | 175 |
| Natural cheeses, 1½ oz | | 110–450 |
| Process cheeses, 2 oz | | 600 |
| **Nuts, seeds, and legumes** | | |
| Peanuts, salted, ⅓ cup | | 120 |
| Peanuts, unsalted, ⅓ cup | | 0–5 |
| Beans, cooked from dried or frozen, without salt, ½ cup | | 0–5 |
| Beans, canned, ½ cup | | 400 |
| **Lean meats, fish, and poultry** | | |
| Fresh meat, fish, poultry, 3 oz | | 30–90 |
| Tuna canned, water pack, no salt added, 3 oz | | 35–45 |
| Tuna canned, water pack, 3 oz | | 230–350 |
| Ham, lean, roasted, 3 oz | | 1020 |

*Whole grains are recommended for most grain servings.

**Source:** USDHHS, NIH, NHLBI (2006). Your Guide to Lowering Your Blood Pressure with DASH. NIH Publication No. 06-4082.

| BOX 20.2 | TIPS FOR CONTROLLING SODIUM INTAKE WHILE EATING OUT |
|---|---|

- Request that food not be salted, if possible.
- Choose fruit juice instead of soup for an appetizer.
- Use oil and vinegar or fresh lemon instead of regular salad dressing.
- Choose foods that are grilled, baked, or roasted.
- Order plain meat and vegetables without gravy or sauce, or order them "on the side" and use sparingly.
- Choose plain baked potatoes and season sparingly with sour cream, butter, or pepper.
- Select fresh fruit for dessert. If the client is going to splurge, ice cream or sherbet is a better choice than pie, cake, cookies, or other desserts.
- Avoid fast food restaurant meals, which usually are high in sodium. If you have to go, order a child-sized meal.
- Order sandwiches without mayonnaise, sauces, or condiments; load with lettuce, tomato, and onion.

| TABLE 20.4 | 2000-Calorie Dash Menus at two Sodium Levels | | |
|---|---|---|---|
| **2400-mg Sodium Menu** | **Sodium (mg)** | **Substitutions to ↓ Sodium to 1500 mg** | **Sodium (mg)** |
| **Breakfast** | | The same as the 2400-mg sodium menu except: | |
| ¾ cup wheat flakes cereal | 199 | 2 cups puffed wheat cereal | 1 |
| 1 slice whole-wheat bread | 149 | | 149 |
| 1 medium banana | 1 | | 1 |
| 1 cup nonfat milk | 126 | | 126 |
| 1 cup orange juice | 5 | | 5 |
| 1 tsp soft margarine | 51 | 1 tsp soft margarine, unsalted | 1 |
| **Lunch** | | | |
| Beef sandwich: | | | |
| 2 oz ham, low sodium | 101 | 2 oz beef, eye of round | 35 |
| 1 tbsp Dijon mustard | 360 | 1 tbsp low-fat mayonnaise | 101 |
| 2 slices cheddar cheese, reduced fat | 260 | 2 slices Swiss cheese, natural | 109 |
| 1 sesame roll | 319 | | 319 |
| 1 large leaf romaine lettuce | 1 | | 1 |
| 2 slices tomato | 22 | | 22 |
| 1 cup low-fat, low-sodium potato salad | 12 | | 12 |
| 1 medium orange | 0 | | 0 |
| **Dinner** | | | |
| 3 oz cod with lemon juice | 90 | | 90 |
| ½ cup brown rice | 5 | | 5 |
| ½ c cooked spinach | 88 | | 88 |
| 1 small corn bread muffin | 363 | 1 small dinner roll | 146 |
| 1 tsp soft margarine | 51 | 1 tsp soft margarine, unsalted | 1 |
| **Snacks** | | | |
| 1 cup fruit yogurt, fat free, no added sugar | 107 | | 107 |
| ¼ cup dried fruit | 6 | | 6 |
| 2 large graham cracker rectangles | 156 | | 156 |
| 1 tbsp peanut butter, reduced fat | 101 | 1 tbsp peanut butter, unsalted | 3 |
| **Total sodium (mg)** | **2228** | | **1539** |

sodium intake raises blood pressure more when potassium intake is low (Appel et al., 2006). It is recommended that people consume 4.7 g potassium/day, the AI set by the IOM (IOM, 2004). This amount can be obtained by following the DASH guidelines of 4 to 5 servings/day of both fruits and vegetables, eating whole grains, and 4 to 5 servings/ week of nuts, seeds, and legumes.

**QUICK BITE**

**Selected sources of potassium**

| | *Potassium (mg)* | | *Potassium (mg)* |
|---|---|---|---|
| 1 medium potato | 926 | ½ cup cooked lentils | 370 |
| 1 medium sweet potato | 540 | ⅓ cup roasted almonds | 310 |
| ½ cup cooked soybeans | 440 | ½ cup cooked spinach | 290 |
| 1 medium banana | 420 | ½ cup zucchini | 280 |
| ¼ cup apricots | 380 | 1 medium orange | 237 |

***Source:*** USDHHS, NIH, NHLBI. (2006). *Your guide to lowering your blood pressure with DASH.* Available at www.nhlbi.nih.gov/health/public/heart/hbp/dash/new_dash.pdf. Accessed on 7/16/08.

## Alcohol

Observational studies and clinical trials show a direct dose-dependent relationship between alcohol and blood pressure, especially when alcohol intake is more than 2 drinks/day (Xin et al., 2001). If people chose to drink, alcohol intake should be limited to 2 drinks or less per day for men and 1 drink or less per day for women (Appel et al., 2006).

## ▶ ATHEROSCLEROSIS

**Atherosclerosis:** the formation of plaques along the smooth inner walls of arteries, which results in progressive narrowing and diminished blood flow to the tissue they supply.

**Coronary Heart Disease:** damage to the heart resulting from inadequate supply of blood to the heart.

**Plaque:** deposits of fatty material, cholesterol, calcium, and other blood components that are covered with connective tissue and embedded in the artery wall.

**Atherosclerosis**, or "hardening of the arteries," is the underlying cause of the most common CVDs such as **coronary heart disease**, ischemic stroke, and peripheral arterial disease. It is a progressive process that begins in childhood or adolescence and may continue for decades before symptoms occur.

Initially, a microscopic but chronic injury to the artery wall—such as from smoking, hypertension, or hyperglycemia—causes an immune response that attracts monocytes and platelets to the injured area. These cells trap low-density lipoprotein (LDL) cholesterol and grow to become fatty streaks (Fig. 20.2). Over time, deposits of smooth muscle cells, connective tissue cells, calcium, and cholesterol cause the fatty streak to enlarge and harden into **plaque**. Narrowing inside the artery lumen restricts blood flow to the surrounding tissue. Figure 20.3 illustrates the relationship between hypertension and atherosclerosis.

Complications of atherosclerosis depend on the size, stability, and location of the plaque. Plaques can grow large enough to completely block an artery. More often, complications are from an unstable plaque rupturing, which triggers the formation of a blood clot (thrombus) that may break away (embolus) and travel to a smaller artery where it can cause a myocardial infarction (coronary arteries) or stroke (brain). Diet has a significant effect on the progression of atherosclerosis and CVD (Jung et al., 2008).

## ▶ CORONARY HEART DISEASE

Coronary heart disease is usually caused by atherosclerosis in the large and medium-sized coronary arteries. Most plaques are unstable; blood clots that form after these plaques rupture are responsible for causing ischemia and tissue damage. Most heart attacks occur in people whose coronary arteries are less than 50% blocked (Libby, 2000).

Numerous risk factors have been identified as the cause of CHD. Genetics, gender, and advancing age are risk factors that cannot be modified; major modifiable risk factors are listed in Box 20.3. Hu and Willet estimate that 74% of coronary "events" among nonsmokers might have been prevented with a heart healthy diet, maintaining a healthy body weight, exercising regularly, and consuming a moderate amount of alcohol (Hu & Willet, 2002). Prospective cohort studies show that approximately 90% of people with CHD have at least one of the following major risk factors: high blood cholesterol levels (or are taking medication for it), hypertension (or are taking medication for it), current cigarette smoking, and diabetes (AHA, 2008). High blood cholesterol levels, cigarette smoking, and metabolic syndrome (MetS) are discussed next.

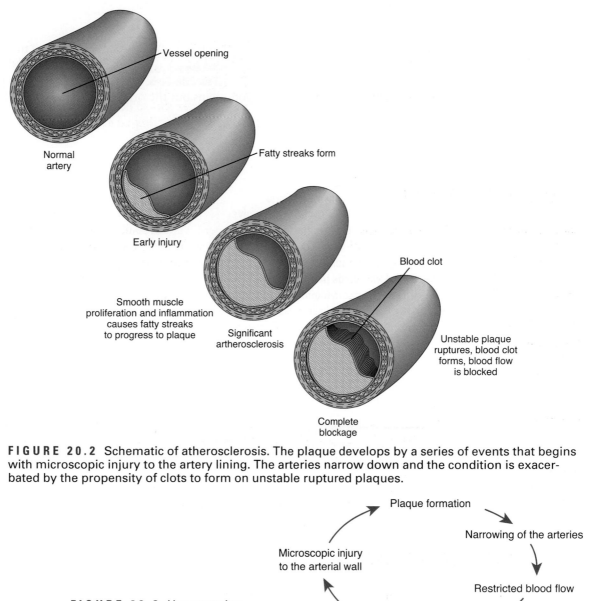

**FIGURE 20.2** Schematic of atherosclerosis. The plaque develops by a series of events that begins with microscopic injury to the artery lining. The arteries narrow down and the condition is exacerbated by the propensity of clots to form on unstable ruptured plaques.

**FIGURE 20.3** Hypertension and atherosclerosis (plaque formation) are intertwined.

Plaque formation

Narrowing of the arteries

Restricted blood flow

Increased blood pressure

Microscopic injury to the arterial wall

---

**BOX 20.3**    **MAJOR MODIFIABLE RISK FACTORS FOR CHD**

- High blood LDL cholesterol
- Low blood HDL cholesterol
- High blood pressure
- Obesity, especially abdominal obesity
- Physical inactivity

- Cigarette smoking
- An atherogenic (meaning likely to cause atherosclerosis) diet, namely, a diet high in saturated fat, trans fat, and cholesterol and low in vegetables, fruits, and whole grains.

*Source:* Expert Panel on Detection, Evaluation, and Treatment of High Blood Cholesterol in Adults (Adult Treatment panel III). (2001). *Third report of the National Cholesterol Education Program (NCD)* (NIH Publication No. 02-5215), Bethesda, MD: National Heart, Lung, Blood Institute, 2002.

## High Blood Cholesterol Levels

**Lipoprotein:** clusters of lipids (cholesterol, phospholipids, and triglycerides) encased in protein for transport through the blood and lymph.

Because cholesterol and other fats are insoluble in water, they are transported through watery blood in lipoprotein molecules. Of the four major types of **lipoproteins**, LDL and high-density lipoprotein (HDL) impact risk of heart disease. It is not the cholesterol, per se, that differs between these two types of lipoproteins but the origins of the cholesterol within.

### QUICK BITE

The four major types of lipoproteins

Chylomicrons: transport dietary fat (triglycerides) from the intestine to the rest of the body via the lymph system

Very low-density lipoproteins (VLDL): contain cholesterol and lipids made in the liver and triglycerides from chylomicrons; transport cholesterol and lipids to the tissues

Low-density lipoproteins (LDL): originate from VLDL that have lost much of their triglycerides so they are approximately 50% cholesterol; transport cholesterol to the tissues

High-density lipoproteins (HDL): transport cholesterol (and smaller quantities of fatty acids) from the tissues back to the liver for metabolism and excretion

Approximately half of each LDL molecule is composed of cholesterol that has been produced in the liver (Lichtenstein et al., 2006). As the level of LDL increases, so does the risk of developing CVD (Expert Panel on Detection, Evaluation, and Treatment of High Blood Cholesterol in Adults, 2001). Conversely, a large number of randomized controlled clinical trials have shown that lowering LDL reduces the risk for major CVD events (Grundy et al., 2004).

Diet and lifestyle changes to lower LDL are the focus of public health efforts to prevent CHD; they are also an integral component of treatment for managing CHD. LDL goals are determined by the number of major independent risk factors an individual has, with a goal of <70 for the highest risk group and a goal of <160 for the lowest (Table 20.5). Diet and lifestyle changes are appropriate for all people, whether the goal is preventing or treating heart disease and regardless of the LDL level. Cholesterol-lowering medications are added for high-risk people.

Cholesterol accounts for only about 25% of each HDL molecule, and it is cholesterol that has been "picked up" from tissues and is on the way back to the liver for breakdown and excretion. Levels of HDL, the "good cholesterol," are inversely correlated to CHD risk

---

**TABLE 20.5** **Classification of Cholesterol Levels**

|  | Total Cholesterol (mg/dL) | LDL cholesterol (mg/dL) | HDL cholesterol (mg/dL) |
|---|---|---|---|
| Desirable | <200 | <100* | ≥60 |
| Borderline risk | 200–239 | 130–159 | |
| High risk | ≥240 | 160–189† | |

*Less than 70 is desirable for people at very high risk.

†Greater than 190 is considered very high risk.

**Source:** National Cholesterol Education Program, National Heart, Lung, and Blood Institute, National Institutes of Health. (2002). *Third report of the expert panel on detection, evaluation, and treatment of high blood cholesterol in adults (Adult Treatment Panel III)* (NIH Publication No. 02-5215). Washington, DC: Government Printing Office.

Grundy, S. M., Cleeman, J. I., Merz, C. N., Brewer, H. B. Jr., Clark, L. T., Hunninghake, D. B., et al. (2004). Implications of recent clinical trials for the National Cholesterol Education Program Adult Treatment Panel III Guidelines. *Circulation, 111,* 227–239.

(Lichtenstein et al., 2006). However, it is not known if raising HDL reduces the risk of CHD, so there are no goal levels for increasing HDL. The best strategy for people with low HDL is to lower their LDL, lose weight if overweight, avoid smoking, and exercise—factors that lower CHD risk independent of their effect on HDL (Singh et al., 2007).

## Cigarette Smoking

Smoking harms almost every organ in the body (Surgeon General, 2004). It contributes to the development of atherosclerosis, increases heart rate, narrows arteries, increases blood pressure, lowers HDL, and promotes clot formation. On average, male smokers die 13.2 years earlier than male nonsmokers and female smokers die 14.5 years earlier than female nonsmokers (Surgeon General, 2004). According to the CDC's Health Effects of Cigarette Smoking Fact Sheet (2008):

- People who smoke have a 2 to 4 times greater risk of CHD than nonsmokers. Smoking low-tar or low-nicotine does not appear to reduce the risk for CHD.
- People who smoke have approximately double the risk of stroke as nonsmokers. The risk of stroke steadily decreases after smoking cessation; former smokers have the same stroke risk as nonsmokers after 5 to 15 years (Surgeon General, 2004).
- People who smoke are 10 times more likely to develop peripheral arterial disease than nonsmokers.
- Smoking causes abdominal aneurysm (USDHHS, CDC, National Center for Chronic Disease Prevention and Health Promotion, Office on Smoking and Health, 2004).

## Metabolic Syndrome

MetS is a cluster of metabolic abnormalities that appear to promote a relatively high long-term risk for both atherosclerotic CVD and type 2 diabetes (Grundy et al., 2005). Diagnostic criteria appear in Table 20.6. The primary objective of controlling MetS is to reduce the risk

| TABLE 20.6 | Diagnostic Criteria for Metabolic Syndrome | |
|---|---|---|
| **Risk Factor** | **Defining Level** | |

| | |
|---|---|
| Metabolic syndrome is confirmed by the presence of three of the following five risks: | |
| 1. Abdominal obesity* | |
|    Men | >40 in. waist |
|    Women | >35 in. waist |
| 2. Elevated triglycerides | ≥150 mg/dL |
| 3. Low HDL | |
|    Men | <40 mg/dL in men |
|    Women | <50 mg/dL in women |
| 4. Elevated blood pressure | ≥130 mmHg systolic blood pressure |
| | or |
| | ≥85 mmHg diastolic blood pressure |
| | or |
| | Drug treatment for hypertension |
| 5. Elevated fasting glucose | ≥100 mg/dL |

*Some white, black, and Hispanic American adults may benefit from lifestyle changes to reduce waist circumference, due to strong genetic contribution to insulin resistance. Because Asian Americans appear to be at risk with smaller waist sizes, 35 in. in Asian men and 31 in. in Asian women are appropriate cut points.

***Source:*** Grundy, S. M., Cleeman, J. I., Daniels, S. R., Donato, K. A., Eckel, R. H., Franklin, B. A., et al. (2005). *Diagnosis and management of the metabolic syndrome.* An American Heart Association/National Heart, Lung, and Blood Institute scientific statement. Executive summary. Available at http://www.circulationaha.org. Accessed on 6/19/08.

for atherosclerotic CVD (Grundy et al., 2005). Goals include smoking cessation, losing weight, and controlling blood pressure and glucose levels.

# ▶ HEART HEALTHY DIET AND LIFESTYLE

A heart healthy diet is a balanced, varied, and nutritionally adequate eating plan intended to help people achieve and maintain healthy weight, normal blood lipid levels, blood glucose control, and normal blood pressure. It is part of a healthy lifestyle that includes regular physical activity and the avoidance of tobacco products. With few exceptions, the recommendations to lower the risk of CHD are the same as the ones made to lower the blood pressure (Table 20.2).

## Calories, Activity, and Weight

Attaining and maintaining healthy weight to reduce the risk of CVD is an appropriate goal throughout the lifecycle in the general population (Lichtenstein et al., 2006). Excess body weight increases the risk of CHD, heart failure (HF), stroke, and cardiac arrhythmias by raising LDL and blood glucose levels; increasing blood pressure; and lowering HDL levels. A decrease in calorie intake and an increase in physical activity are recommended to promote weight loss. A physically active lifestyle with minimal sedentary activities (e.g., TV watching, playing computer games) is appropriate for all people, regardless of their weight status.

## Fruits and Vegetables

Diets rich in fruits and vegetables have been shown to lower blood pressure and improve other CVD risk factors in short-term, randomized trials (Obarzanek et al., 2001). In long-term observational studies, people who have a high intake of fruits and vegetables are at lower risk of developing CVD, especially stroke (Hung et al., 2004). It is not known if they reduce the risk of CVD because of the nutrients and substances they provide or because they displace other foods that are not as beneficial (Lichtenstein et al., 2006). A variety of fruits and vegetables are recommended. Preparation methods should preserve the fiber and nutrient content without adding saturated fat, trans fat, sugar, or salt.

## Whole Grains

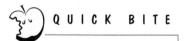 **Q U I C K   B I T E**

**Sources of soluble fibers**
Barley
Dried peas and beans
Flax seed
Fruit
Oats

Diets high in whole-grain products are associated with decreased risk of CVD (Hu & Willet, 2002; Jensen et al., 2004). Soluble fibers modestly lower LDL levels beyond the effects of a low saturated fat, low trans fat, low cholesterol diet (Brown et al, 1999). Insoluble fiber is also associated with decreased risk of CVD (Lichtenstein et al., 2006). Consistent with the Dietary Guidelines for Americans and MyPyramid, the AHA recommends at least half of grain choices be whole grains.

**EPA:** eicosapentaenoic acid.

**DHA:** docosahexaenoic acid.

## Fatty Fish

Increased intake of omega-3 fatty acids, namely, **EPA** and **DHA**, the polyunsaturated fatty acids found in fish oils, reduces the risk of CVD, including myocardial infarction, cardiac arrhythmias,

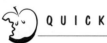

## QUICK BITE

**"Fatty" fish is a relative term**

| Fatty fish: | Fat (g) per ounce |
|---|---|
| Atlantic herring | 3.5 |
| Atlantic salmon | 3 |
| Rainbow trout | 2 |
| Swordfish | 1.3 |
| Fatty meats: | |
| Fresh pork spareribs | 8.7 |
| Lamb (ribs) | 8.3 |
| Beef ribs | 8.3 |
| Beef and pork bologna | 7 |

*Source: USDA National Nutrient Database for Standard Reference, Release 20.* Available at www.nal.usda.gov/fnic/foodcomp. Accessed on 7/25/08.

**ALA:** alpha-linolenic acid.

sudden cardiac death, atherosclerosis, and hypertension (Jung et al., 2008). Although it is not known exactly how omega-3 fatty acids help prevent CVD, it may be through a combination of factors that include preventing arrhythmias, lowering triglycerides, lowering blood pressure, decreasing platelet aggregation, and decreasing inflammation. The American Heart Association recommends 2 servings (~8 ounces) of fatty fish per week, prepared in ways that do not add saturated or trans fats.

ALA is an omega-3 fatty acid found in flaxseed, canola, soybeans, and walnuts. Only very small quantities are converted to EPA and DHA in the body. Although some studies show that ALA may also lower CVD risk, there is not enough evidence to suggest that it can be used as a replacement for seafood to prevent CHD or sudden cardiac death (Mozaffarian, 2008).

## Saturated Fat

## QUICK BITE

**Sources of monounsaturated and polyunsaturated fats**

Monounsaturated fats:
  Olive oil
  Canola oil
  Peanut oil
Polyunsaturated fats:
  Safflower oil
  Sunflower oil
  Corn oil
  Soybean oil

Saturated fat increases LDL and total cholesterol levels, the ratio of LDL to HDL cholesterol, and the risk for CHD (Mesnick et al., 2003; Oh et al., 2005). The majority of saturated fat in the typical American diet comes from meat and dairy products. Coconut oil and palm oil are high in saturated fat, but their overall contribution to the diet is relatively small. Choosing lean meats and trimming away visible fat lower saturated fat intake. Skinless chicken and fish are frequently used in place of red meats. Because even lean meats, poultry, and fish provide saturated fat and cholesterol, portion sizes are limited to 6 ounces or less per day. Dry peas and beans and tofu are recommended as substitutes for animal proteins. Low- or nonfat milk, cheese, and yogurt are used in place of full-fat varieties. Butter is replaced with trans fat–free margarine.

Monounsaturated and polyunsaturated fats are inversely related to CHD (Pietinen et al., 1997), but optimal intake level of each is currently unknown and actively debated (Lichtenstein, 2006). The American Heart Association recommends total fat provide 25% to 35% of total calories, a range compatible with recommendations from the Institute of Medicine (IOM, 2005) and National Cholesterol Education Program (NCEP, 2001).

## Trans Fat

Like saturated fats, trans fats increase LDL and total cholesterol levels, the ratio of LDL to HDL cholesterol, and the risk of CHD (Mesnick et al., 2003), but the magnitude may be greater (Merchang et al., 2008). Trans fats also increase inflammation (Mozaffarian et al., 2006). Man-made trans fats are found in partially hydrogenated fats (e.g., stick margarine, shortening) used to make commercially fried and baked products. Mandatory trans fat labeling, which began in January 2006, enables consumers to identify and limit their intake of trans fats. The AHA recommends trans fat intake be less than 1% of total calories, and the Institute of Medicine recommends trans fat intake be as low as possible in the context of a nutritionally adequate diet (IOM, 2005). That means using "trans fat free" margarines or oils in place of stick margarine and avoiding commercially prepared products containing partially hydrogenated fat such as baked products, processed foods, and shortenings.

## Cholesterol

Dietary cholesterol raises LDL levels, especially in people who are lean (Katan, 2005). Cholesterol is found only in foods originating from animals, such as meat, diary products, and eggs. Efforts made to reduce saturated fat, namely, replacing animal fats with vegetable fats; limiting portion sizes of meat and using only lean varieties; eating occasional meatless meals; and using low-fat or nonfat milk and dairy products also lower cholesterol intake.

## Added Sugars

The purpose of limiting the intake of beverages and foods with added sugars is to lower calorie intake and help ensure nutritional adequacy. Food and beverages high in added sugars tend to provide calories with few nutrients.

## Sodium

As previously discussed, as the intake of salt increases, so does blood pressure; high blood pressure is a major risk factor for CVD. The AHA acknowledges that an achievable goal for reducing sodium intake may be 2300 mg, not 1500 mg that may be the upper level of ideal intake (Lichtenstein, 2006). Mean sodium intake of Americans aged 19 and older is 3964 mg in men and 2853 mg in women (Moshfegh et al., 2005).

## Alcohol

**Moderate Alcohol Consumption:** 2 drinks/day for men; 1 drink or less/day for women.

### QUICK BITE

**Sodium content of selected foods**

| | Sodium (mg) |
|---|---|
| 1 packet dry onion soup mix | 3132 |
| 1 tsp salt | 2325 |
| 1 six-inch fast food sub | 1651 |
| 1 fast food single cheeseburger with condiments and bacon | 1314 |
| 1 large fast food taco | 1233 |
| 2 fast food pancakes with syrup | 1104 |
| 1 cup canned macaroni and cheese | 1061 |
| 1 fast food beef chimichanga | 910 |

*Source:* USDA National Nutrient Database for Stand Reference, Release 20. Available at www.nal.usda.gov/fnic/foodcomp. Accessed on 7/25/08.

**Moderate alcohol consumption** from any source—beer, wine, or distilled liquor—is associated with a reduced risk of CVD (Lichtenstein et al., 2006), possibly because alcohol raises HDL, reduces platelet aggregation, and reduces inflammation (Merchang et al., 2008). Despite its potential cardiac benefits, health professionals do not encourage nondrinkers to drink as a means of reducing their risk of CVD. Alcohol can be addictive, and high intakes are associated with high triglyceride (TG) levels, hypertension, liver damage, physical abuse, vehicular and work accidents, and increased risk of breast cancer (Lichtenstein, 2006). People who do drink should do so in moderation.

| BOX 20.4 | **UNPROVEN STRATEGIES TO LOWER CVD RISK** |
| --- | --- |

**Antioxidant Supplements**

• Although observational studies indicate that a high intake of antioxidant vitamins from food and supplements lowers CVD risk, clinical trials using antioxidant supplements have not confirmed any benefit and some have shown harm.

• Food sources of antioxidant vitamins are recommended from a variety of fruits, vegetables, whole grains, and vegetable oils

**Soy Protein**

• Studies have not confirmed earlier reports that soy protein lowers LDL and CVD risk factors.

• Soy protein used in place of high-fat dairy products may have an indirect effect on CVD by replacing saturated fat and cholesterol

**Folate and Other B Vitamins**

• Folate, vitamin $B_6$, and vitamin $B_{12}$ lower homocysteine levels; in observational studies, high homocysteine levels increase the risk for CVD. Trials of homocysteine-lowering vitamins have been disappointing.

• There is insufficient evidence to recommend folate and other B vitamin supplements for CVD risk reduction.

**Phytochemicals**

• Although phytochemicals may lower the risk of CVD, not enough is known about sources and actions of phytochemicals to recommend supplements. A variety of plant foods is the best way to obtain phytochemicals.

*Source:* Lichtenstein, A. H., Appel, L. J., Brands, M., Carnethon, M., Daniels, S., Franch, H. A., et al. (2006). *Diet and lifestyle recommendations revision 2006.* A scientific statement from the American Heart Association Nutrition Committee. *Circulation, 114*, 82–96.

## Other Dietary Components that Influence CVD Risk

Fish oil supplements and plant sterols/stanols are additional options that may be used in the treatment of heart disease. Unproven strategies to lower the risk of CVD are summarized in Box 20.4.

## Fish Oil Supplements

For people who do not have CVD, the AHA recommends two servings of fatty fish per week; approximately 1 g of EPA + DHA per day is recommended for people with documented CHD, either through fish or supplements, upon the physician's approval (Lichtenstein et al., 2006).

Fish is not a staple menu item for many Americans; for them, fish oil supplements may be a viable alternative. Because the decrease in CHD death and sudden cardiac death associated with eating fish are related to the omega-3 fatty acid content and not other components in the fish, any source of EPA and DHA, including supplements, will likely provide similar benefits (Mozaffarian, 2008). In most cases, 1 capsule per day of a 1 g fish oil supplement contains 200 to 800 mg of total omega-3, enough to meet the recommendations of approximately 1500 to 2000 mg/week to prevent CHD.

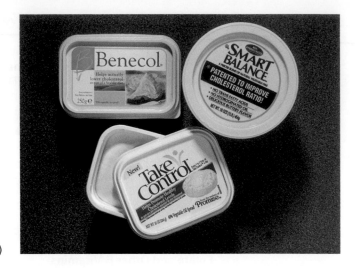

**FIGURE 20.4** Margarine-based products marketed to lower cholesterol. (***Source:*** Photo by Keith Weller, USDA, Agricultural Research Service.)

## Plant Stanols/Sterols

**Plant Stanols/Sterols:** compounds derived from soybeans and pine-tree oils; plant sterols are plant stanols that have been commercially hydrogenated to be used as a food additive. They reduce intestinal absorption of cholesterol from food and bile.

For people with high LDL levels, **plant stanols/sterols** can be used as a therapeutic option to help lower LDL levels by up to 15% (Grundy, 2005). Maximum benefits occur when intake is approximately 2 g/day and a daily intake is necessary to achieve sustained results. Sterol-fortified margarines were the first products available (Fig. 20.4). More newly added sources include orange juice, granola bars, cheese, and chocolates.

## Putting Recommendations into Practice

Two examples of eating plans that can be used to implement a heart healthy diet are the DASH-sodium diet and the therapeutic lifestyle changes (TLC) diet put forth by the National Cholesterol Education Program's Adult Treatment Panel (ATP III). Table 20.3

---

| BOX 20.5 | **TIPS FOR EATING A HEART HEALTHY DIET** |
|---|---|

- Limit lean meats, poultry, and fish to 5 to 6 oz/day. Use the "plate method" to get the proportion right: cover ≥⅔ of the plate with plant foods (vegetables, fruit, whole grains, dried peas, and beans) and ≤⅓ with fish, poultry, meat, or low-fat dairy products.
- Trim away visible fat from meats before cooking; drain ground beef after browning.
- Bake, broil, grill, or poach meat, poultry, or fish instead of frying.
- Drain off fat that appears during cooking.
- Skip high-fat sauces and gravies.
- Eat occasional meatless meals that feature dried peas and beans, tofu, or vegetables.
- Prepare foods from "scratch" instead of purchasing convenience foods and mixes, which tend to be high in saturated fat.
- Use recommended oils to season cooked vegetables and in the preparation of salad dressings, marinades, and barbecue sauces.
- Make fat-free soup stock by preparing the stock a day ahead and refrigerating it overnight. The fat will harden and can be removed easily from the surface. Also use this method to make fat-free gravies thickened with cornstarch.
- Use herbs and spices, lemon juice, and flavored vinegars to flavor foods without fat.
- Use these low-fat snack ideas: low-fat yogurt, fresh fruits and vegetables, dried fruit, unbuttered popcorn, unsalted pretzels, bread sticks, melba toast, frozen juice bars, low-fat crackers.

illustrates each of these plans for a 2000-calorie diet with representative foods. Each plan can be adjusted to provide more or fewer calories, depending on the client's requirements. Tips for implementing a heart healthy diet are listed in Box 20.5.

A "Mediterranean" type diet is another eating style option that comes close to the American Heart Association guidelines for a "heart healthy" diet (Fig. 20.5). It is generally a plant-based diet rich in unrefined grains, fruit, and vegetables. Olive oil is used liberally. Red meats constitute the apex of the horizontal pyramid, with only 4 servings per month recommended. The diet is higher in fat than the AHA recommendations, but more than half the fat calories come from heart healthy monounsaturated fat (AHA, 2007). The incidence of heart disease and death rate are lower in Mediterranean countries than in the United States, but other lifestyle factors in addition to diet may also be credited.

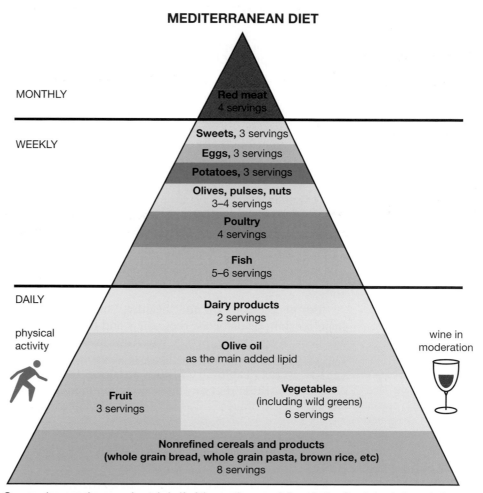

**MEDITERRANEAN DIET**

MONTHLY — Red meat, 4 servings

WEEKLY — Sweets, 3 servings; Eggs, 3 servings; Potatoes, 3 servings; Olives, pulses, nuts 3–4 servings; Poultry 4 servings; Fish 5–6 servings

DAILY — Dairy products 2 servings; Olive oil as the main added lipid; Fruit 3 servings; Vegetables (including wild greens) 6 servings; Nonrefined cereals and products (whole grain bread, whole grain pasta, brown rice, etc) 8 servings

physical activity

wine in moderation

One serving equals approximately half of the portions as defined in the Greek market regulations (portions served in restaurants)

Also remember to:
• drink plenty of water
• avoid salt and replace it with herbs (e.g., oregano, basil, thyme, etc.)

**FIGURE 20.5**
Mediterranean diet pyramid. (***Source:*** Supreme Scientific Health Council, Hellenic Ministry of Health.)

| TABLE 20.7 | Diet for Other Cardiac Conditions | |
| --- | --- | --- |
| Condition | Other Nutrition Recommendations in Addition to a Heart Healthy Diet with Exercise and Weight Loss As Appropriate | Rationale |
| Hypertriglyceridemia | A slightly lower percentage of calories from carbohydrate, slightly higher percentage of calories from unsaturated fat<br>2–4 g of supplemental fish oil may be used<br>Alcohol is limited or eliminated | Hypertriglyceridemia, independent of LDL level, may increase the risk heart disease; it is a characteristic of metabolic syndrome |
| | If triglycerides are >500 mg/dL, a very low-fat diet is used to prevent pancreatitis | Very high triglyceride levels (>1000 mg/dL) increase the risk of pancreatitis |
| Status post coronary artery bypass graft | High protein, adequate calories | The need for healing increases protein and calorie requirements. The goal of weight loss may be postponed until healing is complete |
| Cerebrovascular accident | A National Dysphagia Diet, as appropriate (Chapter 17) | Texture modification or enteral feeding may be necessary depending on the patient's ability to chew and swallow |

"Heart healthy diet" is less than 7% saturated fat, trans fat intake as low as possible, less than 200 mg cholesterol, 2 servings of fatty fish/week, high fiber, possibly the use of plant sterols. Sodium intake should range from 1500 to 2300 mg/day.

**Source:** American Dietetic Association. (2008). *Nutrition care manual.* Available at http://www.nutritioncaremanual.org. Accessed on 7/21/08.

## Is a "Heart Healthy" Diet and Lifestyle for Everyone?

For "healthy" people, the DASH-sodium diet and TLC diet may help prevent heart disease, stroke, type 2 diabetes, and obesity if calories are appropriate. These diets are consistent with the Dietary Guidelines for Americans and MyPyramid eating plans. There are few situations in which this "diet" and the recommendations to lose weight if overweight, and exercise more are inappropriate. Smoking cessation is *always* an appropriate lifestyle choice.

For people who are not "healthy," such as those who are being treated for CHD, hypertension, or diabetes, these diets and lifestyle changes are an integral part of management. Even among people who have had complications of CVD, such as a heart attack or stroke, these diet and lifestyle changes are recommended to prevent subsequent cardiac events (Table 20.7). With attention to cultural considerations, as appropriate (Box 20.6), these diet and lifestyle recommendations come close to being "one size fits all."

## ▶ HEART FAILURE

HF is a major and growing public health problem in the United States and is the most common Medicare diagnosis–related group (Hunt et al., 2005). It is a syndrome characterized by specific symptoms, namely, shortness of breath, fatigue, and edema. CHD and high blood pressure are prevalent causes; arrhythmias and valve disorders may also cause HF. Obesity, diabetes, MetS, and previous heart attack increase the risk for HF.

| BOX 20.6 | **CULTURAL CONSIDERATIONS** |

For all cultural groups, emphasize the positive aspects of their eating styles and suggest modifications to lower the fat and sodium content of traditional foods.

**African-American Tradition**

Traditional soul foods tend to be high in fat, cholesterol, and sodium. On the positive side, there is a heavy emphasis on vegetables and complex carbohydrates.

Changes in cooking techniques can improve fat, cholesterol, and sodium content, such as

- Using nonstick skillets sprayed with cooking spray when pan-frying eggs, fish, and vegetables
- Using small amounts of liquid smoke flavoring in place of bacon, salt pork, or ham
- Using more seasonings such as onion, garlic, and pepper, in place of some of the salt
- Substituting fat-free mayonnaise for regular mayonnaise in biscuits
- Using turkey ham or turkey sausage in place of bacon
- Using "lite" or sugar-free syrups
- Using egg substitutes or egg whites in pancakes and biscuits

**Mexican-American Tradition**

The traditional diet is primarily vegetarian with a heavy emphasis on fruits, vegetables, rice, and dried peas and beans. Processed foods are used infrequently.

Cooking techniques rely on frying and stewing with liberal amounts of oil or lard. An alternative is to sauté or stew with small amounts of canola or olive oil. High-fat meats and lard are commonly used. Using less meat, choosing lower-fat varieties, trimming visible fat, and substituting oil for lard are heart healthy alternatives.

**Chinese-American Tradition**

Traditional Chinese cooking relies heavily on vegetables and rice with plants providing the majority of calories. Meat is used more as a condiment than an entrée. Cooking techniques tend to preserve nutrients. Sauces add little fat.

Sodium intake is high related to heavy use of soy sauce, MSG, and salted pickles. Reduced sodium soy sauce is available, but it is still high in sodium. Because of the difficulty in eliminating the use of soy sauce, a more practical approach is to gradually use less.

**Native-American/Alaska-Native Traditions**

Widely diverse eating styles make useful generalizations difficult.

In general

- Encourage traditional cooking methods such as baking, roasting, boiling, and broiling
- Encourage the use of traditional meats such as fish, deer, and caribou
- Remove fat from canned meats
- Use vegetable oil for frying instead of lard or shortening

**Jewish Tradition**

Many traditional foods are high in sodium such as *kosher* meats (salt is used in the koshering process), herring, lox, pickles, canned chicken broth or soups, and delicatessen meats (e.g., corned beef, *pickled tongue*, pastrami).

*Pareve* (neutral) nondairy creamers are often used as a dairy substitute at meat meals but they are high in fat. Encourage light and fat-free versions.

Encourage methods to lower fat in traditional recipes such as

- Baking instead of frying potato pancakes
- Limiting the amount of schmaltz (chicken fat) used in cooking
- Using reduced-fat or fat-free cream cheese on bagels
- Using low-fat or nonfat cottage cheese, sour cream, and yogurt in kugels and blintzes

## Nutrition Therapy

For people at risk of HF, the goals of therapy are to control underlying risks. A DASH-sodium diet is appropriate for people with CHD or hypertension, although there is no direct evidence that controlling sodium intake prevents the development of HF (Hunt et al., 2005). Regular exercise and smoking cessation are encouraged; alcohol is discouraged.

For people with stage C heart failure, defined as structural heart disease with prior or current symptoms of HF, sodium is limited to 2 g of sodium/day or less (Box 20.7). Other diet modifications are made as appropriate, such as:

- A fluid restriction of 1.5 L/day for patients with hyponatremia.
- A low-calorie diet for patients who are overweight because losing weight decreases cardiac workload.
- Small frequent meals to limit gastric distention and pressure on the heart.
- Soft easy to chew foods for patient with fatigue.
- Increased potassium intake for patients who are taking thiazide (potassium-wasting) diuretics or digitalis.

---

| BOX 20.7 | **2000-mg SODIUM-RESTRICTED DIET** |
| --- | --- |

Although a 2000-mg sodium diet is considered "restricted," it is more than the Adequate Intake (AI) of 1500 mg, the level that may be optimal for preventing and treating hypertension. It is a restriction when compared to the typical American intake.

Sometimes sodium is more severely restricted, such as to 1000 mg; diets that are severely restricted in sodium are unpalatable, extremely difficult to follow, and likely to be inadequate in some nutrients. To promote compliance and allow greater flexibility, exchange lists featuring the sodium content of high- and low-sodium foods may be used.

### General Guidelines:
- Eliminate processed and prepared foods and beverages high in sodium; use fresh, frozen, and canned low-sodium products.
- Do not use salt in cooking or at the table.
- Read Nutrition Facts labels; most foods eaten should provide less than 300 mg sodium per serving. Foods that fall under these guidelines include:
  - Most breads; many ready-to-eat cereals, cooked cereals, pasta, rice, and other starches cooked without salt.
  - Fresh and frozen vegetables; low-sodium or sodium-free canned vegetables and soups.
  - Fresh and canned fruit.
  - Low-fat and nonfat milk and yogurt; small amounts of low-fat natural cheese.
  - Fresh and frozen meats; low-sodium canned tuna, dried peas and beans, eggs.
  - Baked goods made without baking soda, angel food cake.
  - Tub or liquid margarine; vegetable oils.

### Patient Teaching
Provide general information:

- Reducing sodium intake will help the body rid itself of excess fluid and help lower high blood pressure.
- Sodium appears in the diet in the form of salt and, to some degree, in almost all foods and beverages. Most unprocessed, unsalted foods are low in sodium; they account for approximately 12% of usual sodium intake.
- Approximately 77% of the sodium in a typical American diet comes from processed foods. Sodium-containing compounds are used extensively as preservatives (sodium propionate, sodium sulfite, and sodium benzoate), leavening agents (sodium bicarbonate, baking soda, and baking powder), and flavor enhancers (e.g., salt, monosodium glutamate) [MSG] and are found in foods that may not taste salty.

| BOX 20.7 | **2000-mg SODIUM-RESTRICTED DIET** (continued) |
|---|---|

- Salt substitutes replace sodium with potassium or other minerals. "Low-sodium" salt substitutes are not sodium free and may contain half as much sodium as regular table salt. Use neither type without a physician's approval.
- The preference for salt taste eventually will decrease.
- When an occasional food containing >300 mg/serving is eaten, balance it out with low-sodium foods the rest of the day.
- Try to make low-sodium choices while dining out (see Box 20.2).

Teach the client food preparation techniques to minimize sodium intake:

- Make foods from "scratch" whenever possible.
- Experiment with sodium-free seasonings such as herbs, spices, lemon juice, vinegar, and wine. Fresh ingredients are more flavorful than dried ones.
- Try a commercial "salt alternative" for sodium-free flavor enhancement.
- Consult a low-sodium cookbook.

Teach the client how to read labels:

- Salt, MSG, baking soda, and baking powder contain significant amounts of sodium. Other sodium compounds such as sodium nitrite, benzoate of soda, sodium saccharin, and sodium propionate add less sodium to the diet.
- "Sodium free," "low sodium," "very low sodium," and "reduced" or "less" sodium are reliable terms.
- A variety of low- and reduced-sodium products are available, such as bread and bread products, cereal, crackers, cakes, cookies, pastries, soups, bouillon, canned vegetables, tomato products, meats, entrées, processed meats, hard and soft cheeses, condiments, nuts and peanut butter, butter, margarine, salad dressings, and snack foods. The difference in taste between some low-sodium products and their high-sodium counterparts is barely noticeable; others taste flat and may need to have herbs or spices added.

Malnutrition among CHF patients, known as cardiac cachexia, may occur with poor nutritional intake and long-term use of medication. Nutritional deficiencies can have a severe impact on the heart. Patients with cardiac cachexia need a high-calorie, high-protein, high-nutrient diet while maintaining a low-sodium diet. Caloric and nutrient density is important to maximize intake. Often these patients do not tolerate enteral feedings because of access to the thoracic cavity and decreased blood flow to the gastrointestinal tract.

## NURSING PROCESS: *Heart Failure*

Mrs. Gigante is a 79-year-old widow admitted with stage C heart failure, with a long-standing history of hypertension and one previous myocardial infarction. She lives alone. She relies heavily on convenience foods such as canned and packaged soups, frozen dinners, canned pasta, and tuna fish sandwiches because she is too tired to cook. She appears frail with significant lower extremity edema.

### Assessment

| Medical-Psychosocial History | |
|---|---|
| | - Medical history and comorbidities including diabetes, hypertension, myocardial infarction, alcohol abuse, and other CHD risk factors |
| | - Use of medications that affect nutrition such as diuretics, antihypertensives, antidiabetics, and lipid-lowering medications; adherence to prescribed drug therapy |

*(nursing process continues on page 506)*

## NURSING PROCESS: *Heart Failure* (continued)

|  |  |
|---|---|
|  | • Complaints including activity intolerance, fatigue, and shortness of breath |
|  | • Observe behavior for restlessness, anxiety, or confusion |
|  | • Psychosocial and economic issues such as living situation, cooking facilities, financial status, education, and eligibility for the Meals on Wheels program |
|  | • Understanding of the relationship between sodium, fluid accumulation, and symptoms of CHF |
|  | • Motivation to change eating style |
| Anthropometric Assessment | • Height, weight; BMI |
|  | • Recent weight history, especially rapid weight gain |
| Biochemical and Physical Assessment | • Blood pressure |
|  | • Measure of edema |
|  | • Lab values related to comorbidities, such as total cholesterol, LDL, HDL, and triglycerides |
|  | • Serum osmolality, serum sodium, BUN/creatinine ratio, and hematocrit |
|  | • Intake and output |
|  | • Lung sounds for crackles |
|  | • Respirations for effort |
| Dietary Assessment | • How many meals and snacks do you usually eat? |
|  | • What is your usual 24-hour food intake like? |
|  | • What cooking methods do you use to prepare your food? |
|  | • How is your appetite? |
|  | • Do you feel full quickly after you start to eat? |
|  | • Have you ever been advised to follow a certain kind of diet in the past? If so, how did you change your eating habits? |
|  | • Do you watch the kind of fats you eat? |
|  | • Do you try to limit your intake of salt? |
|  | • How many glasses of fluid do you drink in a day? |
|  | • Do you have health impairments that impact your ability to shop, cook, or eat? |
|  | • Do you have any cultural, religious, or ethnic influences on your food preferences or eating habits? |
|  | • Do you take any vitamins, minerals, and nutritional supplements? If so, what are the reasons? |
|  | • Do you use alcohol or caffeine? |

### Diagnosis

| | |
|---|---|
| Possible Nursing Diagnoses | Excess fluid volume related to impaired excretion of sodium and water as evidenced by 3+ peripheral edema |

*(nursing process continues on page 507)*

## NURSING PROCESS: *Heart Failure* (continued)

| **Planning** | |
|---|---|
| Client Outcomes | The client will<br>• Attain and maintain normal fluid balance<br>• Consume a varied and nutritious diet with adequate calories to attain healthy body weight<br>• Limit sodium intake<br>• Explain how and why sodium is limited in her diet |

| **Nursing Interventions** | |
|---|---|
| Nutrition Therapy | • Provide a 2-g sodium diet as ordered<br>• Provide five to six small meals to limit gastric distention and pressure on the heart<br>• Monitor input and output for need for fluid restriction |
| Client Teaching | Instruct the client:<br>• On the roles of sodium, fluid, and medication, managing HF<br>• On the availability of the Meals on Wheels program. Explain that Meals on Wheels can provide her with the appropriate diet after discharge to ensure that she gets the proper foods even on days when she feels short of breath or too tired to cook (Notify the discharge planner that the client may be a candidate for Meals on Wheels.)<br>On eating plan essentials such as<br>• Eliminating the use of salt in cooking and at the table<br>• Using low-sodium canned foods when available<br>• Avoiding other high-sodium foods<br>• Limiting milk intake to 2 cups daily<br>• Increasing intake of high-potassium foods<br>• Avoiding alcohol<br>• Adhering to fluid restriction if appropriate<br>On behavioral matters including<br>• How to read labels to identify and avoid foods that provide >300 mg sodium/serving<br>• That a gradual reduction in sodium intake may be easier to comply with than an abrupt withdrawal of sodium. Because the preference for salt gradually diminishes when intake is limited, following a low-sodium diet tends to get easier with time<br>• Timing meals and snacks to avoid shortness of breath and fatigue<br>• Physical activity goals if applicable and appropriate |

| **Evaluation** | |
|---|---|
| Evaluate and Monitor | • Monitor weight daily for rapid weight gain<br>• Monitor edema and other signs and symptoms of fluid retention<br>• Tolerance to small meals<br>• Need for additional diet counseling |

## ▶ How Do You Respond?

**How long do I have to be on this diet for my heart?** The term "diet" commonly implies a short-term change in eating habits that deprives people of their favorite foods. People often "follow a diet" for as long as they can, "fall off" the diet, then dismiss it as impractical or unachievable. Encourage clients to gradually change their usual habits into a more heart healthy "eating style." A person cannot "fall off" an eating style. Ongoing group nutrition classes may help clients maintain motivation and commitment.

**My doctor put me on a pill to lower my cholesterol. Do I still need to change what I eat now that my cholesterol level is normal?** Cholesterol lowering medications like Lipitor, Zocor, Mevacor, and Pravachol are not meant to be used in place of healthy eating and other lifestyle modifications. Although these drugs are very powerful, their effectiveness can be undermined by a "bad" diet. Urge clients to commit to lifestyle changes to give their medication the greatest chance of success.

**Hypercholesterolemia:** generic term to describe high levels of cholesterol in the blood.

**I do everything right and still my LDL cholesterol is sky high. Why?** People with a genetic form of **hypercholesterolemia** generally have an LDL ≥190 mg/dL. For them, diet will not effectively lower LDL to acceptable levels. Still, diet, exercise, and weight loss are important—maybe even more important than for other people— because of the potential beneficial effects on other risks, such as blood pressure and insulin sensitivity.

## ▶ Case Study

Matt is 34 years old. His BMI is 28 and has steadily increased over the last few years when he accepted a position with his company that requires frequent travel. It is hard for him to exercise and he eats out the majority of time. He is a "steak and potatoes" kind of guy who wouldn't dream of eating lunch or dinner without meat as the centerpiece of the meal. At his most recent annual employee physical, Matt's total cholesterol was 245 mg/dL, his HDL was 50, fasting glucose was 92, and his blood pressure was 154/85. His father died of a heart attack at age 49. Matt feels doomed by genetics and is resistant to going on medication because of the potential side effects. He is willing to try to change his diet and lifestyle, but is skeptical it will help.

- What risks does Matt have for heart disease?
- Knowing that he is willing to change his diet and lifestyle, what additional information would you ask of Matt before devising a teaching plan?
- What diet recommendations would you prioritize in helping Matt initiate a heart healthy diet? What suggestions could you offer him to help him meet these recommendations?
- How would you respond to Matt's skepticism that diet and lifestyle factors will probably not lower his risk of heart disease?

1. Which statement indicates the patient understands the instruction about a heart healthy diet?
   a. "The most important thing about a heart healthy diet is to eat less cholesterol. No egg yolks for me."
   b. "I need to limit my intake of meat and make sure I make lean choices."
   c. "As long as I don't add salt to my food while cooking or at the table, I will be able to achieve a low-sodium diet."
   d. "Trans fats are found only in foods that come from animals."

2. The client asks if he can continue using butter on his heart healthy diet. Which of the following would be the nurse's best response?
   a. "No, butter does not fit into a heart healthy diet."
   b. "Butter is not limited in a heart healthy diet because most people only use small amounts."
   c. "You can use small amounts of butter if you are willing to compromise on other foods, such as eating meatless meals occasionally."
   d. "You can use small amounts of butter if you give up meat entirely."

3. When developing a teaching plan for a client on a DASH-sodium diet, which of the following foods would the nurse suggest to meet increase in the client's intake of potassium?
   a. Potatoes and sweet potatoes
   b. Rice and pasta
   c. Chicken and fish
   d. Canola and olive oils

4. The nurse knows her instructions for a heart healthy diet have been effective when the client verbalizes she should eat more
   a. Salmon and herring
   b. Tofu and soymilk
   c. Diet soda and diet desserts
   d. Italian bread and cornflakes

5. Which of the following recommendations would be most appropriate to limit trans fats?
   a. Avoid red meats
   b. Avoid egg yolks and shellfish
   c. Avoid salad dressings and mayonnaise
   d. Avoid commercially made sweets and stick margarines

6. A client asks why whole grains are so important for a heart healthy diet. Which of the following is the nurse's best response?
   a. "Whole grains are rich in B vitamins that help lower homocysteine levels which lowers the risk of heart disease."
   b. "Whole grains help raise the good cholesterol in your blood."
   c. "Whole grains are a better choice than refined grains because they are lower in sodium."
   d. "Whole grains help lower the bad cholesterol."

7. When teaching a client diagnosed with heart failure about her nutritional needs, which of the following types of diet should the nurse discuss?
   a. Low cholesterol
   b. Low fat
   c. Low sodium
   d. Low potassium

8. A rule-of-thumb guideline for helping clients read labels to lower their sodium intake recommends choosing mostly foods that provide less than
   a. 50 milligram/serving
   b. 100 milligram/serving
   c. 300 milligram/serving
   d. 500 milligram/serving

## KEY CONCEPTS

- Dietary factors play a prominent role in blood pressure regulation. The DASH-sodium diet effectively lowers blood pressure and cholesterol levels. It is low in sodium; rich in fruits, vegetables, whole grains, and nuts and dried peas; and limited in saturated fat, trans fat, cholesterol, and total fat.

- Other lifestyle factors that help control blood pressure include losing weight if overweight and using alcohol moderately, if at all.

- Atherosclerosis is a progressive disease that may begin in childhood or adolescence and continue for decades before symptoms develop. CHD is the most common athero-sclerotic CVD and the leading cause of death in the United States.

- The primary focus of preventing and managing CHD is to lower LDL. An individual's LDL goal is based on the presence of independent risk factors such as smoking, age, family history, low HDL level, and hypertension.

- Smoking greatly increases the risk of CHD, stroke, peripheral arterial disease, and aneurysm. Smoking cessation improves risk factors for CVD, such as increasing HDL and decreasing the risk of blood clots.

- MetS is a cluster of metabolic abnormalities that increase the risk of diabetes and heart disease. Treatment focuses on controlling risks for CVD, such as lowering blood glucose levels, controlling blood pressure, and losing weight.

- Lifestyle modifications recommended to lower total cholesterol and LDL include weight loss, increasing physical activity, smoking cessation, and a heart healthy diet.

- A heart healthy diet is rich in fruits and vegetables and whole grains. Two servings of fatty fish are recommended weekly.

- A heart healthy is limited in saturated fat, trans fat, and cholesterol. Limiting the meat to 5 to 6 oz/day, choosing only lean varieties, using low-fat or nonfat milk and dairy products, and using oils or soft tub margarines are strategies that lower the intake of unhealthy fats.

- The optimal intake of monounsaturated and polyunsaturated fats is not known. Total fat in a heart healthy diet is consistent with the Acceptable Macronutrient Distribution Range of 25% to 35% of total calories.

- Food and beverages high in added sugars should be avoided because they contribute empty calories that may promote excess weight.

- A heart healthy diet provides 2300 mg/day or less of sodium to prevent/treat hypertension, a major risk factor for CHD. An intake of 1500 mg may be ideal, but it is not likely to be achieved without major changes to the typical American eating pattern.

● Moderate alcohol consumption is considered heart healthy. Moderate is defined as less than or equal to 2 drinks/day for men and less than or equal to 1 drink/day for women.

● The American Heart Association does not endorse the use of fish oil supplements for healthy people but other experts assert that one 1 g capsule/day is a reasonable substitute for eating two servings of fatty fish/week.

● Foods fortified with plant sterols/stanols are a therapeutic option for lowering cholesterol, but they must be consumed every day to be effective.

● Changing eating patterns can be difficult. Gradual and sequential changes may improve the chance of long-term success.

● A heart healthy eating plan is appropriate for the general population over the age of 2 as well as for people who are being treated for CHD. It is relatively consistent with the Dietary Guidelines for Americans and the MyPyramid eating plans. A heart healthy diet is also recommended for prevention of subsequent cardiac events in people who have had coronary artery bypass graft surgery, a heart attack, or a stroke. A modified heart healthy diet is used for people with elevated triglycerides.

● A 2000-mg sodium restricted diet is often used to manage heart failure. It is not known if a low-sodium diet can prevent heart failure in high-risk people. A fluid restriction may be necessary for patients with hyponatremia.

## ANSWER KEY

1. **FALSE** The DASH-sodium diet *is* low in sodium, but it is also low in saturated fat, cholesterol, and total fat and high in fruits, vegetables, and foods high in fiber that provide nutrients that are thought to be protective against high blood pressure.

2. **FALSE** Approximately 77% of sodium in the typical American diet comes from sodium added to food during processing. Only 11% is added during cooking or eating, with the remaining 12% from sodium naturally found in foods.

3. **TRUE** Weight loss lowers high blood pressure, even if healthy weight is not achieved.

4. **FALSE** The primary focus of preventing and treating CHD is to lower LDL.

5. **FALSE** Total fat is not restricted in a heart healthy diet but particular kinds of fat are: saturated fat, trans fat, and cholesterol.

6. **TRUE** Diets high in fiber are linked to lower risk of CVD. Soluble fibers modestly lower LDL cholesterol. Insoluble fibers are also associated with lower CVD risk.

7. **FALSE** It is relatively certain that it is the omega-3 fatty acid content of fish, and not any other components, that is heart healthy.

8. **TRUE** Moderate alcohol intake is associated with a lowered risk of CVD. Because of other risks associated with alcohol, the AHA does not recommend that people who do not drink start consuming alcohol.

9. **TRUE** Plant sterols must be consumed daily for them to effectively lower blood cholesterol levels.

10. **FALSE** The diet and lifestyle recommendations issued by the American Heart Association are intended for the general public over the age of 2.

## WEBSITES

American Heart Association at **www.americanheart.org**
Heart and Stroke Foundation of Canada at **www.hsf.ca**
National Heart, Lung and Blood Institute at **www.nhlbi.nih.gov** to estimate your risk of heart disease, go to www.nhlbi.nih.gov/guidelines/cholesterol/index.htm and click on 10-year Risk Calculator—online version.

## REFERENCES

American Heart Association (AHA). (2007). *Mediterranean diet.* Available at www.americanheart .org/print_presenter.jhtml?identifier=4644%3EMediterranean. Accessed on 7/26/08.

American Heart Association (AHA). (2008). *Heart disease and stroke statistics—2008 update.* Available at www.americanheart.org/downloadable/heart/1200078608862HS_Stats% 202008.final.pdf. Accessed on 7/16/08.

Appel, L. J., Brands, M. W., Daniels, S. R., et al. (2006). Dietary approaches to prevent and treat hypertension. A scientific statement from the American Heart Association. *Hypertension, 47,* 296–308.

Brown, L., Rosner, B., Willett, W. W., et al. (1999). Cholesterol-lowering effects of dietary fiber: A meta-analysis. *The American Journal of Clinical Nutrition, 69,* 30–42.

CDC. (2008). *Smoking & tobacco use fact sheet. Health effects of cigarette smoking.* Available at www.cdc.gov/tobacco/Data_statistics/fact_sheets/health_effects/health_effects.htm. Accessed on 7/21/08.

Expert Panel on Detection, Evaluation, and Treatment of High Blood Cholesterol in Adults (Adult Treatment Panel III). (2001). *Third report of the National Cholesterol Education Program (NCD)* (NIH Publication No. 02-5215), Bethesda, MD: National Heart, Lung, Blood Institute, 2001.

Grundy, S. (2005). Stanol esters as a component of maximal dietary therapy in the National Cholesterol Education Program Adult Treatment Panel III report. *The American Journal of Cardiology, 96,* 47D–50D.

Grundy, S. M., Cleeman, J. I., Daniels, S. R., et al. (2005). *Diagnosis and management of the metabolic syndrome. An American Heart Association/National Heart, Lunch, and Blood Institute scientific statement. Executive summary.* Available at www.circulationaha.org. Accessed on 6/19/07.

Grundy, S. M., Cleeman, J. I., Merz, C. N., et al. (2004). Implications of recent clinical trials for the National Cholesterol Education Program Adult Treatment Panel III Guidelines. *Circulation, 110,* 227–239.

Hu, F., & Willett, W. (2002). Optimal diets for prevention of coronary heart disease. *The Journal of the American Medical Association, 288,* 2569–2578.

Hung, H. C., Josipura, K. J., Jiang, R., et al. (2004). Fruit and vegetable intake and risk of major chronic disease. *Journal of the National Cancer Institute, 96,* 1577–1584.

Hunt, S. A., Abraham, W. T., Chin, M. H., et al. (2005). ACC/AHA 2005 Guidelines update for the diagnosis and management of chronic heart failure in the adult. *Circulation, 112,* 1825–1852.

Institute of Medicine. (2004). *Dietary reference intakes for water, potassium, sodium, chloride, and sulfate.* Washington, DC: National Academy Press.

Institute of Medicine (IOM). (2005). *Dietary reference intakes for energy, carbohydrates, fiber, fat, fatty acids, cholesterol, protein, and amino acids (macronutrients).* Washington, DC: National Academy Press.

Jensen, M. K., Koh-Banerjee, P., Hu, F. B., et al. (2004). Intakes of whole grain, bran, and germ and the risk of coronary heart disease among men. *The American Journal of Clinical Nutrition, 80,* 1492–1499.

Jung, U. J., Torrejon, C., Tighe, A. P., et al. (2008). N-3 Fatty acids and cardiovascular disease: Mechanisms underlying beneficial effects. *The American Journal of Clinical Nutrition, 87*(Suppl.), 2003S–2009S.

Katan, M. (2005). The response of lipoproteins to dietary fat and cholesterol in lean and obese persons. *Current Atherosclerosis Reports, 7,* 460–465.

Libby, P. (2000). Changing concepts of atherogenesis. *The Journal of International Medical Research, 247,* 349–358.

Lichtenstein, A. H., Appel, L. J., Brands, M., et al. (2006). Diet and lifestyle recommendations revision 2006. A scientific statement from the American Heart Association Nutrition Committee. *Circulation, 114,* 82–96.

Merchang, A. T., Kelemen, L. E., de Koning, L., et al. (2008). Interrelation of saturated fat, trans fat, alcohol intake, and subclinical atherosclerosis. *The American Journal of Clinical Nutrition, 87,* 168–174.

Mesnick, R. P., Zock, P. L., Kester, A. D., et al. (2003). Effects of dietary fatty acids and carbohydrates on the ratio of serum total to HDL cholesterol and on serum lipids and apolipoproteins: A meta-analysis of 60 controlled trials. *The American Journal of Clinical Nutrition, 77,* 1146–1155.

Moshfegh, A., Goldman, J., & Cleveland, L. (2005). *What we eat in America, NHANES, 2001–2002: Usual nutrient intakes from food compared to dietary reference intakes.* USDA, Agricultural Research Service.

Mozaffarian, D. (2008). Fish and n-3 fatty acids for the prevention of fatal coronary heart disease and sudden cardiac death. *The American Journal of Clinical Nutrition, 87*(Suppl.), 1991S–1996S.

Mozaffarian, D., Katan, M. B., Ascherio, A., et al. (2006). Trans fatty acids and cardiovascular disease. *The New England Journal of Medicine, 354,* 1601–1613.

National Cholesterol Education Program. (2001). *Third report of the expert panel on detection, evaluation, and treatment of high blood cholesterol in adults (Adult Treatment Panel III). Executive summary* (NIH Publication No. 01-3670). Bethesda, MD: U.S. Department of Health and Human Services, Public Health Service, National Institutes of Health.

Obarzanek, E., Sacks, F. M., Vollmer, W. M., et al. (2001). Effects on blood lipids of a blood pressure-lowing diet: The Dietary Approaches to Stop Hypertension (DASH) trial. *The American Journal of Clinical Nutrition, 74,* 80 89.

Oh, K., Hu, F. B., Manson, J. E., et al. (2005). Dietary fat intake and risk of coronary heart disease in women: 20 years of follow-up of the nurses' health study. *American Journal of Epidemiology, 161,* 672–679.

Pietinen, P., Ascherio, A., Korhonen, P., et al. (1997). Intake of fatty acids and risk of coronary heart disease in a cohort of Finnish men. The Alpha-Tocopherol, Beta-Carotene Cancer Prevention Study. *American Journal of Epidemiology, 145,* 876–887.

Singh, I., Shishehbor, M., & Ansell, B. (2007). High-density lipoprotein as a therapeutic target. *The Journal of the American Medical Association, 298*(7), 786–798.

Stevens, V. J., Obarzanek, E., Cook, N. R., et al. For the Trials for the Hypertension Prevention Research Group. (2001). Long-term weight loss and changes in blood pressure: Results of the Trials of Hypertension Prevention, phase II. *Annals of Internal Medicine, 134,* 1–11.

The Trials of the Hypertension Prevention Research Group. (1997). Effects of weight loss and sodium reduction intervention on blood pressure and hypertension incidence in overweight people with high-normal blood pressure: The Trials of Hypertension Prevention, phase II. *Annals of Internal Medicine, 157,* 657–667.

USDHHS, CDC, National Center for Chronic Disease Prevention and Health Promotion, Office on Smoking and Health. (2004). *The health consequences of smoking: A report of the surgeon general.* Available at www.cdc.gov/tobacco/data_statistics/sgr/sgr_2004/index.htm. Accessed on 7/21/08.

USDHHS, NIH, NHLBI. (2006). *DASH eating plan. Lower your blood pressure* (NIH Publication No. 06-4082). Bethesda, MD: U.S. Department of Health and Human Services, Public Health Service, NIH, NHLBI. Available at www.nhlbi.nih.gov/health/public/heart/hbp/dash/new_dash.pdf. Accessed on 7/16/08.

Vasan, R. S., Beiser, A., Seshadri, S., et al. (2002). Residual lifetime risk for developing hypertension in middle-aged women and men: The Framingham Heart Study. *The Journal of the American Medical Association, 287,* 1003–1010.

Whelton, P. K., He, J., Cutler, J. A., et al. (1997). Effects of oral potassium on blood pressure: Meta-analysis of randomized controlled clinical trials. *The Journal of the American Medical Association, 277,* 1624–1632.

Xin, X., He, J., Frontini, M. G., et al. (2001). Effects of alcohol reduction on blood pressure: A meta-analysis of randomized controlled trials. *Hypertension, 38,* 1112–1117.

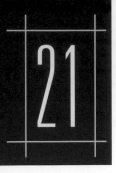

# 21

# Nutrition for Patients with Kidney Disorders

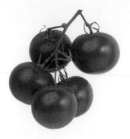

| TRUE | FALSE | | |
|------|-------|---|---|
| ☐ | ☐ | **1** | Early in the course of chronic kidney disease, limiting protein may help to preserve kidney function. |
| ☐ | ☐ | **2** | Foods high in protein tend to be high in phosphorus. |
| ☐ | ☐ | **3** | Milk is an excellent source of high–biologic value protein for people with chronic kidney disease. |
| ☐ | ☐ | **4** | All people with kidney impairments need to limit their sodium intake. |
| ☐ | ☐ | **5** | People with chronic renal disease tend to have accelerated atherosclerosis and may benefit from eating a heart healthy diet. |
| ☐ | ☐ | **6** | Dialysis causes protein requirements to increase about 50% above normal. |
| ☐ | ☐ | **7** | People receiving peritoneal dialysis absorb calories from the dialysate. |
| ☐ | ☐ | **8** | People who have gained more than 2 pounds between dialysis treatments have eaten too many calories. |
| ☐ | ☐ | **9** | People with calcium oxalate renal stones should avoid calcium. |
| ☐ | ☐ | **10** | Increasing fluid intake can effectively prevent kidney stones from forming, eliminating the need for any other nutrition or medical interventions. |

## UPON COMPLETION OF THIS CHAPTER, YOU WILL BE ABLE TO

- Explain nutrition therapy recommendations for nephrotic syndrome.
- Describe the impact chronic kidney disease (CKD) has on nutritional status and requirements.
- Compare nutrient recommendations for CKD to the DRI for healthy people.
- Calculate the calorie and protein requirements of an individual with CKD on the basis of age, stage of CKD, and weight.
- Develop a teaching plan to help a client with CKD adhere to nutrient recommendations.
- Compare nutrient recommendations for stages 1 to 4 CKD to those for patients on dialysis.
- Compare nutrient recommendations for dialysis to those for posttransplant patients.
- Compare nutrient recommendations for diabetic kidney disease with those for people with CKD only.
- Explain why nutrient recommendations for acute renal failure are elusive.
- Teach nutrition therapy recommendations to a client with a history of calcium oxalate kidney stones.

**Nitrogenous Wastes:**
wastes produced from nitrogen—namely, ammonia, urea, uric acid, and creatinine.

**Rennin:** an enzyme secreted by the kidneys in response to a reduced blood flow that stimulates the release of aldosterone.

**Erythropoietin:** a hormone secreted by the kidneys that stimulates the bone marrow to produce red blood cells.

The kidneys perform many vital functions. They maintain normal blood volume and composition by reabsorbing needed nutrients and excreting wastes through urine; urinary excretion is the primary method by which the body rids itself of excess water, **nitrogenous wastes,** electrolytes, sulfates, organic acids, toxic substances, and drugs. The kidneys help to regulate acid–base balance by secreting hydrogen ions to increase pH and excreting bicarbonate to lower pH. The kidneys are involved in blood pressure regulation through the action of **rennin** and in red blood cell production through the action of **erythropoietin.** Because vitamin D is converted to its active form in the kidneys, they have an important role in maintaining normal metabolism of calcium and phosphorus.

Kidney diseases can have a profound impact on metabolism, nutritional status, and nutritional requirements. In 2005, kidney diseases were the ninth leading cause of death in the United States (NCHS, 2008). This chapter presents nutrition therapy for nephrotic syndrome, chronic kidney disease (CKD), acute renal failure (ARF), and urolithiasis.

## ▶ NEPHROTIC SYNDROME

**Nephrotic Syndrome:**
a collection of symptoms that occurs when increased capillary permeability in the glomeruli allows serum proteins to leak into the urine.

**Proteinuria:** protein in the urine; also known as albuminuria.

**Hypoalbuminemia:** low blood levels of albumin, the most abundant plasma protein.

**Hyperlipidemia:** abnormally high level of lipids in the blood, such as LDL cholesterol and triglycerides.

**Nephrotic syndrome** is a generic term that refers to a kidney disorder characterized by urinary protein losses greater than 3.0 g/day. **Proteinuria, hypoalbuminemia, hyperlipidemia,** and edema are major symptoms. Increased urinary losses of proteins such as albumin, transferrin, immunoglobulins, vitamin D-binding protein, and anti-blood clotting proteins may lead to protein-calorie malnutrition, anemia, increased risk of infection, vitamin D deficiency, and increased clotting, respectively. Hyperlipidemia increases the risk of cardiovascular disease and progressive renal damage.

Causes of nephrotic syndrome include diabetes, autoimmune diseases (e.g., lupus, IgA nephropathy), infection, and certain chemicals and medications. In some cases, treating the underlying disorder corrects nephrotic syndrome. In others, especially diabetes, nephrotic syndrome may be the beginning of CKD.

### Nutrition Therapy

The goals of nutrition therapy are to minimize edema, proteinuria, and hyperlipidemia; replace nutrients lost in the urine; and reduce the risk of progressive renal damage and atherosclerosis.

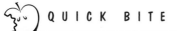

**QUICK BITE**

Putting protein in perspective
Adult RDA: 0.8 g/kg
Average American adult intake: 1.2 g/kg

A mild protein "restriction" of 0.8 to 1.0, along with the use of an angiotensin-converting enzyme (ACE) inhibitor, decreases urinary protein losses. The benefits of minimizing proteinuria include an increase in serum albumin, a decrease in serum lipid levels, a slower progression of kidney disease, and less edema (Kopple, 2006). Several studies suggest that soy protein is better than high–biologic value proteins in reducing proteinuria, lowering lipid levels, and slowing progression of kidney disease (Velasquez & Bhathena, 2001). Table 21.1 lists other nutrition therapy recommendations for nephrotic syndrome.

| TABLE 21.1 | **Nutrition Therapy for Nephrotic Syndrome** | |
|---|---|---|
| **Dietary Component** | **Recommendation** | **Rationale** |
| Protein | 0.8–1.0 g/kg/day; soy protein may be more beneficial than animal proteins | To minimize proteinuria; soy protein may decrease proteinuria more than high–biologic value proteins |
| Calories | 35 cal/kg | To maintain weight and spare protein<br>A lower calorie intake to promote weight loss is recommended if blood pressure or hyperlipidemia are problems |
| Sodium | 1000–2000 mg | To help control edema; fluid restriction is generally not necessary |
| Fat and cholesterol | <30% of calories from total fat, <7% of calories from saturated fat, <200 mg cholesterol, and low trans fats | To improve hyperlipidemia<br>12 g of fish oil/day may be useful for IgA nephropathy |
| Vitamins and minerals | DRI amounts unless otherwise indicated | A multiple vitamin may be used to prevent nutrient deficiencies because many vitamins are bound to protein and are lost through proteinuria<br>Vitamin D and calcium are given if vitamin D is deficient<br>Iron is given if deficient |

*Source:* Kaysen, G. & Yeun, J. (2005). Nephrotic syndrome: Nutritional consequences and dietary management. In: Mitch, W., Klahr, S. (Eds.). Nutrition and the Kidney, 5th ed. Philadelphia, PA: Lippincott Williams and Wilkins; American Dietetic Association. (2006). *Nutrition care manual.* (Online subscription). Available at www. nutritioncare manual.com. Accessed on 7/29/08.

# ▶ CHRONIC KIDNEY DISEASE

**Glomerular Filtration Rate (GFR):** the rate at which the kidneys form filtrate estimated from the amount of creatinine excreted per 24 hours. Normal GRF is about 120 to 130 mL/min.

CKD is a syndrome of progressive kidney damage and loss of function. Over time, a decrease in the number of functioning nephrons overburdens the remaining nephrons, and the kidney's ability to filter blood deteriorates, as measured by a decrease in **glomerular filtration rate (GFR).** The National Kidney Foundation defines the stages of CKD on the basis of GFR (Table 21.2) (NKF, 2002). CKD is associated with premature mortality and decreased quality of life (CDC, 2007).

| TABLE 21.2 | **Classification of Chronic Kidney Disease Stages** | |
|---|---|---|
| **Stage** | **Description** | **GFR (mL/min/1.73 m$^2$)** |
| 1 | Kidney damage with normal or increased GFR | ≥90 |
| 2 | Kidney damage with mildly decreased GFR | 60–89 |
| 3 | Moderately decreased GFR | 30–59 |
| 4 | Severely decreased GFR | 15–29 |
| 5 | Kidney failure | <15 or dialysis |

*Source:* National Kidney Foundation. (2002). K/DOQI clinical practice guidelines for chronic kidney disease: Evaluation, classification and stratification. *American Journal of Kidney Disease, 39(suppl 1)*:S246. (Permission requested.)

**Stages 1 to 4 CKD:** the stages of kidney disease when kidney function is impaired but not to the degree where dialysis or transplant is required. GFR defines each stage, with stage 1 characterized by a normal or increased GFR; stage 4 has a severe impairment of GFR with a rate of 15 to 29.

CKD progresses slowly and may not be apparent until 50% to 70% of function is lost. For **stages 1 to 4**, medical and nutrition therapy can potentially delay the progression to stage 5. Smoking cessation, an increase in physical activity, and controlling blood lipid levels are modifiable risk factors that have the potential to reduce CKD damage (Beto & Bansal, 2004). People with CKD that progresses to stage 5 require dialysis or kidney transplant for survival.

Diabetes is the leading cause of CKD, accounting for approximately 40% of cases. Other risk factors include cardiovascular disease, hypertension, and obesity (CDC, 2007). Compared with whites, African-Americans, Native Americans, and Hispanics are at increased risk for CKD.

## The Impact on Nutrition

**Uremic Syndrome:** a cluster of symptoms related to the retention of nitrogenous substances in the blood such as fatigue, decreased mental acuity, muscle twitches, cramps, anorexia, unpleasant nausea, vomiting, diarrhea, itchy skin, gastritis, and GI bleeding.

**Active Form of Vitamin D:** 1,25-dihydroxycholecalciferol.

The loss of kidney function produces widespread effects. As urine output decreases, fluid and electrolytes accumulate in the blood, producing symptoms of overhydration such as increased blood pressure, weight gain, edema, shortness of breath, and lung crackles. The retention of nitrogenous wastes leads to **uremic syndrome**. Acidosis occurs because the kidneys are unable to excrete excess acid produced through normal metabolic processes. Reabsorption of some nutrients is impaired, which causes them to be lost in the urine. Gastrointestinal (GI) absorption of some minerals, such as calcium and iron, is impaired. Impaired synthesis of rennin, erythropoietin, and the **active form of vitamin D** can lead to high blood pressure, anemia, and bone demineralization, respectively. Certain peptide hormones, such as insulin, parathyroid hormone, and glucagon, are not adequately inactivated, which contributes to altered metabolism. Accelerated atherosclerosis increases the risk of coronary heart disease, myocardial infarction, and further renal damage. Poor intake related to dietary restrictions, anorexia, alterations in taste, nausea, vomiting, stomatitis, depression, or anxiety is common. Drug therapy, dialysis, or renal transplantation may cause nutrient losses. In short, the disruption to homeostasis is profound.

## Nutrition Therapy

The goals of nutrition therapy are to

- Reduce workload on the kidneys to delay or prevent further kidney damage
- Restore or maintain optimal nutritional status
- Control the accumulation of uremic toxins such as urea, phosphorus, sodium, and sometimes potassium.

The optimal interventions needed to meet these objectives vary among individuals and according to the nature, severity, and stage of the disease. Generally, diet modifications are made in response to symptoms and laboratory values and require frequent monitoring and adjustment. Alterations in the intake of protein, calories, sodium, fluid, potassium, phosphorus, calcium, and other vitamins and minerals are necessary initially or eventually. The diet is both complex and dynamic. Table 21.3 summarizes the nutrient recommendations issued by the National Kidney Foundation (NKF, 2000).

## Protein

As kidney function declines, the ability to excrete nitrogenous and other wastes also declines. Restricting protein helps lessen workload on the kidneys. Results from the Modification of Diet in Renal Disease (MDRD) study showed tight control of blood pressure and a restricted protein

| TABLE 21.3 | Nutrient Recommendations for Chronic Kidney Disease | | | |
|---|---|---|---|---|
| Nutrient | Stages 1–4 Chronic Kidney Disease | Stage 5 Hemodialysis | Stage 5 Peritoneal Dialysis | Transplant |
| Protein (g/kg/day) | 0.6–0.75; 50% HBV | 1.2; 50% HBV | 1.2–1.3; 50% HBV | Initial: 1.3–1.5 Maintenance: 1.0 |
| Calories (cal/kg/day) | 35 if <60 years 30–35 if ≥60 years | 35 if <60 years 30–35 if ≥60 years | 35 if <60 years 30–35 if ≥60 years | Initial: 30–35 Maintenance: 25–30 |
| Fat | Heart healthy guidelines | Heart healthy guidelines | Heart healthy guidelines | Heart healthy guidelines |
| Sodium (mg/day) | 1000–3000 | 1000–3000 | 2000–4000 | Unrestricted; monitor effects of medication |
| Fluid (mL/day) | Unrestricted with normal urine output | 1000 + urine output | 1500–2000 (monitor) | Generally unrestricted |
| Potassium (mg/day) | Usually unrestricted unless serum level is high | 2000–3000 | 3000–4000 | Unrestricted; monitor effects of medication |
| Phosphorus (mg/day) | 800–1000 when serum phosphorus >4.6 mg/dL or PTH is high | 800–1000 | 800–1000 | Generally unrestricted |
| Calcium (mg/day) | 1000–1500 | ≤2000 from diet and medications | ≤2000 from diet and medications | 1200 |

*Source:* National Kidney Foundation-K/DOQI, 2000; K/DOQI, 2002; K/KOQI, 2003. Beto, J. and Bansal, V. (2004). Medical nutrition therapy in chronic kidney failure: Integrating clinical practice guidelines. *Journal of American Diet Association, 104,* 404–409.

QUICK BITE

Sources of high–biologic value protein
Eggs
Meat, fish, poultry
Milk, yogurt, cheese
Soy

**Dialysate:** the dialysis solution used to extract wastes and fluid from the blood.

intake of 0.6 g/kg/day helped delay the progression of kidney disease by 41% (Levey et al., 1996). High–biologic value proteins are emphasized because they provide a higher percentage of essential amino acids, which may promote reuse of circulating nonessential amino acids for protein synthesis and by doing so minimizes urea production.

For stages 1 to 4, the recommended daily protein intake is 0.6 to 0.75 g/kg, a level that can be difficult to implement because most Americans generally consume almost twice this level. Protein allowance may be liberalized to maintain appropriate body protein stores or because the severity of restriction is too difficult to follow (Beto & Bansal, 2004). Protein allowance in stage 5 is 50% higher than the recommended daily allowance (RDA) to account for the loss of serum proteins and amino acids in the **dialysate**. Achieving this level of intake within the confines of other restrictions, especially phosphorus restriction, is difficult. Box 21.1 illustrates a menu at two different protein levels.

## Calories

Whenever protein intake is restricted, it is vital to consume adequate calories to spare protein from being used for energy, enabling it to be used for protein synthesis. For all stages of CKD, calorie recommendations are 35 cal/kg for adults under 60 years of age and 30 to 35 cal/kg for those who are older. People who undergo peritoneal dialysis absorb a large amount of calories daily through the dialysate (approximately 340 to 680 cal/day), which needs to be considered. Calories from the dialysate impair the natural sense of hunger and

| BOX 21.1 | SAMPLE CKD DIET: WITHOUT AND WITH DIALYSIS |
|---|---|

| Sample CKD without Dialysis (50 g Protein Diet) | Sample CKD with Dialysis (90 g Protein Diet) |
|---|---|
| **Breakfast** | |
| ½ cup apricot nectar | ½ cup apricot nectar |
| 1 English muffin | 1 English muffin |
| At least 1 tbsp margarine | 1 tbsp margarine |
| Jelly | 2 eggs fried in margarine |
| Coffee | Jelly |
| Sugar | 1 cup coffee |
| Nondairy creamer | Sugar |
| | Nondairy creamer |
| **Lunch** | |
| Sandwich made with | Sandwich made with |
|   2 oz turkey |   4 oz turkey |
|   2 slices whole wheat bread |   2 slices whole wheat bread |
|   Salad dressing |   Salad dressing |
|   Lettuce and 1 slice tomato |   Lettuce and 1 slice tomato |
| 1 small apple | 1 small apple |
| ½ cup low-fat milk | ½ cup low-fat milk |
| **Snack** | |
| 2 fruit rollups | |
| **Dinner** | |
| 2 oz roast beef | 4 oz toast beef |
| Low-sodium gravy | Low-sodium gravy |
| ½ cup unsalted noodles with margarine | ½ cup unsalted noodles with margarine |
| ½ cup carrots with margarine | ½ cup carrots |
| Lettuce, onions, cucumbers, green salad with olive oil and vinegar dressing | Lettuce, onions, cucumbers, green pepper salad with olive oil and vinegar dressing |
| ⅛ blueberry pie | ⅛ blueberry pie |
| Ginger ale | 1 cup ginger ale |
| **Snacks** | |
| Carbonated beverages* | |
| Marshmallows, gum drops, hard candy | Marshmallows, gum drops, hard candy |

*As allowed, depending on fluid needs.

---

### QUICK BITE

Examples of pure sugars and pure fats
Pure sugars: cotton candy, fruit rollups, jelly beans, lollipops, marshmallows, honey, jam, maple syrup, sweetened beverages (within fluid allowance)
Pure fats: butter, margarine, mayonnaise, oils, shortening

generally prevent a fall in blood glucose levels between meals. Although they may look well fed, they may actually have protein malnutrition (Beto & Bansal, 2004).

Unlike the general population, clients who must limit their intake of protein may be advised to increase their intake of pure sugars and pure fats to meet their calorie requirements while keeping protein intake low, even though they are not considered "nutritious." In this population in whom diabetes and hyperlipidemia are common, an increased intake of pure sugars and pure fats is seemingly contraindicated. The best protein-free calorie option is to choose foods rich in monounsaturated fats such as canola oil, olive oil, and trans fat–free margarines.

## Sodium and Fluid

> **QUICK BITE**
>
> Sodium perspective
> Adequate intake (AI) for healthy adults: 1200 to 1500 mg
> Upper limit (UL) for adults: 2300 mg
> Daily value listed on the "Nutrition Facts" label: 2400 mg
> Mean intake among U.S. adults 19 and older[*]: 2853 mg (women); 3964 mg (men)
>
> ***Source:*** Moshfegh, A., Goldman, J., Cleveland, L. (2005). What we eat in America, NHANES 2001–2002: Usual nutrient intakes from food compared to Dietary Reference Intakes. USDA, Agricultural Research Service.

Sodium restriction begins when fluid retention occurs (Beto & Bansal, 2004). For stages 1 to 4 and hemodialysis, 1000 to 3000 mg/day are recommended; the range is 2000 to 4000 mg for peritoneal dialysis. Fluid is unrestricted in stages 1 to 4 with normal urine output. For people on hemodialysis, fluid allowance equals the volume of any urine produced plus 1000 mL. Fluid intake is monitored by weight gain: anuric hemodialysis patients should not gain more than approximately 2 pounds/day between treatments. Peritoneal dialysis patients usually have fewer problems with fluid retention.

For many clients on hemodialysis, limiting fluid intake is the biggest challenge. Teaching clients *why* the fluid restriction is important is only half the battle; teaching them *how* to control their intake and thirst is vital. Strategies to relieve thirst are listed in Box 21.2.

## Potassium

Normally, potassium consumed in excess of need is excreted in the urine. With loss of kidney function, potassium excretion is impaired and hyperkalemia is a risk. GI bleeding, acidosis, catabolism, and hyperglycemia also increase the risk of hyperkalemia. Conversely, hypokalemia is a risk for people who receive continuous ambulatory peritoneal dialysis, take potassium-wasting diuretics, or experience vomiting or diarrhea. For all CKD stages, potassium allowance is based on the individual's serum potassium levels.

Unlike sodium, potassium cannot be tasted and rarely appears on the "Nutrition Facts" label, making it difficult to comply with a potassium-restricted eating plan.

---

**BOX 21.2** **STRATEGIES TO RELIEVE THIRST**

- Use ice or popsicles within the fluid allowance—very cold things are better at relieving thirst.
- Suck on hard candy or mints.
- Chew gum.
- Rinse your mouth without swallowing using refrigerated water.
- Rinse your mouth occasionally with refrigerated mouthwash.
- Suck on a lemon wedge.
- Eat bread with applesauce or jelly with margarine.
- Control blood glucose levels, as appropriate.
- Try frozen low-potassium fruit, such as grapes.
- Use small glasses instead of large ones.
- Apply petroleum jelly to the lips.

## Phosphorus and Calcium

**QUICK BITE**

Phosphorus and calcium intakes (mean intakes in Americans aged 19 and older)

|         | Phosphorus (mg) | Calcium (mg) |
|---------|-----------------|--------------|
| Males   | 1552            | 984          |
| Females | 1109            | 735          |

***Source:*** Moshfegh, A., Goldman, J., Cleveland, L. (2005). What we eat in America, NHANES 2001–2002: Usual nutrient intakes from food compared to Dietary Reference Intakes. USDA, Agricultural Research Service.

As kidney function deteriorates, the conversion of vitamin D to its active form is impaired. Without active vitamin D, the metabolism of calcium, phosphorus, and magnesium is altered and leads to hyperphosphatemia, bone demineralization, and bone pain. Hyperphosphatemia stimulates parathyroid hormone (PTH) secretion, creating secondary hyperparathyroidism and further aggravating loss of bone mass and increasing the risk that damaging deposits of calcium and phosphorus will form in the kidneys and other soft tissues such as the eyes, skin, heart, lungs, and blood vessels.

The National Kidney Foundation recommends both phosphorus and calcium intake be controlled, not just phosphorus as was done in the past (NKF, 2003). In stages 1 to 4, phosphorus allowance is based on laboratory values and calcium is limited to 1000 to 1500 mg/day. A low phosphorus intake is relatively easy to achieve because protein intake is also restricted in these stages and protein and phosphorus share similar dietary sources. When dialysis begins and protein allowance increases, phosphorus intake correspondingly increases yet the recommendation is to limit intake to 800 to 1000 mg. Phosphate binders, which decrease GI absorption of phosphorus and promote fecal excretion, along with a dietary restriction, are necessary to control serum phosphorus levels for the majority of patients. Phosphate binders must be taken with all meals and snacks. Table 21.4 lists the calcium, phosphorus, and protein contents of selected foods.

## Other Vitamins and Minerals

The original studies on vitamin and mineral requirements in CKD remain the cornerstone for recommendations today; very few recent studies have been published to address nutrient needs in this population (Beto & Bansal, 2004). Specially formulated vitamin supplements are available with the appropriate levels of essential vitamins for people with CKD because routine multivitamin preparations may provide too much of some vitamins (e.g., vitamin A) and too little of others (e.g., folic acid). In general

- Deficiencies of water-soluble vitamins may be caused by inadequate intake related to anorexia or dietary restrictions, altered metabolism related to uremia or medications, or increased losses related to dialysis. The requirement for some water-soluble vitamins increases, such as vitamins $B_6$ and $B_{12}$ (for protein synthesis) and folic acid (for red blood cell production).
- Fat-soluble vitamins A and E have been shown to accumulate in CKD and are not recommended for supplementation (Beto & Bansal, 2004). The need for vitamin D is determined on an individual basis.
- Clients who are undergoing dialysis may develop a deficiency of zinc, which could contribute to anorexia and taste alterations. Supplements are recommended if a zinc deficiency is identified.
- Oral iron supplementation has largely been replaced with IV iron for people receiving hemodialysis. Iron and erythropoietin are used to treat anemia of CKD (Beto & Bansal, 2004).

| TABLE 21.4 | Calcium, Phosphorus, and Protein Content of Selected Foods | | | |
|---|---|---|---|---|
| Item | Amount | Calcium (mg) | Phosphorus (mg) | Protein (g) |
| **Grains** | | | | |
| White bread | 1 slice | 27 | 24 | 2 |
| Whole wheat bread | 1 slice | 20 | 64 | 3 |
| Long-grain rice | ½ cup | 10 | 81 | 3 |
| Corn tortilla | 1 med | 44 | 79 | 1 |
| **Vegetables** | | | | |
| Artichoke, boiled | 1 med | 135 | 258 | 3 |
| Kale, frozen, boiled | ½ cup | 90 | 18 | 2 |
| Spinach, boiled | ½ cup | 122 | 50 | 3 |
| Turnip greens, boiled | ½ cup | 99 | 21 | 1 |
| **Fruits** | | | | |
| Orange juice, calcium fortified | ¾ cup | 200 | 25 | 0 |
| Avocado, raw | 1 med | 13 | 45 | 2 |
| **Milk** | | | | |
| Skim | 1 cup | 302 | 247 | 8 |
| 2% | 1 cup | 297 | 232 | 8 |
| Chocolate milk (with 1% milk) | 1 cup | 287 | 256 | 8 |
| Low-fat fruit-flavored yogurt | 1 cup | 314 | 247 | 8 |
| Cheddar cheese | 1 oz | 214 | 145 | 7 |
| **Meat and Beans** | | | | |
| Ground beef, broiled | 3½ oz | 12 | 191 | 27 |
| Ham, cured, roasted | 3½ oz | 6 | 224 | 19 |
| Chicken breast, roasted | ½ | 13 | 196 | 27 |
| Salmon, Chinook | 3 oz | 24 | 316 | 22 |
| Refried beans, canned | ½ cup | 45 | 109 | 7 |
| Great northern beans, canned | ½ cup | 70 | 178 | 7 |
| Egg, poached | 1 | 25 | 89 | 6 |
| Almonds, blanched | 1 oz | 73 | 150 | 6 |
| Peanut butter | 2 tbsp | 13 | 101 | 7 |
| Sunflower seeds, dry roasted | 1 oz | 20 | 327 | 6 |

## Translating Recommendations into Meals

The diet for CKD is complex; modifications can be numerous, extensive, and lifelong, and changes are frequent. It is a difficult task to design a meal plan that balances what the individual needs with what the individual can tolerate—and will accept. Getting the client to make permanent changes in eating habits and food choices can be an ongoing challenge. Box 21.3 lists strategies that may help promote dietary adherence.

A "choice" system, similar to the diabetic exchange system, may be used to help clients implement dietary restrictions. An individualized meal plan that corresponds as closely as possible to the client's food preferences and habits details the number of choices permitted from each list for each meal. Portion sizes are specified to help ensure relative consistency in nutrient intake. Table 21.5 shows choice lists with examples of representative foods. The composition and complexity of the choice list system differs with the type of treatment used (e.g., no dialysis, hemodialysis, or peritoneal dialysis). For instance, people not receiving dialysis may not need to limit their intake of potassium and would be free to choose among low-, medium-, and high-potassium fruits and vegetables, whereas people undergoing hemodialysis

| BOX 21.3 | STRATEGIES THAT MAY HELP PROMOTE DIETARY ADHERENCE TO CKD DIET |
|---|---|

- Provide positive messages about what to eat rather than emphasizing food restrictions.
- Encourage social support from family and friends.
- Foster the client's perception as successfully adhering to the plan. People who are more confident in their ability to adhere to the eating plan make better choices.
- Provide feedback on self-monitoring and laboratory data. Correlation of records with laboratory data enables the client to see cause and effect, reinforces the importance of nutrition therapy, and opens the door for problem solving.
- For clients who must restrict their intake of protein, encourage the use of low-protein breads, cereals, cookies, gelatin, and pastas. Acceptability varies greatly among low-protein products, so if a client does not like one brand, it does not mean he will not like another.

| TABLE 21.5 | Choice Lists and Examples of Representative Foods |
|---|---|

| Choice Lists | Examples of Representative Foods |
|---|---|
| High-protein foods | Beef, fish, eggs, poultry, shellfish |
| High protein and high phosphorus | Cheese, dried peas and beans, milk, yogurt, tofu |
| High protein and high sodium | Canned tuna and salmon; cottage cheese; deli beef or turkey; vegetarian burgers |
| Vegetables | |
|   Low potassium | Cabbage, carrots, corn, eggplant, green beans, onions |
|   Medium potassium | Asparagus, broccoli, celery, peas, turnips, zucchini |
|   High potassium | Avocado, Brussels sprouts, "greens," okra, potatoes, pumpkin, spinach, sweet potatoes, tomatoes, yams |
| Bread, cereal, and grain | Bagel, bread, pita, flour tortilla, low-salt ready-to-eat cereals, pasta, rice, unsalted crackers |
| Bread, cereal, and grain with added salt and phosphorus | Muffins, oatmeal, most ready-to-eat cereals, pancakes, waffles |
| Fruit | |
|   Low potassium | Apples, blueberries, grapes, pineapples, watermelon |
|   Medium potassium | Cherries, cantaloupe, papaya, prunes, raisins |
|   High potassium | Apricots, bananas, nectarines, orange juice, prune juice |
| Fluids | Beverages, ice, soup, gelatin; ice cream and ice milk (each melt to ½ initial volume) |
| Calorie and flavoring | Gumdrops, hard candy, jelly, jelly beans, lifesavers, margarine, mayonnaise, sugar, syrup, vegetable oil |
| Salt | 2 tbsp ketchup, 1/8 dill pickle, 1/8 tsp salt, ¾ tsp soy sauce, 3 tbsp taco sauce |

*Source:* American Dietetic Association. (2008). Chronic kidney disease nutrition therapy for people not on dialysis. In *Nutrition care manual* (Online subscription). Available at www.nutritioncaremanual.com. Accessed 8/5/08.

may need to eat only low-potassium fruits and vegetables. Despite the term "choice lists," selections can be severely limited. Tips for implementing nutrition therapy recommendations for CKD are featured in Box 21.4.

## Diabetic Kidney Disease

Formerly known as diabetic nephropathy, diabetic kidney disease (DKD) refers to CKD believed to have resulted from diabetes. The National Kidney Foundation recently published clinical practice guidelines and clinical recommendations for improving outcomes

| BOX 21.4 | **TIPS FOR IMPLEMENTING NUTRITION THERAPY FOR CKD STAGES 1 TO 4** |

- Initially weigh or measure portion sizes and, thereafter, periodically spot-check portion sizes for accuracy because either too little or too much protein in the diet can cause uremic symptoms to return.
- Be sure to eat a good breakfast if appetite decreases as the day progresses, which may occur secondary to uremia.
- Limit meat intake to less than 5 to 6 oz/day for most men and less than 4 oz/day for most women. Think of meat as a side dish, not the main entrée.
- Spread protein allowance over the whole day instead of saving it all for one meal.
- Limit dairy products, including milk, yogurt, ice cream, and frozen yogurt, to ½ cup/day. Nondairy creamers are a low-phosphorus alternative, but they can be high in saturated fat.
- Limit cheese to 1 oz hard cheese/day or ⅓ cup cottage cheese/day.
- Limit high-phosphorus foods to 1 serving or less/day. High-phosphorus foods include beer, chocolate, cola, nuts, peanut butter, dried peas and beans, bran, bran cereals, and some whole grains.
- Do not add salt during cooking or at the table. Avoid processed foods, regular canned vegetables, convenience foods, and seasonings that contain salt (e.g., onion salt, lemon pepper, MSG).
- Eat heart healthy by choosing lean meats, nonfat milk and dairy products, trans fat–free margarines, and canola and olive oils.
- Try highly seasoned or strongly flavored foods if uremia has caused a change in the sense of taste.
- Eat a consistent intake of carbohydrate with regularly timed meals to control blood glucose levels, if appropriate.
- Seek physician approval before using any vitamin, mineral, or supplement.

| BOX 21.5 | **NUTRITION RECOMMENDATION GUIDELINES FOR DIABETIC KIDNEY DISEASE** |

| | |
|---|---|
| Protein | 0.8 g/kg |
| Sodium | 2300 mg/day |
| Lipids | ≤30% calories from fat, <10% calories from saturated fat, 200 mg cholesterol/day |
| Carbohydrates | 50–60% of total calories |
| Phosphorus | 1700 mg/day for stages 1 and 2<br>800 to 1000 mg/day for stages 3 and 4 |
| Potassium | <4000 mg/day for stages 1 and 2<br>2400 mg/day for stages 3 and 4 |

*Source:* Burrowes, J. (2008). New recommendations for the management of diabetic kidney disease. *Nutrition Today, 43,* 65–69.

in patients with diabetes and CKD, stages 1 to 4 (NKF, 2007). Risk factors for DKD are hyperglycemia, hypertension, and altered lipid levels. Nutrition therapy seeks to control these risks to slow or prevent the progression of kidney disease and reduce the risk of cardiovascular disease.

General nutrition guidelines for DKD are listed in Box 21.5. One notable difference between guidelines for DKD compared with nondiabetic guidelines is that protein allowance is slightly higher, based on studies that show this level of protein stabilizes or reduces albuminuria, slows the deterioration of GFR, and may possibly prevent kidney failure (Burrowes, 2008). Also, when protein decreases, the amount of carbohydrate and/or fat increases, which may not be ideal for diabetic control or managing the risk of heart disease, respectively. Recommended levels of intake for phosphorus and potassium are specified according to the stage of CKD. For people with diabetes, hypertension, and CKD stages 1 to 2, a DASH-type diet (Chapter 20) that stresses non–red meat sources of protein may be a reasonable alternative to a lower protein intake (Marcason, 2008).

## Kidney Transplantation

Kidney transplantation is a treatment option for people with stage 5 CKD. As with all major surgeries, the immediate postoperative diet is high in protein and calories to promote healing; nutrient needs gradually decrease after the initial postoperative period (Table 21.3). Most dietary parameters are removed when the new kidney functions normally; side effects from immunosuppressant drugs may require some dietary modifications (Beto & Bansal, 2004). A lifelong commitment to a "healthy" eating is important to decrease the risk of obesity, hypertension, diabetes, and hyperlipidemia, and maximizes bone density.

# ▶ ACUTE RENAL FAILURE

ARF is the sudden loss of renal function characterized by an acute increase in serum creatinine and decrease in urine output. It can develop over a period of hours or days, and the impairment can range from mild to severe. Among the many causes of ARF are shock, severe infection, trauma, medications, and obstruction. In most cases, patients who recover from the underlying illness are able to recover from ARF (Kopple, 2006). The estimated 50% mortality rate is attributed to the degree of underlying hypercatabolism and infection. The primary focus of treatment is to correct the underlying disorder to prevent permanent renal damage.

## Nutrition Therapy

It has not been proven that nutrition therapy for ARF promotes recovery of kidney function or improves survival, but it is a way of supporting the patient until the underlying illness is controlled (ADA, 2008). The goal is to provide adequate amounts of calories, protein, and other nutrients to prevent or minimize malnutrition; however, the metabolic abnormalities that occur in hypercatabolic patients with ARF, such as accelerated protein breakdown, increased energy expenditure, and an inability to use protein and calories efficiently, make it difficult to achieve nutritional goals with oral, enteral, or parenteral nutrition (Kopple, 2006).

Data on the optimal nutrition therapy for ARF are scarce and contradictory, leading to the conclusion that "it is not possible to justify strongly any treatment plan for such patients" (Kopple, 2006). One approach is to strictly limit fluid, electrolytes, and protein to reduce the need for dialysis. Conversely, for patients who are malnourished and hypercatabolic, the approach may be to give ample amounts of protein and nutrients and provide dialysis as needed. Between these two extremes is a range of scenarios, approaches, and opinions.

A list of nutrients of concern and factors that influence an individual's allowance are featured in Table 21.6. Whenever possible, patients are fed orally. Enteral products may be used orally or given via tube if oral intake is inadequate. Parenteral nutrition is often the only effective means of providing adequate nutrition (Kopple, 2006).

| TABLE 21.6 | Nutrition Guidelines for Acute Renal Failure | |
| --- | --- | --- |
| **Nutrient** | **Recommendations** | **Factors that Impact Actual Allowance** |
| Protein | 0.6–2.0 g/kg | Degree of catabolism<br>Renal function<br>Use of dialysis |
| Calories | 35–50 cal/kg | Degree of stress<br>Nutritional status |
| Sodium | 1.1–3.3 g/day | Serum sodium levels<br>Blood pressure<br>Edema<br>Urinary losses (in diuretic phase)<br>Use of dialysis |
| Potassium | 2.0–3.0 g/day | Serum potassium levels<br>Urinary losses (in diuretic phase) |
| Phosphorus | Individualized | Serum phosphorus levels |
| Calcium | Individualized | Serum calcium levels |
| Fluid | 500 mL + urine output | Urine output<br>Type of dialysis, if any |
| Vitamins and minerals | DRI amounts | Level of catabolism |

*Source:* American Dietetic Association. (2008). Nutrition prescription for acute renal failure. *Nutrition care manual* (Online subscription). Available at www.nutritioncaremanual.com. Accessed on 7/29/08.

# ▶ KIDNEY STONES

Kidney stones form when insoluble crystals precipitate out of urine. They vary in size from sandlike "gravel" to large, branching stones, and although they form most often in the kidney, they can occur anywhere in the urinary system.

Approximately 75% of kidney stones are made of calcium oxalate (Reynolds, 2005). The remaining stones are composed of calcium phosphate, uric acid, or **struvite**. Cystine (an amino acid) stones are rare and occur only in people with cystinuria, an autosomal recessive disorder.

Certain factors increase the risk of kidney stones, including dehydration or low urine volume, urinary tract obstruction, gout, chronic inflammation of the bowel, and intestinal bypass or ostomy surgery. Nutritionally, inadequate fluid intake and excessive intakes of oxalate, calcium, protein, and sodium may increase the risk of calcium oxalate stones in susceptible people.

*Fluid.* A low fluid intake concentrates the urine, increasing the likelihood of chemicals precipitating out to form kidney stones—regardless of the composition of the stone. An adequate fluid intake helps keep urine dilute.

*Oxalate.* Normally only 6% to 14% of **oxalate** consumed is absorbed (Marcason, 2006). People who have **hyperoxaluria**, known as "super absorbers," can absorb 50% more oxalate than nonstone formers (Reynolds, 2005). Hyperoxaluria can be caused by genetic disorders, to altered bowel function, or a high oxalate intake.

Hyperoxaluria is a primary risk factor for the formation of calcium oxalate kidney stones (Chai et al., 2004). In fact, hyperoxaluria is more of a risk for stone formation than

**Struvite:** magnesium ammonium phosphate crystals formed by the action of bacterial enzymes.

**Oxalate:** a salt of oxalic acid. Oxalate can form strong bonds with various minerals; when combined with calcium, it forms a nearly insoluble compound.

**Hyperoxaluria:** elevated levels of oxalate in the urine.

---

**BOX 21.6**  **FOODS HIGH IN OXALATE**

Nuts: peanuts, almonds, pecans, cashews, walnuts

Nut butters

Tea

Instant coffee (more than 8 oz/day)

Rhubarb

Beets

Beans: green, wax, baked, and dried, such as kidney beans, garbanzo beans, pinto beans

Berries: blackberries, raspberries, strawberries, gooseberries

Chocolate

Concord grapes

Dark leafy greens

Oranges

Tofu

Sweet potatoes

Draft beer

**Sources:** National Kidney Foundation. (2005). Diet and kidney stones. Available at http://www.kidney.org/ atoz/ atozPrint.cfm?id=41. Accessed on 7/31/08.

American Dietetic Association. Urolithiasis/Urinary Stones Nutrition Therapy. Nutrition Care Manual. (Online subscription). Available at www.nutritioncaremanual.com. Accessed on 8/5/08.

---

**Hypercalciuria:** elevated levels of calcium in urine.

**Megadoses:** amounts at least 10 times greater than the DRI.

hypercalciuria (Mendonca et al., 2003). People who form calcium oxalate stones are advised to limit their intake of oxalate, which is found primarily in plants (Box 21.6). Because **megadoses** of vitamin C increase both oxalate absorption and oxalate synthesis in people prone to calcium oxalate stones, daily doses should be limited to less than 2000 mg/day (Chai et al., 2004).

*Calcium.* Dietary calcium favorably binds with dietary oxalate in the intestines, forming an insoluble compound that the body cannot absorb. When calcium intake is low, more oxalate is available for absorption and the risk of stone formation increases. A normal calcium intake consumed throughout the day is recommended to prevent stone formation.

*Protein.* High intakes of animal protein increase urinary excretion of calcium, oxalate, and uric acid, and reduce urinary pH (Seiner et al., 2003). Protein intake in excess of the RDA is not recommended for people with a history of calcium oxalate kidney stones.

*Sodium.* A high sodium intake promotes urinary calcium excretion by decreasing calcium reabsorption by the kidney (Seiner et al., 2003). Patients with hypercalciuria should limit their intake of sodium.

## Nutrition Therapy

None of the diet recommendations made to prevent kidney stones are effective when used alone (Box 21.7), yet nutrition therapy is considered the cornerstone in kidney stone management, whether or not medication is needed.

---

**BOX 21.7**  **NUTRITION RECOMMENDATIONS FOR CALCIUM OXALATE KIDNEY STONES**

- Drink 3 to 4 quarts of fluid throughout the day, with most in the form of water.
- Avoid high-oxalate foods (Box 21.6) and megadoses of vitamin C.
- Maintain adequate calcium intake that is balanced throughout the day.
- Avoid high intakes of animal protein and sodium.

**Source:** National Kidney Foundation. (2005). Diet and kidney stones. Available at http://www.kidney.org/atoz/ atozPrint.cfm?id=41. Accessed on 7/31/08.

## NURSING PROCESS: *Chronic Kidney Disease*

arlos is 66 years old and has had type 2 diabetes for 20 years. He is 5 ft. 7 in. tall and weighs 181 pounds. His A1c was 8.2; he takes insulin twice a day. He has a history of hypertension and mild anemia and complains of sudden weight gain and "swelling." His blood urea nitrogen (BUN) and creatinine have been steadily increasing over the last several years, and his GFR is currently 83. During his last appointment, the doctor told Carlos to watch his protein intake and avoid salt. At this visit, Carlos' chief complaint is that he does not have an appetite anymore; he attributes his change in taste to not salting his food. The doctor has asked you to talk to Carlos about his diet.

| Assessment |
|---|

| | |
|---|---|
| Medical–Psychosocial History | • Medical history including cardiovascular disease, hypertension, diabetes, and renal disease |
| | • Medications that affect nutrition such as diuretics, insulin, and lipid-lowering medications |
| | • Physical complaints such as fatigue, taste changes, anorexia, nausea, vomiting, diarrhea, muscular twitches, and muscle cramps |
| | • Psychosocial and economic issues such as living situation, cooking facilities, financial status, employment, and education |
| | • Understanding of the relationship between diet and renal function |
| | • Motivation to change eating style |
| Anthropometric Assessment | • Current height, weight, and BMI |
| | • Recent weight history |
| Biochemical and Physical Assessment | • Blood values of: |
| | • BUN and creatinine |
| | • Sodium, potassium, and other electrolytes |
| | • Phosphorus and calcium |
| | • Glucose |
| | • Lipid profile |
| | • Hemoglobin and hematocrit |
| | • GFR |
| | • Urinalysis for volume, urea, protein, etc. |
| | • Blood pressure |
| Dietary Assessment | • What kind of nutrition counseling have you had in the past? |
| | • How many meals and snacks do you usually eat? |
| | • What is a typical day's intake for you? |
| | • Do you follow a diet for diabetes? What gives you the most difficulty? |
| | • How is your appetite? |
| | • Do you have any food allergies or intolerances? |
| | • Do you have any feeding issues, such as difficulty chewing or swallowing? |
| | • What kind of protein do you eat most often? What is a typical serving size? Is it spread out over the day? |

*(nursing process continues on page 529)*

## NURSING PROCESS: Chronic Kidney Disease (continued)

- Do you drink milk and, if so, how much per day?
- How successful were you "watching your protein and avoiding salt"?
- How often do you eat high-sodium foods, such as cold cuts, bacon, frankfurters, smoked meats, sausage, canned meats, chipped or corned beef, buttermilk, cheese, crackers, canned soups and vegetables, convenience products, pickles, and condiments?
- Do you use a salt substitute?
- Do you regularly eat fruits and vegetables? How many servings of each do you take in an average day?
- How much fluid do you drink daily? What is your favorite beverage?
- Do you have any cultural, religious, and ethnic food preferences?
- Do you use vitamins, minerals, or nutritional supplements? If so, what, how much, and why do you use them?
- Do you drink alcohol?
- How often do you eat out?

### Diagnosis

Possible Nursing Diagnosis

Imbalanced nutrition: less than body requirements r/t anorexia, taste changes, dietary restrictions.

### Planning

Client Outcomes

The client will:
- Consume adequate calories to prevent weight loss
- Attain and maintain adequate nutritional status
- Experience improved appetite
- Practice self-management strategies especially self-monitoring protein and sodium intake
- Achieve normal or near-normal electrolyte levels
- Maintain adequate glucose control
- Achieve and maintain normal blood pressure
- Maintain normal urinary output
- Describe the rationale and principles of nutrition therapy for CKD and implement appropriate dietary changes
- Prevent further kidney damage

### Nursing Interventions

Nutrition Therapy

Provide a 2400-calorie carbohydrate-controlled diet with 65 g protein and 2300 mg sodium, as ordered.

*(nursing process continues on page 530)*

## NURSING PROCESS: *Chronic Kidney Disease* (continued)

| | |
|---|---|
| Client Teaching | Instruct the client on: |

1. The role of nutrition therapy in the treatment of CKD
2. Eating plan essentials, including
   - Limiting protein, emphasizing high-quality proteins, spreading protein allowance over the whole day
   - Consuming adequate calories
   - Limiting high-sodium foods, not adding salt during cooking or at the table
   - Using sodium-free seasonings and salt alternatives to improve the flavor of food
3. Behavioral matters including
   - How to weigh and measure foods to ensure accurate portion sizes
   - To self-monitor protein intake
   - To weigh oneself at approximately the same time every day with the same scale while wearing the same amount of clothing. Unexpected weight gain or loss should be reported to the physician.
   - That renal diet cookbooks are available to increase variety
4. Changing eating attitudes
   - Learn to view the diet as an integral component of treatment and a means of life support
   - Strict adherence to the diet can improve the quality of life and decrease the workload on the kidneys

### Evaluation

| | |
|---|---|
| Evaluate and Monitor | • Monitor weight |
| | • Monitor lab values, blood pressure, and urine output |
| | • Monitor appetite |
| | • Evaluate food records, if available |
| | • Provide periodic feedback and reinforcement |

▶ How Do You Respond?

**Does cranberry juice prevent urinary tract infections?** Although conclusive evidence is lacking, cranberry juice may be effective against urinary tract infections by preventing bacteria from adhering to the lining of the urinary tract, thereby promoting their excretion. However, the effects are transitory, so regular, perhaps daily, intake is necessary. Clients who are prone to urinary tract infections and like cranberry juice should be encouraged to consume it regularly.

**Are omega-3 fish oil supplements beneficial for people on hemodialysis?** In addition to their beneficial effects on the heart, supplements of omega-3 fats may help benefit people on hemodialysis by preventing itching (uremic pruritus), decreasing vascular access graft thrombosis, and decreasing the dose of erythropoietin needed to maintain hemoglobin level within the goal range. The American Heart Association recommends people with or at risk of heart disease consume 1 g of EPA and DHA per day, but people on dialysis may need as much as 2 g daily (Vergili, 2007). Because omega-3 fatty acids decrease platelet aggregation, clients should talk to their physician before using them, especially if they are taking anticoagulants. Fish oil supplements should be stored in the refrigerator to prevent rancidity.

▶ CASE STUDY

Dorothea is a 72-year-old black woman who is 5 ft. 5 in. tall and weighs 149 pounds. She has coronary heart disease and a long-standing history of hypertension with progressive loss of kidney function. She recently started receiving hemodialysis and is gaining about 4 pounds between treatments. She has convinced herself that because she is on dialysis, she can eat and drink whatever she wants and "the machine will take care of it."

Yesterday she ate the following:

| **Breakfast:** | Grits with cheese |
| | Bacon |
| | Biscuit with butter |
| | Coffee |
| **Lunch:** | Hamburger on bun with ketchup and mustard |
| | Potato chips |
| | Banana |
| | Sweetened tea |
| **Dinner:** | Fried chicken |
| | Macaroni and cheese |
| | Collard greens |
| | Pound cake |
| | Sweetened tea |

- What risk factors does Dorothea have for CKD?
- Based on her age, weight, and use of hemodialysis, what should the composition of her diet be (e.g., number of calories, grams of protein, gram of sodium)?
- Why is she gaining 4 pounds between treatments? What is a more reasonable goal? What would you suggest she do to achieve the goal?
- Evaluate her protein intake and recommend changes she could make to achieve her protein goals.
- What foods is she eating that are not heart healthy? What substitutions would you recommend?
- Evaluate her sodium intake and recommend changes she could make to limit her sodium intake.
- What foods is she eating that are high in potassium? What alternatives would you suggest?
- What foods is she eating that are high in phosphorus? Is her calcium intake adequate?
- What would you tell Dorothea about the use of dialysis and her theory about eating anything she wants?
- Which is the lesser risk: getting enough calories and protein by eating non–heart healthy foods or adhering to the sodium and other restrictions but not getting enough calories and protein?

1. Which statement indicates the patient needs further instruction about diet for nephrotic syndrome?
   a. "I know I need to eat a high-protein diet to replace the protein lost in urine."
   b. "I need to limit my intake of saturated fat and cholesterol."
   c. "I should not use salt in cooking or at the table, and avoid foods high in sodium such as processed foods, fast foods, convenience foods, condiments, and canned meat and vegetables."
   d. "I am going to try substituting soy protein for animal sources of protein because it may be better for me."

2. The client with stage 4 CKD asks if it is okay that she saves all her meat allowance for her evening meal. Which of the following would be the nurse's best response?
   a. "You cannot have any meat on a stage 4 diet."
   b. "It doesn't matter when you eat your meat allowance, so if you prefer to save it all for dinner, that is fine."
   c. "If you want to eat your meat allowance all at one time, it would be better to eat it for breakfast so that your body has all day to metabolize it."
   d. "It is best if you spread your meat allowance out over the whole day."

3. When developing a teaching plan for a client who in on dialysis, which of the following protein sources would the nurse suggest for a client who must also limit her intake of phosphorus?
   a. Beef
   b. Cheese
   c. Tofu
   d. Kidney beans

4. The nurse knows her instructions about preventing future calcium oxalate stones have been effective when the client verbalizes he should:
   a. Avoid milk, cheese, and other sources of calcium
   b. Take megadoses of vitamin C
   c. Avoid draft beer, beans, berries, chocolate, and other high-oxalate foods
   d. Eat a high-protein diet

5. How do the protein recommendations for chronic kidney disease differ from those for diabetic kidney disease?
   a. Protein is more restricted for chronic kidney disease than for diabetic kidney disease.
   b. Protein is more restricted for diabetic kidney disease than for chronic kidney disease.
   c. The protein recommendations are the same for chronic kidney disease and diabetic kidney disease.
   d. There are no specific protein recommendations for diabetic kidney disease because carbohydrates and fat are the priority concerns.

6. A client on hemodialysis asks if she can use popsicles to help relieve her thirst. Which of the following is the nurses' best response?
   a. "That's a great idea as long as you deduct the equivalent amount of fluid from your total daily fluid allowance."
   b. "Popsicles are empty calories. You are better off drinking just plain water."
   c. "Popsicles are great at relieving thirst, and because they are solid, they do not count as fluid so you can eat them as desired."
   d. "Hot things are better at relieving thirst than cold things. Try small amounts of hot tea or coffee to relieve your thirst."

**7.** One of the factors that influence protein allowance during acute renal failure is the individual's:
   **a.** Level of activity
   **b.** Degree of catabolism
   **c.** Blood pressure
   **d.** Serum albumin concentration

**8.** The client asks if she will need to follow a diet after she recovers from her kidney transplant. Which of the following is the nurses' best response?
   **a.** "You will always have to limit protein and phosphorus intake to help preserve the health of the new kidney."
   **b.** "After recovery, all restrictions are lifted and you can eat anything you want."
   **c.** "You may need to modify some aspects of your diet because of side effects from the medications you will be taking, and you should continue to eat a heart healthy diet to decrease the risks of diabetes, hypertension, heart disease, and obesity."
   **d.** "All the restrictions you followed before dialysis will resume after you recover from the transplant."

## KEY CONCEPTS

- Loss of renal function profoundly affects metabolism, nutritional status, and nutritional requirements. The nutrients most affected are protein, calcium, phosphorus, vitamin D, fluid, sodium, and potassium.

- People with nephrotic syndrome lose protein, mostly albumin, in the urine. Hypoalbuminemia and hyperlipidemia are other characteristics. Protein intake should be limited to 0.8 to 1.0, an amount consistent with the RDA for protein, to minimize protein loss in the urine. Sodium intake is limited; a fluid restriction is usually not necessary.

- Diet modifications for CKD are complex, unpalatable, and frequently adjusted according to the client's laboratory values and symptoms.

- Protein restriction remains the cornerstone of nutrition therapy for stages 1 to 4 of CKD because limiting protein has the potential to lessen renal workload and slow disease progression.

- There is a narrow margin of error regarding protein intake: too little protein results in body protein catabolism, which has the same effect as eating too much protein, namely, an increase in BUN and creatinine levels.

- A high-calorie diet is indicated whenever protein intake is restricted to ensure that the protein consumed will be used for specific protein functions, not for energy requirements.

- Usually clients with stages 1 to 4 CKD need to limit phosphorus and, if blood pressure is a problem, sodium. Potassium and fluid are usually not restricted.

- Calcium metabolism is impaired because of faulty vitamin D metabolism, impaired intestinal absorption, and hyperphosphatemia as a result of loss of renal function. A high calcium intake from food is not achievable when phosphorus is restricted.

- When dialysis is instituted, a high protein intake is recommended to compensate for protein lost through the dialysate. Calories need to be adequate to spare protein.

- People on hemodialysis generally have more severe restrictions (e.g., fluid, sodium, potassium) than people on peritoneal dialysis.

- Clients who experience renal transplantation may need to alter their diets to lessen the side effects of immunosuppressant therapy. They should commit to a lifestyle of healthy eating to reduce the risk of diabetes, hypertension, obesity, and heart disease.

- ARF represents an even greater nutritional challenge than CKD. Protein, sodium, potassium, phosphorus, and fluid are adjusted according to laboratory data, use of dialysis, renal function, and degree of catabolism.

- Clients with a history of calcium oxalate kidney stones should consume 3 to 4 quarts of fluid daily, avoid megadoses of vitamin C, eat a normal calcium intake spread out over the day, and avoid foods high in oxalate.

## ANSWER KEY

1. **TRUE** Early in the course of chronic kidney disease, limiting protein may help to preserve kidney function, but there are no guarantees and the optimal level of protein intake is not known.

2. **TRUE** Foods high in protein tend to be high in phosphorus. Other high-phosphorus foods include cola, chocolate, beer, bran, and bran cereal.

3. **FALSE** Although milk is an excellent source of high–biologic value protein, it is high in phosphorus and so it can only be consumed in limited amounts (½ cup/day).

4. **FALSE** Some people with advanced kidney failure are unable to conserve sodium, and a sodium deficit may occur if sodium intake is restricted.

5. **TRUE** People with chronic renal disease tend to have accelerated atherosclerosis and may benefit from eating a heart healthy diet–namely, less saturated fat, cholesterol, and trans fat.

6. **TRUE** Dialysis causes protein requirements to increase about 50% above normal because proteins and amino acids are lost in the dialysis.

7. **TRUE** People receiving peritoneal dialysis may absorb 100 to 200 g of glucose from the dialysate, which is 340 to 680 calories.

8. **FALSE** Weight gain between dialysis treatments reflects fluid retention. Excessive weight gain between dialysis treatments means the intake of sodium and fluid is too high, not that calorie intake is too high.

9. **FALSE** Most people with hypercalciuria should consume a normal calcium intake. Restricting calcium intake does not decrease the risk of calcium stones because it increases urinary oxalate concentration.

10. **FALSE** No single component of nutrition therapy, including increasing fluids, can effectively prevent kidney stones from forming.

## WEBSITES

American Association of Kidney Patients at **www.aakp.org**
American Kidney Fund at **www.kidneyfund.org**
National Institute of Diabetes and Digestive and Kidney Diseases at **www.niddk.nih.gov**
National Kidney and Urologic Diseases Information Clearinghouse (NKUDIC)
    at **http://kidney.niddk.nih.gov**
National Kidney Foundation at **www.kidney.org**
Nephron Information Center at **www.nephron.com**
**www.ikidney.com**
Oxalosis and Hyperoxaluria Foundation at **www.ohf.org**

## REFERENCES

Beto, J., & Bansal, V. (2004). Medical nutrition therapy in chronic kidney failure: Integrating clinical practice guidelines. *Journal of the American Dietetic Association, 104*, 404–409.

Burrowes, J. (2008). New recommendations for the management of diabetic kidney disease. *Nutrition Today, 43*, 65–69.

Centers for Disease Control (CDC). (2007). Prevalence of chronic kidney disease and associated risk factors—United States, 1999–2004. *Morbidity and Mortality Weekly Report, 56*(08), 161–165. Available at http://www.cdc.gov/MMWR/preview/mmwrhtml/mm5608a2.htm. Accessed on 8/7/08.

Chai, W., Liebman, M., Kynast-Gales, S., et al. (2004). Oxalate absorption and endogenous oxalate synthesis from ascorbate in calcium oxalate stone formers and in non-stone formers. *American Journal of Kidney Diseases, 44*, 1060–1069.

Kopple, J. (2006). Nutrition, diet, and the kidney. In M. Shils, M. Shike, A. Ross, et al. (Eds.), *Modern Nutrition in Health and Disease.* Philadelphia: Lippincott Williams & Wilkins.

Levey, A. S., Adler, S., Caggiula, A. W., et al. For the Modification of Diet in Renal Disease Study Group. (1996). Effects of dietary protein restriction on the progression of advanced renal disease in the Modification of Diet in Renal Disease Study. *American Journal of Kidney Diseases, 27*, 652–663.

Marcason, W. (2006). Where can I find information on the oxalate content of foods? *Journal of the American Dietetic Association, 106*, 627–628.

Marcason, W. (2008). What does the term "diabetic kidney disease" mean and what is the dietary intervention? *Journal of the American Dietetic Association, 108*, 1268.

Mendonca, C. O. G., Martini, L. A., Baxman, A. C., et al. (2003). Effects of oxalate load on urinary oxalate excretion in calcium stone formers. *Journal of Renal Nutrition, 13*, 39–46.

National Center for Health Statistics (NCHS). (2008). *Fast stats: Kidney disease.* Available at http://www.cdc.gov/nchs/fastats/kidbladd.htm. Accessed on 8/5/08.

National Kidney Foundation (NKF). (2000). K/DOQI Clinical practice guidelines for nutrition in chronic renal failure. *American Journal of Kidney Diseases, 35*(6), S1–S104.

National Kidney Foundation (NKF). (2002). K/DOQI Clinical practice guidelines for chronic kidney disease: Evaluation, classification, and stratification. *American Journal of Kidney Diseases, 39*(Suppl. 1), S1–S75.

National Kidney Foundation (NKF). (2003). K/DOQI Clinical practice guidelines for managing bone metabolism in chronic kidney disease. *American Journal of Kidney Diseases, 42*(Suppl. 1), S1–S92.

National Kidney Foundation (NKF). (2007). *KDOQI clinical practice guidelines and clinical practice recommendations for diabetes and chronic kidney disease.* Available at http://www.kidney.org/professionals/KDOQI/guideline_diabetes/pdf/guidelineRevDiabetesFull.pdf. Accessed on 8/4/08.

Reynolds, T. (2005). ACP Best Practice No. 181: Chemical pathology clinical investigation and management of nephrolithiasis. *American Journal of Clinical Pathology, 58*, 134–140.

Seiner, R., Ebert, D., Nicolay, C., et al. (2003). Dietary risk factors for hyperoxaluria in calcium oxalate stone formers. *International Society of Nephrology, 63*, 1037–1043.

Velasquez, M., & Bhathena, S. (2001). Dietary phytoestrogens: A possible role in renal disease protection. *American Journal of Kidney Diseases, 37*(5), 1056–1068.

Vergili, J. (2007). *Are fish oil supplements right for you?* Kidney Times. Available at http://www.kidneytimes.com/article.php?id=20071015191039. Accessed on 8/6/08.

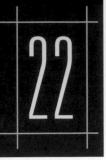

# 22

# Nutrition for Patients with Cancer or HIV/AIDS

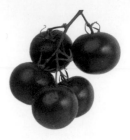

| TRUE | FALSE | |
|---|---|---|
| ☐ | ☐ | **1** People who are obese are at increased risk of several types of cancer. |
| ☐ | ☐ | **2** Weight loss is an indicator of poor prognosis in people with cancer. |
| ☐ | ☐ | **3** Clients who are adequately nourished may be better able to withstand the effects of cancer treatment. |
| ☐ | ☐ | **4** Cachexia is directly related to the amount of calories consumed. |
| ☐ | ☐ | **5** The appetite of clients with anorexia tends to improve as the day progresses. |
| ☐ | ☐ | **6** Cancer survivors are urged to follow diet recommendations to reduce the risk of cancer in the future. |
| ☐ | ☐ | **7** Lipodystrophy can be prevented with a low-fat diet. |
| ☐ | ☐ | **8** Clients with HIV who are experiencing malabsorption always have diarrhea. |
| ☐ | ☐ | **9** Clients with HIV/AIDS have problems with appetite and intake similar to those of cancer clients. |
| ☐ | ☐ | **10** Nutritional counseling of clients with HIV/AIDS should include how to avoid foodborne illnesses. |

## UPON COMPLETION OF THIS CHAPTER, YOU WILL BE ABLE TO

- Evaluate a person's usual diet according to dietary recommendations to reduce the risk of cancer.
- Summarize how cancer and cancer therapies affect nutritional status.
- Give examples of ways to modify the diet to alleviate side effects of anorexia, nausea, fatigue, taste changes, mouth sores, dry mouth, and diarrhea.
- Discuss three ways to increase a client's calorie and protein intake.
- Calculate the calorie and protein requirements of a patient with cancer based on clinical status and weight.
- Explain how HIV/AIDS affects nutritional status.
- Compare cancer cachexia with HIV-related wasting.
- Teach a person living with HIV/AIDS guidelines for a healthy diet.

ancer and HIV/AIDS can cause devastating weight loss and malnutrition. Although nutrition therapy cannot cure either disease, it has the potential to maximize the effectiveness of drug therapy, alleviate the side effects of the disease and its treatments, and improve overall quality of life.

# ► CANCER

Cancer, the second leading cause of death in the United States (CDC, 2008), is a group name for more than 100 different diseases characterized by the uncontrolled growth of cells. Individual cancers differ in where they develop, how quickly they grow, the type of treatment they respond to, and how much they impact nutritional status.

The relationship between nutrition and cancer is multifaceted:

- Nutrition may play a role in cancer prevention. As many as one-third of all cancer deaths are related to dietary factors (WCRF, AICR, 2007), such as eating substances that may promote cancer or failing to eat foods that may protect against cancer. The general population as well as cancer survivors are urged to follow dietary recommendations to reduce the risk of cancer.
- Nutrient intake or utilization can be impaired from the local effects of tumors, particularly those of the gastrointestinal (GI) tract. For instance, head and neck cancers can interfere with swallowing.
- Nutrient utilization can be altered from tumor-induced changes in metabolism. It is possible for people with cancer to eat an adequate calorie intake and still lose weight because of altered nutrient absorption or metabolism.
- Nutrient intake, absorption, or need can be impacted by cancer treatments. While some effects may be relatively short term, such as the increased need for protein and calories to heal from surgery, others may be more long lasting, such as altered sense of taste, which may persist for months after radiation to the head and neck area is completed.
- Nutrition therapy during the course of cancer treatment may improve tolerance to treatment, enhance immune function, aid in recovery, and maximize quality of life.
- Palliative nutrition for terminally ill patients with cancer may improve quality of life and enhance well-being.

## Nutrition in Cancer Prevention and Promotion

The *Second Expert Report on Food, Nutrition, Physical Activity, and the Prevention of Cancer* is the culmination of 5 years of rigorous and thorough review of the literature on diet and cancer (WCRF, AICR, 2007). Contained within the report are the overriding guidelines to maintain a healthy weight, be physically active, and eat a mostly plant-based diet. A more detailed set of practical recommendations focuses on an overall eating pattern to reduce the risk of cancer (Box 22.1). Table 8.2 (Chapter 8) outlines the American Cancer Society's dietary recommendations to reduce the risk of cancer.

Some of the strongest links to cancer risk are excess body weight and physical inactivity. The Report found convincing evidence that higher body fatness increase the risk of cancer of the esophagus, colon/rectum, postmenopausal breast, endometrium, and kidney (WCRF, AICR, 2007). The evidence that colorectal cancer is related to abdominal obesity is also convincing (WCRF, AICR, 2007). There are a few possible mechanisms by which fat may increase cancer risk: by increasing hormones that promote cancer cell growth; by promoting insulin resistance and hyperinsulinism, which increases the risk of certain cancers; or by promoting low levels of chronic inflammation which can promote cancer cell growth and development (WCRF, AICR, 2007). Physical activity on its own appears to protect against colon cancer and probably postmenopausal breast and endometrial cancers (WCRF, AICR, 2007). Physical activity provides an added benefit of helping avoid excess body weight. The connection between weight and cancer risk is so strong that the Report lists a public health goal of maintaining body mass index (BMI) between 21 and 23, even though the "healthy" range extends to 24.9.

| BOX 22.1 | AMERICAN INSTITUTE FOR CANCER RESEARCH RECOMMENDATIONS FOR CANCER PREVENTION |
|---|---|

- Be as lean as possible without becoming underweight.
- Be physically active for at least 30 minutes every day.
- Avoid sugary drinks. Limit consumption of energy-dense foods, particularly processed foods that are high in added sugar, low in fiber, or high in fat.
- Eat more of a variety of vegetables, fruits, whole grains, and legumes such as beans.
- Limit consumption of red meats, such as beef, pork, and lamb. Avoid processed meats.
- If consumed at all, limit alcohol to 2 drinks/day for men and 1 drink/day for women.
- Limit consumption of foods high in salt.
- Don't use supplements to protect against cancer.

Additionally,

- Exclusive breast feeding for up to 6 months is recommended.
- Cancer survivors should follow these guidelines after treatment is completed.
- Do not smoke or chew tobacco.

## The Impact of Cancer on Nutrition

Cancer impacts nutrition through local effects caused by the tumor and by altering metabolism. It has been shown that at the time of diagnosis, 80% of patients with upper GI cancer and 60% of patients with lung cancer have already experienced significant weight loss, defined as more than or equal to 10% of body weight in 6 months (NCI, 2008a, b). Weight loss is an indicator of poor prognosis in people with cancer.

### Local Tumor Effects

Local tumor effects occur when the tumor impinges on surrounding tissue, impairing its ability to function. The effects vary with the site and size of the tumor and are most likely to impact nutrition when the GI tract is involved (Table 22.1). GI obstruction can cause anorexia, dysphagia, early satiety, nausea, vomiting, pain, or diarrhea, leading to weight loss and malnutrition.

| TABLE 22.1 | Potential Local Effects of Cancer on Nutrition |
|---|---|

| Site | Potential Effects |
|---|---|
| Brain/CNS | Eating disabilities<br>Chewing and swallowing difficulties |
| Head and neck | Difficulty in chewing and swallowing |
| Esophagus | Dysphagia related to obstruction<br>Gastroesophageal reflux disease |
| Stomach | Early satiety, nausea, vomiting<br>Impaired motility<br>Obstruction which may necessitate tube feeding or TPN |
| Bowel | Maldigestion and malabsorption<br>Obstruction which may necessitate tube feeding or TPN |
| Liver | Watery diarrhea related to an increase in serotonin, histamines, and other substances |
| Pancreas | Maldigestion and malabsorption<br>Diabetes |

| BOX 22.2 | CATEGORIES OF MEDICATIONS THAT MAY HELP MANAGE SYMPTOMS TO IMPROVE INTAKE AND WEIGHT |
|---|---|

- Prokinetic or antiemetic agents to prevent nausea and vomiting
- Antidiarrheals to control diarrhea
- Pancreatic enzymes to improve nutrient digestion
- Bulk-forming agents or stool softeners to ease constipation
- Saliva stimulants for dry mouth
- Topical oral anesthetics for mouth pain
- Pain medications for pain relief

*Source:* NCI. (2008). *Nutrition in cancer care (PDQ).* Available at http://www.cancer.gov/cancertopics/pdq/supportivecare/nutrition/healthprofessional/allpages. Accessed on 8/14/08.

## Metabolic Changes

Tumors can induce changes in metabolism that alter the body's use of fuels and promote loss of lean body mass and weight (NCI, 2008a, b). Metabolic alterations may include glucose intolerance and insulin resistance, increased energy expenditure, increased body protein turnover, reduced muscle protein synthesis, and accelerated fat breakdown. Hormone-like substances produced by the tumor can alter nutrient absorption and metabolism. People with solid tumors of the lung, pancreas, and upper GI tract are more susceptible to tumor-induced weight loss than are people with breast cancer or cancer of the lower GI tract (NCI, 2008a, b).

Changes in metabolism can also be attributed to the body's response to cancer. Immune cells involved in the inflammatory response cause an increase in metabolism and protein catabolism. Calories and nutrients are diverted from fueling the body to supporting the growth of the tumor. Nutrient requirements are high but availability may be low.

## Anorexia

Anorexia is a common symptom in people with cancer and a contributing factor to weight loss and malnutrition. Anorexia, which may be intermittent or continuous, tends to be multifactorial. Potential causes include pain, depression/anxiety, early satiety, fatigue, nausea, and vomiting. Cancer treatments may contribute to anorexia by causing taste alterations, loss of taste, sore mouth, dry mouth, thick saliva, esophagitis, and fatigue. Modifications in texture, temperature, and eating schedule, as well as administering medications to control side effects, may optimize intake (Box 22.2).

## Cachexia

**Cachexia:** a wasting syndrome marked by weakness and progressive loss of body weight, fat, and muscle.

**Wasting:** generally described as an unintentional loss of more than 10% of body weight.

**Lean Body Mass:** the weight of the body minus the weight of fat.

Cancer **cachexia** is a progressive **wasting** syndrome characterized by anorexia, fatigue, with preferential loss of **lean body mass** and weight loss (NCI, 2008a, b). Although altered metabolism and anorexia are involved, the etiology of cancer cachexia is not completely understood. It appears to be unrelated to tumor size, type, or extent and occurs in both metastatic cancer and localized disease (NCI, 2008a, b). Cachexia is estimated to be present in 80% of cancer deaths (Nelson, 2000).

Once wasting and weight loss begin, they are hard to reverse. Medications may be used to stimulate appetite and promote weight gain, depending on the client's wishes, medical condition, and life expectancy (Table 22.2). Nutrition therapy, aimed at preserving lean muscle mass and fat stores, improves quality of life but does not guarantee increased length of survival (NCI, 2008a, b).

| TABLE 22.2 | Drugs Commonly Used to Stimulate Appetite and Promote Weight Gain in People with Cancer | | |
|---|---|---|---|
| **Drug Category** | **Common Drugs Used** | **Comments** | |
| Progestational agents | Megestrol acetate Medroxyprogesterone | Appetite stimulant activity and weight gain with use, but weight gain is from an increase in fat stores, not lean body tissue | |
| Glucocorticoids | Dexamethasone Methylprednisolone Prednisolone | Stimulate appetite. Studies show positive but short-term effects on appetite and quality of life but minimal or no effect on weight gain. Risks limit suitability for long-term use | |
| Cannabinoids | Dronabinol | Inconsistent evidence of effectiveness. Has not been shown superior benefit in promoting weight gain and appetite | |
| Antihistamines | Cyproheptadine | Not well studied in cancer patients. Side effect of sedation may limit usefulness | |
| Antidepressants/ antipsychotics | Mirtazapine Olanzapine | Clinical data supporting routine use are lacking | |
| Antiimflammatory agents | Thalidomide Pentoxifylline Melatonin Omega-3 fatty acids (EPA) | Mixed results regarding weight gain and appetite stimulation in clinical trials | |
| Metabolic inhibitors | Hydrazine sulfate | Not approved by the FDA for marketing in the United States | |
| Anabolic agents | Oxandrolone Nandrolone Decanoate Fluoxymesterone | Limited reports of successful appetite stimulation in cancer patients | |

*Source:* National Cancer Institute (NCI). (2008). *Nutrition in cancer care (PDQ).* Available at http://www.cancer.gov. Accessed on 8/11/08.

## The Impact of Cancer Treatments

Cancer treatments include surgery, chemotherapy, radiation, immunotherapy, hemopoietic and stem cell transplantation, or a combination of therapies. Each treatment modality can contribute to progressive nutritional deterioration related to localized or systemic side effects that interfere with intake, increase nutrient losses, or alter metabolism. Nutritional therapy, used as an adjuvant to effective cancer therapy, helps to sustain the client through adverse side effects and may reduce morbidity and mortality. Conversely, inadequate nutrition can contribute to the incidence and severity of treatment side effects and increase the risk of infection, thereby reducing the chance for survival (Vigano et al., 1994).

### Surgery

Surgery is often the primary treatment for cancer; approximately 60% of people diagnosed with cancer undergo some type of cancer-related surgery (ACS, 2007). People who are malnourished prior to surgery are at higher risk of morbidity and mortality. If time allows, nutritional deficiencies are corrected before surgery.

Postsurgical nutritional requirements increase for protein, calories, vitamin C, B vitamins, and iron to replenish losses and promote healing. Physiological or mechanical barriers

| TABLE 22.3 | Potential Complications of Surgery |
| --- | --- |
| **Type** | **Potential Complications** |
| Head and neck resection | Impaired ability to speak, chew, salivate, swallow, smell, taste, and/or see<br>Tube feeding dependency |
| Esophagectomy or esophageal resection | Early satiety<br>Regurgitation<br>Fistula formation<br>Stenosis<br>Vagotomy→decreased stomach motility, decreased gastric acid production, diarrhea, steatorrhea |
| Gastric resection | "Dumping syndrome": crampy diarrhea that develops quickly after eating; accompanied by flushing, dizziness, weakness, pain, distention, and vomiting<br>Hypoglycemia<br>Esophagitis<br>Decreased gastric motility<br>Fat malabsorption and diarrhea<br>Deficiencies in iron, calcium, and fat-soluble vitamins<br>Vitamin $B_{12}$ malabsorption related to lack of intrinsic factor |
| Intestinal resection | Malnutrition related to generalized malabsorption<br>Fluid and electrolyte imbalance<br>Diarrhea<br>Increased risk of renal oxalate stone formation and increased excretion of calcium<br>Metabolic acidosis |
| Massive bowel resection | Steatorrhea<br>Malnutrition related to severe generalized malabsorption<br>Metabolic acidosis<br>Dehydration |
| Ileostomy or colostomy<br>Pancreatic resection | Fluid and electrolyte imbalance<br>Generalized malabsorption<br>Diabetes mellitus |

to good nutrition can occur depending on the type of surgery, with the greatest likelihood of complications arising from GI surgeries. Table 22.3 outlines potential side effects and complications incurred for various types of surgery.

## Chemotherapy

More than 90 different chemotherapy drugs are approved for use in the United States (NCI, 2008a, b). Given alone or in combination, chemotherapy drugs damage the reproductive ability of both malignant and normal cells, especially rapidly dividing cells such as well-nourished cancer cells and normal cells of the GI tract, respiratory system, bone marrow, skin, and gonadal tissue. Cyclic administration of multiple drugs is given in maximum tolerated doses.

The side effects of chemotherapy vary with the type of drug or combination of drugs used, dose, rate of excretion, duration of treatment, and individual tolerance. Chemotherapy side effects are systemic and, therefore, potentially more numerous than the localized effects seen with surgery or radiation. The most commonly experienced nutrition-related side effects are anorexia, nausea and vomiting, taste alterations, sore mouth or throat, diarrhea, early satiety, and constipation (NCI, 2008a, b). Side effects increase the risk of malnutrition and

| TABLE 22.4 | **Potential Complications of Radiation** |
|---|---|
| **Area** | **Potential Complications** |
| Head and neck | Altered or loss of taste (mouth blindness)<br>Xerostomia (dry mouth)<br>Thick salivary secretions<br>Difficulty swallowing and chewing<br>Loss of teeth<br>Mucositis<br>Stomatitis |
| Lower neck and midchest | Acute: esophagitis with dysphagia<br>Delayed: fibrosis, esophageal stricture, dysphagia<br>Nausea<br>Edema |
| Abdomen and pelvis | Acute or chronic bowel damage can cause diarrhea, nausea, vomiting, enteritis, and malabsorption<br>Bowel constriction, obstruction, or fistula formation<br>Chronic blood loss from intestine and bladder<br>Pelvic radiation can cause increased urinary frequency, urgency, and dysuria |
| CNS | Nausea<br>Dysgeusia |

weight loss, which may prolong recovery time between treatments. When subsequent chemotherapy treatments are delayed, successful treatment outcome is potentially threatened.

## Radiation

Radiation causes cell death; particles of radioactive energy break chemical bonds, disrupting reproductive ability. Although radiation injures all rapidly dividing cells, it is most lethal for the poorly differentiated and rapidly proliferating cells of cancer tissue. Recovery from sublethal doses of radiation occurs in the interval between the first dose and subsequent doses. Normal tissue appears to recover more quickly from radiation damage than cancerous tissue does.

The type and intensity of radiation side effects depend on the type of radiation used, the site, the volume of tissue irradiated, the dose of radiation, the duration of therapy, and individual tolerance. Patients most at risk for nutrition-related side effects are those who have cancers of the head and neck, lungs, esophagus, cervix, uterus, colon, rectum, and pancreas (Table 22.4). Side effects usually develop around the second or third week of treatment and then diminish 2 or 3 weeks after radiation therapy is completed. Some side effects may be chronic. Managing side effects helps improve intake and quality of life.

## Immunotherapy

Immunotherapy seeks to enhance the body's immune system to help control cancer. The most common side effects include fever, which increases protein and calorie requirements, and nausea, vomiting, diarrhea, and fatigue. Left untreated, symptoms can cause weight loss and malnutrition, which impedes recovery.

## Hemopoietic and Peripheral Blood Stem Cell Transplantation

Hemopoietic and stem cell transplants are preceded by high-dose chemotherapy and possibly total-body irradiation to suppress immune function and destroy cancer cells.

| BOX 22.3 | STRATEGIES TO REDUCE THE RISK OF FOODBORNE ILLNESS |
|---|---|

- Wash hands before and after handling food and eating and after using the restroom.
- Cook all meat, fish, and poultry to the well-done stage.
- Do not eat raw or undercooked eggs such as soft boiled eggs, "over easy" eggs, or Caesar salads with raw eggs in the dressing.
- Do not eat sushi, raw seafood, raw meats, or unpasteurized milk or dairy products.
- Do not drink water unless it is known to be safe.
- Refrigerate foods immediately after purchase.
- Avoid cross-contamination by using separate cutting boards and work surfaces for raw meats and poultry; keep work surfaces clean.
- Wash fruits and vegetables thoroughly in clean water.
- Do not use moldly or damaged fruits and vegetables.
- Thaw food in the refrigerator, never at room temperature.
- If the microwave is used to thaw frozen meat, cook the meat immediately after it is defrosted.
- Refrigerate leftovers immediately after eating; thoroughly reheat before eating.
- Discard leftovers after 3 days.
- Keep hot foods >140° F and cold food <40° F.
- Use expiration dates on food packaging to discard foods that may be unsafe to eat.
- Avoid salad bars and buffets when eating out.

Nutritional side effects arise from high-dose chemotherapy, total body irradiation, and immunosuppressant medications, which are given before and after the procedure. Anorexia, taste alterations, nausea, vomiting, dry mouth, thick saliva, constipation, stomatitis, esophagitis, and intestinal damage that causes severe diarrhea and malabsorption may occur. Total parenteral nutrition (TPN) may be needed for 1 to 2 months after bone marrow transplantation.

When an oral diet resumes, a liquid diet restricted in lactose, fiber, and fat is given to minimize malabsorption and improve tolerance. Solid foods are gradually reintroduced. **Neutropenia** leaves the patient susceptible to infection, so precautionary measures must be taken to prevent foodborne illness (Box 22.3). Initially, most fresh fruit and vegetables and ground meats may be excluded to reduce the risk of foodborne illness. A high-protein, high-calorie, high-calcium diet is needed to counter the negative nitrogen and calcium balances caused by immunosuppressant medications.

**Neutropenia:** abnormally low number of neutrophils in the blood, which increases the risk of infection.

## Nutrition Therapy during Cancer Treatment

The focus of nutrition therapy for people being treated for cancer is to prevent weight loss (even in overweight patients), maintain lean body mass, and prevent unintentional weight gain in certain groups of people, such as women treated for breast cancer (ADA, 2008). Adequate nutrition may improve tolerance to treatment, improve immunocompetence, promote wound healing, and improve quality of life.

A "typical" cancer client does not exist. Whereas some clients present with weight loss and malnutrition at the time of cancer diagnosis, others are well nourished and asymptomatic. The course of treatment may be aggressive or palliative; it may include surgery, chemotherapy, radiation, or a combination of treatments. The effect on nutritional status and intake may be mild or dramatic. Nutrition intake and status should be routinely monitored so nutrition therapy interventions can be adjusted accordingly.

| BOX 22.4 | CALORIE AND PROTEIN GUIDELINES COMMONLY USED FOR PEOPLE WITH CANCER |
|---|---|

| Calories | Protein |
|---|---|
| 25–30 cal/kg for nonambulatory or sedentary adults | 1.0–1.2 g/kg for nonstressed patients |
| 30–35 cal/kg for slightly hypermetabolic patients or for weight gain | 1.2–1.5 g/kg for patients undergoing treatment |
| 35 cal/kg for hypermetabolic or severely stressed patients or for people with malabsorption | 1.5–2.5 for patients with protein-losing enteropathies or wasting |

*Source:* American Dietetic Association (ADA). (2008). *Nutrition care manual.* Available at http://www.nutritioncaremanual.com. Accessed on 8/13/08.

## Nutrient Needs

There are no validated parameters for determining the nutrition needs of patients with cancer (ADA, 2008). Small frequent snacks may be better tolerated than three large meals. Nutritional formulas can supplement a regular diet or replace meals as needed. A regular diet is used as a starting point and individualized as needed.

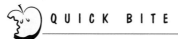 **QUICK BITE**

Selected high-calorie, high-protein, nutritional formulas

| | Calories (per 240 mL) | Proteins (g/240 mL) |
|---|---|---|
| Ensure High Protein | 230 | 12 |
| Boost | 240 | 10 |
| Boost High Protein | 240 | 15 |
| Carnation Instant Breakfast (made with 8 oz whole milk) | 300 | 12 |
| Ensure Plus | 360 | 13 |
| Carnation Instant Breakfast Plus | 375 | 12 |
| Resource Shake Plus | 480 | 15 |

## Calories and Protein

Commonly used calorie and protein guidelines are outlined in Box 22.4. Calories and protein are adjusted to meet the individual's needs. An increase in protein and calories can be achieved by having the client

- Eat more food, which is not a realistic option for most people experiencing anorexia, nausea, or other side effects of cancer or cancer treatments.
- Eat food that has been modified to be more protein- and calorie-dense. This approach can be effective if the client or caregiver understands how to increase the protein and calorie density of a variety of foods. Suggestions for increasing protein and calorie density appear in Box 22.5.
- Consume high-protein, high-calorie nutritional supplements, which may be the easiest and most consistent way to achieve a high-calorie, high-protein intake.
- A combination of the above.

| BOX 22.5 | **WAYS TO INCREASE THE PROTEIN AND CALORIE DENSITY OF FOODS** |
|---|---|

**To Increase Protein and Calories**
- Add skim milk powder to milk to make double-strength milk; chill well before serving.
- Use double-strength milk on hot or cold cereals and in scrambled eggs, soups, gravies, casseroles, milk shakes, and milk-based desserts.
- Substitute whole milk for water in recipes.
- Add grated cheese to soups, casseroles, vegetable dishes, rice, and noodles.
- Use peanut butter as a spread on slices of apple, banana, pear, crackers, or waffles; use as a filling for celery.
- Add finely chopped, hard-cooked eggs to sauces; add cream to soups and casseroles.
- Choose desserts made with eggs or milk such as sponge cake, angel food cake, custard, and puddings.
- Dip meat, poultry, and fish in eggs or milk and coat with bread or cereal crumbs before baking, broiling, or pan frying.
- Use yogurt as a topping for fruit, plain cakes, or other desserts; use in gravies and dips.

**To Increase Calories**
- Mix cream cheese with butter and spread on hot bread and rolls.
- Whenever possible, add butter to hot foods: breads, pancakes, waffles, soups, vegetables, potatoes, cooked cereal, rice, and pasta.
- Substitute mayonnaise for salad dressing in salads, eggs, casseroles, and sandwiches.
- Add dried fruit, nuts, or granola to desserts and cereal.
- Use whipped cream on pies, fruit pudding, gelatin, ice cream, and other desserts and in coffee, tea, and hot chocolate.
- Use marshmallows in hot chocolate, on fruits, and in desserts.
- Top baked potatoes, vegetables, and fruits with sour cream.
- Snack frequently on nuts, dried fruit, candy, buttered popcorn, cheese, granola, and ice cream.
- Use honey on toast, cereal, and fruit and in coffee and tea.

## Managing Nutrition-Related Symptoms

In a study of patients with advanced cancer, some degree of impairment in taste and/or smell was reported by 86% of patients and approximately 50% reported that the impairments interfered with their enjoyment of eating (NCI, 2008a, b). Patients may experience a decreased threshold for urea (bitter) and an increased threshold for sucrose (sweet), although these changes are not universal among all people with cancer (Schattner & Shike, 2006). Poor appetite, nausea, early satiety, and impairments in taste and smell often occur together and are significantly linked to decreased calorie intake (NCI, 2008a, b). Managing nutrition-related symptoms has the potential to improve calorie intake and maintain weight (Box 22.6).

## Enteral and Parenteral Nutrition Support

For both physiologic and psychological reasons, an oral diet is preferred whenever possible. When oral intake is inadequate or contraindicated, enteral or parenteral nutrition can nourish critically ill cancer patients. A client may be a candidate for nutrition support if one or more of the following criteria are met (NCI, 2008a, b):

- Weight of less than 80% of ideal or a recent unintentional weight loss of more than 10% of usual weight
- Malabsorption of nutrients related to disease, short bowel syndrome, or cancer treatments

| BOX 22.6 | **TIPS FOR MANAGING NUTRITION-RELATED PROBLEMS** |

**Anorexia**
- Overeat during "good" days.
- Eat a high-protein, high-calorie, nutrient-dense breakfast if appetite is best in the morning.
- Eat small, frequent, meals (e.g., every 2 hours by the clock).
- Add extra protein and calories to food.
- Eat nutrient-dense foods first.
- Limit liquids with meals to avoid early satiety and bloating at mealtime.
- Use nutrition formulas (instant breakfast mixes, milk shakes, commercial supplements) in place of meals when appetite deteriorates or the client is too tired to eat.
- Make eating a pleasant experience by eating in a bright, cheerful environment, playing soft music, and enjoying the company of friends or family.
- Avoid strong food odors if they contribute to anorexia. Cook outdoors on a grill, serve cold foods rather than hot foods, or use takeout meals that do not need to be prepared at home. In the hospital, the tray cover should be removed before the tray is placed in front of the client so that food odors can dissipate.

**Nausea**
- Eat frequently.
- Slowly sip fluids throughout the day.
- Eat foods served cold, such as chicken salad instead of hot baked chicken or deli roast beef instead of pot roast.
- Eat high-carbohydrate, low-fat easy to digest foods such as toast, crackers, yogurt, sherbet, cooked cereal, soft or canned fruits, watermelon, bananas, fruit juices, and angel food cake.
- Avoid fatty, greasy, fried, or strongly seasoned foods.
- Keep track of and avoid foods that cause nausea.
- Avoid eating 1 to 2 hours before chemotherapy or radiotherapy.
- Take antiemetics as prescribed even when symptoms are absent.

**Fatigue**
- Eat a hearty breakfast because fatigue may worsen as the day progresses.
- Engage in regular exercise if possible.
- Consume easy-to-eat foods that can be prepared with a minimal amount of effort, such as frozen dinners, take out foods, sandwiches, instant breakfast mixes, and liquid formulas, cheese and crackers, peanut butter on crackers, yogurt, and pudding.
- Enlist the help of friends and family to provide meals.

**Taste Changes**
- Use sugar-free lemon drops, gum, or mints to counter a metallic or bitter taste in the mouth.
- Brush your teeth or rinse with a mouthwash before eating.
- Eat small frequent meals.
- Use plastic utensils if food has a metallic taste.
- Experiment with tart foods such as citrus juices, cranberry juice, pickles, or relishes to help overcome metallic taste.
- Substitute poultry, eggs, cheese, and mild fish for beef and pork if they have a "bad," "rotten," or "fecal" taste.
- Add coffee to a sweet, milk-based beverage or buttermilk to a smoothie to cut sweetness.
- Avoid foods that are offensive; stick to those that taste good.
- Try new foods, such as lemon yogurt in place of strawberry.

| BOX 22.6 | **TIPS FOR MANAGING NUTRITION-RELATED PROBLEMS** (continued) |

### Sore Mouth (Stomatitis)
• Practice good oral hygiene (thorough cleaning with a soft-bristle toothbrush or cotton swabs plus frequent mouth rinses with normal saline and water or baking soda and water). Commercial mouthwashes containing alcohol may irritate and burn the oral mucosa.
• Eat soft, nonirritating foods that are easy to chew and swallow, such as bananas, applesauce, watermelon, canned fruit, cottage cheese, yogurt, mashed potatoes, macaroni and cheese, puddings, milkshakes, instant breakfast mixes, scrambled eggs, oatmeal, and other cooked cereals.
• Add gravy, broth, or sauces to increase the fluid content of foods, as appropriate.
• Cut food into small portions.
• Numb the mouth with frozen bananas, ice chips, ice cream, or popsicles.
• Avoid spices, acidic foods, coarse foods, salty foods, alcohol, and smoking that can aggravate an already irritated oral mucosa.
• Use a straw to drink liquids.
• Avoid wearing ill-fitting dentures.

### Xerostomia (Dry Mouth)
• Rinse mouth before eating.
• Drink fluids with meals and all day long.
• Eat moist foods softened with gravies or sauces. Casseroles and stews are easier to eat than baked or roasted meats.
• Avoid dry, coarse foods.
• Avoid foods that stick to the roof of the mouth such as peanut butter.
• Avoid sugary food and beverages that promote dental decay.
• Drink high-calorie, high-protein liquids between meals.
• Stimulate secretions with sugar-free fluids containing citric acid such as lemonade and popsicles.
• Use ice chips and sugar-free hard candies and gum between meals to relieve dryness.
• Use a straw to drink liquids.
• Apply a moisturizer to the lips to help prevent drying.
• Brush after every meal and snack.

### Diarrhea
• Replace fluid and electrolytes with broth, soups, sports drinks, and canned fruit.
• Drink at least 1 cup of liquid after each loose bowel movement.
• Limit caffeine, hot or cold liquids, and high-fat foods because they aggravate diarrhea.
• Avoid gassy foods and liquids such as dried peas and beans, cruciferous vegetables, carbonated beverages, and chewing gum.
• Try foods high in pectin and other soluble fibers to slow transit time, such as oatmeal, cooked carrots, bananas, peeled apples, and applesauce.
• Avoid sugar-free candy or gum containing sorbitol because it can contribute to osmotic diarrhea.
• Unless tolerance to lactose has been confirmed, limit or avoid milk.

• Fistulas or draining abscesses
• Inability to eat or drink for more than 5 days
• Moderate or high nutritional risk as determined by nutritional screening or assessment
• Client or caregiver demonstrate competency in nutrition support for discharge planning

Although enteral nutrition therapy may prevent or treat malnutrition in people with cancer, it is not routinely used in well-nourished patients undergoing chemotherapy or surgery.

| BOX 22.7 | SUPPORTIVE MEASURES FOR PALLIATIVE NUTRITION THERAPY |
| --- | --- |

- Control unpleasant side effects, such as pain, constipation, nausea, vomiting, and heartburn, with medication.
- Respect the client's wishes regarding the level of nutritional support desired.
- Provide adequate mouth care to control dryness and thirst.
- Respect the client's personal tastes and preferences.
- Ensure a pleasant eating environment and serve attractive food.
- Serve food of appropriate textures.
- Use a team approach that includes physician, dietitian, and nurse.

Data from randomized trials studying the efficacy of enteral nutrition for patients receiving chemotherapy for a variety of different cancers failed to show a clear benefit with regard to survival or response to treatment (Schattner & Shike, 2006). A notable exception is the routine use of enteral nutrition for patients undergoing chemoradiation to the head or neck. In this population, enteral nutrition has been shown to prevent dehydration and treatment interruptions resulting from an impaired oral intake related to mucositis (Schattner & Shike, 2006). For all other cases, the decision to use enteral nutrition is individualized and should be limited to malnourished patients with a functional GI tract who are unable to consume an adequate intake of nutrients orally.

Parenteral nutrition can be a lifesaving therapy because it can deliver nutrients to patients who have a nonfunctional GI tract. However, studies evaluating the use of parenteral nutrition in cancer patients have found no improvement in nutritional parameters with an increase in complications, especially infections (ADA, 2008). Yet parenteral nutrition may be appropriate for patients who are unable to tolerate oral or enteral feedings for more than 7 to 10 days, who need to improve their nutritional status before beginning chemotherapy or surgery, or who are undergoing bone marrow transplantation (Schattner & Shike, 2006).

## Palliative Nutrition Therapy

For clients with terminal cancer who are not being aggressively treated, nutrition therapy is an integral component of palliative care, with the goals of providing comfort and relieving side effects. Eating is encouraged as a source of pleasure, not as an adjunct to treatment. The client's requests and preferences are more important than the nutritional quality of the diet. Box 22.7 lists supportive measures for palliative nutrition therapy.

# ▶ NUTRITION AND IMMUNODEFICIENCY

Nutritional status and immunity are interrelated. The inflammatory, hormonal, and immune response to infection increases nutrient requirements, promotes loss of lean body tissue, and alters nutrient storage and availability (ADA, 2008). Conversely, nutrient deficiencies and sometimes excesses can impair immune system function and the ability to fight infection. Nutritional status, particularly maintaining body weight and protein stores, affects a person's ability to survive HIV disease (ADA, 2004).

## HIV-Associated Weight Loss and Wasting

When the AIDS epidemic began, severe malnutrition and weight loss were common. Despite major advances in the treatment and survival of people living with HIV and AIDS (PLHA), weight loss and wasting remain common problems and occur in people successfully treated

**Highly Active Antiretroviral Therapy (HAART):** a combination of antiretroviral therapy medications that are typically used to control and reduce viral load.

**Lipodystrophy:** also called fat redistribution syndrome; a condition characterized by changes in body shape (loss of subcutaneous fat in the limbs and face and fat accumulation in the abdomen and breast areas) and metabolism (increased resistance to insulin and abnormally high levels of blood cholesterol and triglycerides). Characteristics may occur separately or in any combination. Weight change is not always present.

with **highly active antiretroviral therapy (HAART)**, in people in whom HAART has failed, and in people who have not used HAART (Mangili et al., 2006). HAART has significantly improved morbidity and mortality related to HIV infection, but has not eliminated the issue of weight loss. The prevalence of weight loss and wasting are as common now as they were in 1997 (Tang et al., 2005).

HIV-associated wasting, an AIDS-defining condition (ADC), is defined by the CDC as unintentional weight loss more than 10% of baseline weight plus either diarrhea, fever, or weakness for more than or equal to 30 days in the absence of a concurrent illness (CDC, 1987). Shortcomings with this definition are that (1) it assumes that baseline weight, which may have been reported not measured, was the patient's usual or ideal weight and (2) the rate of weight loss is not considered (Mangili et al., 2006). Rapid or significant weight loss may be a risk even if BMI stays within the normal range (Mangili et al., 2006).

"Wasting" is a vague term referring to weight loss; it is not specific as to the type of weight lost. Body weight alone does not reveal changes in body composition, such as loss of lean body mass or **lipodystrophy**. Studies suggest that the type of weight loss in HIV-associated wasting varies with baseline body composition and that women may lose primarily fat, whereas men preferentially lose lean body mass until their body composition changes and then fat becomes preferentially lost (ADA, 2008). However, weight loss is a stronger predictor of death than loss of lean body mass and baseline BMI is important; people with a baseline BMI $\geq 25$ have a much lower risk of dying than those with a baseline BMI of $<25$, even though 25 is the beginning of the "overweight" range (Mangili et al., 2006).

Like cancer cachexia, the etiology of HIV-associated wasting is multifactorial and may be related to socioeconomic status, access to healthcare, cultural practices, psychological factors, and medical complications of and therapies for HIV infection (Mangili et al., 2006). Although the majority of weight loss currently seen in PLHA cannot be explained, impaired intake and altered metabolism may be at least partially responsible.

## Impaired Intake

Results from the Nutrition for Healthy Living Cohort study show that impaired intake among PLHA may be related to diet itself, GI symptoms, or malabsorption and GI dysfunction (Mangili et al., 2006). For instance:

- Men in the lowest CD4+ cell count percentile need the most calories per kilogram of body weight to maintain a lower BMI yet their total daily calorie intake was not different than that of men of similar age in the general population. This suggests that nutritional need is high and intake falls short.
- Episodes of acute weight loss, defined as more than or equal to 5% of body weight, were associated with oral symptoms and difficulty swallowing, but not anorexia. Even in the absence of an opportunistic infection, many people may have GI symptoms related to HIV infection or HIV medications that increase the risk of weight loss.
- Eighty eight percent of the cohort had at least one abnormality in GI function, such as malabsorption. Because malabsorption can occur in the absence of diarrhea, malabsorption cannot be excluded on the basis of normal bowel patterns alone. Uncorrected, malabsorption can lead to malnutrition, wasting, and impaired quality of life.
- In many cases, socioeconomic factors, not clinical factors, may be blamed for poor intake. Almost 8% of participants did not have access to adequate food.

## Changes in Metabolism

**Viral Load:** the level of virus or viral markers measured in the blood.

**Viral load** and HAART have been found to independently increase resting energy expenditure (REE), the amount of calories used to fuel the involuntary activities of the body (Roubenoff et al., 2002; Shevitz et al., 1999). This increase may account for weight loss and

**Cytokines:** a group name for more than 100 different proteins involved in immune responses; they are also critical for normal growth and development. Prolonged production of proinflammatory cytokines promotes hypercatabolism (hyper = excessive; catabolism = breaking down phase of metabolism).

wasting as well as changes in metabolism and body shape and occur in PLHA (Mangili et al., 2006). Opportunistic infections or malignancies may also contribute to altered metabolism and weight loss, although they are not the major cause of wasting in PLHA. Excessive production of **cytokines** has also been implicated in HIV associated weight loss.

## Nutrition Therapy

Nutrition therapy begins with an individualized assessment that determines the client's level of risk based on weight, weight change, changes in body composition, biochemical markers of malnutrition, clinical signs of malnutrition, dietary intake, and symptoms of HIV or side effects of treatment that impact intake or nutritional status. An individualized plan of care is designed that takes into account the client's socioeconomic, cultural, and ethnic background. Ideally, nutrition therapy begins before the client exhibits any symptoms of HIV disease even if intake appears adequate, because the effectiveness of nutrition therapy may be limited once the client is ill enough to need hospital care. Nutrition therapy for PLHA seeks to meet the client's nutrient needs, alleviate symptoms, and manage complications of the disease or medication intolerance.

## Nutrient Needs

Although scientific knowledge about the role of nutrition in HIV is incomplete, it is apparent that the nutrient needs of PLHA differ from those of noninfected people, even before the onset of symptoms (e.g., weight loss). There are no unanimously agreed upon recommendations for calories or nutrients despite the universal goals of maintaining body weight and lean body mass. Tips for healthy eating with HIV are outlined in Box 22.8.

**Calories.** Because REE increases in PLHA, the WHO recommends calorie intakes increase by 10% for asymptomatic clients so that body weight can be maintained (WHO, 2003). When HIV is symptomatic, calorie needs are estimated to increase by 20% to 30% above normal. Realistically, a high calorie intake may not be possible during periods of acute illness or infection so during the recovery period, clients should strive to consume 30% more calories than normal.

Calorie recommendations from HIV Research of the Nutrition Infection Unit at Tufts University School of Medicine are as follows (the "normal" healthy adult standard commonly used is 30 cal/kg) (Woods et al., 2008):

- 37 to 45 cal/kg if the client's weight is stable and there are no secondary infections
- 45 cal/kg if the client has an opportunistic infection
- 55 cal/kg if the client is losing weight

| BOX 22.8 | HEALTHY EATING TIPS FOR PATIENTS WITH HIV |
| --- | --- |

- Eat a diet rich in whole grains, vegetables, fruits, and legumes with lean sources of protein.
- Make at least half of all grain choices whole grains.
- Eat at least 3 cups/day of a variety of fruits and vegetables.
- Choose skinless poultry, fish, extra-lean cuts of pork and beef, and low-fat milk and dairy products.
- Avoid sweetened beverages and foods high in added sugar.
- Choose monounsaturated fats, such as nuts, seeds, canola oil, olive oil, and avocado.
- Avoid foods high in saturated fat, such as fatty meat, poultry skin, butter, whole milk dairy foods, and products made with coconut or palm oils.
- Eat some carbohydrate, protein, and fat at each meal and snack.

*Source:* Woods, M., Potts, E., & Connors, J. (2008). *Building a high-quality diet.* Available at http://www.tufts.edu/med/nutrition-infection/hiv/health_high_quality_diet.html. Accessed on 8/18/08.

**Protein.** PLHA may have increased protein requirements to maintain or build lean body mass. A protein intake of 1.2 to 2.0 g/kg is frequently recommended, although there are no data to support this recommendation. This recommendation translates to a rule-of-thumb guideline of 100 to 150 g/day for men and 80 to 100 g/day for women (Woods et al., 2008).

**Fat.** There is no evidence HIV/AIDS increases total fat requirements. A high saturated fat intake contributes to hypertriglyceridemia in PLHA who have lipid abnormalities (Joy et al., 2007). A low saturated fat diet, not a low total fat diet, is indicated (see "Metabolic Alterations of Lipodystrophy").

**Vitamins and Minerals.** Observational studies suggest that low blood levels and inadequate intakes of some vitamins and minerals are associated with faster HIV disease progression and mortality (WHO, 2003). Nutrient deficiencies may occur from poor intake, malabsorption, infections, or diet–medication interactions. Although food is the preferred source for nutrients, multivitamin and mineral supplements are usually recommended at levels of 100% to 200% of the Dietary Reference Intakes (DRI). Some evidence suggests that supplements of vitamin A, zinc, and iron can produce adverse outcomes in PLHA (WHO, 2003).

## Enteral and Parenteral Nutrition Support

Clients who are unable to consume an adequate oral intake may require tube feeding for supplemental or complete nutrition. The same guidelines for use apply in HIV as in other populations, with extra attention to ensure sanitary conditions (ADA, 2008). The use of sterile water may be necessary for patients who have severe immune function impairments. Parenteral nutrition is reserved for clients whose GI tract is nonfunctional. Hydrolyzed formulas consumed orally may be just as effective as parenteral nutrition (PN) in preventing weight loss in patients with severe malabsorption—with none of the risk associated with PN.

## Alleviate Symptoms

Clients with HIV/AIDS may experience problems with appetite and intake similar to those of cancer clients. Nutrition therapy recommendations in Box 22.6 for managing nutrition-related problems are appropriate for PLHA as well as for people with cancer. As in the case of cancer, nutritional formulas are frequently used because they tend to leave the stomach quickly, are easy to consume, and provide significant quantities of calories and protein. Small frequent feedings (e.g., six to nine times daily) are encouraged.

## Metabolic Alterations of Lipodystrophy

Lipodystrophy is not life threatening, but emotional distress caused by the significant changes in body shape and social stigmatization may cause clients to decrease or stop their antiretroviral therapies because they are believed to be involved in its cause. Some studies show that unless HIV-infected people with altered lipid levels have other risk factors for heart disease (e.g., hypertension, smoking, obesity), they are at no greater risk for heart attack than noninfected people (Kressy et al., 2008).

Nutrition therapy and exercise may help reverse some changes in body shape and improve the metabolic abnormalities of glucose intolerance, hypertriglyceridemia, and hypercholesterolemia (Kressy et al., 2008). A Mediterranean diet low in saturated fat, refined sugar, and alcohol, and high in fiber-rich whole grains, vegetables, and fruit may help to improve lipoprotein profiles and glucose tolerance. Fiber alone may help promote abdominal fat loss and improve insulin resistance. Resistance exercise, with or without an aerobic component, is recommended because it increases lean body mass and improves insulin resistance (Leyes et al., 2008), and may also lower triglycerides and decrease abdominal fat (Kressy et al., 2008).

| TABLE 22.5 | | | | |
|---|---|---|---|---|
| **HIV Medications and Timing of Food Intake** | | | | |
| Generic Name (Brand Name) | Take with Food | Take on Empty Stomach | Take without Regard to Food | |
| **Fusion Inhibitor** | | | | |
| Enfuvirtide (Fuzeon) | | | ✓ | |
| **Nucleoside Reverse Transcriptase Inhibitors (NRTI)** | | | | |
| Abacavir (Ziagen) | | | ✓ | |
| Didanosine (Videx) | | ✓ | | |
| Emtricitabine (Emtriva) | | | ✓ | |
| Lamivudine (Epivir) | | | ✓ Fewer side effects if taken with meals | |
| Stavudine (Zerit) | | | ✓ Avoid alcohol | |
| Tenefovir (Viread) | ✓ | | | |
| Zalcitabine (Hivid) | | ✓ | | |
| Zidovudine (Retrovir) | | | ✓ Do not take with high-fat meal | |
| **Nonnucleoside Reverse Transcriptase Inhibitors (NNRTI)** | | | | |
| Delavirdine (Rescriptor) | | | ✓ | |
| Efavirenz (Sustiva) | | ✓ | | |
| Nevirapine (Viramune) | | | ✓ | |
| **Protease Inhibitors** | | | | |
| Amprenavir (Agenerase) | | | ✓ Do not take with high-fat meal | |
| Atazanavir (Reyataz) | ✓ | | | |
| Darunavir (Prezista) | ✓ | | | |
| Fosamprenavir (Lexiva) | | | ✓ | |
| Indinavir (Crixivan) | | ✓ | | |
| Lopinavir (Kaletra) | ✓ | | | |
| Nelfinavir (Viracept) | ✓ | | | |
| Ritonavir (Norvir) | ✓ | | | |
| Saquinavir (Invirase) | ✓ Take within 2 hours of a high-calorie, high-fat meal | | | |

*Source:* Skidmore-Roth, L. (2008). Nursing *drug reference*. St. Louis, Missouri: Mosby, Inc.

## Food and Drug Interactions

Due to food/drug interactions, medication schedules and food restrictions are both complex and strict. Some clients stop antiretroviral therapies because they are convinced that the drugs' side effects and complicated regimens are not worth the effort. Maximum effectiveness of drug therapy is dependent on compliance with the medication schedule and food restrictions. Table 22.5 lists drugs that should be taken on an empty stomach and those that need to be taken with food.

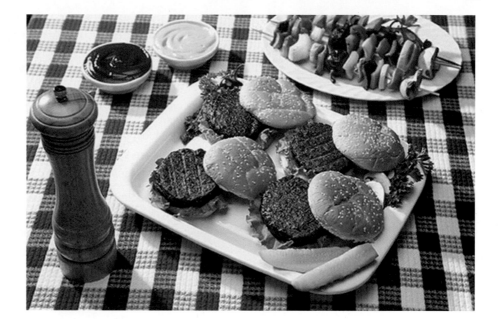

**FIGURE 22.1** Cooking ground beef to 160 degrees eliminates any danger from pathogenic bacteria such as *Escherichia coli.* (***Source:*** USDA. Photo by Stephen Ausmus.)

## Food Safety

Because PLHA have compromised immune systems, steps should be taken to reduce the risk of foodborne illness (Fig. 22.1). Food safety strategies are listed in Box 22.3 (see Chapter 9 for more on foodborne illness).

## NURSING PROCESS: *Cancer*

Karen is a 59-year-old former smoker who now calls herself a "health nut." She was recently diagnosed with lung cancer. She had surgery to remove her right lung and is receiving chemotherapy for cancerous "spots" on the left lung and stomach. She has lost 28 pounds and complains of nausea, vomiting, and a bad taste in her mouth. Because she has followed a healthy diet to prevent cancer for years, she is reluctant to now change her eating habits and eat more protein, fat, and calories. Right now she is eating mostly fruit, sherbet, and skim milk.

| Assessment |
| --- |

| Medical-Psychosocial History | • Medical history such as diabetes, heart disease, or hypertension<br>• Types of drugs the client is receiving through chemotherapy; other prescribed medications that affect nutrition<br>• Physician's goals and plan of treatment<br>• Pattern of nausea and vomiting<br>• Client's understanding of increased nutritional needs related to cancer and cancer therapies<br>• Willingness to change her attitudes toward food and nutrition<br>• Psychosocial and economic issues such as financial status, employment, and outside support system<br>• Usual activity patterns |
| --- | --- |

*(nursing process continues on page 554)*

## *NURSING PROCESS: Cancer* (continued)

| | |
|---|---|
| Anthropometric Assessment | • Height, current weight, usual weight |
| | • Rate of weight loss; % of usual body weight loss |
| | • BMI |
| Biochemical and Physical Assessment | • Laboratory data: serum albumin, serum transferrin, thyroxine-bound prealbumin, retinol-binding protein, serum electrolytes, and other abnormal values |
| | • Nitrogen balance study, if available |
| | • General appearance/evidence of muscle wasting |
| Dietary Assessment | • How many daily meals and snacks are you eating? |
| | • What is a typical day's intake for you? |
| | • How is your appetite? When is your appetite the best? |
| | • What things do you do to alleviate nausea? |
| | • How has your sense of taste changed? What things do you do to cope with the changes? |
| | • Do you have any food allergies or intolerances? |
| | • Do you have any cultural, religious, or ethnic food preferences? |
| | • Do you use vitamins, minerals, or nutritional supplements? |
| | • Do you use liquid formulas, such as instant breakfast mixes or commercial products? |
| | • How much liquid do you consume in a day? |
| | • Do you use alcohol? |

## Diagnosis

| | |
|---|---|
| Possible Nursing Diagnoses | Imbalanced nutrition: less than body requirements related to nausea, vomiting, and taste changes secondary to cancer/cancer therapy as evidenced by 28-pound weight loss |

## Planning

| | |
|---|---|
| Client Outcomes | The client will: |
| | • Eat 6–8 times daily |
| | • Add to the protein and calorie density of foods she eats |
| | • Drink at least 16 oz of a high-calorie, high-protein supplement daily |
| | • Switch from skim milk to whole milk, as tolerated |
| | • Verbalize interventions she will try to help alleviate nausea and taste alterations |
| | • Verbalize the importance of consuming adequate protein and calories and the role of fat in providing calories |
| | • Maintain present weight until chemotherapy is completed |
| | • Maintain/improve health status as evidenced by a prealbumin value within normal limits |

*(nursing process continues on page 555)*

# NURSING PROCESS: *Cancer* (continued)

## Nursing Interventions

| | |
|---|---|
| Nutrition Therapy | Provide regular diet as ordered with high-protein, high-calorie in-between meal supplements |
| Client Teaching | Instruct the client: |

- That an adequate nutritional status reduces the side effects of treatment, may make cancer cells more receptive to treatment and may improve quality of life. Poor nutritional status may potentiate chemotherapeutic drug toxicity
- That a preventative eating style is no longer appropriate. Consuming adequate protein and calories (even fat calories) is the major priority

On eating plan essentials, including

- Protein sources the client may tolerate despite nausea and taste changes such as eggs, cheese, mild fish, nuts, dried peas and beans, milk shakes, eggnogs, puddings, ice cream, instant breakfast mixes, and commercial supplements
- How to increase the protein and calorie density of foods eaten (see Box 22.5)
- To eat small, frequent "meals" to help maximize intake but to avoid eating 12 hours before chemotherapy
- To drink ample fluids 1 to 2 days before and after chemotherapy to enhance excretion of the drugs and to decrease the risk of renal toxicity

On interventions to minimize nausea such as

- Eating foods served cold or at room temperature
- Eating high-carbohydrate, low-fat foods such as toast, crackers, yogurt, sherbet, cooked cereal, soft or canned fruits, watermelon, bananas, fruit juices, and angel food cake
- Avoiding fatty, greasy, fried, and strongly seasoned foods

On behavior to help maximize intake, including

- Viewing food as a medicine, rather than a social pleasure, that must be "taken" even when the desire to eat is lacking
- Keeping track of and avoiding foods that cause nausea
- Taking antiemetics as prescribed even when symptoms are absent
- Sucking on sugarless hard candy during chemotherapy and using plastic utensils and dishes to mitigate the "bad taste" in her mouth
- Avoiding anything that tastes unpleasant

## Evaluation

| | |
|---|---|
| Evaluate and Monitor | - Monitor weight |
| | - Monitor food intake records |
| | - Monitor management of side effects; suggest additional interventions, as needed |
| | - Monitor laboratory values |

▶ HOW DO YOU RESPOND?

**Why do cancer prevention recommendations suggest red meat intake be limited?** Some of the most convincing evidence in the report issued by the World Cancer Research Fund and the American Institute for Cancer Research is the link between red meat and colorectal cancer. The risk of colorectal cancer clearly rises when more than 18 oz/week of cooked red meat are eaten (WCRF, AICR, 2007). The risk may be related to substances that occur naturally in red meat and substances that are produced when red meat is processed or cooked. Although more research is needed to fully explain the relationship between red meat and cancer, it is prudent to eat less red meat and processed meat and to avoid cooking red meat at high temperatures.

**Doesn't canola oil cause cancer?** The rumors that canola oil causes cancer stem from the fact that canola is derived from rapeseed. Rapeseed is naturally high in erucic acid, a fatty acid shown to be harmful to animals. However, in the 1970s, traditional plant breeding methods led to the creation of a low–erucic acid rapeseed, which is used to make canola oil. There are no human health risks associated with canola oil.

▶ CASE STUDY

Steve is a 39-year-old male who has been HIV positive for 6 years. His waistline is expanding and he blames that for his recent onset of heartburn. Based on a physical examination and insulin resistance, his doctor diagnosed lipodystrophy syndrome. Steve is 6 ft. tall and weighs 190 pounds. His weight has been stable for the last several years, although he feels "fatter." He is on HAART but is thinking of discontinuing the medication if it is the cause of his change in shape. He is willing to exercise but wants maximum benefit from minimum effort. He is also willing to change his eating habits, but relies heavily on eating out. A typical day's intake is as follows:

| | |
|---|---|
| **Breakfast:** | A fast-food egg, bacon, and cheese sandwich on an English muffin |
| | Hash browns |
| | Large black coffee |
| **Lunch:** | Double hamburger |
| | French fries |
| | Cola |
| **Dinner:** | Grilled steak |
| | Baked potato with sour cream |
| | Water |
| **Snacks:** | Chips |

- Evaluate Steve's current weight. Would you recommend weight loss?
- How does Steve's weight impact heartburn and insulin resistance?
- How does his usual intake impact lipodystrophy, insulin resistance, and heartburn?
- What are Steve's nutrition-related problems? What nutrition therapy recommendations would you make?
- What would you tell Steve about exercise?
- What criteria would you monitor to evaluate the effectiveness of nutrition therapy?

1. The nurse knows her instructions about healthy eating to reduce the risk of cancer have been understood when the client states
   a. "If I follow those healthy eating guidelines I will not get cancer."
   b. "To reduce the risk of cancer I have to eat a vegetarian diet."
   c. "There is not enough known about diet and cancer to make informed choices about what to eat to reduce the risk of cancer."
   d. "A mostly plant-based diet may reduce the risk of cancer."

2. Which of the following metabolic changes often occur from cancer? Select all that apply.
   a. Increased fat synthesis
   b. Increased body protein turnover
   c. Insulin resistance
   d. Increased energy expenditure
   e. Decreased muscle protein synthesis

3. Which of the following strategies would the nurse suggest to help the client increase the protein density of his diet?
   a. Top baked potatoes with sour cream
   b. Mix cream cheese with butter and spread on hot bread
   c. Substitute milk for water in recipes
   d. Add whipped cream to coffee

4. Which of the following meals would be most appropriate for a patient whose only cancer treatment symptom that impacts intake is neutropenia?
   a. Baked macaroni and cheese with cooked green beans
   b. Cottage cheese and fresh fruit plate
   c. Soft cooked eggs with toast
   d. Caesar salad with Caesar salad dressing

5. The client asks what foods she can eat for protein because meat tastes "rotten" to her. Which of the following would be the nurse's best response?
   a. Cheese omelet, cold chicken sandwich, shrimp salad
   b. Vegetable soup, pulled pork sandwich, meatloaf with gravy
   c. Spaghetti with meat balls, tacos, peanut butter and jelly sandwich
   d. Hot dogs, hamburgers, vegetable pizza

6. A client asks if it is okay to drink nutrition formulas in place of eating solid food because it seems to be the only thing she tolerates. Which of the following is the nurse's best response?
   a. "Nutrition formulas are okay to use as a supplement in your diet but they do not provide enough nutrition to use it in place of a meal."
   b. "Nutrition formulas are rich in nutrients and can be used in place of meals if they are what you are able to tolerate best."
   c. "It is fine to rely on nutritional supplements but vary the brand to ensure you are getting adequate nutrition."
   d. "Nutrition formulas generally are too high in calories and protein to use in place of meals."

7. Which statement indicates the client with HIV needs further instruction about healthy eating?
   a. "Eating fat increases my chances of getting fat around my middle so I am trying to choose all nonfat or low-fat food."
   b. "Eating carbs makes insulin resistance worse so I am eating a very low-carbohydrate diet."
   c. "Protein is the most important nutrient so I am eating extra red meat at every meal."
   d. "Monounsaturated fats in olive oil, canola oil, nuts, and avocado are healthiest. I am eating more of them and less of other types of fats."

**8.** When should nutrition become part of the care plan for a client with HIV?
 a. Before the onset of symptoms.
 b. When the client begins to lose weight.
 c. After an acute episode of illness.
 d. When weight loss is more than 5% of initial weight.

## KEY CONCEPTS

- Cancer is a group name for different diseases that differ in their impact on nutrition.

- As many as 30% of cancers may be related to dietary factors. Eating a plant-based diet, being physically active, and avoiding excess weight may reduce the risk of cancer. A BMI goal of 21 to 23 is recommended.

- Tumors in the GI tract are more likely than other tumors to produce local effects that impact nutrition.

- Cancer may alter metabolism by causing glucose intolerance and insulin resistance, increasing energy expenditure, increasing protein catabolism, increasing fat catabolism, and increasing the use of fat for energy.

- Anorexia, a common problem in people with cancer, may lead to weight loss and malnutrition. Pain, depression/anxiety, early satiety, taste changes, fatigue, and nausea caused by cancer or its treatment may be contributing factors.

- Cancer cachexia is a progressive wasting syndrome characterized by preferential loss of lean body mass. Altered metabolism and anorexia are involved. The severity of cachexia is not directly related to calorie intake or tumor weight.

- Nutrition therapy may help sustain the client through adverse side effects of cancer treatments and may reduce morbidity and mortality.

- Requirements for protein, calories, vitamin C, B vitamins, and iron increase after surgery to replenish losses and promote healing. GI surgeries have the greatest chance of impacting nutrition.

- Unlike surgery and radiation, chemotherapy produces systemic side effects. Anorexia, nausea and vomiting, taste alterations, sore mouth or throat, diarrhea, early satiety, and constipation are the most common nutrition-related side effects of chemotherapy.

- Nutrition-related side effects from radiation are most likely to occur in people who have cancers of the head and neck, lungs, esophagus, cervix, uterus, colon, rectum, and pancreas.

- People who have bone marrow transplantation may need total parenteral nutrition (TPN) for 1 to 2 months or longer after the procedure.

- The goal of nutrition therapy for people being treated for cancer is to prevent weight loss (even in overweight patients) and maintain lean body mass. Avoiding unintentional weight gain is a goal for women treated for breast cancer.

- There are no validated parameters for determining the nutrition needs of patients with cancer. Generally a high-calorie, high-protein diet with small frequent meals is recommended. The diet is modified to alleviate nutrition-related side effects.

- Increasing the calorie and protein densities of the diet is generally more acceptable than increasing the volume of food served.

- An oral diet is used whenever possible. Enteral and parenteral nutrition are options in specific situations.

- Malnutrition may speed the progression from HIV disease to AIDS.

- Weight loss and wasting remain common problems in PLHA, despite major advances in the treatment and survival.

● The cause of HIV-associated wasting is multifactorial. Impaired intake and altered metabolism may be at least partially responsible.

● The exact nutritional requirements of PLHA are not known. Generally, calorie requirements increase 10% to 30% depending on the phase of the disease. There are no data to support an increased need for protein. Saturated fat, added sugars, and alcohol should be limited in cases of lipodystrophy syndrome.

● PLHA may experience side effects similar to those of people with cancer. Nutrition therapy can help alleviate side effects to promote an adequate intake.

● Drugs used for HIV/AIDS may interact with food or certain foods. Complex and strict dietary restrictions may be necessary to maximize drug effectiveness.

● PLHA should practice food sanitation and safety to decrease the risk of foodborne illness.

## ANSWER KEY

1. **TRUE** Convincing evidence links obesity with several types of cancer, such as pancreatic, kidney, and postmenopausal breast.

2. **TRUE** Weight loss is an indicator of poor prognosis in cancer patients.

3. **TRUE** Clients who are adequately nourished are better able to withstand the effects of cancer treatments.

4. **FALSE** Although anorexia can contribute to the development of cachexia, neither the incidence nor the severity of cachexia can be related directly to calorie intake.

5. **FALSE** The cancer patient's appetite is generally better in the morning and tends to deteriorate as the day progresses.

6. **TRUE** Cancer survivors are urged to follow diet recommendations to reduce the risk of cancer in the future.

7. **FALSE** A low-fat diet cannot prevent lipodystrophy, but following a Mediterranean type diet that is low in saturated fat, added sugar, and alcohol may improve blood lipid levels and glucose tolerance. Fiber may promote loss of abdominal fat and improves insulin resistance.

8. **FALSE** Diarrhea does not necessarily accompany malabsorption caused by HIV infection. Malabsorption cannot be ruled out on the basis of bowel movements alone.

9. **TRUE** Patients with HIV/AIDS may well experience problems related to appetite and intake similar to those of cancer patients.

10. **TRUE** The risk of foodborne infections in patients with HIV/AIDS can be reduced by educating them on food and water safety such as the importance of refrigerating foods, washing fruit and vegetables, and cooking meats thoroughly.

## WEBSITES

*Websites related to cancer*

American Botanical Council at **www.herbalgram.org**
American Cancer Society at **www.cancer.org**
American Institute for Cancer Research at **www.aicr.org**
American Society for Clinical Oncology at **www.asco.org**
National Cancer Institute at **www.cancer.gov**
National Center for Complementary and Alternative Medicine (NCCAM) at **www.nccam.nih.gov**
Oncology Nursing Society at **www.ons.org**

*Websites related to HIV/AIDS*

AIDS Education Global Information System (AEGIS) at **www.aegis.com**
Association of Nutrition Services Agencies at **www.aidsnutrition.org**

AIDSinfo (A Service of the U.S. Department of Health and Human Services) at
**www.aidsinfo.nih.gov**
HIV Research of the Nutrition Infection Unit at Tufts University School of Medicine at
**www.tufts.edu/med/nutrition-infection/hiv/**
Center for HIV Information from the University of California San Francisco School of Medicine at
**www.hivinsite.org**
Centers for Disease Control (CDC), Division of HIV/AIDS Prevention (DHAP)
**http://www.cdc.gov/hiv/dhap.htm**
Community Programs for Clinical Research on AIDS, CPCRA (Government-funded research) at
**http://www.cpcra.org/**
Food and Drug Administration HIV/AIDS Page at **http://www.fda.gov/oashi/aids/hiv.html**
Health Resources and Services Administration (HRSA) HIV/AIDS Services at
**http://hab.hrsa.gov**
National Institute of Allergy and Infectious Diseases (NIAID), Division of Acquired
Immunodeficiency Syndrome (DAIDS) at **http://www.niaid.nih.gov/daids/default.htm**
National Institutes of Health, National Center for Complementary and Alternative Therapies at
**http://nccam.nih.gov**
National Institutes of Health Office of AIDS Research at **http://www.nih.gov/od/oar/**

# REFERENCES

American Cancer Society (ACS). (2007). *Nutrition and cancer*. Available at
www.cancer.org. Accessed on 8/11/08.
American Dietetic Association (ADA). (2004). Position of the American Dietetic Association and
Dietitians of Canada: Nutrition intervention in the care of persons with human immunodefi-
ciency virus infection. *Journal of the American Dietetic Association, 104*, 1425–1441.
American Dietetic Association (ADA). (2008). *Nutrition care manual*. Available online at
www.nutritioncaremanual.com. Accessed on 8/19/08.
Center for Disease Control (CDC). (1987). Revision of the CEC surveillance case definition for ac-
quired immunodeficiency syndrome: Council of state and territorial epidemiologists; AIDS Program,
Center for Infectious Diseases. *Morbidity and Mortality Weekly Report, 36* (Suppl. 1), 1S–15S.
CDC, NCHS. (2008). *Deaths-leading causes*. Available at www.cdc.gov/nchs/fastats/lcod.htm.
Accessed on 8/13/08.
Joy, T., Keogh, H. M., Hadigan, C., et al. (2007). Dietary fat intake and relationship to serum lipid
levels in HIV-infected patients with metabolic abnormalities in the HAART era. *AIDS, 21*,
1591–1600.
Kressy, J., Wanke, C., & Gerrior, J. (2008). *Lipodystrophy*. Available at www.tufts.edu/
med/nutrition-infection/hiv/health_lipo.html. Accessed on 8/11/08.
Leyes, P., Martinez, E., & Forga Mde, T. (2008). Use of diet, nutritional supplements and exercise
in HIV-infected patients receiving combination antiretroviral therapies: A systematic review.
*Antiviral Therapy, 13*, 149–159.
Mangili, A., Murman, D. H., Zampini, A. M., et al. (2006). Nutrition and HIV infection: Review of
weight loss and wasting in the era of highly active antiretroviral therapy from the Nutrition for
Healthy Living Cohort. *Clinical Infectious Diseases, 42*, 836–842.
National Cancer Institute (NCI). (2008a). *Surveillance epidemiology and end results stat fact sheets*.
Available at www.seer.cancer.gov/statfacts/html/all_print.html. Accessed on 8/11/08.
National Cancer Institute (NCI). (2008b). *Nutrition in cancer care (PDQ): Supportive care*.
Available at www.nci.nih.gov. Accessed on 8/11/08.
Nelson, K. (2000). The cancer anorexia-cachexia syndrome. *Seminars in Oncology, 27*, 64–68.
Roubenoff, R., Grinspoon, S., Skolnik, P. R., et al. (2002). Role of cytokines and testosterone in
regulating lean body mass and resting energy expenditure in HIV-infected men. *American
Journal of Physiology Endocrinology Metabolism, 283*, E138–E145.
Schattner, M., & Shike, M. (2006). Nutrition support of the patient with cancer. In: M. Shils, M.
Shike, A. Ross, et al. (Eds.), *Modern nutrition in health and disease*. Philadelphia: Lippincott
Williams & Wilkins.
Shevitz, A. H., Know, T. A., Spiegelman, D., et al. (1999). Elevated resting energy expenditure
among HIV-seropositive persons receiving high active antiretroviral therapy. *AIDS, 12*,
1351–1357.

Tang, A. M., Jacobson, D. L., Spiegelman, D., et al. (2005). Increasing risk of 5% of greater unintentional weight loss in a cohort of HIV-infected patients, 1995 to 2003. *Journal of Acquired Immune Deficiency Syndromes, 40,* 70–76.

Vigano, A., Watanabe, S., & Bruera, E. (1994). Anorexia and cachexia in advanced cancer patients. *Cancer Surveillance, 21,* 99–115.

Woods, M., Potts, E., & Connors, J. (2008). *Building a high quality diet.* Available at www.tufts.edu/med/nutrition-infection/hiv/health_high_quality_diet.html. Accessed on 8/18/08.

World Cancer Research Fund, American Institute for Cancer Research (WCRF, AICR). (2007). *Food, nutrition, physical activity, and the prevention of cancer: A global perspective.* Washington, DC: AICR.

World Health Organization (WHO). (2003). *Nutrient requirements for people living with HIV/AIDS.* Available at www.who.int/nutrition/publications/Content_nutrient_requirements.pdf. Accessed on 8/20/08.

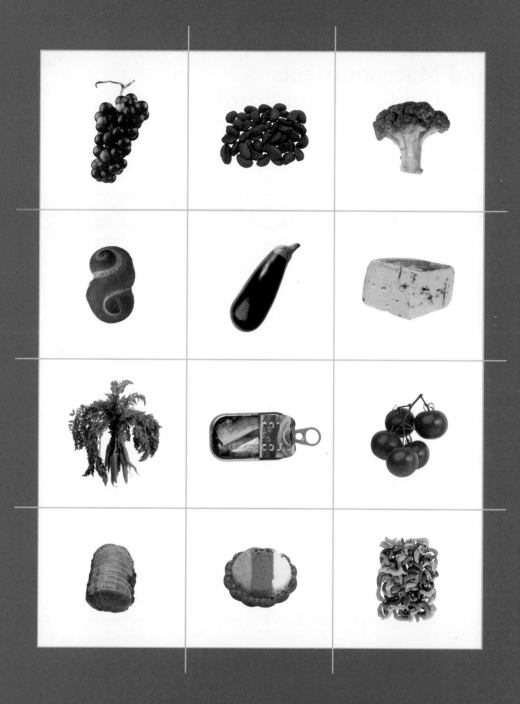

APPENDICES

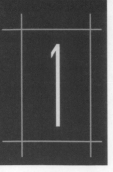

# 1 Dietary Reference Intakes (DRIs): Recommended Dietary Allowances and Adequate Intakes, Total Water and Macronutrients

Food and Nutrition Board, Institute of Medicine, National Academies

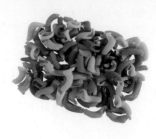

| Life Stage Group | Total Water[a] (L/d) | Carbohydrate (g/d) | Total Fiber (g/d) | Fat (g/d) | Linoleic Acid (g/d) | α-Linolenic Acid (g/d) | Protein[b] (g/d) |
|---|---|---|---|---|---|---|---|
| **Infants** | | | | | | | |
| 0–6 mo | 0.7* | 60* | ND | 31* | 4.4* | 0.5* | 9.1* |
| 7–12 mo | 0.8* | 95* | ND | 30* | 4.6* | 0.5* | **11.0+** |
| **Children** | | | | | | | |
| 1–3 y | 1.3* | **130** | 19* | ND[c] | 7* | 0.7* | **13** |
| 4–8 y | 1.7* | **130** | 25* | ND | 10* | 0.9* | **19** |
| **Males** | | | | | | | |
| 9–13 y | 2.4* | **130** | 31* | ND | 12* | 1.2* | **34** |
| 14–18 y | 3.3* | **130** | 38* | ND | 16* | 1.6* | **52** |
| 19–30 y | 3.7* | **130** | 38* | ND | 17* | 1.6* | **56** |
| 31–50 y | 3.7* | **130** | 38* | ND | 17* | 1.6* | **56** |
| 51–70 y | 3.7* | **130** | 30* | ND | 14* | 1.6* | **56** |
| >70 y | 3.7* | **130** | 30* | ND | 14* | 1.6* | **56** |
| **Females** | | | | | | | |
| 9–13 y | 2.1* | **130** | 26* | ND | 10* | 1.0* | **34** |
| 14–18 y | 2.3* | **130** | 26* | ND | 11* | 1.1* | **46** |
| 19–30 y | 2.7* | **130** | 25* | ND | 12* | 1.1* | **46** |
| 31–50 y | 2.7* | **130** | 25* | ND | 12* | 1.1* | **46** |
| 51–70 y | 2.7* | **130** | 21* | ND | 11* | 1.1* | **46** |
| >70 y | 2.7* | **130** | 21* | ND | 11* | 1.1* | **46** |
| **Pregnancy** | | | | | | | |
| 14–18 y | 3.0* | **175** | 28* | ND | 13* | 1.4* | **71** |
| 19–30 y | 3.0* | **175** | 28* | ND | 13* | 1.4* | **71** |
| 31–50 y | 3.0* | **175** | 28* | ND | 13* | 1.4* | **71** |
| **Lactation** | | | | | | | |
| 14–18 y | 3.8* | **210** | 29* | ND | 13* | 1.3* | **71** |
| 19–30 y | 3.8* | **210** | 29* | ND | 13* | 1.3* | **71** |
| 31–50 y | 3.8* | **210** | 29* | ND | 13* | 1.3* | **71** |

*Note:* This table (taken from the DRI reports, see www.nap.edu) presents Recommended Dietary Allowances (RDA) in **bold type** or Adequate Intakes (AI) in ordinary type followed by an asterisk (*). An RDA is the average daily dietary intake level sufficient to meet the nutrient requirements of nearly all (97–98 percent) healthy individuals in a group. It is calculated from an Estimated Average Requirement (EAR). If sufficient scientific evidence is not available to establish an EAR, and thus calculate an RDA, an AI is usually developed. For healthy breastfed infants, the AI is the mean intake. The AI for other life stage and gender groups is believed to cover the needs of all healthy individuals in the group, but lack of data or uncertainty in the data prevent being able to specify with confidence the percentage of individuals covered by this intake.

[a]*Total* water includes all water contained in food, beverages, and drinking water.

[b]Based on g protein per kg of body weight for the reference body weight, e.g., for adults 0.8 g/kg body weight for the reference body weight.

[c]Not determined.

*Sources:* Dietary Reference Intakes for Energy, Carbohydrate, Fiber, Fat, Fatty Acids, Cholesterol, Protein, and Amino Acids (2002/2005); Dietary Reference Intakes for Water, Potassium, Sodium, Chloride, and Sulfate (2005). These reports may be accessed via http://www.nap.edu.

Reprinted with permission from the National Academies Press, Copyright 2005, National Academy of Sciences.

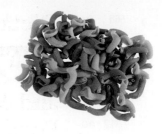

# 2

## Dietary Reference Intakes (DRIs): Recommended Dietary Allowances and Adequate Intakes, Vitamins
Food and Nutrition Board, Institute of Medicine, National Academies

| Life Stage Group | Vitamin A (μg/d)[a] | Vitamin C (mg/d) | Vitamin D (μg/d)[b,c] | Vitamin E (mg/d)[d] | Vitamin K (μg/d) | Thiamin (mg/d) |
|---|---|---|---|---|---|---|
| **Infants** | | | | | | |
| 0–6 mo | 400* | 40* | 5* | 4* | 2.0* | 0.2* |
| 7–12 mo | 500* | 50* | 5* | 5* | 2.5* | 0.3* |
| **Children** | | | | | | |
| 1–3 y | **300** | **15** | 5* | **6** | 30* | **0.5** |
| 4–8 y | **400** | **25** | 5* | **7** | 55* | **0.6** |
| **Males** | | | | | | |
| 9–13 y | **600** | **45** | 5* | **11** | 60* | **0.9** |
| 14–18 y | **900** | **75** | 5* | **15** | 75* | **1.2** |
| 19–30 y | **900** | **90** | 5* | **15** | 120* | **1.2** |
| 31–50 y | **900** | **90** | 5* | **15** | 120* | **1.2** |
| 51–70 y | **900** | **90** | 10* | **15** | 120* | **1.2** |
| >70 y | **900** | **90** | 15* | **15** | 120* | **1.2** |
| **Females** | | | | | | |
| 9–13 y | **600** | **45** | 5* | **11** | 60* | **0.9** |
| 14–18 y | **700** | **65** | 5* | **15** | 75* | **1.0** |
| 19–30 y | **700** | **75** | 5* | **15** | 90* | **1.1** |
| 31–50 y | **700** | **75** | 5* | **15** | 90* | **1.1** |
| 51–70 y | **700** | **75** | 10* | **15** | 90* | **1.1** |
| >70 y | **700** | **75** | 15* | **15** | 90* | **1.1** |
| **Pregnancy** | | | | | | |
| 14–18 y | **750** | **80** | 5* | **15** | 75* | **1.4** |
| 19–30 y | **770** | **85** | 5* | **15** | 90* | **1.4** |
| 31–50 y | **770** | **85** | 5* | **15** | 90* | **1.4** |
| **Lactation** | | | | | | |
| 14–18 y | **1,200** | **115** | 5* | **19** | 75* | **1.4** |
| 19–30 y | **1,300** | **120** | 5* | **19** | 90* | **1.4** |
| 31–50 y | **1,300** | **120** | 5* | **19** | 90* | **1.4** |

*Note:* This table (taken from the DRI reports, see www.nap.edu) presents Recommended Dietary Allowances (RDA) in **bold type** or Adequate Intakes (AI) in ordinary type followed by an asterisk (*). An RDA is the average daily dietary intake level sufficient to meet the nutrient requirements of nearly all (97–98 percent) healthy individuals in a group. It is calculated from an Estimated Average Requirement (EAR). If sufficient scientific evidence is not available to establish an EAR, and thus calculate an RDA, an AI is usually developed. For healthy breastfed infants, the AI is the mean intake. The AI for other life stage and gender groups is believed to cover the needs of all healthy individuals in the group, but lack of data or uncertainty in the data prevent being able to specify with confidence the percentage of individuals covered by this intake.

[a]As retinol activity equivalents (RAEs). 1 RAE = 1 μg retinol, 12 μg β-carotene, 24 μg α-carotene, or 24 μg β-cryptoxanthin. The RAE for dietary provitamin A carotenoids is two-fold greater than retinol equivalents (RE), whereas the RAE for preformed vitamin A is the same as RE.

[b]As cholecalciferol. 1 μg cholecalciferol = 40 IU vitamin D.

[c]In the absence of adequate exposure to sunlight.

[d]As α-tocopherol. α-Tocopherol includes *RRR*-α-tocopherol, the only form of α-tocopherol that occurs naturally in foods, and the *2R*-stereoisomeric forms of α-tocopherol (*RRR*-, *RSR*-, *RRS*-, and *RSS*-α-tocopherol) that occur in fortified foods and supplements. It does not include the *2S*-stereoisomeric forms of α-tocopherol (*SRR*-, *SSR*-, *SRS*-, and *SSS*-α-tocopherol), also found in fortified foods and supplements.

| Riboflavin (mg/d) | Niacin (mg/d)[e] | Vitamin $B_6$ (mg/d) | Folate (µg/d)[f] | Vitamin $B_{12}$ (µg/d) | Pantothenic Acid (mg/d) | Biotin (µg/d) | Choline (mg/d)[g] |
|---|---|---|---|---|---|---|---|
| 0.3* | 2* | 0.1* | 65* | 0.4* | 1.7* | 5* | 125* |
| 0.4* | 4* | 0.3* | 80* | 0.5* | 1.8* | 6* | 150* |
| 0.5 | 6 | 0.5 | 150 | 0.9 | 2* | 8* | 200* |
| 0.6 | 8 | 0.6 | 200 | 1.2 | 3* | 12* | 250* |
| 0.9 | 12 | 1.0 | 300 | 1.8 | 4* | 20* | 375* |
| 1.3 | 16 | 1.3 | 400 | 2.4 | 5* | 25* | 550* |
| 1.3 | 16 | 1.3 | 400 | 2.4 | 5* | 30* | 550* |
| 1.3 | 16 | 1.3 | 400 | 2.4 | 5* | 30* | 550* |
| 1.3 | 16 | 1.7 | 400 | 2.4[h] | 5* | 30* | 550* |
| 1.3 | 16 | 1.7 | 400 | 2.4[h] | 5* | 30* | 550* |
| 0.9 | 12 | 1.0 | 300 | 1.8 | 4* | 20* | 375* |
| 1.0 | 14 | 1.2 | 400[i] | 2.4 | 5* | 25* | 400* |
| 1.1 | 14 | 1.3 | 400[i] | 2.4 | 5* | 30* | 425* |
| 1.1 | 14 | 1.3 | 400[i] | 2.4 | 5* | 30* | 425* |
| 1.1 | 14 | 1.5 | 400 | 2.4[h] | 5* | 30* | 425* |
| 1.1 | 14 | 1.5 | 400 | 2.4[h] | 5* | 30* | 425* |
| 1.4 | 18 | 1.9 | 600[j] | 2.6 | 6* | 30* | 450* |
| 1.4 | 18 | 1.9 | 600[j] | 2.6 | 6* | 30* | 450* |
| 1.4 | 18 | 1.9 | 600[j] | 2.6 | 6* | 30* | 450* |
| 1.6 | 17 | 2.0 | 500 | 2.8 | 7* | 35* | 550* |
| 1.6 | 17 | 2.0 | 500 | 2.8 | 7* | 35* | 550* |
| 1.6 | 17 | 2.0 | 500 | 2.8 | 7* | 35* | 550* |

[e]As niacin equivalents (NE). 1 mg of niacin = 60 mg of tryptophan; 0–6 months = preformed niacin (not NE).

[f]As dietary folate equivalents (DFE). 1 DFE = 1 µg food folate = 0.6 µg of folic acid from fortified food or as a supplement consumed with food = 0.5 µg of a supplement taken on an empty stomach.

[g]Although AIs have been set for choline, there are few data to assess whether a dietary supply of choline is needed at all stages of the life cycle, and it may be that the choline requirement can be met by endogenous synthesis at some of these stages.

[h]Because 10 to 30 percent of older people may malabsorb food-bound $B_{12}$, it is advisable for those older than 50 years to meet their RDA mainly by consuming foods fortified with $B_{12}$ or a supplement containing $B_{12}$.

[i]In view of evidence linking folate intake with neural tube defects in the fetus, it is recommended that all women capable of becoming pregnant consume 400 µg from supplements or fortified foods in addition to intake of food folate from a varied diet.

[j]It is assumed that women will continue consuming 400 µg from supplements or fortified food until their pregnancy is confirmed and they enter prenatal care, which ordinarily occurs after the end of the periconceptional period—the critical time for formation of the neural tube.

**Sources:** *Dietary Reference Intakes for Calcium, Phosphorous, Magnesium, Vitamin D, and Fluoride* (1997). *Dietary Reference Intakes for Thiamin, Riboflavin, Niacin, Vitamin $B_6$, Folate, Vitamin $B_{12}$, Pantothenic Acid, Biotin, and Choline* (1998); *Dietary Reference Intakes for Vitamin C, Vitamin E, Selenium, and Carotenoids* (2000); *Dietary Reference Intakes for Vitamin A, Vitamin K, Arsenic, Boron, Chromium, Copper, Iodine, Iron, Manganese, Molybdenum, Nickel, Silicon, Vanadium, and Zinc* (2001); *and Dietary Reference Intakes for Water, Potassium, Sodium, Chloride, and Sulfate* (2005). These reports may be accessed via http://www.nap.edu.

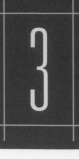

# 3

## Dietary Reference Intakes (DRIs): Recommended Dietary Allowances and Adequate Intakes, Elements

Food and Nutrition Board, Institute of Medicine, National Academies

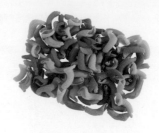

| Life Stage Group | Calcium (mg/d) | Chromium (µg/d) | Copper (µg/d) | Fluoride (mg/d) | Iodine (µg/d) | Iron (mg/d) | Magnesium (mg/d) | Manganese (mg/d) | Molybdenum (µg/d) | Phosphorus (mg/d) | Selenium (µg/d) | Zinc (mg/d) | Potassium (g/d) | Sodium (g/d) | Chloride (g/d) |
|---|---|---|---|---|---|---|---|---|---|---|---|---|---|---|---|
| **Infants** | | | | | | | | | | | | | | | |
| 0–6 mo | 210* | 0.2* | 200* | 0.01* | 110* | 0.27* | 30* | 0.003* | 2* | 100* | 15* | 2* | 0.4* | 0.12* | 0.18* |
| 7–12 mo | 270* | 5.5* | 220* | 0.5* | 130* | 11 | 75* | 0.6* | 3* | 275* | 20* | 3 | 0.7* | 0.37* | 0.57* |
| **Children** | | | | | | | | | | | | | | | |
| 1–3 y | 500* | 11* | 340 | 0.7* | 90 | 7 | 80 | 1.2* | 17 | 460 | 20 | 3 | 3.0* | 1.0* | 1.5* |
| 4–8 y | 800* | 15* | 440 | 1* | 90 | 10 | 130 | 1.5* | 22 | 500 | 30 | 5 | 3.8* | 1.2* | 1.9* |
| **Males** | | | | | | | | | | | | | | | |
| 9–13 y | 1,300* | 25* | 700 | 2* | 120 | 8 | 240 | 1.9* | 34 | 1,250 | 40 | 8 | 4.5* | 1.5* | 2.3* |
| 14–18 y | 1,300* | 35* | 890 | 3* | 150 | 11 | 410 | 2.2* | 43 | 1,250 | 55 | 11 | 4.7* | 1.5* | 2.3* |
| 19–30 y | 1,000* | 35* | 900 | 4* | 150 | 8 | 400 | 2.3* | 45 | 700 | 55 | 11 | 4.7* | 1.5* | 2.3* |
| 31–50 y | 1,000* | 35* | 900 | 4* | 150 | 8 | 420 | 2.3* | 45 | 700 | 55 | 11 | 4.7* | 1.5* | 2.3* |
| 51–70 y | 1,200* | 30* | 900 | 4* | 150 | 8 | 420 | 2.3* | 45 | 700 | 55 | 11 | 4.7* | 1.3* | 2.0* |
| >70 y | 1,200* | 30* | 900 | 4* | 150 | 8 | 420 | 2.3* | 45 | 700 | 55 | 11 | 4.7* | 1.2* | 1.8* |
| **Females** | | | | | | | | | | | | | | | |
| 9–13 y | 1,300* | 21* | 700 | 2* | 120 | 8 | 240 | 1.6* | 34 | 1,250 | 40 | 8 | 4.5* | 1.5* | 2.3* |
| 14–18 y | 1,300* | 24* | 890 | 3* | 150 | 15 | 360 | 1.6* | 43 | 1,250 | 55 | 9 | 4.7* | 1.5* | 2.3* |
| 19–30 y | 1,000* | 25* | 900 | 3* | 150 | 18 | 310 | 1.8* | 45 | 700 | 55 | 8 | 4.7* | 1.5* | 2.3* |
| 31–50 y | 1,000* | 25* | 900 | 3* | 150 | 18 | 320 | 1.8* | 45 | 700 | 55 | 8 | 4.7* | 1.5* | 2.3* |
| 51–70 y | 1,200* | 20* | 900 | 3* | 150 | 8 | 320 | 1.8* | 45 | 700 | 55 | 8 | 4.7* | 1.3* | 2.0* |
| >70 y | 1,200* | 20* | 900 | 3* | 150 | 8 | 320 | 1.8* | 45 | 700 | 55 | 8 | 4.7* | 1.2* | 1.8* |
| **Pregnancy** | | | | | | | | | | | | | | | |
| 14–18 y | 1,300* | 29* | 1,000 | 3* | 220 | 27 | 400 | 2.0* | 50 | 1,250 | 60 | 12 | 4.7* | 1.5* | 2.3* |
| 19–30 y | 1,000* | 30* | 1,000 | 3* | 220 | 27 | 350 | 2.0* | 50 | 700 | 60 | 11 | 4.7* | 1.5* | 2.3* |
| 31–50 y | 1,000* | 30* | 1,000 | 3* | 220 | 27 | 360 | 2.0* | 50 | 700 | 60 | 11 | 4.7* | 1.5* | 2.3* |
| **Lactation** | | | | | | | | | | | | | | | |
| 14–18 y | 1,300* | 44* | 1,300 | 3* | 290 | 10 | 360 | 2.6* | 50 | 1,250 | 70 | 13 | 5.1* | 1.5* | 2.3* |
| 19–30 y | 1,000* | 45* | 1,300 | 3* | 290 | 9 | 310 | 2.6* | 50 | 700 | 70 | 12 | 5.1* | 1.5* | 2.3* |
| 31–50 y | 1,000* | 45* | 1,300 | 3* | 290 | 9 | 320 | 2.6* | 50 | 700 | 70 | 12 | 5.1* | 1.5* | 2.3* |

***Note:*** This table (taken from the DRI reports, see www.nap.edu) presents Recommended Dietary Allowances (RDA) in **bold type** or Adequate Intakes (AI) in ordinary type followed by an asterisk (∗). An RDA is the average daily dietary intake level sufficient to meet the nutrient requirements of nearly all (97–98 percent) healthy individuals in a group. It is calculated from an Estimated Average Requirement (EAR). If sufficient scientific evidence is not available to establish an EAR, and thus calculate an RDA, an AI is usually developed. For healthy breastfed infants, the AI is the mean intake. The AI for other life stage and gender groups is believed to cover the needs of all healthy individuals in the group, but lack of data or uncertainty in the data prevent being able to specify with confidence the percentage of individuals covered by this intake.

***Sources:*** *Dietary Reference Intakes for Calcium, Phosphorous, Magnesium, Vitamin D, and Fluoride* (1997); *Dietary Reference Intakes for Thiamin, Riboflavin, Niacin, Vitamin B₆, Folate, Vitamin B₁₂, Pantothenic Acid, Biotin, and Choline* (1998); *Dietary Reference Intakes for Vitamin C, Vitamin E, Selenium, and Carotenoids* (2000); *Dietary Reference Intakes for Vitamin A, Vitamin K, Arsenic, Boron, Chromium, Copper, Iodine, Iron, Manganese, Molybdenum, Nickel, Silicon, Vanadium, and Zinc* (2001); and *Dietary Reference Intakes for Water, Potassium, Sodium, Chloride, and Sulfate* (2005). These reports may be accessed via http://www.nap.edu.

Reprinted with permission from the National Academies Press, Copyright 2005, National Academy of Sciences.

# Answers to Study Questions

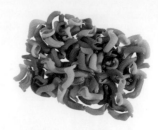

## Chapter 1
1. a
2. d
3. b
4. b
5. b
6. d

## Chapter 2
1. c
2. a
3. b
4. d
5. c
6. a
7. c
8. d

## Chapter 3
1. a
2. b
3. d
4. d
5. c
6. a
7. c
8. a

## Chapter 4
1. b
2. d
3. b
4. b
5. a
6. c
7. d
8. a

## Chapter 5
1. b
2. c
3. c
4. c
5. d
6. b
7. c
8. a

## Chapter 6
1. b
2. a
3. c
4. b
5. c
6. a
7. d
8. c

## Chapter 7
1. c
2. b
3. c
4. b
5. c
6. b
7. a
8. b

## Chapter 8
1. a
2. c
3. c
4. a
5. c
6. a
7. a
8. b

## Chapter 9
1. b
2. c
3. c
4. d
5. a, c, d
6. c
7. a
8. a

## Chapter 10
1. b
2. c
3. b
4. a, d, e
5. a, b, d, e
6. d
7. b
8. a

## Chapter 11
1. b
2. a
3. b, d, e, f
4. c
5. b
6. a
7. a
8. c

## Chapter 12
1. d
2. a
3. b
4. b
5. a, b, c
6. c
7. a
8. d

## Chapter 13
1. d
2. c
3. a
4. b
5. a
6. a, b, d, d, e
7. c
8. a, c, d, e

## Chapter 14
1. b
2. a
3. a
4. b, c, d
5. a, b, c, d
6. a
7. c
8. b

## Chapter 15
1. b, c, d
2. d
3. c
4. a
5. b
6. a, b, c, d, e
7. a, b, d
8. c

## Chapter 16
1. a
2. a
3. d
4. c
5. c
6. c
7. d
8. a

## Chapter 17

1. a
2. a
3. c
4. b
5. b
6. b
7. d
8. d

## Chapter 18

1. a
2. a
3. b
4. b
5. b
6. a
7. a
8. b

## Chapter 19

1. c
2. d
3. d
4. d
5. a
6. b
7. c
8. a, b, c

## Chapter 20

1. b
2. c
3. a
4. a
5. d
6. d
7. c
8. c

## Chapter 21

1. a
2. d
3. a
4. c
5. a
6. a
7. b
8. c

## Chapter 22

1. d
2. b, c, d, e
3. c
4. a
5. a
6. b
7. d
8. a

# INDEX

▲

*Note*: Page numbers followed by *b* indicate a box; those followed by *f*, an illustration; and those followed by *t*, a table.

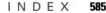

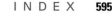

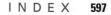